Pediatric Psychosocial Oncology: Textbook for Multidisciplinary Care

To our mentors and colleagues who have taught us invaluable lessons about being present with and caring for patients and families.

To the children living with cancer and their family members who have allowed us to share in their journey. You inspire us with your strength, courage, and resilience.

To those who have not survived. We carry your stories with us.

To Marty, Lulu, Rachel, and Charlie whose love and support keep me grounded
For my parents who inspire me by the lives they lead

Annah Abrams

To Theo, Sam, and Karen who remind me of what is most important

Nina Muriel

With love and gratitude to Marilyn and Walter Wiener who provided me with deep roots and flexible wings
To Sylvan who provides loving arms to come home to
For Marisa and Brett whose gifts of spirit, wisdom, and resilience have nourished my soul

Lori Wiener

In Memoriam
Robert Arceci, MD, PhD
1950–2015
Scientist, physician, colleague, patient advocate, friend and champion for children and adolescents with cancer and the field of pediatric psycho-social oncology. You will be missed.

Foreword

Many of us who work in the field of pediatric psychosocial oncology have had the experience of meeting someone for the first time at a cocktail party or other social gathering and being asked what we do for a living. Disclosing that we work with children who have cancer and their families in order to help them manage the stresses and challenges of this illness may bring a number of common responses: often an awkward pause; sometimes an expression of admiration suggesting that we must be saintlike to do such work; and not infrequently a question – "Isn't that depressing?" We each must develop our own response to that question, and while mine varies depending on the circumstances, it always includes a definitive statement, "No, it's not depressing, it's actually quite rewarding." And because most of us are not saints (not even close in my case), it behooves us to reflect on why it is that this work is, in fact, so rewarding. From whence comes the uplift?

My introduction to work with the childhood cancer population began during my postdoctoral fellowship training nearly 30 years ago. At that time, great strides had already been made in the treatment of pediatric cancer and survival rates were improving rapidly, while the areas of supportive and psychosocial care were earlier in development and just beginning to catch up. I remember vividly one of my first patient care experiences. An 11-year-old boy with relapsed lymphoma was having a bone marrow transplant. He had had his first dose of total body irradiation (TBI) that morning and suffered a panic attack during the procedure. This was a major concern for his treatment team, not only for his distress but because he needed to maintain some degree of self-control for the treatment to be administered properly. His second dose of TBI was scheduled for later that afternoon, and we were consulted urgently to help him get through the process. I felt ill-prepared for this challenge and rather apprehensive with the enormity of this responsibility. Then I met him. He was a pleasant young man who appeared to be developing normally and adjusting well in most spheres of his life, although he was notably and understandably anxious about his current predicament. Given his level of anxiety, we agreed to postpone the discussion of his upcoming procedure while we talked about more pleasant things. I learned that he loved baseball, and gathered quite a bit of information about the exploits of his little league team. Talking about this appeared to be a good distraction and he became less anxious. Thus, we hatched our initial treatment plan to get him through that afternoon's procedure. Using the intercom system in the radiation suite to continue our baseball dialogue, I suggested he could close his eyes and picture himself back on the baseball field, so that he could describe the game to me. He was able to engage in this imagery, and before we knew it, the procedure was over. My own relief was palpable. Then, the radiation doors opened and he walked out slowly, dressed in the full "space suit" in use at that time. He came directly to me and gave me a hug saying, "Thanks for helping me." Although I honestly wasn't sure that anything I had done had contributed to this improved outcome, the experience of his gratitude was something I will never forget. It engendered a lot of feelings, but depression was not one of them.

Now I will not pretend that all my subsequent clinical experiences have been as successful or rewarding as that one. But they need not be. To have just the occasional satisfaction of knowing that something we have done may have helped to reduce the distress of a child or ease the worry of an anxious parent is sufficient to remind us of why we do this work and maintain our commitment to it. I have experienced more than my share of failures and frustrations along the way, as most of us do, but the positive experiences keep us going, even if occurring infrequently. Of course, our goal is to have all of our clinical encounters result in positive outcomes, and to move toward that goal we want to ensure that our work is guided by the most up to date and comprehensive information available, as developed by the leading experts in this field. To make that knowledge available in a single volume has been the ambitious goal of the editors of this book, an aim that I am pleased to say has been admirably achieved.

Since those early days of my postdoctoral experience, the progress across multiple areas of supportive and psychosocial care of the child with cancer has been remarkable, and exciting developments and new approaches are currently being studied, as described in many of the following chapters. Looking back, it is impressive to reflect on how far we've come. It is hard for me to believe it has been two decades since the publication of an earlier volume on pediatric psychooncology, edited by my close colleague and longtime Division Chief, the late Raymond Mulhern, along with David Bearison, summarizing progress in the field up to that date. A decade later, a special issue of the *Journal of Pediatric Psychology* focused on childhood cancer (Mulhern and Bearison 1994), and the editors of that special issue, Andrea Patenaude and Mary Jo Kupst, along with Anne Kazak, provided comprehensive reviews of recent progress in the field (Patenaude and Kupst 2005; Kazak 2005). Notably, the focus had changed somewhat over that decade, with a much greater emphasis on survivorship, as mortality continued to decline and pediatric cancer was becoming conceptualized as a chronic illness. Thus, much research addressed the recognition of late effects of cancer and anticancer therapy – psychosocial, physical, functional, and neuropsychological – and interventions to prevent or ameliorate them. In the past decade, there has been increased emphasis on the development of evidence-based treatment and empirically supported interventions, again focused largely on survivorship issues but with continued attention to acute care issues and end-of-life care as well. With all this emphasis on intervention, I would be remiss if I didn't also mention research pointing to the resilience demonstrated by so many children and families facing this challenge, which has been the focus of my own recent work (Phipps et al. 2014). The positive adjustment observed in this setting provides another example of the remarkable human capacity to adjust, and even thrive in the face of adversity, and provides another source of inspiration for many working in the field.

The great progress that we have seen over the past decades is the result of the dedication, creativity, and perseverance of many individual investigators and clinicians across multiple disciplines. One of the many strengths of this volume is the multidisciplinary nature of the authors, which includes contributions not only from leaders in pediatric psychology and psychiatry but also oncology, behavioral pediatrics, nursing, child life, social work, and pastoral care, along with the consumer view of both patients and parents. The challenge of providing effective and comprehensive psychosocial care to children with cancer and their families requires a multidisciplinary team effort, which is illustrated so persuasively in the following chapters. Progress in psychosocial care has also been augmented by the support of the Children's Oncology Group (COG), the national cooperative group for clinical trials in childhood cancer (Noll et al. 2013). The COG has provided a forum for investigators from multiple disciplines to develop research and translate empirically supported interventions from research to practice. Thus, for a young person entering the field today, there is a much broader knowledge base and wider repertoire of empirically supported techniques and treatments available than when I began my training years ago. This volume provides a comprehensive compendium of that progress and a manual for the current state of the art in supportive and psychosocial care in pediatric oncology. I am very grateful to the editors for the opportunity to provide this foreword and hope that this volume will serve as a reference for all working in this field and as a guide to promote future research that will maintain and accelerate our progress in the future.

Memphis, TN, USA — Sean Phipps, PhD

References

Kazak AE (2005) Evidence-based interventions for survivors of childhood cancer and their families. J Pediatr Psychol 30:29–39.

Mulhern RK, Bearison DJ (eds) (1994) Pediatric psychooncology: psychological perspectives on children with cancer. Oxford University Press, New York.

Noll RB, Patel SK, Embry L et al (2013) Children's Oncology Group 2013 blueprint for research: behavioral science. Pediatr Blood Cancer 60:1048–1054.

Patenaude AF, Kupst MJ (2005) Psychosocial functioning in pediatric cancer. J Pediatr Psychol 30:9–27.

Phipps S, Klosky JK, Long A et al (2014) Posttraumatic stress and psychological growth in children with cancer: has the traumatic impact of cancer been overestimated? J Clin Oncol 32:641–646.

Preface

We are pleased to offer the first edition of *Pediatric Psychosocial Oncology: Textbook for Multidisciplinary Care*. It has been written to provide up-to-date clinical information and resources addressing the many aspects of exemplary psychosocial care for children, adolescents, and young adults living with cancer and their family members.

We have assembled this textbook into practical readable chapters covering the breadth of psychosocial care in pediatric oncology. Sixty four authors, from 37 centers, share their expertise to help clinicians assess, anticipate, and respond to the emotional issues that arise in the context of treating children and adolescents with cancer. We are hopeful that the chapters will be useful for new clinicians in the field of pediatric oncology as well as for those who are more experienced. We anticipate the chapters will be used in the classroom, as reference material, and in inpatient and outpatient clinical settings.

Each chapter includes case material that brings the clinical challenges and opportunities to life. Clinical pearls are also provided at the end of each chapter to highlight the key points for each topic covered. The last chapter in the textbook includes a comprehensive resource guide that can be copied and shared with colleagues.

All cases described in this textbook are a compilation of patient experiences, and names have been changed to protect the identities of children and families. You will note that we use he or she interchangeably throughout the book and the material applies to either gender. We use parents as a general term as opposed to caregivers while recognizing that many children receive primary care from other family members.

We acknowledge that not every child and family will have access to the full range of psychosocial services described here. This book highlights the ideal psychosocial care that oncology programs can provide and how to access resources online or through cancer networks when comprehensive psychosocial care is not available locally.

We hope the textbook conveys the warm spirit of collegiality and mutual respect that exists among pediatric oncology care providers including, but not limited to, psychologists, social workers, psychiatrists, chaplains, child life specialists, nurses, and oncologists. We also value the chapter contributions from parents, advocates, and survivors, who help us better understand and appreciate the patient and family experience.

Pharmacological dosage information provided in this textbook is a guideline, and prior to prescribing medications, one should consult drug manufacturers' current indications, dosage recommendations, and drug interactions as well as warnings.

We extend wholehearted thanks to our chapter authors who not only share their expertise in this textbook but who also provide thoughtful clinical care to children with cancer and their families in pediatric oncology settings. We greatly appreciate the support of our respective pediatric oncology programs which value the role of psychosocial care. And most of all, we are grateful to our patients and their families who teach and inspire us every day.

Boston, MA, USA — Annah N. Abrams, MD
Anna C. Muriel, MD, MPH
Bethesda, MD, USA — Lori Wiener, PhD

Contents

Contributors

Robert J. Arceci†, MD, PhD Department of Child Health, Ronald Matricaria Institute of Molecular Medicine at Phoenix Children's Hospital, University of Arizona College of Medicine, Phoenix, AZ, USA

Caroline H. Armington, MS, CCLS Division of Pediatric Hematology and Oncology, MassGeneral Hospital for Children, Boston, MA, USA

Abraham S. Bartell, MD Departments of Pediatrics and Psychiatry & Behavioral Sciences, Memorial Sloan Kettering, New York, NY, USA

Daniel Benedetti, MD Department of Pediatric Hematology/Oncology, Dana Farber/Boston Children's Cancer and Blood Disorders Center, Boston, MA, USA

Kristin Bingen, PhD Division of Hematology/Oncology/Blood and Marrow Transplant, Department of Pediatrics, Medical College of Wisconsin, Milwaukee, WI, USA

Sarah R. Brand, PhD Department of Psychosocial Oncology and Palliative Care, Dana-Farber Cancer Institute, Boston, MA, USA

Reverend Mark Brown, MDiv, BCC Department of Chaplain Services, St. Jude Children's Research Hospital, Memphis, TN, USA

Peter J. Brown, MBA Mattie Miracle Cancer Foundation, Arlington, VA, USA

Candice Chow, PhD Department of Psychosocial Oncology and Palliative Care, Dana-Farber Cancer Institute, Boston, MA, USA

Stephen DiDonato, MS Nemours Biomedical Research, Center for Pediatric Traumatic Stress at the Nemours / Alfred I. duPont Hospital for Children, Wilmington, DE, USA

Reverend Kathleen Ennis-Durstine, MDiv, BCC Department of Family Services, Children's National Health System, Washington, DC, USA

Cynthia A. Gerhardt, PhD Department of Pediatrics and Psychology, The Ohio State University, Columbus, OH, USA

Center for Biobehavioral Health, The Research Institute at Nationwide Children's Hospital, Columbus, OH, USA

Mitch Golant, PhD Cancer Support Community, Washington, DC, USA

Alexandra Gubin, MSW, LCSW-C Department of Pediatric Oncology, The Sidney Kimmel Comprehensive Cancer Center at Johns Hopkins, Baltimore, MD, USA

Ulman Cancer Fund for Young Adults, Johns Hopkins Bloomberg Children's Center, Baltimore, MD, USA

Jennifer A. Hoag, PhD Division of Hematology/Oncology/Blood and Marrow Transplant, Department of Pediatrics, Medical College of Wisconsin, Milwaukee, WI, USA

Marilyn Hockenberry, PhD, RN, PPCNP-BC, FAAN Duke University School of Nursing, Durham, NC, USA

Ruth I. Hoffman, MPH American Childhood Cancer Organization, Kensington, MD, USA

Stephanie Hopkinson, MA, CCLS Child Life Services, Development and Continuing Education, Allied Health, Sidra Medical and Research Center, Doha, Qatar

Barbara L. Jones, PhD, MSW School of Social Work, University of Texas at Austin, Austin, TX, USA

The Institute for Grief, Loss, and Family Survival, UT Austin School of Social Work, Austin, TX, USA

The Institute for Palliative Care and Family Survival, UT Austin School of Social Work, Austin, TX, USA

Cynthia W. Karlson, PhD Department of Pediatrics, Division of Hematology/Oncology, University of Mississippi Medical Center, Jackson, MS, USA

Anne E. Kazak, PhD, ABPP Nemours Biomedical Research, Nemours Center for Healthcare Delivery Science/Alfred I. duPont Hospital for Children, Wilmington, DE, USA

Julia Kearney, MD Departments of Pediatrics and Psychiatry & Behavioral Sciences, Memorial Sloan Kettering, New York, NY, USA

Natalie C. Kelly, PhD, ABPP Department of Supportive Care Medicine, City of Hope Medical Center, Duarte, CA, USA

Jennifer C. Kesselheim, MD, MBE, EdM Department of Pediatric Hematology/Oncology, Dana Farber/Boston Children's Cancer and Blood Disorders Center, Boston, MA, USA

Mary Jo Kupst, PhD Department of Pediatrics, Medical College of Wisconsin, Milwaukee, WI, USA

Vicky Lehmann, PhD Department of Pediatrics, The Ohio State University, Columbus, Ohio, USA

Center for Biobehavioral Health, The Research Institute at Nationwide Children's Hospital, Columbus, OH, USA

Cori C. Liptak, PhD Department of Psychosocial Oncology and Palliative Care, Dana-Farber Cancer Institute, Boston, MA, USA

Jennifer W. Mack, MD, MPH Department of Pediatric Hematology/ Oncology, Dana-Farber/ Boston Children's Cancer and Blood Disorders Center, Boston, MA, USA

Hilary McClafferty, MD, FAAP Departments of Pediatrics and Medicine, University of Arizona, Tucson, AZ, USA

Larry L. Mullins, PhD Department of Psychology, Oklahoma State University, Stillwater, OK, USA

Ahna L.H. Pai, PhD Department of Behavioral Medicine and Clinical Psychology, Blood Diseases Institute, Cincinnati Children's Hospital Medical Center, Cincinnati, Ohio, USA

Tonya M. Palermo, PhD Department of Anesthesiology and Pain Medicine, University of Washington and Seattle Children's Research Institute, Seattle Children's Hospital Research Institute, Seattle, WA, USA

Maryland Pao, MD Office of the Clinical Director, National Institutes of Mental Health, Bethesda, MD, USA

Sunita K. Patel, PhD Departments of Population Sciences and Supportive Care Medicine, City of Hope Medical Center, Duarte, CA, USA

Andrea Farkas Patenaude, PhD Department of Psychosocial Oncology and Palliative Care, Dana-Farber Cancer Institute, Boston, MA, USA

Pandora Patterson, PhD CanTeen Australia and Cancer Nursing Research Unit, Sydney University, Sydney, NSW, Australia

Heather E. Peach, MS, CCLS Division of Pediatric Hematology and Oncology, MassGeneral Hospital for Children, Boston, MA, USA

Catherine C. Peterson, PhD Department of Psychology, Eastern Michigan University, Ypsilanti, MI, USA

Farya Phillips, PhD, CCLS School of Social Work, The University of Texas at Austin, Austin, TX, USA

Christopher J. Recklitis, PhD, MPH Perini Family Survivors' Center, Dana-Farber Cancer Institute, Boston, MA, USA

Stacy S. Remke, MSW, LICSW, ACHP-SW School of Social Work, University of Minnesota, Paul, MN, USA

Cheryl Rodgers, PhD, RN, CPNP, CPON Duke University School of Nursing, Durham, NC, USA

Marilyn A. Rosen, MLS Research Librarian (ret) Edward G. Miner Library, University of Rochester Medical Center, Rochester, NY, USA

Abby R. Rosenberg, MD, MS Seattle Children's Hospital Cancer and Blood Disorders Center, Seattle, WA, USA

Clinical Research Division, Fred Hutchinson Cancer Research Center, Seattle, WA, USA

Treuman Katz Center for Pediatric Bioethics, Seattle Children's Research Institute, Seattle, WA, USA

Olle Jane Z. Sahler, MD Division of Hematology/Oncology, Golisano Children's Hospital @ Strong, University of Rochester School of Medicine & Dentistry, Rochester, NY, USA

Christina G. Salley, PhD Department of Psychiatry & Behavioral Sciences, Memorial Sloan Kettering Cancer Center, New York, NY, USA

Sheila Judge Santacroce, PhD, MSN School of Nursing, The University of North Carolina at Chapel Hill, Chapel Hill, NC, USA

Victoria A. Sardi-Brown, PhD, LPC Mattie Miracle Cancer Foundation, Arlington, VA, USA

Stephanie J. Schneider, MS Nemours Biomedical Research, Nemours / Alfred I duPont Hospital for Children, Wilmington, DE, USA

Fiona Schulte, PhD, RPsych Departments of Oncology and Paediatrics, University of Calgary, Calgary, AB, Canada

Haematology, Oncology and Transplant Program, Alberta Children's Hospital, Calgary, AB, Canada

Sandra E. Smith American Childhood Cancer Organization, Kensington, MD, USA

Amii C. Steele, PhD Department of Pediatric Hematology, Oncology, and BMT, Levine Children's Hospital at Carolinas Medical Center, Charlotte, NC, USA

Kristina I. Suorsa, MS Department of Psychology, Oklahoma State University, Murray Stillwater, OK, USA

Alayna P. Tackett, MS Department of Psychology, Oklahoma State University, Stillwater, OK, USA

Michael H. Tang, MD Department of Pediatrics, The Dimock Center, Roxbury, MA, USA

Sarah Tarquini, PhD Department of Psychosocial Oncology and Palliative Care, Dana-Farber Cancer Institute, Boston, MA, USA

Christine L. Trask, PhD, ABPP Department of Psychiatry and Human Behavior, Rhode Island Hospital/The Warren Alpert Medical School of Brown University, Providence, RI, USA

Department of Psychiatry and Human Behavior, School of Brown University, Providence, RI, USA

Rachel Tunick, PhD Boston Children's Primary Care at Longwood, Boston Children's Hospital, Boston, MA, USA

Janice Withycombe, PhD, RN, MN, CCRP Emory University, Nell Hodgson Woodruff School of Nursing, Atlanta, GA, USA

Joanne Wolfe, MD, MPH Department of Psychosocial Oncology and Palliative Care, Center for Outcomes and Policy Research, Dana-Farber Cancer Institute, Boston, WA, USA

Department of Psychosocial Oncology and Palliative Care, Dana-Farber Cancer Institute, Boston, WA, USA

Boston Children's Hospital, Boston, WA, USA

Sima Zadeh, PsyD Pediatric Oncology Branch, National Institutes of Health, National Cancer Institute, Bethesda, MD, USA

Brad Zebrack, PhD, MSW, MPH University of Michigan School of Social Work, Ann Arbor, MI, USA

Eric S. Zhou, PhD Perini Family Survivors' Center, Dana-Farber Cancer Institute, Boston, MA, USA

1 Pediatric Oncology: Psychosocial Care in Context

Robert J. Arceci †

Origins and Evolution

Cancer in children has always been inexorably linked to feelings of unfathomable unfairness, urgent pleas for cures, and the psychological challenges for patients and their families. While the incidence of childhood cancer represents only about 2 % of all cancers, the impact of its treatment extends beyond the child and includes the family and the community. The worldwide incidence of childhood cancer has been estimated to be about 200,000 cases annually. Approximately 80 % of children are cured in developed countries, but that cure rate is inversed in resource-poor countries where often less than 20 % of children are cured. The incidence of cancer also appears to be slowly increasing (Rodriguez-Galindo et al. 2013; Spector et al. 2013; Pritchard-Jones et al. 2013).

The origins of the fight to cure children with cancer arose in the seemingly contradictory efforts of war and welfare with the adoption of nitrogen mustard for the treatment of adult patients with lymphoma. However, the true entry of children with cancer onto this stage had its beginning in the late 1940s with the publication of the Farber and Diamond study entitled "Temporary Remissions in Acute Leukemia in Children Produced by Folic Acid Antagonist, 4-amenopteroyl-Glutamic Acid (Aminopterin)" (Farber and Diamond 1948). Farber went on to establish the Children's Cancer Research Foundation, later the Sidney Farber Cancer Institute (now Dana Farber Cancer Institute), with the conviction that basic scientists and physicians could work together to eradicate these dreaded diseases.

The promise of finding curative therapies for children and adults with cancer ignited much enthusiasm and hope that in turn led to several important initiatives. These included the engagement of the federal government, culminating, in large part through the efforts of Ms. Mary Lasker and the Citizen's Committee for the Conquest of Cancer, in substantial financial support through the "War on Cancer" channeled through the National Cancer Act (National Cancer Institute 1971). Subsequent efforts led to the development of more integrated, comprehensive cancer centers, broad-based anti-cancer drug screening (something Farber anticipated early on), preclinical models, pediatric and medical oncology specialty training, as well as the beginnings of cooperative clinical trial groups.

† Author was deceased at the time of publication

R.J. Arceci, MD, PhD
Department of Child Health, Ronald Matricaria Institute of Molecular Medicine at Phoenix Children's Hospital, University of Arizona College of Medicine, 445 N. 5th Street, TGen Building, 3rd Fl, Room 322, Phoenix, AZ 85004, USA

A.N. Abrams et al. (eds.), *Pediatric Psychosocial Oncology: Textbook for Multidisciplinary Care*,
DOI 10.1007/978-3-319-21374-3_1

In many ways, the work that focused on curing children with cancer pioneered many of the optimal approaches to understanding and optimizing the treatment of all patients with cancer. One of these lessons was the realization that there was strength in numbers and that progress would depend on trained pediatric specialists working together. The emergence of the Children's Cancer Group followed by the Pediatric Oncology Group, the National Wilms Tumor Study Group, and the Intergroup Rhabdomyosarcoma Group all paved the course for their merger into the Children's Oncology Group, well before the clinical trial groups focused on adults began to integrate their work.

Other key approaches took advantage of new scientific insights and the exploitation of older drugs, as many newer drugs lagged behind or were never approved for children. Pediatric investigators and caregivers pioneered the need for optimal supportive care and they established integrated, multidisciplinary care teams. Further, the development of carefully designed national and sometimes international cooperative group clinical trials, has clearly played a fundamental role in improving survival rates to what they are today.

Ongoing Challenges

The progress that has been made is clearly momentous, and, yet, there are several important realities that temporize enthusiasm and provide significant challenges. The first is the acknowledgement that cancer remains the leading cause of death by disease in children. Further, there remain several types of cancer with either extremely poor or universally fatal outcomes such as brainstem gliomas and metastatic sarcomas. The unfortunate underside of modern therapeutic approaches, including more intensive treatment regimens and expanded use of radiation therapy and bone marrow transplantation, have resulted in significant adverse, late effects in survivors (Meadows 2003). Oeffinger et al. reported that about 66 % of survivors of childhood cancer had at least one related adverse condition and about 25 % had one serious and potentially life-threatening condition (Oeffinger et al. 2006). Such reports have focused on the physical consequences of survivorship, and as noted throughout this textbook, psychosocial issues constitute an equally enormous challenge. The high survival rates are offset by significant rates of adverse late effects. Thus, if one considers what a true cure rate is, i.e., having a child cured of their cancer without the encumbrances of adverse effects, I believe a recalculation is indicated that results in a figure less than 20 % (80 % minus the 66 % noted above).

Another critical issue is that of the "adolescent gap" of clinical trial participation (Bleyer 2005). The adolescent and young adult populations have low rates of participation in clinical trials, and they have not had the same increases in survival as younger and older patients with cancer. Similarly, data demonstrates that approximately 85 % of children with cancer are in resource-poor countries, without access to clinical trials or often without access to basic treatments. There also remain areas within developed countries in which children have lower survival rates. Both groups of patients represent underserved populations and this must be addressed.

Finally, an issue that may not be commonly considered as problematic is that of our inability to predict whether a new treatment is more likely than not to improve responses and outcomes (Kumar et al. 2005). While this provides caretakers with equipoise when speaking to families about whether to enter a randomized clinical trial, it nevertheless remains a substantial limitation. Essentially, the question arises as to why we are not better at predicting whether a new drug will improve outcomes or not?

Future Advances in Pediatric Oncology

A possible solution to such predictive ambiguity may reside in the development of "omic" and refined drug sensitivity testing. The ability to integrate such information in terms of the contextual, biological complexity of a cancer and in a form that would significantly improve our ability to predict meaningful clinical responses from single and combination therapies in individual patients may be one of our greatest challenges. Further, there are also the legitimate concerns for patients and their immediate and extended family members concerning the genomic implications of these approaches, as not infrequently, they result in findings of potentially important inherited disease predisposition in otherwise healthy members of the family. In addition, methodologies to determine how best to define success with such personalized approaches to therapy, resulting in small numbers of patients treated, are in need of development, along with agreement from investigators, drug developers, legislators, and regulatory agencies.

Thus, while there are significant challenges to achieving success in this investigative area, such approaches have extraordinary potential to profoundly change current treatment paradigms. The future of effective in silico predictive testing of drugs prior to treating patients is likely to change the very core of how medicine, and pediatric oncology, is practiced in the future. A direct consequence of these advances is whether there will be equitable access to patients from different socioeconomic and geographic settings. This latter point will clearly be a key issue as to how effective such new technologies and approaches are utilized and judged.

Without invoking the quatrains of Nostradamus, one might envision a future in which you or your child would sense something is wrong, such as a lump in the neck, and go to your physician, in this scenario, an android-based integrative system. The visit would involve an android making automated decisions based on extensive neural networks that would lead to an integrated omic analysis and a diagnosis of a particular type of lymphoma and treatment plan. During this entire scenario, no human would ask you how you feel or what concerns or fears you have if this treatment does not work. While the challenges of the biology are daunting enough, addressing such psychosocial issues represent an equally challenging area, in which, however, many of us find ourselves quite inadequate.

A Pediatric Oncologist's View

To that end, I admit that I am not a psychiatrist, psychologist, or social worker. Instead, I work as a pediatric hematologist/oncologist and translational scientist with the strong conviction that a complete, quantitative analysis of cancer and the host in which it arises will provide the path to eradicating cancer. And yes, maybe the above scenario will be all that is needed. Thus, at least on the surface, there would appear to be an inherent conflict between the analytical assessment of cancer and the often-considered less analytical, "scientifically softer" world of psychosocial assessment of patient needs and outcomes. But maybe that conflicting point of view misses the essence of the issue.

In the *Plague*, Albert Camus strikes at the heart of such issues and apparent conflicting sides (Camus 1947). In the last third of the novel, a magistrate's child is dying a horrific death from the plague with the key characters at his bedside: Paneloux, a priest; Castel, an experimental investigator trying a new treatment; and Jean Tarrou, a chronicler and companion of Rieux, the protagonist and physician.

When the child dies, Tarrou reflects, "Must we start all over again?" Castel aptly responds, "Perhaps. After all, he did fight it for a long time."

Rieux abruptly walks away, brushing by Paneloux, who queries, "Come now doctor."

Rieux turns to the priest and says, "Ah, now that one, at least, was innocent, as you very well know!"

He walks away, but the priest persists: "Why did you speak to me with such anger just now? I, too, found that unbearable to watch."

In response, Rieux says, "That's true. Forgive me. But tiredness is a form of madness. And there are times in this town when I can only feel outrage and revolt."

The debate deepens with Paneloux responding, "I understand. It is outrageous because it is beyond us. But perhaps we should love what we cannot understand."

Rieux counters, "No, Father, I have a different notion of love; and to the day I die I shall refuse to love this creation in which children are tortured."

Paneloux retreats a bit and states, "Ah, doctor, I have just understood what is meant by God's grace."

Rieux, who will have none of this, retorts, "Which I don't have, I know. But I don't want to discuss this with you. We are working together for something that unites us at a higher level than prayer or blasphemy, and that's all that counts."

The priest concedes, "Yes, yes, you too are working for the salvation of mankind."

A bit sardonically, Rieux moves back to reality with, "Salvation is too big a word for me. I don't go that far. What interests me is man's health, his health first of all."

Sensing defeat, the priest says, "Yet, I have not managed to convince you!"

Rieux concedes, "What does it matter? What I hate is death and evil, as you know. And whether you accept this or not, we are together in enduring them and fighting against them. You see, even God himself cannot separate us now."

Biology and Psychology

And so this complex mix of biology and psychology represents an inseparable weave. What happens in one part inexorably links to and impacts the other. But how does one articulate the right questions to study and the methodological approaches to use? Being at a loss for answers, such considerations in part led me to conceive of using the approach of narrative to help define some of the key questions better than I might otherwise do. To provide immediacy, I concluded that documentary film would provide the substrate to engage patients and their families during all stages of their treatment and in various physical settings, such as while in clinic, the hospital, at school, home, and in transit. Their stories would highlight the complexity of decision-making on their part as well as on that of caretakers, the nuances of research and clinical trials, the difficult issue of patient/caretaker boundaries, access to care and health-care disparities, the hope and fears of survivorship, and the brutal reality of accepting the end-of-life transition. Two incredible documentary filmmakers, Steven Bognar and Julia Reichert, agreed to actualize such a documentary with the film, "A Lion in the House" (http://www.lioninthehouse.com) (Reichert et al. 2011). While not providing definitive answers, I believe the film does accurately phrase key questions and provides a path for thinking together about defining credible answers. So while the quantitative analysis of host and cancer genomes, transcriptomes, epigenomes, proteomes, metabolomes, and kinomes is pursued, the response of patients and families to such catastrophe adds other profoundly complex venues for analysis and support. Most of these challenges are discussed in this book. However, bearing witness to them here is not intended to be redundant, but rather to highlight the continuum of challenges that require preventive and therapeutic intervention while demanding continued investigation.

The first issue that is strikingly evident is that pediatric patients with cancer have profound differences in neurocognitive and psychological capabilities. Pediatric patients also come with immediate and extended families who must grapple with the nuances of the impact of a child's age on the response to diagnosis, treatment, pain, separation, altered body image, and uncertainty. Such considerations are clearly going to be extremely different for a newborn vs. a 2-year-old vs. an 8-year-old or a teenager. Rigorous tools to study neurocognitive and psychological adaption are still lacking for many of these ages.

The timing of evaluations and interventions also constitutes a continuously changing target. Critical events and responses present at diagnosis (disease description, treatment options, research trial considerations, guilt, fear, hope), during the initiation and continuation of treatment (dealing with adverse effects, including body image, neurocognitive changes, psychological adaption to isolation, pain, fear of dying, separation), and with new challenges that accompany end of treatment and survivorship (fear of recurrence, achieving normalcy and peer acceptance, dealing with resulting treatment and disease-related limitations, questions of fertility, issues of insurability, school, employment). As noted in Koocher and O'Malley's insightful analogy in "Damocles Syndrome" (Koocher and O'Malley 1981), the realized fear of recurrence and its intense redefining of all the issues previously experienced represent a further challenge for patients, families, caretakers, and investigators.

Access to Quality Care for All

In a speech to the Medical Committee for Human Rights in 1966, Dr. Martin Luther King Jr. stated, "Of all the forms of inequality, injustice in health care is the most shocking and inhumane." Many people have concluded that the catastrophic nature of a diagnosis of cancer in a child should automatically result in equality of care. Unfortunately, there also exists the reality that unequal treatment and supportive care remain problems. Consider the difference of a young teenage patient from a less fortunate socioeconomic environment taking a bus or taxi by himself for an appointment to receive chemotherapy compared to a child being taken to clinic by his parents in the family car. Consider a single mother balancing the time spent keeping a job while caring for other children and challenged to spend time with her dying, hospitalized child, compared to parents spending that time with their hospitalized child while extended family care for other children and adjustments are made for missed work. There is also the issue of access to new treatments on clinical trials depending upon one's socioeconomic status. A large percentage of children with cancer have Medicaid or similar insurance plans, which often preclude access to certain treatments or clinical trials if they require travel to another state. The issue becomes even more poignant for patients and their families who live in resource poor countries, where abandonment of treatment, often based on economic considerations, remains a significant impediment to cure. These realities are extraordinarily challenging from a healthcare delivery perspective, including psychosocial support, but they also raise important investigative questions in terms of how they impact patient and family adjustment and well-being.

Integrating Care and Discovery

We are left with what might be considered an overwhelming set of problems that involve the total care of patients and their families, including the integration of physical and psychological interventions. There is an essential need to define the methodological approaches to study key psychosocial questions and turn such studies into solutions. William Osler aptly stated in Aequanimitas (Osler 1910) that "Every patient you see is a lesson in much more than the malady from which he suffers." The challenges of caring for the physical and psychosocial needs of all patients, including children with cancer, are enormous, and, yet, they are magnified by our lack of knowledge concerning the mechanisms that underlie the biology of cancer as well as the human response to disease. The development of new and more effective treatment regimens should include the study and assessment of such psychological, sociological, and quality-of-life responses to therapy. The complexity of such questions should not be a deterrent, but a challenge to be solved. If we had all receded from these challenges in the past, we would still be debating the paradox illustrated by Castel, Paneloux, and Rieux. Such debate should only serve to focus the questions and the potential solutions as achieved through compassionate care and rigorous investigation.

References

Bleyer A (2005) The adolescent and young adult gap in cancer care and outcome. Curr Probl Pediatr Adolesc Health Care 35(5):182–217

Camus A (1991), The plague. (Trans: Buss R, 2001). First Vintage International Edition. Random House, Inc., NY, USA

Farber S, Diamond LK (1948) Temporary remissions in acute leukemia in children produced by folic acid antagonist, 4-aminopteroyl-glutamic acid. N Engl J Med 238(23):787–793

King ML Jr. (1966) Medical Committee for Human Rights Convention; Chicago

Koocher GP, O'Malley JJ (1981) Damocles syndrome: psychosocial consequences of surviving childhood cancer. McGraw-Hill, Inc., New York

Kumar A, Soares H, Wells R, Clarke M, Hozo I, Bleyer A, Reaman G, Chalmers I, Djulbegovic B, Children's Oncology G (2005) Are experimental treatments for cancer in children superior to established treatments? Observational study of randomised controlled trials by the Children's Oncology Group. BMJ 331(7528):1295

Meadows AT (2003) Pediatric cancer survivors: past history and future challenges. Curr Probl Cancer 27(3):112–126

National Cancer Institute (1971) The National Cancer Act of 1971. http://legislative.cancer.gov/history/phsa/1971

Oeffinger KC, Mertens AC, Sklar CA, Kawashima T, Hudson MM, Meadows AT, Friedman DL, Marina N, Hobbie W, Kadan-Lottick NS, Schwartz CL, Leisenring W, Robison LL, Childhood Cancer Survivor Study (2006) Chronic health conditions in adult survivors of childhood cancer. N Engl J Med 355(15):1572–1582

Osler W (1910) Aequanimitas, 2nd edn. P. Blakiston's Son & Co, Philadelphia, pp 1–12. http://www.medicalarchives.jhmi.edu/osler/aequessay.htm

Pritchard-Jones K, Pieters R, Reaman GH, Hjorth L, Downie P, Calaminus G, Naafs-Wilstra MC, Steliarova-Foucher E (2013) Sustaining innovation and improvement in the treatment of childhood cancer: lessons from high-income countries. Lancet Oncol 14(3):e95–e103

Reichert J, Bognar S, Greenberg LW, Godoy M, Durgans KY (2011) New educational modules offer tough case studies around humanistic issues. J Cancer Educ 26(2):386–387

Rodriguez-Galindo C, Friedrich P, Morrissey L, Frazier L (2013) Global challenges in pediatric oncology. Curr Opin Pediatr 25(1):3–15

Spector LG, Ross JA, Olshan AF, C.O.G.Epidemiology Committee (2013) Children's Oncology Group's 2013 blueprint for research: epidemiology. Pediatr Blood Cancer 60(6):1059–1062

Communication in the Pediatric Oncology Setting

2

Sarah R. Brand, Sarah Tarquini, and Jennifer W. Mack

Case Vignette

Charlie is a 13-year-old boy with newly diagnosed Ewing sarcoma. He is the youngest of three children and is very close with his older brothers and his parents. From the time of diagnosis, Charlie's parents requested that Charlie be given minimal information about his disease. This dynamic quickly became difficult for the clinicians involved in Charlie's care. They felt that by not being able to freely speak with Charlie and answer his questions, they were not providing appropriate care. Charlie started experiencing multiple symptoms of anxiety including panic attacks and began to withdraw, often refusing to participate in aspects of medical care.

Introduction

Communication skills and relational abilities are essential core competencies in patient-centered care and are associated with improved patient health outcomes, better patient adherence, fewer malpractice claims, and enhanced satisfaction with care (Meyer et al. 2009). However, for communication to contribute to healing and reduce suffering, clinicians must have the skills necessary to engage in patient-centered communication. When caring for pediatric patients, clinicians must not only find ways to effectively communicate with the child or adolescent patient but also engage meaningfully with the parents or caregivers. In the United States, parents have the legal authority to make medical decisions for a child under the age of 18. The American Academy of Pediatrics Committee on Bioethics recommends that healthcare providers communicate information to pediatric patients in a way that is truthful and developmentally appropriate and include them in medical decision-making to the greatest extent possible; however, there is limited guidance about how to translate these recommendations into clinical practice. This lack of guidance results in significant stress for patients, parents, and providers and large variations in care, as each member of the triad may have differing ideas about what their own role and the role of the other members should be.

S.R. Brand, PhD (✉) • S. Tarquini, PhD
Department of Psychosocial Oncology and Palliative Care, Dana-Farber Cancer Institute, 450 Brookline Avenue, Boston, MA 02215, USA
e-mail: SarahR_Brand@dfci.harvard.edu; sarah_tarquini@dfci.harvard.edu

J.W. Mack, MD, MPH
Department of Pediatric Hematology/Oncology, Dana-Farber/ Boston Children's Cancer and Blood Disorders Center, 450 Brookline Avenue, Boston, MA 02215, USA
e-mail: Jennifer_mack@dfci.harvard.edu

A.N. Abrams et al. (eds.), *Pediatric Psychosocial Oncology: Textbook for Multidisciplinary Care*,
DOI 10.1007/978-3-319-21374-3_2

Effective communication with pediatric oncology patients and their caregivers is critical to improving the disease outcome and emotional well-being of these vulnerable patients (Rutishauser 2003). Effective communication has been shown to be related not only to parent satisfaction with medical services but also adherence to medical treatment. In fact, insufficient and inadequate doctor/patient/family communication is one of the most important causes of medical nonadherence in pediatric patients (Spinetta et al. 2002). There are noted benefits in providing pediatric cancer patients with age-appropriate information, to both the patient and the family, and doing so fulfills the ethical responsibility of the provider (Mack and Joffe 2014).

Psychosocial clinicians can play a crucial role as an active member of the clinical care team for pediatric oncology patients. Unique contributions by psychosocial providers include helping the medical team understand the family context, including individual and family preferences around communication with the care team, identifying complicated family dynamics that may serve as a barrier to communication, and developing skills in facilitating group and family discussions that honor the preferences of the patient and family while also ensuring a productive conversation. In addition, psychosocial clinicians can enhance communication through providing education to medical providers about the issues discussed below.

General Principles of Communication

Goals and Purposes of Communication

Communication between pediatric patients, caregivers, and clinicians involves the sharing of words, thoughts, and feelings. Communication moves both ways, to and from the clinician, so that patients and families can both take in new information and also feel heard and understood. Because of this, one of the most critical communication skills for all clinicians is *listening*. *Telling*, which is sometimes perceived as the core communication skill, is nearly always secondary.

Communication Has Three Central Purposes, No Matter the Forum or Clinical Scenario

1. To allow for the development of shared knowledge
2. To build a relationship
3. To facilitate shared decision-making

The *development of shared knowledge*, often thought of as the central purpose of communication, starts with learning about the child and family. Doing so allows the clinician to understand the unique history and experiences of the child and family and to understand the state of the child and family's present knowledge about the medical situation, both of which help when the time comes to provide information and make decisions about care.

Initial communication between the medical provider and the family, which usually takes place in the context of the shock associated with a new cancer diagnosis, is often focused on learning about the child and caregivers. The presence of a psychosocial clinician can be helpful during such conversations to ensure that information is obtained regarding the developmental needs of the child, challenges to understanding and learning new information, and other relevant information. The clinician may start with general questions about how the child would describe herself as a person, questions that affirm the clinician's caring for the child as an individual and begin to create a relationship in which the child feels known. Caregivers, too, can provide their perspective on what makes their child unique. This information helps the clinician to understand core values for the child and family and offers the opportunity to reinforce those values over time. For example, a child who is most focused on friends and school as central aspects of identity may need additional acknowledgment and support if treatment disrupts these critical areas.

Because these conversations often occur over time, a continued relationship allows the clinician to deepen conversations over the ensuing days or months, to consider issues such as the meaning of illness for this child and family, religious and spiritual beliefs, and sources of both psychological resilience and distress. The opportunity to be part of a child's and family's search for meaning is often quite powerful for the clinician as well. Building a relationship over time is particularly helpful when it comes to communication with children; the relationships and mutual understanding that develop often require an experience of clinician presence, constancy, and trustworthiness over time. Clinicians also need to be alert to opportunities to build on relationships, especially moments in which a child opens a door to important information that can be explored.

Listening also allows the clinician to understand caregivers' and children's perceptions of the child's medical condition. This can help the clinician know where to start when it comes to sharing medical information. Thus, we often suggest opening conversations by asking a question such as, "Can you tell me what your understanding of the medical situation is so far?" Some families and children will begin with a level of knowledge that only requires confirmation of their own statements; others will have misconceptions or limited knowledge, even if information has been previously shared. In addition, hearing information directly from the child and family first allows the clinician to hear their own words, which can be instrumental to communication going forward. For example, within oncology, some families feel worried about using the word "cancer" around a child; others will use it freely, and the clinician can usually discover which strategy they have chosen with that simple first question. While the clinician may then wish to suggest greater openness about the diagnosis, understanding the parents' own phrasing can help clinicians to be respectful in this conversation, rather than wandering into this difficult territory thoughtlessly.

Once this information has been established, the medical clinician can move forward toward the sharing of important medical information, which we address more fully in the section below (General Strategies for Communication).

The second primary purpose of communication is *building a relationship*. Many of the tasks described above, especially eliciting information about the child and family, form the basis for this relationship. Along with this work, clinicians can develop relationships by identifying emotions and creating an atmosphere of emotional understanding and empathy. Relatively simple techniques can allow clinicians to bring emotion into the conversation. For example, naming an emotion can help children and families to feel that their feelings are understood and also allow for conversation about that emotion. Alternatively, especially when emotions are not clear, clinicians may wish to ask the child or caregiver how they are feeling. Once emotions have been shared and explored, clinicians may wish to respond by acknowledging emotions and expressing empathy. Although words are important, listening is often more important; in addition to empathic words, the clinician may wish to respond with a listening silence and attention. Words are not the only way to help children and families to feel known, respected, and understood.

The final core purpose of communication is *facilitation of shared decision-making*. Once medical information has been shared, children and families often have to use that information to make decisions about care going forward. But children and families need not be alone in that process; medical and psychosocial clinicians who know them well and understand what is most important to them can join in that process with recommendations and support.

Caregivers and children have a variety of preferences for the decision-making process, ranging from wanting to hold primary responsibility for decision-making themselves, to wanting to share in decision-making with the medical team, to preferring to delegate all decision-making to the clinician. In addition to asking about what framework feels best to the family, a second important approach is to use goals to inform recommendations from the medical team. The clinician may first wish, for example, to ask about values and goals for the future – "As you think about your future, what is most important to you? What are you most worried about? What are you hoping for the most?" Near diagnosis, goals typically center on cure, but asking about all of the child's and family's goals can help the clinician to understand what matters and also establish a framework for goal-oriented decision-making over time.

Once the child's and family's goals are understood, the clinician can provide recommendations about decisions to be made, with an eye toward supporting personal values. For example, a clinician may be able to say, "I understand that supporting your child's quality of life is very important to you. Here are some ways that I feel we can do that." Making such statements affirms to the child and family that what is important to them has been heard and is important to the medical team (Beale et al. 2005).

General Strategies for Communication

Many general strategies for communication have been developed. For example, Walter Baile's SPIKES model (Baile et al. 2000) is thoughtful and lends itself well to pediatric communication. This model suggests that clinicians first *S*et up the interview, letting children and families know that an important conversation is to take place. For example, one might say, "Tomorrow, I'd like to spend some time hearing about how the treatment is affecting you, so that we can think together about how to best get you through this." Second, once the conversation has begun, the clinician can assess the patient's *P*erceptions: "Can you start by telling me about what you think is the hardest part of treatment?" A third step is to obtain the patient's *I*nvitation, asking for permission to give information and recommendations. One might ask, for example, "Would it be okay for me to give you some of my thoughts and suggestions about how to deal with this?" Next, with the child's and parent's permission, the clinician can give *K*nowledge and information to the patient. A fifth step suggests that the clinician address the patient's *E*motions: "This can be a hard topic; what is it like for you to hear this information?" Finally, offering *S*trategy and summary reminds the child and family of the important points of the conversation and allows for a shared agreement on next steps. This model can be especially effective for teaching less experienced clinicians (both medical and psychosocial) to consider all of the relevant steps in preparing for important communication tasks.

Box 2.1: SPIKES Model of Communication

1. *S*et up the interview
2. *P*erceptions
3. *I*nvitation
4. *K*nowledge
5. *E*motions
6. *S*trategy

A related model proposed by Back et al. (2005) and others presents a somewhat simpler way to approach these difficult communication scenarios: Ask, then tell, and then ask again. For example, one might first ask for a child's understanding of medical information; then provide information, correcting any misconceptions; and then ask again for the child to tell the clinician what he will be taking away from the conversation, in his own words.

When disclosing medical information, the clinician may first wish to seek permission to embark on these topics ("Would it be helpful to hear more about what is happening medically?"). Although in some cases medical disclosure is a necessity rather than an option, children and families may still wish for the opportunity to negotiate the timing and extent of disclosure. In such cases, the clinician may wish to say something like, "Our medical team would like to discuss more of the medical information with you. We can do that now or later today and with just the four of us or with others. What do you think would be the most helpful to you?" Caregivers may also wish for the opportunity to discuss whether the child will be present for these conversations; as we discuss later in this chapter, allowing for a separate discussion with the parents in advance can allow the clinician to identify and address their fears.

Special Dynamics in Pediatric Oncology

Multidisciplinary Collaboration

Effective communication and collaboration between multidisciplinary team members are essential in providing high-quality clinical care within the pediatric oncology setting. Implementing mechanisms for ensuring ongoing, accurate communication can assist in maintaining a cohesive, well-informed team of clinicians. Concretely, the effectiveness of multidisciplinary collaboration can be maximized by providing documentation of clinical encounters in a thorough and timely manner, coordinating team meetings when appropriate, and seeking consultation prior to or after encounters when discussion of case material is warranted.

Triadic Communication and Decision-Making

When caring for pediatric oncology patients, clinicians must not only find ways to effectively communicate with the patient but also negotiate the triadic communication with the patient and the caregiver. "Patient-centered care" in this setting is best conceptualized as family-centered care, as children exist within families (as defined as any system of caregivers who participate in the child's care), and each member of the family plays a critical role in the patient's adjustment and ability to cope with treatment. For effective communication to occur, it is essential that providers are able to communicate with the child, the caregiver(s), and the family as a unit. As noted in the previous section, effective communication not only allows for the successful exchange of information but also serves as the foundation of the relationship between the clinician and the family and is essential for the execution of shared decision-making.

Clinician-Caregiver Communication

For clinicians to communicate effectively with caregivers, they must recognize that caregivers know their child best and are the experts on their child and their family. Naming this for caregivers can often be helpful as it provides them with a specific role as an essential member of their child's healthcare team. This framework allows clinicians the opportunity to learn about the patient and their family, who they are as individuals outside of the hospital setting, their beliefs and dreams, their hopes, their goals, and their fears. It also allows for open discussion about family communication and decision-making style.

Within pediatric illness, caregivers often act as gatekeepers, managing the information their child has given about their illness (Ranmal et al. 2008). Caregivers want to be involved in the decision regarding how their child is informed about their illness (Levetown 2008). While some prefer that medical information come from them, others prefer that medical providers have these discussions with the child, either alone or in their presence. In general, communication is most straightforward when the medical provider communicates serious medical information directly to the child in the presence of the parents. Clinicians can share the language that they plan to use with the parents ahead of time and even offer to role-play conversations with parents so the parent is comfortable with the information that will be delivered. While the majority of caregivers acknowledge the benefit of open communication with their child about their medical illness (Young et al. 2011), many are uncertain about how to initiate and engage in these conversations. As noted by Mack and colleagues (2006), there may be a natural reluctance to share serious information with a child due to a caregiver's fear about the child's emotional reaction or fear that the child will lose hope about the situation. Clinicians are able to help caregivers understand that research has demonstrated improved adherence to the plan and resultant health outcomes when the child is treated as a partner, included in treatment planning, and provided accurate and developmentally appropriate information (Sawyer and Aroni 2005).

Clinician-Child Communication

There is a strong ethical and legal obligation for medical providers to discuss information about health and illness with the pediatric patient. The principle of self-determination applies to children as well as adults. Involving children in communication about their illness and in treatment decisions demonstrates respect for their capacities and may provide opportunities for further development (McCabe 1996). National and international policies (e.g., American Academy of Pediatrics, International Society of Pediatric Oncology) recommend that best practice for providers includes encouraging all pediatric patients to express their views and to participate in their own healthcare (Spinetta et al. 2009). Research has uniformly shown that better information leads to lower levels of general distress including lower levels of symptoms of depression and anxiety (Clarke et al. 2005) and that children report feeling valued and less anxious about their medical condition when they are included in discussions about their healthcare treatment (Dixon-Woods et al. 2002; Kelsey et al. 2007; Moore and Kirk 2010).

However, children are often not treated as active participants in their own medical care. A review on triadic communication in the pediatric primary care setting found that children often had little involvement in the consultations. Their involvement was often limited to the history and examination phases of the encounter, with very little participation during the explanation and planning phases (Cahill and Papageorgiou 2007). Research examining the type of communication between pediatric patients and doctors has found that communication often seems to be restricted to the affective domain, typified by some researchers as a "joking relationship" (Aronsson and Rundström 1989; Tates and Meeuwesen 2001). While there is not a robust literature about communication preferences of pediatric patients, observational studies have shown many children express a desire to be more involved in the communication process and decision-making (Björk et al. 2006; Lambert et al. 2008). The act of engaging children in decision-making and treatment planning can be complicated, but thoughtful consideration of their developmental stage and experience with illness may help both clinicians and caregivers in decisions regarding specific language used in conversations, frequency of conversations, and depth of material covered (Bluebond-Langner et al. 2010).

Enhancing Triadic Communication and Decision-Making through Shuttle Diplomacy

Communication in pediatric oncology requires providers to delicately balance the often overlapping but sometimes distinct needs of both the patient and their caregivers. While it is understood that the clinical team has a legal, moral, and ethical obligation to include children in discussions about their own healthcare, there is limited guidance about how to translate these recommendations into clinical practice. This lack of guidance creates challenges for patients, caregivers, and clinicians and large variations in care, as each member of the triad may have differing ideas about what their own role and the role of the other members should be. Furthermore, existing family dynamics and the natural difference in authority between children and caregivers can complicate the treatment decision-making process. Clinicians must continually assess the extent to which children are granted their own "voice" within the family system, the degree to which children are aware of and wish to support their caregivers' preferences, and the possible discrepancy in amount and type of information provided to both parties, as all factors can significantly influence the outcome of the decision-making process.

Shuttle diplomacy, coined in the pediatric illness context by Bluebond-Langner and colleagues (2005), is an approach for involving children in the decision-making process that both formally and respectfully recognizes three participants: the clinician, the caregivers, and the child. In political shuttle diplomacy, a diplomat conducts discussions with each of the parties (e.g., countries, political groups) separately before moving on to negotiations between the parties. This strategy can be particularly helpful when discrepancies arise within the triad. Within the context of pediatric oncology, clinicians can serve as the diplomat, meeting with caregivers and the child to understand their preferences about communication. These meetings provide the framework for exploration of how decisions have historically been made in the family from the perspective of the caregiver(s) and the child. It provides an opportunity for clinicians to understand any caregiver concerns about providing the child with information about their illness and to address common misconceptions. For the child, it provides an opportunity for the clinician to get to know them better, to provide honest and developmentally appropriate information in a manner that is consistent with family values and preferences, and to understand their perspective on the current circumstance. Within this approach, clinicians are better able to understand the preferences of all participants involved and "negotiate" an individualized plan for ongoing communication and decision-making.

Principles for Communicating with Parents

1. Build a relationship with parents. Factors predictive of effective communication between providers and parents include perception of interest, caring, warmth, and responsiveness (as cited in Levetown 2008).
2. Solicit information about family communication style, past decision-making experiences, and cultural considerations.
3. Recognize the parent as the expert on their child.
4. Openly discuss child involvement from day 1:
   (a) Provide information to the child:
      (i) Consider the order of delivery (all together, parents first, then child).
      (ii) Consider the delivery of information to the child (by parent, provider).
      (iii) Consider what information is delivered.
   (b) Respect the role of the child in treatment decision-making.

Plan in advance for challenging circumstances: What if the child's preference and the parent's preference are different?

Developmental Considerations

Infants and Toddlers (Ages 0–3)

The period between birth and age three is a critically formative time when children are developing attachment and trust through their relationships with their primary caregivers. Separation, pain, exposure to strange people and unfamiliar situations, and disruption of normal routines can all impact the child's ability to cope with their illness. Very young children do not have the ability to comprehend verbal explanations or the idea of "cancer." Intervention should focus on helping parents establish (or reestablish) a daily routine including feeding, baths, naptime, and bedtime, which will help maximize consistency and predictability, increase the family's sense of agency and control, and decrease stress for both the children and their parents.

Preschool Children (Ages 3–5)

Cognitive development during this period is characterized by egocentric and magical thinking, along with associative logic. Therefore, preschoolers will benefit from receiving simple and consistent explanations about their illness and treatment. It should be made very clear to preschoolers that nothing they did or said caused the illness, as in the absence of this information they

Principles for Communication with Pediatric Patients

1. Never underestimate the importance of taking time to establish rapport and build a relationship with the patient.
2. Elicit from the patient what is important to them (e.g., attending school, minimizing needle sticks, playing soccer).
3. Ask the patient (every time) who they would like to be present during the conversation.
4. If the parent is in the room, focus attention on the patient. Look at them, speak directly to them, and elicit their opinion.
5. Listen actively. Children are attuned to when they do not have an adult's undivided attention.
6. Consider the use of communication tools – iPads, drawing, etc. Many children are visual and may benefit from the use of multiple modalities to help them understand information.
7. Put information into a context that resonates with the patient (importance of pearl 1 in section "Clinical Pearls for Communicating with Patients and Caregivers in distress"):
   (a) If the patient's main desire is to attend school as much as possible, discuss the treatment within this frame (e.g., you should be able to attend school on these days; one of the side effects of the medicine is feeling tired, so to keep this from interfering with school, we are going to do X, Y, Z).

are capable of creating their own, likely egocentric, explanations such as "I didn't listen to Mommy and that is why I got sick." It is important to include factual information such as the name of the illness, basic and concrete information about the treatment, and the expected impact on the child's normal routine. For example, "You have a tumor called neuroblastoma, which is why your stomach has been hurting. You need special medicine called chemotherapy to make the tumor go away and this will be given at the clinic. You will get the chemotherapy through your tube. On days that you are getting the medicine you will not go to daycare." Children at this age can report on situation-specific symptoms (e.g., what hurts right now). The use of play or other communication techniques such as drawing can be both very helpful to communicate information to preschool children and also serve as a way of helping them report on their subjective experience. Stuffed animals or dolls with a central line or a port (e.g., Chemo Duck; www.chemoduck.org) are also useful tools for facilitating communication for clinicians, parents, and children.

School-Age Children (Ages 6–12)

School-age children have an increased capacity to think logically and to differentiate between themselves and the outside world. Thinking patterns continue to be relatively concrete with a focus on cause and effect and on fairness. When talking to school-age children, it is again important to clearly state that nothing they did caused them to get cancer and that their cancer is not a punishment for something they did. Children may have heard the word cancer before, and asking them about their understanding of what cancer is and what causes it can be helpful so that any misconceptions can be addressed directly. As children will vary widely in their desire for information, participation in discussions about their illness, and their role in the decision-making process, it is important to address each of these topics specifically with the child and their family.

Adolescents (Ages 13–18)

Adolescence is a period of great cognitive development, with a transition from concrete thinking to formal logical operations. As the ability to understand and to use abstract concepts begins to develop, adolescents become increasingly capable of making independent and informed decisions. Adolescent patients should be given a say in how they would like to receive information and what role they would like to have in the decision-making process (McCabe 1996). It is helpful to encourage providers to routinely meet with adolescent patients individually, giving them a time to discuss their own feelings without worry about parental reaction.

Special Topics

Discussing Bad News

At Diagnosis

Delivering news about a child's cancer diagnosis often comes in phases – first, when a cancer diagnosis is suspected but not confirmed, or when the details of the pathologic diagnosis are still in question, and then again later when the specifics of the diagnosis and treatment are known. At each phase, a commitment to honesty and timely disclosure of medical information is critical; at the same time, disclosing a probable diagnosis before it is final can also create unnecessary distress. Thus, during the initial phase of uncertainty, clinicians must find a balance between disclosing what is known and waiting to discuss information that holds significant uncertainty. This time period tends to be particularly difficult for children and families, who often express relief when clear information is available, no matter how difficult the content of that information may be.

Once a diagnosis and treatment plan or clear options for treatment are known with greater certainty, the clinician can sit down with the child and family for what is termed the Day One Talk (Mack and Grier 2004). As in other important conversations, the team (including medical providers and the psychosocial clinician) start by asking the child and family about their understanding of the child's illness. This helps us to understand where the conversation should start and whether there are misconceptions we should correct. In addition, this sets the stage for listening as one of our most important roles.

As we begin to share information, we focus our communication on three major points. Although these conversations can be quite long, we emphasize the three main aspects of the Day One Talk as the issues we want them to hear and remember:

1. The diagnosis – that we know what this is. This is particularly important because, as noted, this conversation tends to follow a period of uncertainty. In addition, we make sure to use the word cancer, to ensure that families understand that the child has cancer, even if the name of the type of cancer is something like Hodgkin's disease or leukemia, where cancer is not explicit. In addition, the word cancer has history and meaning in many families, and using that word allows us to ask about and address that meaning, which may or may not apply to their child.
2. We have treatment for the child's cancer. Along with this, we detail the goals of treatment. Often, for children with newly diagnosed cancer, we have good treatment and the goal of the treatment is cure. When cure is not possible, however, we explain that also. Along with this, we ask families whether they would like to hear any prognostic information. Research has shown that most families do indeed wish to hear about prognosis (Mack et al. 2006), and offering them the most accurate information possible can help them to make good decisions for their children going forward.
3. Cause of the child's cancer. Although much of the time no known cause exists, families often try to understand why this event would have happened in their lives and blame themselves. Making this an explicit part of the discussion allows us to address this as clearly as possible. We therefore tell children and families that childhood cancer has very few known causes and that we know of nothing that they or their child did, or didn't do, to cause this. In rare cases where potential causality exists, such as a genetic cause for the cancer, we explain this directly as well. Along similar lines, caregivers often wonder if they should have come in

sooner for evaluation or if other physicians should have recognized signs of cancer sooner. Most of the time, we are able to reassure caregivers that everything they (and the pediatrician) did was appropriate and that finding this even sooner would not have changed what we would have done for the child or her prognosis. In the rare cases where we know there has been a delay, we acknowledge that fact. While we cannot know whether a child's outcome would have been different if the cancer had been found sooner, we can at least acknowledge their sadness and fear. Of note, children, like their parents, also need to hear that the cancer is not their fault; if the child was not present for this conversation, we make sure to address this issue with him or her later.

After we have addressed these three main points, we then turn to the details of the child's cancer and its treatment. We describe where the cancer begins, how it can spread, and what we know about whether the tumor has spread to other parts of the body. A treatment plan can be introduced, with written information for the child and family to follow, so that they can review the information again later. If a research study is an option, we explain what taking part in the research means and what the standard treatment is. Because families often believe that research studies offer improved outcomes (Cousino et al. 2012), we also explain that the purpose of research is to benefit future patients, but that it could be better, worse, or the same as existing standard treatment.

We discuss treatment in general terms with an emphasis on the phases of treatment (e.g., induction or local control) and its expected impact on the child's life during the different phases, such as time in the hospital or when the child may return to school. We describe side effects of chemotherapy in general, with an emphasis on common side effects, such as myelosuppression and hair loss, and then discuss more specific side effects of each medication. We tell children and families that everyone gets some side effects, but no one gets all of the possible side effects; we also make sure to discuss which side effects are expected, which are unlikely, which could be permanent or life-threatening, and which are reversible.

Once the basic medical information has been discussed, the psychosocial clinician will discuss other important issues, such as sources of support, ways that friends and family can be helpful (and the ways they sometimes are not), information resources, and the structure of our team. Finally, after this very long conversation, we return to our first three points as those that should be remembered – we know what this is, we have treatment for it, and the cancer diagnosis is neither the child's nor the family's fault.

At Relapse

When children experience a cancer relapse, they and their families come to a very similar conversation with greater experience with cancer and its treatment and also new worries about whether the recurrent cancer can be cured. Because a recurrence means that all the child already went through was not effective, and because recurrent cancer can be much harder to treat, these conversations can be particularly painful. However, in most cases, the clinical team now has a longstanding relationship with this child and family. This can therefore be a particularly important time to come together with a shared history and deep caring.

The structure of the Day One Talk remains appropriate at the time of relapse, but with some changes. The clinical team again starts by telling the child and family that we know what this is, and we offer them a name for the cancer. This is usually a name that they know, as it is the same tumor, but because it can recur in new locations, it is important to confirm that we are indeed talking about the same cancer type. Second, we discuss treatment and its goals, including whether it may be possible to cure the child's recurrent cancer or whether treatment can offer symptom palliation and longer life. Finally, we again review the topic of causation, this time discussing the fact that we usually never know why cancer recurs for some children but not for others. Nonetheless, whenever possible, we reaffirm that the child and family did everything they possibly could and everything we asked them to do. Sometimes families question whether the cancer was treated properly in the first place, and we discuss those worries openly. When our own opinion is not enough to dispel fears, we offer families the chance to seek a second opinion and hear this information from others.

At the Transition to Palliative Care

Ideally palliative care is integrated early for all children with cancer, soon after diagnosis, with attention to symptom management, personal goals and values, and quality of life throughout care. Even in these cases, however, children and families who move away from curative measures to palliation have special communication needs.

One issue is that of communication about prognosis. While most families want to hear about prognosis even from the time of diagnosis, knowledge of prognosis is particularly salient for decision-making about end-of-life care; caregivers (and children) who do not know the child is dying are more likely to continue to pursue aggressive measures, even near death. Thus, rather than deferring to caregiver preferences about prognosis communication, clinicians may have special obligations to discuss prognosis even if caregivers find it painful. Reflecting on whether prognosis communication is essential, and the best timing for this discussion, is important before the conversation starts. The medical providers might then either offer prognostic information ("Would it be helpful to hear more about your child's prognosis?") or, alternatively, express the importance of such a conversation ("I think it's important that we talk about his future, including his prognosis.") Prognosis can then be stated in clear and unambiguous terms, albeit with caring and empathy (e.g., "I am so sorry to say this, but we no longer have a way to cure his cancer. We expect that it will continue to come back, no matter what we do, and that eventually he will not be able to survive it.")

Caregivers and children who understand a child's poor prognosis can begin to make decisions about care, with support and input from the clinical team. We suggest focusing on their goals as a path toward value-driven decision-making. A conversation about goals can begin with questions for the child and family – "as you think about the future, what is most important to you? Is there anything you are especially worried about? Is there anything you are especially hoping for?" Some families may continue to express hopes for cure, even when it is no longer possible. In this case, it can be helpful to ask, "and what else are you hoping for?" or, alternatively, "And what if what you are hoping for were no longer possible? What kind of things might you hope for in that situation?" Asking gently about alternative hopes can allow parents to express a full range of hopes, without forcing them to acknowledge that cure will never be.

Once goals are known, then recommendations for care can be made that reflect those goals. For example, if a child values being at home and in school, the medical team might recommend against intensive chemotherapy, which could detract from those goals. Alternatively, a family who wishes to prolong life may wish to use more intensive measures, even if they are associated with greater symptoms. Understanding goals can help to frame each decision and allows affirmation of the patient's and parent's goals all along the trajectory of care.

A final issue in palliative care communication is what to expect at the end of life. For many children and families, understanding what is ahead can take away some of the painful uncertainty of this period of time. Please see Chap. 14 on Palliative Care for further details. Although this is a difficult topic, some find that this information offers a sense of control and, for caregivers, an ability to anticipate the needs of the child even during her last days. As the clinical team, we therefore offer this information "Would it be helpful to talk about what to expect as the end of life grows closer?" to those who are looking ahead to this phase.

For children and adolescents, the conversation can begin with a focus on fears, worries, and hopes. The clinician might ask, for example, "As you think about the time ahead, is there anything you are most worried about? Anything you are hoping for?" Understanding worries and hopes can then serve as a starting point for talking about what is likely to happen and how symptoms will be managed. This can also be an opportunity for understanding wishes for the location of care near death and for addressing worries about loved ones and a desire to be remembered beyond death. Tools such as "Voicing My CHOICES" can offer adolescents and young adults the opportunity to think about their wishes for end-of-life care and make those wishes known to loved ones (Wiener et al. 2012; Zadeh and Wiener 2014).

For families who are interested in knowing more about what to expect, we similarly discuss topics such as location of death (eliciting their preferences) and avenues of support (such as home hospice, inpatient hospice, or inpatient hospital care.) In addition, family members may find it helpful to understand changes that the child may go through in her last days. This includes discussion of decreased perfusion of extremities, decreased urine output, and decreased consciousness, as well as respiratory depression, noisy breathing, and irregular breathing patterns. We talk about signs of discomfort or distress and how we will ensure the child is as comfortable as possible during this time. Finally, we also try to offer some discussion about autopsy before death occurs, as well as care of the body after death, to help parents prepare for those moments after the child has died. Not every family wishes for this information, but many do, and of those, many are afraid to ask (Wiener et al. 2014).

Communication with Patients and Caregivers in Distress

Cancer diagnoses and associated care planning are inherently stressful and understandably distressing for patients and their caregivers. In this context, it is likely that patients and caregivers experience strong feelings, such as fear, anger, and sadness, and it is also expected that such feelings will be present and perhaps even heightened, during interactions with clinicians in the position of sharing complex and often unpleasant information. Such strong emotional expression is a complicated component of already delicate interactions. The recommendations in the following sections are designed to assist medical and psychosocial clinicians in navigating interpersonally complex interactions with patients and their caregivers in a manner that maximizes effective communication and prioritizes the execution of high-quality medical care.

Proactive Interventions

We know, even before such situations present themselves, that these types of communication challenges are likely to emerge within our work in pediatric psycho-oncology. Therefore, proactive measures that may positively impact clinician-patient and clinician-caregiver relationships should be implemented whenever possible to maximize understanding of medical information and minimize the likelihood of miscommunication and associated negative feelings.

Relationship Factors

All clinical team members would benefit from making an active effort to develop positive working relationships with patients and their family members as early as possible and to maintain them throughout the course of treatment. The establishment of a positive working relationship characterized by trust, mutual respect, and collaboration should not be underestimated. This relationship will not only facilitate the effective exchange of information throughout one's course of treatment, but it may also aid in the resolution of any strong negative feelings by providing a foundation upon which such feelings can be explored in a supportive, nonjudgmental, and productive manner.

Communication Preferences

Beginning early on in treatment, it would behoove clinicians to discuss, document, and accommodate family preferences in regard to communication. For example, in an effort to minimize anxiety and maximize the extent to which information is understood during important conversations (Schwabe and Wolf 2010), individuals may request, or clinicians may observe, that patients and/or their family members benefit from the following:

- The provision of written information to read and review independently and to reference, as needed (e.g., a summary of information discussed with the medical team, medication teaching sheets, published research papers)
- The presence of a specific family member, close family friend, or spiritual or religious representative
- That meetings be held in a specific location, such as a private conference room, as opposed to a shared clinic space or exam room
- The inclusion of as few clinicians as possible in conversations, which may feel less intimidating or overwhelming than the inclusion of multiple clinicians from the oncology service and perhaps consulting services.

Team-Family Meetings

At any point after the initiation of care, if any member of the multidisciplinary team has a sense that communication may be especially challenging due to patient or caregiver distress, consideration of regularly scheduled team-family meetings may be warranted. The specific purpose, timing, and composition of such meetings can be individualized, but the general goal of a team-family meeting is to provide a scheduled opportunity to review relevant information, to preview upcoming treatment needs and potential interventions, and to address any clinician or family concerns. Such meetings have been shown to be effective in facilitating discussions in the context of intensive care admissions and end-of-life decision-making (Marik et al. 2009; Nelson et al. 2009; Radwany et al. 2009), and such principles can be applied to improving communication at any point in the treatment course.

The nature and structure of the discussion may be similar to that of a routine medical visit, but the distinction as a separate meeting can be valuable in that (1) teams can meet separately prior to the meeting to ensure all providers are on the same page and invite relevant multidisciplinary clinicians and/or consulting services to attend, if appropriate, (2) family members can prepare questions and discussion points in advance that clinicians may not have time to address during routine appointments, and (3) it provides an opportunity to repeat, reinforce, or clarify important information that was presented during routine visits, which can be particularly helpful for patients and caregivers whose distress may in some form interfere with the reception, retention, or understanding of important medical information.

Communication Skills

In addition to such preventive methods, the effective and consistent implementation of the basic communication skills described earlier in this chapter is particularly important during interactions with distressed patients or caregivers.

Utilize Active Listening Skills

During challenging exchanges, active listening, acknowledging emotions, and expressing empathy are essential. In addition, maintaining a nonjudgmental approach and validating a family's experience can help clinicians navigate such interactions in a manner that fosters a positive working relationship. Among adult patients, adopting a warm, empathic, emotionally supportive approach has been associated with reduced anxiety and distress, as well as improved recall of medical information (van Osch et al. 2014); this approach is likely to be helpful when interacting with caregivers and patients in pediatric settings, as well.

Flexibly Maintain Structure

Core components of an effective clinical conversation include establishing the purpose of the conversation, eliciting patient and/or caregiver preferences and involvement in decision-making, reviewing options and recommendations, acknowledging patient/caregiver emotions, and eliciting patient and/or caregiver comprehension. The trajectory of conversations with individuals expressing strong negative emotion may be somewhat unpredictable, so remaining mindful of the key aspects of the interaction while maintaining flexibility will likely result in a more successful and satisfactory exchange from the perspective of both the clinician and the patient/caregiver.

Affective and Cognitive Strategies for Clinicians

It is important to acknowledge that the experience of communicating with individuals in distress, whether they are sad, angry, or anxious, naturally elicits emotional reactions in clinicians. After all, communication is a dynamic process. Therefore, when communicating with individuals in distress, depending on the type and intensity of their emotional response, it may be experienced by clinicians as sad, uncomfortable, awkward, frustrating, or even offensive. In order to utilize the communication strategies described above in a genuine and consistent manner, and to remain nondefensive and fully present and available to offer one's clinical expertise, it is helpful for clinicians to remain cognizant of their internal affective and cognitive experience. A clinician's emotional and cognitive experience may be reflected in verbal and nonverbal expressions and, therefore, may have a significant impact on the ongoing communication process. Clinicians benefit from acknowledging feelings, judgments, and assumptions made about patients and caregivers, especially those that fail to foster productive, patient-centered, mutually respectful communication.

If negative feelings or cognitions are identified, the use of internal statements by clinicians may be helpful in minimizing the extent to which such internal experiences interfere with the genuine expression of empathy. For example, when interacting with a frustrated caregiver who is raising her voice, speaking over the clinician, and ruminating on past events that have been discussed repeatedly over the course of many days, a clinician may feel equally frustrated, defeated, or angry. If the clinician is able to recognize those feelings in the moment, she will be much better prepared to redirect or channel them in a productive way. They may serve as cues to use internal statements that recognize the nature of the family's experience or positive intentions, qualities, or abilities, such as the following: "This mother is petrified that her child is going to die," "This mother is doing the very best that she can," or "This family's life has been devastated by their child's diagnosis." Individualized internal statements may help clinicians empathize with families during the most interpersonally challenging moments. In doing so, a clinician may be more likely to maintain a family-centered perspective, to use active listening skills, and to navigate the conversation toward a collaborative end, as opposed to further escalating a vulnerable patient or caregiver.

Practical Interventions

There are a number of very practical interventions that can be containing and reassuring to patients and families in distress, as well as effective for clinicians and staff.

Ensure Safety

Distress is expected and is completely understandable for patients and family members affected by a cancer diagnosis. While that is always true, safety of patients and staff must always be a top priority. Therefore, if expressions of anxiety, anger, or sadness, on the part of a patient or family member ever pose a physical threat or are interpreted as aggressive or disruptive to patients or staff, steps must be taken immediately to de-escalate the individual and to prevent such events from occurring in the future. At the first sign of potential escalation during conversations with clinical staff, it is helpful to clearly and firmly communicate hospital policies and the rationale for such policies, namely, protecting patients and staff. Ideally, clinicians would be able to do so in a gentle, empathic manner, but boundaries around safety must always be maintained and respected. Joining with the family around a mutual responsibility and shared interest in safety and the provision of high-quality clinical care, above all else, may help in navigating situations in which hospital or clinic policies are referenced and reinforced. A discussion of decision-making around issues of child protection is beyond the scope of this chapter, but would also be highly relevant in circumstances of this nature if child abuse or neglect is suspected or observed by clinical staff.

Psychosocial Referral

As patient or caregiver distress may present at any point along a patient's treatment trajectory, access to specialized psychosocial assessment and intervention services is crucial both for families and medical teams. Mental health clinicians who are well integrated and familiar with both administrative and clinical personnel on medical teams will be best suited to address clinical issues in a timely, thorough, and well-informed manner. When providing psychosocial services to patients and families in this context, particularly those exhibiting significant emotional or behavioral distress, it is essential to have a solid understanding of the medical factors at play, as well as knowledge and experience navigating the complex medical systems within which the family and medical teams are operating. Interventions often involve engaging multiple team members and mobilizing hospital-based supports. Mental health clinicians who are easily accessible, available to meet with patients and families throughout their course of treatment, and who have established collaborative relationships with medical providers will be best equipped to effectively and efficiently meet the mental health needs of the pediatric oncology population.

Lessons from the Case Vignette about Charlie

Charlie, the 13-year-old boy with Ewing sarcoma, whose parents did not want anyone to discuss his care needs with him, demonstrates a situation in which the medical team, the parents, and the patient are not on the same page. The following clinical recommendations may be helpful in situations similar to this:

- Early involvement and inclusion of a psychosocial provider on the clinical team
- Relationship building and understanding multiple perspectives:
  - Learning about the parent's fear regarding giving Charlie medical information and correcting misperceptions
  - At parent's request, provision of written material about this topic
- Team communication and collaboration
  - Identification of effective and ineffective communication strategies for this family
  - Multidisciplinary support for staff around disagreement with parent approach
- Established family meetings above and beyond usual clinic appointments that included key medical, psychosocial, and nursing providers

After establishing a relationship with Charlie's parents, they became more receptive to suggestions from the clinical team about providing developmentally appropriate information to Charlie. As Charlie became a more active participant in his clinic appointments, discussions about treatment and decision-making became more inclusive of Charlie. It was notable that as this was occurring, despite ongoing physical side effects, Charlie's symptoms of anxiety began to decrease and he independently started taking a more active role in his care at home, such as requesting to be in charge of his pill box and scheduling his daily routine.

Clinical Pearls

- Discuss, document, and accommodate family preferences in regard to communication.
- The effective use of active listening skills is essential to maintain rapport, understand the ever evolving patient and family experience, and ultimately navigate the conversation toward a mutually beneficial and productive end.
- If challenges in communication are noted, consider the potential benefits of establishing a regularly scheduled team-family meeting.
- Remain aware of internal affective and cognitive experiences and use internal statements, as needed, in order to consistently approach interactions in a nondefensive, nonjudgmental, and empathic manner.
- If emotional expressions are ever interpreted as aggressive or disruptive, join with the family around the establishment of a safe and healing atmosphere for their child, and adopt a gentle but firm approach to de-escalate the individual and to prevent such events from occurring in the future.

References

Aronsson K, Rundström B (1989) Cats, dogs, and sweets in the clinical negotiation of reality: on politeness and coherence in pediatric discourse. Lang Soc 18(04): 483–504

Back AL, Arnold RM, Baile WF, Tulsky JA, Fryer-Edwards K (2005) Approaching difficult communication tasks in oncology. CA Cancer J Clin 55(3): 164–177

Baile WF, Buckman R, Lenzi R, Glober G, Beale EA, Kudelka AP (2000) SPIKES-A six-step protocol for delivering bad news: application to the patient with cancer. Oncologist 5(4):302–311

Beale EA, Baile WF, Aaron J (2005) Silence is not golden: communicating with children dying from cancer. J Clin Oncol 23(15):3629–3631

Björk M, Nordström B, Hallström I (2006) Needs of young children with cancer during their initial hospitalization: an observational study. J Pediatr Oncol Nurs 23(4):210–219

Bluebond-Langner M, DeCicco A, Belasco J (2005) Involving children with life-shortening illnesses in decisions about participation in clinical research: a proposal for shuttle diplomacy and negotiation. In: Kodish E (ed) Ethics and research with children. Oxford University Press, New York, USA. pp 323–344

Bluebond-Langner M, Belasco JB, DeMesquita Wander M (2010) "I want to live, until I don't want to live anymore": involving children with life-threatening and life-shortening illnesses in decision making about care and treatment. Nurs Clin North Am 45(3):329–343

Cahill P, Papageorgiou A (2007) Triadic communication in the primary care paediatric consultation: a review of the literature. Br J Gen Pract 57(544):904–911

Clarke SA, Davies H, Jenney M, Glaser A, Eiser C (2005) Parental communication and children's behaviour following diagnosis of childhood leukaemia. Psychooncology 14(4):274–281

Cousino MK, Zyzanski SJ, Yamokoski AD, Hazen RA, Baker JN, Noll RB, Rheingold SR, Geyer JR, Alexander SC, Drotar D, Kodish ED (2012) Communicating and understanding the purpose of pediatric phase I cancer trials. J Clin Oncol 2012;30(35):4367– 4372

Dixon-Woods M, Anwar Z, Young B, Brooke A (2002) Lay evaluation of services for childhood asthma. Health Soc Care Community 10(6):503–511

Kelsey J, Abelson-Mitchell N, Skirton H (2007) Perceptions of young people about decision making in the acute healthcare environment. Paediatr Nurs 19(6):14–18

Lambert V, Glacken M, McCarron M (2008) 'Visibleness': the nature of communication for children admitted to a specialist children's hospital in the Republic of Ireland. J Clin Nurs 17(23):3092–3102

Levetown M (2008) Communicating with children and families: from everyday interactions to skill in conveying distressing information. Pediatrics 121(5):e1441–e1460

Mack JW, Grier HE (2004) The day one talk. J Clin Oncol 22(3):563–566

Mack JW, Joffe S (2014) Communicating about prognosis: ethical responsibilities of pediatricians and parents. Pediatrics 133(Suppl 1):S24–S30

Mack JW, Wolfe J, Grier HE, Cleary PD, Weeks JC (2006) Communication about prognosis between parents and physicians of children with cancer: parent preferences and the impact of prognostic information. J Clin Oncol 24(33):5265–5270

Marik PE, Callahan A, Paganelli G, Reville B, Parks SM, Delgado EM (2009) Multidisciplinary family meetings in the ICU facilitate end-of-life decision making. Am J Hosp Palliat Med 26(4):295–302

McCabe MA (1996) Involving children and adolescents in medical decision making: developmental and clinical considerations. J Pediatr Psychol 21(4):505–516

Meyer EC, Sellers DE, Browning DM, McGuffie K, Solomon MZ, Truog RD (2009) Difficult conversations: improving communication skills and relational abilities in health care. Pediatr Crit Care Med 10(3):352–359

Moore L, Kirk S (2010) A literature review of children's and young people's participation in decisions relating to health care. J Clin Nurs 19(15–16):2215–2225

Nelson JE, Walker AS, Luhrs CA, Cortez TB, Pronovost PJ (2009) Family meetings made simpler: a toolkit for the intensive care unit. J Crit Care 24(4):626. e627–626. e614

Radwany S, Albanese T, Clough L, Sims L, Mason H, Jahangiri S (2009) End-of-life decision making and emotional burden: placing family meetings in context. Am J Hosp Palliat Care 26(5):376–383

Ranmal R, Prictor M, Scott JT (2008) Interventions for improving communication with children and adolescents about their cancer. Cochrane Database Syst Rev (4):CD002969

Rutishauser C (2003) Communicating with young people. Paediatr Respir Rev 4(4):319–324

Sawyer SM, Aroni RA (2005) Self-management in adolescents with chronic illness. What does it mean and how can it be achieved. Med J Aust 183(8):405

Schwabe L, Wolf OT (2010) Learning under stress impairs memory formation. Neurobiol Learn Mem 93(2): 183–188

Spinetta JJ, Masera G, Eden T, Oppenheim D, Martins AG, van Dongen-Melman J, Siegler M, Eiser C, Weyl M (2002) Refusal, non-compliance, and abandonment of treatment in children and adolescents with cancer. A report of the SIOP Working Committee on Phychosocial Issues in Pediatric Oncology. Med Pediatr Oncol 38(2):114–117

Spinetta JJ, Jankovic M, Masera G, Ablin AR, Barr RD, Arush MWB, D'Angio GJ, Van Dongen-Melman J, Eden T, Epelman C (2009) Optimal care for the child with cancer: a summary statement from the SIOP Working Committee on Psychosocial Issues in Pediatric Oncology. Pediatr Blood Cancer 52(7):904–907

Tates K, Meeuwesen L (2001) Doctor–parent–child communication. A (re) view of the literature. Soc Sci Med 52(6):839–851

van Osch M, Sep M, van Vliet LM, van Dulmen S, Bensing JM (2014) Reducing patients' anxiety and uncertainty, and improving recall in bad news consultations. Health Psychol 33(11):1382

Wiener L, Zadeh S, Battles H, Baird K, Ballard E, Osherow J (2012) Allowing adolescents and young adults to plan their end-of-life care. Pediatrics 130(5): 897–905

Wiener L, Sweeney C, Baird K, Merchant MS, Warren KE, Corner GW, Roberts KE, Lichtenthal WG (2014) What do parents want to know when considering autopsy for their child with cancer? J Pediatr Hematol Oncol 36(6):464–470

Young B, Ward J, Salmon P, Gravenhorst K, Hill J, Eden T (2011) Parents' experiences of their children's presence in discussions with physicians about leukemia. Pediatrics 127(5):e1230–e1238

Zadeh S, Pao M, Wiener L (2014) Opening end-of-life discussions: how to introduce Voicing My CHOiCES™, an advance care planning guide for adolescents and young adults. Palliat Support Care 13(3):591–599

3 Physical Impact of Pediatric Cancer and Its Treatment

Cheryl Rodgers, Janice Withycombe, and Marilyn Hockenberry

Introduction

Childhood cancer survival rates have greatly improved over the last three decades. However, symptoms experienced during treatment often result in complications that may compromise therapy, negatively influence quality of life, and even more notably threaten chances for long-term survival. Each symptom requires careful assessment and appropriate interventions to reduce the distress and improve daily life for the child with cancer and their family.

This chapter discusses the physical impact of cancer and its treatment on the child. The most common symptoms that should be considered during every clinical assessment are reviewed. Discussion includes an overview of each symptom and unique characteristics experienced by children with cancer. Possible causes, risk factors, and important assessment measures for each symptom are examined with specific recommendations for prevention and management.

C. Rodgers, PhD, RN, CPNP, CPON (✉)
M. Hockenberry, PhD, RN, PPCNP-BC, FAAN
Duke University School of Nursing,
307 Trent Drive, Durham, NC 27710, USA
e-mail: cheryl.rodgers@duke.edu; marilyn.hockenberry@duke.edu

J. Withycombe, PhD, RN, MN, CCRP
Emory University, Nell Hodgson Woodruff School of Nursing, 1520 Clifton Rd, Atlanta, GA 30322, USA
e-mail: jwithycombe@emory.edu

Bone Marrow Suppression

Chemotherapy agents and radiation therapy cause myelosuppression, a condition that occurs when bone marrow activity is decreased and produces fewer white blood cells, red blood cells, and platelets. In addition, certain malignancies that metastasize to the bone marrow (e.g., leukemia, lymphoma, neuroblastoma, sarcomas) cause a decrease in the number of normal blood cell precursors. When the myelosuppressive effect is severe enough, the child becomes predisposed to infection, anemia, or bleeding, depending on which blood cell line is affected.

Infection

The risk for serious infection in a child receiving treatment for cancer is related to several factors. Cancer therapy often results in neutropenia which is a decrease in the type of white blood cell (neutrophil) that fights infection. An absolute neutrophil count (ANC) less than 1000 cells/microL is defined as neutropenia. The most common risk factors associated with serious infection include children diagnosed with acute myeloid leukemia (AML) or relapsed leukemia, those receiving highly myelosuppressive chemotherapy for non-hematologic malignancies or undergoing hematopoietic stem cell transplantation, and children with more severe neutropenia (ANC < 500 cells/

A.N. Abrams et al. (eds.), *Pediatric Psychosocial Oncology: Textbook for Multidisciplinary Care*,
DOI 10.1007/978-3-319-21374-3_3

microL) expected to last >7 days (Ahmed and Flynn 2014; Lehrnbecher et al. 2012; Pulsipher 2012). Children with cancer who present with fever are at a lower risk for serious infection when the neutropenia is expected to resolve within a week.

Fever may be the only indication that infection is present; important aspects to consider in the history and physical examination are found in Table 3.1 (Freifeld et al. 2011). The child with fever and neutropenia is at risk for potentially fatal septic shock. Children presenting with an absolute neutrophil count <100/mm^3 and have evidence of focal infection (e.g., mucositis, abdominal pain, cellulitis, upper respiratory infection, perianal tenderness) should be carefully monitored for signs and symptoms of sepsis. Children less than 7 days since receiving intensive chemotherapy with or without dexamethasone, all infants with acute lymphocytic leukemia, patients with leukemia or lymphoma during intensive phases of treatment, patients with Down's syndrome, and those who have experienced a relapse and have fever and neutropenia should be carefully evaluated for sepsis.

Because of the high mortality rate associated with untreated infection, all children with cancer who have severe neutropenia (ANC < 500 cells/microL) and fever are considered at risk for a life-threatening infection until proven otherwise. Families should be taught to contact their healthcare providers at the first signs of infection. Evaluation of a child with fever and neutropenia should be completed as quickly as possible. Immediate medical interventions include: intravenous access to obtain blood specimens and begin hydration, antibiotics that are initiated within 1 hour of assessment of neutropenia and fever, and normal saline bolus for hypotension and blood product support as needed (Lehrnbecher et al. 2012). Medical intervention and antibiotic administration are provided promptly if the child shows any clinical localizing signs of infection regardless of the child's temperature (Koh and Pizzo 2011).

Anemia

Children with cancer may experience anemia that commonly occurs as a consequence of impaired bone marrow production as well as blood loss (Agrawal et al. 2011). Anemia transpires when the body does not have enough red blood cells to carry oxygen to tissues and organs. Anemia can be measured by hemoglobin, the amount of protein in red blood cells, and/or hematocrit, the volume of red blood cells compared to the total blood volume. Normal values of hemoglobin and hematocrit vary according to the child's age and gender. Children are amazingly resilient and tolerate low hemoglobin and hematocrit concentrations well, especially if the decline is gradual.

Signs and symptoms of anemia in the child with cancer are directly related to the severity and onset of anemia as well as the type of cancer.

Table 3.1 History and physical assessment: child with neutropenia

History	Physical assessment
• Date of last treatment and details of therapy (agents, dose, route) • Onset of fever and highest temperature (note: dexamethasone may mask fever) • Other symptoms including nausea, vomiting, diarrhea, pain (e.g., mouth, abdomen, perianal), swelling, redness, drainage • Recent diagnosis of GI or GU tumor • Exposure to infection (e.g., TB, Hx MRSA, recent CVL infection) and seasonal illnesses (i.e., RSV, influenza) • Recent invasive procedure • Recent foreign travel • Renal/hepatic dysfunction	Assess for signs/symptoms of shock: • Entire body for signs, tenderness/pain, induration, redness or discharge from any area; *examine closely the skin, nose, teeth, pharynx, sinuses, joints and extremities, procedure sites, and perineal and perirectal areas* • Central line – if external – note any redness or drainage along tunnel or at exit site • Mental status and changes in the child's awareness of person, place, and surroundings

Symptoms include pallor, headache, dizziness, shortness of breath, fatigue, tachycardia, and heart murmur. Children may complain of tiredness and weakness. Assess the child's level of tolerance for activities of daily living and play, and make adjustments to allow as much self-care as possible without undue exertion.

During times when the child with cancer experiences symptoms related to anemia, advise parents to plan diversional activities that promote rest but prevent boredom and withdrawal. Because short attention span, irritability, and restlessness are common in anemia and increase stress demands on the body, activities such as listening to music, playing games on an electronic devise, reading or listening to stories, working on a favorite hobby, coloring or drawing, playing board and card games, or watching television are appropriate. If the child is in school, it may be necessary for the parents to alert the schoolteacher to the child's physical limitations, particularly in terms of strenuous activity.

Medical interventions for anemia are recommended when the child experiences symptoms that place the child at risk for cardiac decompensation. Packed red blood cell transfusions frequently are required when the hemoglobin falls below 7 g/dL or the hematocrit falls below 21 % (Agrawal et al. 2011). Transfusion of blood products may cause transfusion reactions, manifested by fever, chills, body aches, urticaria, pruritus, and, in severe cases, wheezing, tachycardia, and respiratory compromise. Parents and the child should be educated about the need for blood transfusions and be aware of the possible side effects such as transfusion reactions.

Bleeding

Children with cancer are at risk of bleeding related to thrombocytopenia, described as a drop in the number of platelets that play an important role in blood clotting. Decreased platelet count occurs when treatment given for cancer causes myelosuppression or when platelet production is impaired; the bone marrow produces less platelets and the child is at risk for bleeding. The risk for spontaneous internal hemorrhage does not occur until the platelet count is 20,000 per mm^3 or lower (Agrawal et al. 2011).

Children with low platelets due to cancer or treatment should be carefully assessed for signs and symptoms of bleeding. Healthcare providers should pay close attention for signs of bleeding, inquiring about episodes of bleeding from the nose, mouth, or skin. Presence of blood in the urine and stool is evaluated. If the child has experienced recent vomiting, determine whether there was blood present in the fluid. Healthcare providers should carefully examine the child to determine whether there are signs of active bruising and bleeding on the child's skin; small red or purple spots on the skin are called petechiae and are caused by intradermal hemorrhage. Ecchymoses are larger bruises commonly found on the child's skin when platelets are low.

There are several interventions that minimize bleeding when platelets are low and should be discussed with the family before treatment begins and reinforced during follow-up visits. The family and child should be instructed to avoid ibuprofen, aspirin, and aspirin-containing products. These medications can increase bleeding risks by decreasing the effectiveness of platelets and thereby diminishing their ability to stop bleeding by forming a clot.

Skin punctures are avoided as much as possible because bleeding sites can become easily infected. When finger sticks, venipunctures, intramuscular injections, bone marrow aspirations, or lumbar punctures are performed, aseptic technique must be used along with continued observation for bleeding. The use of razors should be avoided, and a soft toothbrush should be used for dental care. Children should avoid using dental floss and are advised not to eat or chew sharp foods (e.g., tortilla chips, ice) to prevent gingival bleeding. Adolescent female patients may be given oral contraceptives or hormone therapy to suppress menses to decrease the risk of excessive bleeding. Rectal temperatures are avoided to prevent trauma of the gastrointestinal mucosa. When platelets are low, children and parents are advised to avoid activities that might cause injury or bleeding, such as riding bicycles and skateboards, climbing trees and playground equipment, and playing contact sports (Rodgers 2015).

If the child experiences epistaxis (nosebleed), the parents should be instructed to pinch the child's nostrils together with a gauze pad held between the thumb and index finger for at least 10 min. If there is persistent nose bleeding, or if the patient experiences hematuria (blood in the urine) or hematochezia (blood in the stool), the child should be evaluated by their healthcare provider. Platelet transfusions are generally reserved for active bleeding episodes that do not respond to local treatment. These types of transfusions are commonly needed during cancer induction or relapse therapy.

Gastrointestinal Impact

The physiological effects of the cancer diagnosis and/or the related treatment can create a variety of gastrointestinal (GI) issues in pediatric patients. Neurological changes and intestinal obstruction from the disease can create multiple GI symptoms, while destruction of mucosal cells throughout the GI tract from chemotherapy and/or radiation treatment causes multiple side effects. These GI issues are quite common among pediatric oncology patients and are very distressing to the patient and their family. A thorough understanding of these issues, prompt recognition, and comprehensive treatment can assist to minimize the issues and decrease distress.

Mucositis/Esophagitis

Mucositis consists of inflammation or ulceration of the mucous membranes in the oral cavity including the lips, tongue, palate, buccal mucosa, gingiva, or floor of the mouth, while esophagitis involves the mucous membranes of the esophagus (Landers and O'Hanlon-Curry 2008). The prevalence of mucositis and esophagitis among pediatric oncology patients is undetermined because there is no universally recognized definition or assessment tool; however, there is an increased incidence among patients who receive fully ablative chemotherapy, head and neck radiation, or total body irradiation (Hogan 2009). These therapies cause damage or death to the rapidly dividing epithelial mucosal cells and can advance to dysphagia (difficulty swallowing).

Characteristics of mucositis are distinguished according to their etiology. Radiation-induced mucositis typically presents as a whitish discoloration about 2–3 weeks into treatment and develops into deepening erythema with ulcers or inflammation (Hogan 2009). On the other hand, chemotherapy-induced mucositis classically presents 5–8 days after treatment, initially with erythema followed quickly by edema and ulceration (Hogan 2009). Despite the importance of a structured oral assessment, few clinical sites use a formal oral assessment scale (Gibson et al. 2010). Important aspects to consider in assessing the oral cavity include voice, swallow, lips, tongue, saliva, mucous membrane, gingiva, and teeth. A recent systematic review of oral assessment instruments found the Oral Assessment Guide (OAG), as a validated and easy to use scale that was suitable for clinical use (Gibson et al. 2010).

Prevention of mucositis is important because it can cause multiple complications such as pain, infection, malnutrition, dehydration, and decreased quality of life (Hogan 2009). Additionally, severe mucositis may cause a delay and/or reduction of subsequent treatments. Preventative measures include keeping the oral cavity clean with brushing and using nonirritating mouthwashes. Topical and sometimes systemic antifungal, antiviral, and antibiotic medications are used to prevent infections. Research is ongoing to explore methods to decrease saliva production, such as cryotherapy and various medications, to decrease the amount of drug contact with the oral mucous membranes, while additional research is looking at increasing epithelial cell proliferation, such as the use of glutamine, beta-carotene, and prostaglandins (Wohlschlaeger 2004).

Treatment of mucositis and esophagitis primarily focuses on pain control and maintaining nutrition/hydration. Support and close monitoring must be provided for patients with dysphagia, as significant risks are associated with the inability to swallow. In addition to systemic analgesic medication, topical agents such as sucralfate and magnesium hydroxide provide symptomatic relief (Wohlschlaeger 2004). Fluoride rinses and saliva substitutes relieve xerostomia (dry mouth). Fluids and nutrients administered intravenously support the patient's hydration and nutritional requirements during periods of inadequate oral intake. Agents such as vitamin E and granulocyte-macrophage colony-stimulating factor mouthwash are effective in reducing the duration of mucositis among adults but more research is needed with children (Wohlschlaeger 2004).

Anorexia and Cachexia

Anorexia is a loss of appetite and occurs in 6–60 % of all children treated for cancer (Montgomery et al. 2013). Anorexia can be very distressing to the patient and family as eating has cultural, emotional, and religious significance and is often equated as an action of nurturing and caring (Santucci and Mack 2007). Furthermore, anorexia can cause electrolyte disturbances, weight loss, and malnutrition, which can increase morbidities and delays in treatment. Anorexia can be a result of the disease such as brain tumors, poor prognosis or relapsed leukemia, and advanced cancer (Rogers et al. 2008) (see Chap. 14 on palliative care for more information). Taste changes have been reported by children undergoing cancer treatment as one of the primary causes of eating difficulties (Skolin et al. 2006). Other risk factors include mucositis, dysphagia, xerostomia, constipation, pain, and/or a change in environment resulting in the inability of having foods prepared in a culturally familiar manner and eaten in a relaxing environment (Santucci and Mack 2007).

Anorexia can be mild and temporary or can be severe and prolonged. Severe anorexia can lead to cachexia. Cachexia is a multifactorial metabolic syndrome that causes an increase in the catabolic process associated with reduced food intake (Tuca et al. 2013). Cachexia causes a significant loss in weight, muscle mass, and fat that is often not reversible with increased caloric intake (Tuca et al. 2013).

There are multiple methods to assess eating and nutrition in individuals including nutritional history, anthropometric measurements, and laboratory markers. A patient's history is one of the most important methods to obtain data during an assessment and should include an assessment of appetite, 24 hour diet recall or food diary, recent diet changes, food preparation methods, use of vitamins and/or supplements, and gastrointestinal symptoms (Huhmann and August 2008). Anthropometric measurements, such as height and weight, are quick and easy measurements commonly used to evaluate nutritional well-being; however, weight can fluctuate in some patients due to fluid shifts and may not accurately represent a patient's nutritional status. Laboratory measurements are another customary method to assess the nutritional status in patients. Serum protein markers, such as albumin and prealbumin, are traditionally used to evaluate the nutritional status and responses to nutritional interventions. However, conditions such as liver or kidney disease, dehydration, and anemia can affect the accuracy of these tests.

Early intervention of anorexia is important to prevent complications and/or cachexia. Discussions on methods to maintain adequate caloric intake should occur early in treatment and strategies to promote eating are provided in Table 3.2. Food should never be forced on the child and patients report being forced to eat caused them to eat less or not eat at all (Rodgers et al. 2010). Patients who are not interested in eating can benefit from high-calorie oral supplementation but children are often reluctant to drink them because of the taste and consistency. Medications such as progestational drugs, corticosteroids, and cannabinoids can be used to stimulate appetites; however, many of these medications are restricted by the disease and age of the child and can cause unwanted side effects (e.g., hallucinations, irritability, fluid retention) (Santucci and Mack 2007). It is important to educate parents and family caregivers about these potential side effects so they can support the child and make decisions that

Table 3.2 Strategies to promote eating

Symptom	Strategy
Mucositis	Select foods that are easy to chew, such as oatmeal Avoid acidic, spicy, or salty foods Serve foods cold or room temperature
Xerostomia	Chew gum, eat hard candy, or brush teeth prior to meals Offer liquid foods (i.e., soup) or add sauces or gravy on the food Provide small sips of water frequently with a straw while eating Moisten lips with a lip balm
Anorexia	Provide small frequent meals Add extra calories to foods (i.e., cheese, butter) Create homemade smoothies or milkshakes with the child's favorite ingredients Allow the child to prepare the meals Avoid forcing the child to eat Provide meals in a comforting, relaxing environment

Information obtained from Rodgers et al. (2010)

take into account their child's psychological and social needs.

Two traditional methods to provide nutritional support include enteral nutrition (EN) and total parenteral nutrition (TPN). EN can be administered through a tube that is passed from the nose to the stomach (nasogastric tube), through a tube inserted directly into the stomach (gastrostomy) by surgery, or through a tube into the small intestine (jejunostomy). TPN is administered through a central venous catheter. EN is beneficial to patients because it preserves the structure and the function of the GI tract; however, it may not be tolerated because the tube placement and feeds can exacerbate symptoms of nausea, vomiting, and diarrhea (Montgomery et al. 2013). TPN may be better tolerated by patients and can provide more caloric, protein, and vitamin supplementation because the nutrition is received intravenously instead of through an already irritated GI tract; however, TPN has been associated with an increased risk of liver complications and infections (Montgomery et al. 2013). Treatment of cachexia includes appetite stimulants and nutritional support but also requires successful treatment of the malignancy to minimize energy expenditure (Santucci and Mack 2007).

Nausea and Vomiting

Nausea and vomiting are commonly occurring symptoms in pediatric oncology with an incidence as high as 90 % among patients receiving chemotherapy (Phillips et al. 2011) and up to 80 % in patients undergoing radiation therapy (Feyer et al. 2011). These symptoms have very distinct characteristics. Nausea consists of a wavelike sensation of GI distress that may lead to retching or vomiting and is often accompanied by sweating, increased salivation, and weakness, while vomiting is a forcible expulsion of the stomach contents through the mouth that may be accompanied by nausea, rapid breathing, and abdominal cramping (Landers and O'Hanlon-Curry 2008). These symptoms can result from:

- Disease such as brain tumors
- Treatment including chemotherapy, radiation, or anesthesia from surgery
- Side effects from medication(s) such as opioids

The specific emetogenic risk for various radiation sites and chemotherapy agents are listed in Table 3.3. Other factors that may increase the risk of nausea and/or vomiting include prior motion sickness, fatigue, emotional stress such as anxiety or fear, sensitivity to strong odors, and previous bad experiences with nausea or vomiting. Nausea and/or vomiting can occur before the start of treatment, referred to as anticipatory; during administration or within 24 hours after treatment, referred to as acute; or more than 24 hours after completion of treatment, referred to as delayed.

Prompt recognition of these symptoms is crucial as they have significant physical and psychological consequences (Table 3.4). Before treatment begins, an assessment of nausea and vomiting should include type of treatment, prior experience with nausea and

Table 3.3 High and moderate emetogenic potential of radiation sites and common chemotherapy agents

Classification	Radiation sites	Chemotherapy agents
High	Total body irradiation	Carboplatin Carmustine >250 mg/m^2 Cisplatin Cyclophosphamide >1 g/m^2 Cytarabine >3 g/m^2/dose Dactinomycin Methotrexate <12 g/m^2 Procarbazine (oral) Thiotepa >300 mg/m^2
Moderate	Upper abdomen Half-body irradiation Upper-body irradiation	Anthracyclines (daunorubicin, doxorubicin, idarubicin) Amifostine >300 mg/m^2 Arsenic trioxide Busulfan Camustine <250 mg/m^2 Clofarabine Cyclophosphamide <1 g/m^2 or oral Cytarabine 200 mg to <3 g/m^2 Etoposide (oral) Ifosfamide Imatinib (oral) Intrathecal chemotherapy Melphalan >50 mg/m^2 Methotrexate >250 mg to <12 g/m^2

Information from Feyer et al. (2011) and Dupuis et al. (2011)

Table 3.4 Consequences of nausea and/or vomiting

Physical	Psychological
Anorexia	Stress
Malnutrition	Anxiety
Electrolyte imbalances	Worry
Dehydration	Nervousness
Weight loss	Reduced quality of life
Fatigue	Frustration
Insomnia	Irritability

vomiting, and effectiveness of previous interventions. Frequent nausea and vomiting assessments should then occur throughout (acute) and after treatment (delayed). Assessments should include current level of nausea and vomiting, effectiveness of pharmacological and non-pharmacological interventions, and level of emotional stress. Anxiety and psychologically conditioned responses may also contribute to anticipatory nausea and vomiting even before chemotherapy infusion and can be addressed with psychological or pharmacologic interventions.

Additional assessments should consist of a thorough evaluation for complications from the nausea or vomiting including anorexia, malnutrition, dehydration, and electrolyte imbalances.

The goal is to prevent nausea or vomiting from occurring. Prevention and treatment strategies consist of various non-pharmacological and pharmacological interventions, which provide individual levels of relief to patients. Therefore, healthcare providers including psychosocial clinicians should encourage a variety of strategies for patients experiencing nausea or vomiting and evaluate the effectiveness of each strategy. Non-pharmacological interventions (Table 3.5) can often be self-initiated by the patient and have little to no side effects. Pharmacological interventions include a variety of antiemetic medications including 5-HT3 receptor antagonists, NK-1 antagonist, dopamine antagonists, benzodiazepines, cannabinoids, and corticosteroids (Phillips et al. 2011). A recent systematic review found 5-hydroxytryptamine-3 (5-HT3) antagonists are more effective than other antiemetic agents even

Table 3.5 Non-pharmacological interventions for nausea and/or vomiting

Category	Strategy
Diet	Eat small frequent meals; avoid getting hungry Maintain adequate hydration Avoid foods with strong odors Eat foods at room temperature Eat bland foods, such as rice, crackers, and gelatin Avoid greasy, fatty, and spicy foods
Cognitive/behavioral	Relaxation Hypnosis Meditation or guided imagery Progressive muscle relaxation Music or art therapy Distraction
Touch therapies	Acupuncture or acupressure Massage
Herbal remedies	Ginger Aromatherapy
Others	Exercise Social support

Information obtained from Rodgers et al. (2010) and Dupuis et al. (2013)

when combined with a corticosteroid (Phillips et al. 2011) and therefore are the drug of choice for prevention and treatment of therapy-related nausea or vomiting. These medications, such as ondansetron, granisetron, and tropisetron, produce little side effects and are generally well-tolerated. The NK-1 antagonist (aprepitant) is also an effective medication but is currently restricted for use only in children 12 years of age and older (Lexicomp 2014). Despite the legalization of marijuana in several states, the medical use of marijuana for nausea and vomiting is controversial due to potential carcinogens and adverse effects on the cardiovascular, respiratory, and central nervous system and the unidentified outcome evidence (Torado 2012). Synthetic oral cannabinoids once commonly prescribed are now recommended for use only in patients with breakthrough nausea and vomiting due to the development of newer antiemetic medications that cause fewer side effects (Torado 2012).

Case Vignette

Abby is a 16-year-old girl who is undergoing chemotherapy for treatment of her osteosarcoma. Abby has experienced significant nausea with her treatment that has caused her to have a poor appetite. Prior to diagnosis, her body mass index (BMI) was at the 75th percentile and she is now at the 50th percentile. Although her BMI is now within normal limits, her recent weight loss is concerning. Abby's mother reports that she is frustrated because she cooks any type of food that Abby appears interested in and makes her eat it right away but she is still losing weight. Abby reports that she is often nauseous when her mom is cooking and feels that she would start vomiting if she was forced to eat. Healthcare providers discuss ways that Abby may become more interested in eating such as allowing Abby to select favorite foods with minimal smells, go to another room during food preparation, and eat small amounts several times a day in a relaxed environment. Healthcare providers educate Abby's mother about cooking with butter, cheese, or whole milk to add extra calories to food and allowing Abby to eat at her own pace because children who are forced to eat often eat less. Abby's nausea is managed through antiemetic medication taken routinely throughout the day and relaxation techniques to decrease anxiety while eating. Weights are monitored closely at each clinic visit and small weight gains are celebrated with the staff.

Diarrhea

Diarrhea is an increase in quantity, frequency, or fluid content of the stool that is different from usual patterns and can be accompanied by abdominal cramping, flatulence, nausea, vomiting, and fever (Landers and O'Hanlon-Curry 2008). Diarrhea is a result of changes in intestinal absorption and motility caused from a variety of

Table 3.6 Interventions for diarrhea and constipation

Symptom	Pharmacological strategies	Non-pharmacological strategies
Diarrhea	After infection has been ruled out, administer anti-motility agents (e.g., loperamide)	Encourage adequate oral hydration Minimize intake of high-fiber foods Avoid fatty or spicy foods, dairy products, and caffeine
Constipation	Administer stool softeners (e.g., docusate), osmotic agents (e.g., lactulose), and/or stimulants (e.g., senna)	Provide daily access to the toilet and encourage privacy during this time Increase fluid and fiber intake Increase physical activity Resolve pain

Information obtained from Santucci and Mack (2007) and Shaw and Taylor (2012)

triggers including chemotherapy, radiation therapy, infection, and bowel resection. The incidence of diarrhea varies greatly due to the variety of potential etiologies. Treatment is likely the cause of diarrhea once infection is ruled out with multiple testing of the stool.

Patients with diarrhea require a thorough assessment of their stool output and associated symptoms. Diarrhea is classified according to duration and severity. Duration can be classified as acute (occurring less than 2 weeks), persistent (lasting 2–4 weeks), or chronic, which can continue longer than 4 weeks (Pessi et al. 2014). Severity is categorized as uncomplicated, comprised of diarrhea without associated symptoms, and complicated, consisting of diarrhea with associated symptoms or complicating factors (Shaw and Taylor 2012). Diarrhea can deplete fluids, electrolytes, and nutrition; therefore, information regarding hydration and nutrition status, such as food and fluid consumption, weight loss, and urine output, must be obtained to identify complications (Shaw and Taylor 2012).

Treatment of diarrhea consists of diet modifications and pharmacological management (Table 3.6). Foods that are fatty or spicy or contain dairy or caffeine should be avoided (Shaw and Taylor 2012). Small frequent meals are best tolerated, and oral intake of water, sports drinks, broth, etc., is imperative in maintaining adequate hydration (Shaw and Taylor 2012). Inability to maintain adequate hydration results in the immediate need for the administration of intravenous fluid and likely hospitalization (Shaw and Taylor 2012). Antidiarrheal medication is indicated once infections are excluded. Loperamide is a standard medication administered orally for treatment of diarrhea and can be administered to children 2 years of age or older (Lexicomp 2014). For patients unable to tolerate oral medication or with persistent or complicated diarrhea, octreotide can be administered to infants or children subcutaneously or intravenously (Lexicomp 2014). Use of probiotics is likely to be effective for diarrhea related to cancer therapy; however, more research is needed to determine the optimal probiotic strain, dosage, and timing (Shaw and Taylor 2012).

Constipation

Constipation involves the infrequent passage of hard, dry stool that can be accompanied with abdominal cramping, abdominal and/or rectal pain, nausea, vomiting, and blood-streaked stools (Landers and O'Hanlon-Curry 2008). Patients may not realize the importance or feel comfortable discussing their bowel movements with others, so healthcare providers should perform a detailed history and provide education. A thorough assessment includes questions of frequency and consistency of stools, associated symptoms, and any personal concerns. Obtaining a past medical history is also important as patients with a previous history of constipation are more prone to developing constipation during their oncology treatment (Pashankar et al. 2011). Constipation is diagnosed when a child with a developmental age of 4 years meets two or more of the following criteria (Pashankar et al. 2011):

- Two or fewer defecations in the toilet weekly
- At least one fecal incontinence per week

- Retentive posturing or stool retention
- Pain or hard bowel movements
- Large stools that may obstruct the toilet

The cause of constipation in pediatric oncology patients is multifactorial and includes effects from the disease, treatment, medication(s), or problems with mobility, diet, hydration, or psychological adjustment (Phillips and Gibson 2008). The primary or metastatic disease can obstruct portions of the bowel or compress the spinal cord resulting in an inability to defecate. Several chemotherapy agents, radiation therapy especially to the pelvic area, and commonly used medications such as opioids, antiemetics, antidepressants, and anticonvulsants cause a decrease in bowel motility and secretions that can progress to constipation (Santucci and Mack 2007). In addition, a decrease in activity, inadequate intake of fluids and fiber, and issues of anxiety, lack of privacy, or limited access to a toilet can result in constipation (Landers and O'Hanlon-Curry, 2008). If left untreated, constipation can cause significant pain, lack of appetite, nausea, vomiting, and anal fissures (small tears in the skin around the anus).

Prevention is key for constipation (Table 3.6). Maintaining regular exercise, adequate hydration, and a high-fiber diet are important strategies to prevent constipation. Often medications are used in the prevention and treatment of constipation. Medications include stool softeners such as docusate, osmotic agents such as lactulose, and stimulants such as senna or bisacodyl (Santucci and Mack 2007). Enemas are rarely used in pediatric oncology patients because of the risk for mucosal trauma and subsequent infection.

Weight Changes

Weight status in children is measured by body mass index (BMI). Children with a BMI ≥ the 95th percentile based on the Centers for Disease Control and Prevention (CDC) growth charts for age and gender are considered obese (CDC 2014a). The term "overweight" is used to describe children with a BMI between the 85th and 94th percentiles and underweight children are those with BMIs less than the 5th percentile (CDC 2014a).

Table 3.7 Disease/treatment factors associated with weight changes

Associations with weight loss	Associations with weight gain
Medulloblastoma	Acute lymphoblastic leukemia
Head and neck cancers	Cranial radiation
Solid tumors with metastasis	Glucocorticoids
Relapsed leukemia or lymphoma	
Brainstem tumors	
Radiation treatment involving the head, neck, or abdomen	

Children often experience weight changes secondary to the disease and the treatments that they receive (Table 3.7). Baseline BMI and nutritional status should be assessed at diagnosis as patients may present with underlying weight or nutritional issues. Weight trends should be monitored throughout therapy. Changes are very patient specific and variable as people may respond differently to chemotherapy and other medications. It is important to monitor weight trends as being underweight, overweight, or obese can decrease survival in many childhood cancers such as acute lymphoblastic leukemia (Orgel et al. 2014), acute myeloid leukemia (Inaba et al. 2012), and osteosarcoma (Altaf et al. 2013). Abnormal weight status can also have a negative impact on survival in children undergoing hematopoietic stem cell transplant (White et al. 2012).

Weight Loss

It is suggested that up to 46 % of pediatric oncology patients experience malnutrition (Bauer et al. 2011). Marked weight loss may be the symptom that first causes families to seek medical attention and prompt the discovery of a cancer diagnosis. Weight loss, greater than 10 % of a child's bodyweight within 6 months prior to diagnosis, is especially important in Hodgkin and non-Hodgkin lymphoma. This weight loss is considered a "B" symptom, which affects staging and treatment.

A decrease in weight *prior* to therapy is usually associated with the disease process. In the case of solid tumors, the growing mass may exert pressure on structures within the abdomen, central nervous system, or other parts of the gastrointestinal tract that interfere with normal digestion or hunger mechanisms. The presence of pain may also cause decreased appetite. Surgery to remove the tumor often helps to alleviate continued weight loss.

Weight loss *during* therapy is mainly due to the side effects of treatment. Chemotherapy can cause taste changes, dry mouth, nausea, vomiting, anorexia, mucositis, or other conditions which impact appetite and food intake (see Table 3.2 for strategies to promote eating). Depression or mood may also influence eating habits. Radiation that involves the head, neck, or abdominal area also increases the risk for weight loss secondary to esophagitis, mucositis, nausea, vomiting, and diarrhea.

Treatment for weight loss consists of identifying the underlying cause. Side effects of treatment interfering with nutritional intake can often be managed symptomatically. Medications can be administered to decrease nausea and vomiting. Pain medications can also be given to alleviate pain, if that is the underlying cause. If warranted, medications can also be administered to increase appetite.

Weight Gain

It is well documented that children treated for childhood acute lymphoblastic leukemia (ALL) often experience weight gain during and after cancer treatment. One study found that obesity rates increased from 14 % at the beginning of therapy to 23 % by the end of therapy in ALL patients (Withycombe et al. 2009). In addition, weight gain appears to continue after therapy with a meta-analysis of 47 studies showing the prevalence of being overweight/obese in ALL survivors ranging from 29–69 % (Zhang et al. 2013). This is significantly higher than the national childhood obesity rate of approximately 17 % (CDC 2014b).

Some brain tumors, in particular craniopharyngiomas, are also associated with an increased risk for obesity. Tumors or treatments (radiation or surgery) that cause hypothalamic-pituitary axis damage are highly problematic. Hypothalamic obesity is a condition that may occur when the normal hypothalamic center functions are disrupted resulting in imbalances in hunger control, satiety, and energy regulation (Lee and Korner 2009). This condition is often described as intractable weight gain and is present in up to 75 % of children with craniopharyngioma (Lustig 2011).

Currently there is no standard treatment to combat excessive weight gain other than recommending that families watch their diet and engage in physical activity. Prevention of obesity is preferred as it is difficult to reverse once it develops. Having a healthy weight is especially critical for childhood cancer survivors as they may already be at risk for cardiovascular issues due to late effects of chemotherapy. Obesity also increases the risk for hypertension, diabetes, metabolic syndrome, depression, decreased quality of life, and secondary cancers (Berenson and Bogalusa Heart Study Group 2012; Kanellopoulos et al. 2013).

When obesity is present, it is important to refer the family for nutritional counseling. Children are often dependent on their parents for food preparation so it is imperative that the whole family be involved in learning healthy eating habits. Likewise, daily family physical activity should be encouraged. In children with hypothalamic obesity, these interventions are often ineffective in significantly reducing weight and may warrant more invasive treatment options such as gastric bypass surgery.

Sensory Impact

Sensory changes occur frequently during cancer therapy and can be either temporary or permanent in nature depending on the underlying etiology. Although most sensory changes are not life threatening, they can be life changing and can negatively impact a child's quality of life.

Neuropathy

Neuropathy occurs when chemotherapeutic drugs damage the peripheral nerves, which are those outside of the central nervous system such as in the hands and feet (Gilchrist 2012). Neuropathy primarily occurs with drugs that are known to be neurotoxic such as cisplatin, carboplatin, vincristine, and vinblastine. Neuropathy can be sensory in nature and lead to symptoms of burning, tingling, or shooting pain in the hands and feet. Neuropathic jaw pain is also frequently reported in children (McCarthy and Skillings 1992). In addition, neuropathy can impact motor function which can lead to foot drop and problems with balance and coordination. Fine motor skills may also be affected leading to difficulty with grasping objects or performing tasks such as buttoning a shirt. Neuropathy has been reported to occur in up to 18.3 % of children treated for acute lymphoblastic leukemia, brain tumors, and Wilms' tumor (Purser et al. 2014).

Neuropathy can be a dose-limiting toxicity which means that the severity of symptoms may mandate that a reduced dosage of chemotherapy be administered until the neuropathy resolves. There is no treatment for neuropathy, once it occurs, other than symptom management. This management may include pain medicines or other medications specifically for nerve pain. Physical therapy services may be ordered to address balance issues and muscle weakness. In general, neuropathy tends to resolve once the causing agent is stopped but can linger for months to years in a small percentage of patients.

Neuropathy can limit mobility and decrease a child's functional status. Participation in sports and other social activities may decline secondary to physical limitations or pain. Neuropathy may increase a child's reliance on parents as they may be unable to complete tasks such as buttoning a shirt or braiding their hair. For adolescents, this may have greater importance as this is the age at which most begin establishing their independence. Emotional consequences may occur secondary to neuropathy and can range from frustration with the inability to complete tasks independently to anger and/or depression. Emotional changes should be anticipated and mental health professionals should be involved in caring for the child.

Case Vignette

Ben is a 6-year-old boy who received vincristine for treatment of his brain tumor. Ben's parents report that he has become more irritable recently and is difficult to console. He is often seen rubbing his stomach and looking at his fingers. The clinic nurse notices that Ben is having difficulty with his fine motor skills. She uses a pain face scale and Ben points to the sad face, representing pain. After spending time playing and talking with Ben, it is determined that Ben has pain in his abdomen and fingers. Ben is diagnosed with central neuropathy (constipation) and peripheral neuropathy (fingertip numbness). A stool softener medication is started for his constipation along with educating Ben's parents to increase his fluid and fiber intake, while gabapentin medication is given for the fingertip numbness. Ben is monitored closely at subsequent clinic visits for his neuropathy.

Vision

Vision changes, such as blurry vision, have been reported in association with multiple chemotherapeutic agents used to treat childhood cancer. These changes are usually short lived and resolve when the chemotherapy is stopped. More severe vision issues, such as decreased vision, have been reported with the use of cisplatin and etoposide (Hilliard et al. 1997). Ocular nerve and optic motor nerve damage have also been reported in those receiving vinblastine and vincristine (Omoti and Omoti 2006). Ophthalmology evaluations are the optimal method for assessing eye and vision changes during treatment.

Alterations in vision can also be secondary to certain cancers and their location. Diseases such as retinoblastoma, optic gliomas, or leukemia that have spread to the central nervous system can physically invade or destroy optic structures. When disease is the cause, vision changes are usually more severe and may include a decrease or total loss of eyesight. In these cases, treatment options to save or spare vision are limited. Depending on the exact location and size of the tumor, surgery or radiation may be considered in the treatment plan. One potential sequelae of surgery is double vision (called diplopia). Treatment for diplopia may consist of occluding the line of vision in one eye, therefore preventing the overlap of visual fields which causes the double vision. This treatment was traditionally done by patching one eye, but more modern methods of treatment include placing an occlusive patch over the inside of one eyeglass lens which directly blocks the line of sight causing the double vision. Children suffering from diplopia may also benefit from completing a vision rehabilitation program. This type of program teaches people to maximize their eye sight through visual training which may include specialized exercises for the eyes.

Hearing

Hearing loss is variable depending on the treatment received and the individual person. Typically, those treated with chemotherapy such as cisplatin or carboplatin tend to be most at risk for auditory changes. Children undergoing brain surgery and/or cranial radiation may also experience hearing loss.

Hearing issues may be reported by patients as "ringing" in the ears or parents/teachers may observe that the child seems to have difficulty hearing or following instructions. Clinicians should be aware that reports of difficulty in school or apparent lack of attention may be indications of hearing loss. Clinicians are also able to predict which children are at risk for hearing loss by using the Children's Oncology Group Long-Term Follow-Up Guidelines (2013) and screening for the following treatment risk factors: less than 4 years of age during treatment, received a cumulative cisplatin dose of $\geq$360 mg/m^2, received cisplatin after cranial radiation, received higher dose cisplatin (e.g., cisplatin 5 days per course at 40 mg/m^2 per day), received carboplatin for transplant conditioning, or received any carboplatin given prior to 1 year of age. Pediatric oncology diagnoses most associated with hearing loss include neuroblastoma, osteosarcoma, germ cell tumors, and brain tumors. Recommendations for hearing tests following childhood cancer therapy include a hearing exam at least once after finishing therapy for all children who received cisplatin or carboplatin as part of their chemotherapy regime (Children's Oncology Group n.d.). In addition, children who received radiation to the brain (cranial), ear, and infratemporal or nasopharyngeal areas should also undergo hearing exams after ending therapy. This is especially important for those who received radiation doses of 30 Gy or higher. Annual follow-up is recommended if problems are detected during the screening.

Hearing tests can be performed by trained audiologists using headphones which emit various frequencies and volumes of sounds. For children too young to be tested using headphones, a brainstem auditory evoked response (BAER) test can be performed while the child is asleep. This type of test uses electrodes placed on the scalp to measure brain wave activity in response to sound. Behavioral exams can assist with screening in younger children (i.e., testing to see if a child turns his/her head toward voices or noises).

Treatment for hearing loss may include having the child wear hearing aids or teachers using amplification systems in the classroom to increase the volume of sound. Cochlear implants are used for severe cases of hearing loss. A cochlear implant involves surgery to place electrodes that can carry sound signals directly to the auditory nerve. Children with hearing loss may also benefit from early speech therapy services.

Taste

Roughly 16.5 % of children undergoing chemotherapy report alterations in taste (Collins et al. 2000). The perception, or reporting, of taste changes may increase with age as 38–77 % of

Table 3.8 Recommendations to manage taste changes

Strategy	Rationale
Experiment with seasonings/spices/sauces	Seasonings can be added to match taste preferences during therapy
Use plastic silverware	May reduce metallic taste in mouth
Allow food to cool off prior to eating	Changing the temperature may change the taste
Try eating eggs, chicken, and beans along with other protein sources	Avoid beef if it does not taste good, or try marinating the beef prior to cooking to change the flavor
Eat smaller, more frequent meals	Finger foods should always be available
Avoid foods that have a strong odor	Foods such as fish or sauerkraut have strong smells and may be bothersome

Adapted from Rehwaldt et al. (2009)

adult cancer patients note a change in taste after receiving chemotherapy (Rehwaldt et al. 2009). Changes in taste may consist of a metallic taste to food or may present as a change in food preferences. Alterations in taste can be distressing and may lead to food aversion and decreased nutritional intake. This side effect can be especially troubling if it limits their ability to receive adequate nutrition.

Some chemotherapeutic agents are known to have a greater risk for taste disturbances, such as cisplatin, carboplatin, and cyclophosphamide. Although there is no action that prevents taste changes, patients and families can be offered suggestions for how to manage the changes. These strategies include avoiding the use of metal silverware and eating colder food for those who experience a metallic taste (Rehwaldt et al. 2009). Other suggestions include eating smaller amounts of food more frequently or trying the addition/deletion of food seasonings such as salt (Table 3.8).

Musculoskeletal Impact

Changes to the musculoskeletal system usually occur in children who have tumors arising from the bone or muscle. Sarcomas represent 20 % of pediatric solid tumors and include diagnoses such as osteosarcoma, Ewing sarcoma, and rhabdomyosarcoma (Burningham et al. 2012). One of the primary treatment options for these types of tumors is surgery. For those tumors that occur in extremities, the surgery can entail either a limb salvage procedure or an amputation. The decision between these two options is based on whether the tumor can be fully surgically resected and which option allows for the greatest amount of physical functioning post-procedure.

As the chemotherapy regimens change and survival rates increase, the quality of long-term physical functioning becomes increasingly important. Those children with lower extremity involvement have a 50 % higher risk for activity limitations as compared to children with upper extremity involvement (Marina et al. 2013). In general, studies show that amputees and patients with limb-sparing surgery have little reported differences in disabilities (Marina et al. 2013).

Both amputees and those with limb-sparing surgery frequently report long-term pain. Phantom pain occurs in up to 76 % of children with limb amputations, but only 10 % of these patients report pain lasting for greater than 12 months (Burgoyne et al. 2013). Persistence of pain following limb-sparing surgery has also been reported and is most likely related to neuropathy or instability/weakness of the joint or fibrosis around the prosthesis (Anghelescu et al. 2011).

A child's self-image can be impacted by the type of surgery that is completed. Limb salvage is usually the desired option by parents and adolescents. There are multiple types of limb salvage procedures some involving implants and prosthesis. Rotationplasty is one type of surgery considered in children with distal femur tumors. This is a surgery which allows for the lower leg to be partially amputated, the foot rotated 180 degrees, and reattached to the upper femur. This type of surgery allows for the ankle to function in place of the knee joint and works well with special prostheses which can allow for greater participation in sports.

As with all medical decisions related to childhood cancer, parents and age-appropriate children should be allowed to participate in decisions related to surgery options. In addition, conversations should occur prior to surgery to prepare children for amputation and may include the use of pictures or dolls with a similar amputation. Adolescents may benefit from talking to another patient who has had an amputation. Parents also need preparation and guidance for how to support their child before and after the surgery. Individual counseling, support groups, and psychosocial assessments are modalities that can assist families with embracing the changes related to limb amputation or limb-sparing procedures.

Integumentary Impact

Alterations to the integumentary (skin) system are common during cancer treatment. Chemotherapy and radiation damage rapidly dividing cells including rapidly dividing healthy cells such as the hair, skin, and nails. This damage is diverse in presentation ranging from a mild skin rash, to photosensitivity, to a severe hypersensitivity reaction. In addition, surgical procedures such as tumor resection, lumbar punctures, bone marrow aspirates, and implantation of venous access devices alter the integrity of the skin. Factors such as malnutrition and immobility can increase the potential for skin breakdown and/or lengthen the healing process (Norville 2008). Assessment of the integumentary system is an important focus.

Alopecia

Radiation and many chemotherapy agents damage the proliferating cells in the hair follicles, causing thinning or complete loss of hair (Alley et al. 2002). Hair loss can occur on the head, eyebrows, eyelashes, and body. Hair loss related to chemotherapy usually occurs throughout the body, whereas hair loss secondary to radiation only affects a specific area. Hair loss usually appears within 1 week of treatment and new growth usually begins several weeks after the final treatment, although in some cases the hair loss may be permanent. It is important to prepare the child and families for hair loss.

Although alopecia causes no significant medical threats, patients have reported high psychological distress and one of the most feared side effects of cancer treatment (Alley et al. 2002). Distress is often correlated with the patient's age with higher distress reported in adolescents. Research has evaluated strategies to prevent hair loss including scalp tourniquets, hypothermic scalping devices, and topical medications; however, no evidence has supported the use of any of these strategies (Alley et al. 2002; Viale 2006). Management of alopecia consists of the use of wigs, hats, and scarves until the hair returns. Most children and adolescents adapt to temporary alopecia; permanent hair loss or thinning due to scalp radiation is much more distressing and is often in the context of other physical or neurocognitive late effects.

Radiation Recall

Radiation recall is an acute inflammatory reaction that occurs on previously irradiated areas of the skin once triggered by precipitating agents (Burris and Hurtig 2010). Diagnosis occurs after an evaluation of the patient's treatment history, symptoms, and physical examination. Signs of radiation recall range from a mild rash, dry desquamation, or pruritis to swelling, edema, vesicles, and maculopapular eruptions, which are usually confined to a specific area of previous irradiation treatment (Burris and Hurtig 2010). The most common precipitating agents are chemotherapy agents such as bleomycin, dactinomycin, daunomycin, etoposide, melphalan, and methotrexate (Norville 2008); however, not all cases of radiation recall are published and additional unknown agents may be causative factors (Burris and Hurtig 2010). Radiation recall is unpredictable. Most cases occur after an initial dose of the precipitating agent but some patients may experience the effect after several exposures to the precipitating agent.

There is no current therapy specific for the prevention or management of radiation recall, although supportive care may be necessary (Burris and Hurtig 2010). Topical or systemic steroids or antihistamines may be indicated to reduce the inflammation when it occurs. As with any type of irritated skin, good hygiene, sun avoidance, and wearing loose clothing are imperative to the healing process. Resolution of the dermatitis is highly individualized. The precipitating agent should be delayed or withdrawn from the patient's treatment regimen as the skin is healing. Re-exposing the patient to the precipitating agent does not always elicit a second reaction, and determination of restarting the medication depends on individual circumstances and the extent, severity, and location of the reaction (Burris and Hurtig 2010). Steroids can be administered prior to the re-exposure, although there is conflicting evidence about the efficacy of the premedication (Burris and Hurtig 2010).

Palmar-Plantar Erythrodysesthesia (Hand-Foot Syndrome)

Palmar-plantar erythrodysesthesia (PPE, also known as hand-foot syndrome) is a common side effect with certain chemotherapy agents. The syndrome was originally described in patients receiving cytarabine but is now noted to be caused by additional chemotherapy agents such as liposomal doxorubicin, 5-fluorouracil, capecitabine, cisplatin, cyclophosphamide, daunorubicin, etoposide, methotrexate, and thiotepa (Webster-Gandy et al. 2007). Incidence of PPE can range from 3–68 % of patients receiving the high-risk chemotherapy agents (Webster-Gandy et al. 2007). Cause of the syndrome is not well understood, although it has been postulated that either the small capillaries in the palms and soles rupture due to an inflammatory reaction or that the chemotherapy agents are excreted in the sweat making the palms and soles more prone to their large number of sweat glands (Viale 2006; Webster-Gandy et al. 2007).

Regardless of the cause, patients suffering from this syndrome have initial symptoms of tingling in their fingers and toes followed with erythema and swelling of their palms and soles that can continue to progress to rash, ulcerations, desquamation, and burning pain (Webster-Gandy et al. 2007). Although PPE is not life threatening, it can cause considerable pain and interfere with activities of daily living. Patients need to be encouraged to promptly report any of these signs and symptoms to their healthcare provider, so that treatment can be initiated.

Preventative measures consist of cooling of hands and feet with ice packs and using specific topical creams and emollients, such as 99 % dimethyl sulfoxide (DMSO) during treatment; however, studies have yet to prove efficacy of these strategies (Webster-Gandy et al. 2007). The most effective treatment for PPE is stopping the aggravating chemotherapy agent and reducing the dose or lengthening the interval for subsequent administrations (Webster-Gandy et al. 2007), although some patients were able to receive further therapy without changes and experienced no further complications (Viale 2006). Treatment also includes supportive therapies such as the use of lotions and creams, avoidance of extreme temperatures, and avoidance of activities that increase pressure to the palms and soles.

Extravasation

Extravasation refers to the unintentional leakage of a chemotherapy medication from the vessel into surrounding tissue that may be responsible for damage to the skin (Gonzalez 2013). This complication occurs in up to 6 % of patients receiving chemotherapy from peripheral devices and up to 4.7 % of patients receiving chemotherapy from central venous access devices (CVAD) (Gonzalez 2013). Symptoms range from irritation and mild swelling, to ulcerations or blisters, to necrosis of the tissue (Gonzalez 2013).

Damage due to extravasation is related to the amount of leakage and type of medication. Classifications of chemotherapy agents known to cause extravasation include alkylating agents, anthracyclines, other anticancer antibiotics, plant alkaloids, and taxanes (Schulmeister 2011). Factors that increase the risk of extravasation from peripheral devices include small fragile veins, multiple previous venipunctures, and sensory deficits that impair the patient's ability to detect a change in sensation (Schulmeister 2011). Factors that increase the risk of extravasation from CVADs include difficulty during insertion of the device, inadvertent slicing or piercing of the catheter before or during insertion, device misplacement or catheter migration, and presence of a fibrin sheath at the catheter tip (Schulmeister 2011).

Prevention is the focus when administering chemotherapy agents that have the potential to cause extravasation. Guidelines have been developed by professional associations and many institutions to outline appropriate intravenous devices and administration steps. Nurses should educate patients on the potential for extravasation and signs/symptoms to report immediately. Needle placement of the peripheral or CVAD should be verified before and throughout medication administration (Gonzalez 2013).

After prevention, prompt recognition and initial management is the next most important action. The infusion must be stopped immediately upon any signs of extravasation and the nurse should attempt to withdraw as much of the medication as possible through the peripheral device or CVAD (Gonzalez 2013). The nurse should then notify the physician and an antidote and/or warm or cold compresses should be administered if applicable. The event should be thoroughly documented and include photographs of the area for later comparison. Allowing patients to verbalize concerns and feelings about the event can alleviate anxiety and worry. Patients should be educated on caring for the site and follow-up care.

General Skin Variations

General changes to the skin include rash, itching, dryness, acne, skin color changes, and photosensitivity and can occur throughout cancer treatment. These changes can be the result of the disease, treatment, or medication side effects. While not life threatening, any change to the skin can be distressing to patients. It is important for healthcare providers to perform frequent assessments of the skin and discuss how skin changes are affecting the patient. Educating the patient on the use of fragrance-free soaps and laundry detergent, frequent application of moisturizers, adequate sun protection, wearing loose comfortable clothing, and avoiding scrubs and loofahs can minimize most skin changes. Maintaining adequate hydration is also important. For patients who have received surgery, incision sites should be monitored during the healing process and scars should be monitored for keloids or tightness that restricts movement.

Nail Dystrophies

Fingernails and toenails are composed of rapidly proliferating cells that keratinize and make up the nail plate and therefore are sensitive to the effect of chemotherapy (Viale 2006). Anthracyclines and taxanes are associated with more risk for nail changes (Norville 2008). Characteristics of nail changes include:

- Mees' lines – transverse white lines
- Beau's lines – transverse grooves
- Pigmentation changes – pale or dark streaks in the nail plate
- Onycholysis – separation or loosening of the nail plate from the nail bed
- Paronychia – infection

Assessment of the nails should be conducted daily and include assessment for discoloration, ridging, pitting, pain in nail beds, separation or loss of the nail, and infection and if nail changes are interfering with activities of daily life (Viale 2006). There is no current treatment for the prevention or management of nail dystrophies, although antibiotics may be indicated for signs of infection around the nail bed and analgesic medication may be indicated for pain. Patients should be instructed to keep their nails trimmed and clean and avoid nail polish and imitation fingernails until the nails have returned to normal.

Pain

Pain is an unpleasant sensory and/or emotional experience associated with real or potential tissue damage (Krane et al. 2011). It is a common symptom among children with cancer due to the disease, treatment, procedures, infections, or a combination of these factors. Pain can be constant or intermittent and can occur suddenly (acute) or persist for months (chronic). Pain is classified as nociceptive (tissue pain) and neuropathic (nerve pain). Nociceptive pain can be further classified as somatic pain occurring in the bones, joints, muscles, skin, or connective tissue or visceral pain occurring in the visceral organs (Jacob 2008). Neuropathic pain results from nerve damage either in the peripheral or central nerves. In addition to these two pain classifications, pain can occur after surgical amputation of an extremity, referred to as phantom limb pain (Krane et al. 2011).

Pain assessments should be performed at an appropriate developmental level for the child. Measurement of pain in infants consists of assessments of behavior such as facial expressions and physiological measurements such as heart rate and respiratory rate (Hockenberry and Kline 2011). Measurement of pain in toddlers relies on assessment of behavior and physiological measurements but the toddler may provide clues about their pain such as guarding a particular area that is causing pain (Jacob 2008). Around 4 years of age, children are able to convey their pain to others either verbally or in the form of identifying their pain with face scales or photos of children in pain (Krane et al. 2011). Children 8 years and older can rate their pain with verbal or visual analog scales (Krane et al. 2011). In addition to a pain rating score, other pain characteristics such as location, intensity, severity, aggravating factors, and alleviating factors should be assessed.

Procedures are a common part of cancer treatment and may cause pain. Although procedural pain is usually brief, it is often accompanied by fear and anxiety if the child does not have a good experience with the initial procedures that can increase significantly with repeated procedures (Hockenberry et al. 2011; Kennedy et al. 2008). Preparation before the procedure should include providing the child with procedural information in an age-appropriate manner (i.e., medical play for toddlers) and providing training in cognitive behavioral interventions (i.e., distraction, relaxation, guided imagery) for use before, during, and after the procedure (Krane et al. 2011; Hockenberry et al. 2011). Ideally preparation should be initiated in advance for school-age children and adolescents, while toddlers and preschoolers have limited understanding of time and need information immediately before the procedure. Techniques such as cognitive behavioral interventions are often used to support the child during procedures but appropriate analgesia should also be provided. If necessary, analgesia medication should continue after the procedure. The decision for procedural sedation is dependent on a child's past experiences with procedures, their developmental level, and their ability to meet necessary expectations during the procedure (e.g., lying still for radiological exams).

Early intervention in the treatment of pain is important regardless of the cause and often requires multimodal strategies (Jacob 2008). Common pharmacological modalities are listed in Table 3.9 and non-pharmacological strategies are listed in Table 3.10. Electronic technologies are now being used to assess pain, deliver treatment, and enhance communication between patients and healthcare providers (see Chap. 20 for more information). Consideration of the patient's previous pain experiences, cultural and spiritual influences, and current pain assessment will guide the practitioner in determining the most efficacious treatment options. Frequent assessments are necessary to determine the effectiveness of current treatment and current pain levels. In addition, effective management of other symptoms, such as nausea, vomiting, constipation, insomnia, and anxiety, can assist to relieve pain. Interdisciplinary pain management teams as well as palliative care teams are often used in pediatric cancer centers to serve as consultants and provide expertise in pain assessment and management (Hockenberry and Kline 2011). Parents' levels of anxiety and distress can affect the child's pain and related distress; therefore, parents should be educated, supported, and

Table 3.9 Pharmacological interventions for pain

Classification	Medications
Non-opioid agents	Acetaminophen; ibuprofen; aspirin; naprosyn; ketorolac
Opioids	Codeine; fentanyl; hydrocodone; hydromorphone; meperidine; methadone; morphone; oxycodone
Anxiolytic agents	Diazepam; lorazepam
Major sedative agents	Midazolam; ketamine; propofol
Topical agents	EMLA or LMX; lidocaine infiltration
Antiepileptic agents	Gabapentin; pregabalin; topiramate
Antidepressants	Amitriptyline; nortriptyline

Information obtained from Krane et al. (2011) and Hockenberry and Kline (2011)

Table 3.10 Non-pharmacological interventions for pain

Classification	Intervention
Cognitive/behavioral	Relaxation Deep breathing Hypnosis Meditation or guided imagery Progressive muscle relaxation Music or art therapy Distraction
Touch therapies	Acupuncture or acupressure Massage Transcutaneous electrical nerve stimulation (TENS) Therapeutic touch
Activity	Exercise Yoga
Other	Sucrose solution for infants Aromatherapy

Information obtained from Krane et al. (2011) and Hockenberry et al. (2011)

encouraged to use positive support for the patient (Hockenberry and Kline 2011). Please see AYA Chap. 12 for specific issues related to opiate use in teenagers.

Headaches

Forty-one percent of children with brain tumors reported headaches at the time of initial diagnosis and 66 % reported headaches at some time during their treatment (Ullrich 2009). Although headaches are a common symptom among children with brain tumors, there are several other causes of headaches among children with cancer. Infection; fevers; side effects of medications such as antiemetics, antihistamines, and steroids; lumbar puncture procedures; and side effects of treatment including surgery, chemotherapy, and radiation can cause headaches in pediatric oncology patients (Ullrich 2009).

Assessment of headaches should include duration, focalization (i.e., unilateral or bilateral), location, pain quality, severity, associated symptoms (e.g., nausea, vomiting, photophobia), and presence of aura (Trottier et al. 2013). A headache diary is a useful method to obtain accurate and detailed information of the headaches. Reports of a headache that awakens the child from sleep, occurs early in the morning, is worse with coughing or Valsalva maneuvers, is associated with vomiting, and is increasing in frequency or severity are classic characteristics of increased intracranial pressure and a brain tumor and require further evaluation (Ullrich 2009). Neuroimaging should only be performed when abnormalities are noted in the history or physical examination (Bonthius and Lee 2013). Neuroimaging studies include computed tomography (CT) or magnetic resonance imaging (MRI). CT scans without contrast are typically performed in acute situations to quickly identify hemorrhage or space-occupying lesions such as tumors (Bonthius and Lee 2013). MRIs provide a high-resolution image of tissues and organs that is more sensitive than a CT scan for small tumors but are usually performed in non-acute situations due to the need for intravenous contrast and possible sedation. Laboratory tests are rarely helpful in diagnosing headaches; however, lumbar punctures can assist with a diagnosis of intracranial infection, malignancy, and/or intracranial hypertension (Bonthius and Lee 2013).

Prevention strategies primarily focus on procedure-related strategies, such as the prevention of lumbar puncture headaches. Use of a small-size and pencil-point spinal needle that is inserted parallel to the long axis is an established effective strategy to prevent lumbar puncture headaches, while extended bed rest, hydration, and the use of caffeine and ibuprofen have no established efficacy (Rusch et al. 2014). Treatment of headaches depends on the underlying etiology. For example, oncological treatment can assist with resolving disease-related headaches while antibiotics are needed for infection related headaches. Headaches resulting from treatment or side effects of medication may require a change in therapy, analgesic medications, and/or non-pharmacological interventions. Nonsteroidal anti-inflammatory drugs (NSAIDS) such as acetaminophen, ibuprofen, and naproxen are often the initial management strategy. Non-pharmacological interventions include guided imagery, acupuncture, hypnosis, meditation, and massage (Bonthius and Lee 2013). If ineffective, opioid or triptan medications can be used for pain relief (Sheridan et al. 2013).

Fatigue

Fatigue is recognized as one of the most frequent and distressing symptoms experienced by children and adolescents with cancer (Chang et al. 2013; Rodgers et al. 2013). Fatigue among children with cancer has been well characterized and is distinct from everyday tiredness (Hockenberry-Eaton et al. 1998, 1999). Changes in activities of daily living, having no energy, feeling socially isolated, having a difficult time concentrating, needing more rest, and finding it difficult to get up in the morning are common experiences for children with cancer. The experience of fatigue differed by developmental level with school-age children emphasizing the physical sensation of fatigue, while adolescents discussed mental tiredness that changes over time and merges with physical sensations of fatigue (Hockenberry-Eaton et al. 1998, 1999; Hockenberry-Eaton and Hinds 2000; Hockenberry et al. 2003). School-age children described "feeling weak" or "tired," "falling asleep easily," or being "mad" or "sad" when fatigued. Adolescents described fatigue related to cancer as "physical" or "mental exhaustion." It is interesting to note that fatigue descriptions first labeled over 15 years ago hold true today (Hockenberry et al. 2014; Kestler and LoBiondo-Wood 2012; Baggott et al. 2010, 2014).

Table 3.11 Causes of fatigue in children with cancer

Influences	Reasons
Treatment	Chemotherapy, radiation therapy, bone marrow transplant, surgery, biologic response modifiers
Environment	Altered schedules or routines, waiting times in the clinic and hospital, hospital noise, sleep/rest interruptions in the hospital
Child characteristics	Cognitive development, emotions, moods, worry, boredom
Family	Expectations of others (e.g., family, relatives, or friends), absence of a schedule

Causes of fatigue in children with cancer are numerous and described in Table 3.11. Fatigue in children with cancer is unrelated to activity and may not be resolved with rest or sleep. While this symptom develops during cancer treatment, it can continue for years after treatment ends (Bower et al. 2014; Meeske et al. 2005). Survivors of childhood cancer who report chronic fatigue have poorer physical, social, emotional, and school functioning than survivors who were not fatigued (Meeske et al. 2007).

To capture the many characteristics of fatigue, multidimensional instruments are needed. In the clinical setting there are important questions to ask the child and parents during each visit. Fatigue-related questions could be framed using a time period such as in the last week or month:

- Are you feeling tired or weak? If yes, on a scale of 1–5, how bad is the feeling?
- Does feeling tired or weak keep you from playing or doing your usual activities?

There are several instruments that provide valid and reliable measures of fatigue frequency and intensity (Table 3.12).

Preventive measures for fatigue during childhood cancer treatment are not effective. Pharmacological interventions are reviewed in Chap. 8 on Psychiatric Issues. The focus for this symptom is on minimizing the debilitating effects

Table 3.12 Fatigue measures

Instrument	Description
Childhood Fatigue Scale (CFS) (Hinds et al. 2010)	Ten items assessing the experience of fatigue-related symptoms during the past week in children 7–12 years. CFS has three subscales that include Lack of Energy, Not Able to Function, and Altered Mood and is available in English and Spanish
Parent Fatigue Scale (PFS) (Hockenberry et al. 2003)	Seventeen items that ask the parent their perceptions of the amount of fatigue experienced by their child in the past week. Four subscales of the PFS include Lack of Energy, Not Able to Function, Altered Sleep, and Altered Mood. Available in English and Spanish
Fatigue Scale–Adolescent (FS-A) (Mandrell et al. 2011)	Thirteen questions designed to evaluate the intensity of fatigue experienced during the past week. Available in English
Multidimensional Fatigue Scale (Varni et al. 2002)	Eighteen-item scale that has child and parent matching versions. Six of the items measure general fatigue, six measure sleep/rest fatigue, and six items measure cognitive fatigue. Available in 22 languages
Peds FACIT-F (Lai et al. 2007)	Eleven-item scale for children with cancer that has stable measurement properties across age, sex, and cancer types. Available in English and Spanish

of fatigue. Patient and family education concerning the impact cancer and treatment can have on energy level and performance should occur at diagnosis. Developing a plan to minimize energy expenditure with consideration of the child's age and stage of development is important. Patients and families often maintain a diary to track energy level and changes in activity during treatment to review during scheduled clinic visits.

While studies are limited, there is information that exercise is beneficial in relieving fatigue. A recent systematic review (Baumann et al. 2013) confirmed that clinical exercise interventions for childhood cancer patients are promising in their effects on the immune system, body composition, sleep, and activity levels. Greater physical activity is associated with improved sleep quantity and efficiency (Orsey et al. 2013). Exercise that involves rhythmic or repetitive movement of large muscle groups (walking, cycling, swimming) should be encouraged. Patients and families should be reminded that the exercise program should be developmentally appropriate, initiated gradually, and occur several times a week.

Stress and worry contribute to fatigue; teaching patient and family stress reduction techniques such as relaxation therapy, guided imagery, or distraction can facilitate rest. Give reminders that nutrition is important to maintain and that regular exercise may improve appetite and increase nutritional intake. Discuss how improved nutrition can promote increased energy and decrease fatigue.

Sleep disruption is a major influence on the child's fatigue level. Encourage the patient and family to develop a specific bedtime and wake time and emphasize the importance of a schedule and routine prior to bedtime. Sleep interruptions are associated with increased fatigue and determining ways to prevent sleep interruptions during nighttime sleep is essential. Rest periods during the day are encouraged but emphasize the importance of keeping naps and rest times short.

Case Vignette

Julia is an 11-year-old girl who was diagnosed with acute lymphocytic leukemia 3 months ago. Before her diagnosis she was very active in dance classes and gymnastics, taking classes three times a week. Her mom describes her daughter as never lacking energy and always engaged in some type of physical activity before her diagnosis. Since her diagnosis Julia complains of being tired all the time and has had to quit her dance and gymnastic classes. Her mother states that Julia is having trouble sleeping and awakens several times each night to go to the bathroom. Julia returned to school a month ago but continues to miss 1–2 school days a week because she is so tired. Julia and her mother meet with her healthcare provider in the cancer clinic and they discuss these feelings as being common in children on chemotherapy for leukemia. They talk about ways that can help minimize the fatigue including frequent rest periods, daily exercise activities, good nutrition strategies, and ways to reduce stress of treatment.

Sleep Disorders

Approximately 30–45 % of oncology patients experience sleep disorders (Linder and Christian 2012). Sleep disorders consist of difficulty initiating or maintaining sleep (insomnia), sleep-wake cycle disorders (circadian rhythm sleep disorders), and excessive somnolence (hypersomnias). Any of these sleep disorders can cause mood, behavioral, and cognitive difficulties such as decreased ability to pay attention and concentrate and increased irritability, depression, and impulsivity (Linder and Christian 2012). Insomnia and circadian rhythm sleep disorders are caused by the disease, psychological stressors, side effects of treatment and medications, and environmental factors and are characterized by difficulty falling asleep and difficulty staying asleep. Somnolence syndrome is caused by cranial radiation that usually appears 4–8 weeks after completion of therapy (Ryan 2000). Somnolence syndrome symptoms range from mild fatigue and daytime drowsiness to excessive sleep and moderate lethargy (Ryan 2000).

Assessment of sleep disorders usually consists of subjective assessments. Essential components of these assessments include sleep latency, sleep duration including number of awakening episodes, sleep quality, daytime alertness and function, current symptoms, medications, and bedtime routines (Vena et al. 2004). This information can be obtained through a verbal history collected by the provider, a formal questionnaire completed by the patient, or a sleep diary kept by the patient for several days then delivered to the provider. Physical assessments of sleep include a polysomnography or an actigraphy. Polysomnography is the gold standard of sleep that occurs in a sleep laboratory and consists of recording the electrical activity of the brain, muscles, and eye movements to evaluate sleep patterns (Vena et al. 2004). Actigraphy is a less invasive procedure that can be used in any location and consists of a battery-operated wristwatch that records periods of activity and nonactivity (Vena et al. 2004).

Treatment of sleep disorders should focus on alleviating the cause and promoting good sleep hygiene practices. Education of basic sleep hygiene should include sleeping and waking at regular times, relaxing before bedtime including no electronic screens at least 30 minutes prior to bedtime, creating a dark, quiet sleep environment, avoiding naps, limiting caffeine, and participating in regular exercise. Non-pharmacological strategies include cognitive restructuring, behavioral strategies, and relaxation. Most sleep disturbances in children are successfully managed with a combination of good sleep hygiene and non-pharmacological strategies (Owens and Mindell 2011). Although there are many pharmacological interventions available to assist with sleep, the majority of these medications are not recommended by the US Food and Drug Administration for the treatment of sleep disturbances in children. The use of sleep medication is primarily based on clinical experience and empirical data from adult studies (Owens and Mindell 2011). If pharmacological intervention is necessary, the provider should consider the cause of the sleep disturbance, the risks and benefits of the medication, potential drug interactions, and the child's medical history (Owens and Mindell 2011). Herbal remedies may be used for sleep disturbances. Melatonin, a dietary supplement, has been effective for sleep disturbances in children with autism spectrum disorders but has not been established in children undergoing cancer treatment. See Chap. 16, Integrative Care, for more information.

Somnolence syndrome is a self-limiting condition with no known long-term consequences, so education and support are the best management for these children (Ryan 2000).

Conclusion

Childhood cancer, its treatment, and related medical procedures cause multiple physical effects. The disease process can affect multiple sites throughout the body and cause a multitude of physical symptoms. Furthermore, the various procedures and treatments aimed at during the cancer may cause further physical consequences. These physical effects can disrupt a child's life, create additional complications, and compromise treatment. Children with cancer report treatment-related symptoms as the worst part of their cancer experience and were remembered long after treatment ended (Woodgate and Degner 2003). Each issue requires careful assessment and appropriate interventions to minimize further complications, improve outcomes, and enhance the quality of life for children with cancer.

Clinical Pearls

Distressing physical symptoms occur frequently in children with cancer and are caused by the disease, aggressive therapy regimens, and medical procedures.

Chemotherapy agents and radiation therapy cause myelosuppression, a condition that occurs when bone marrow activity is decreased and produces fewer white blood cells, red blood cells, and platelets, which can result in susceptibility to infection, fatigue, and increased bleeding.

Nausea and vomiting are two common yet distinct symptoms that are caused from the disease, treatment, and/or side effects of medications. These symptoms can occur before treatment (anticipatory), during treatment (acute), and/or after treatment (delayed).

A change in weight is common during treatment for childhood cancer and dictates that weight status be monitored frequently to assess for significant shifts. Early referrals for nutritional assessment may assist with preventing significant weight loss or weight gain.

References

Agrawal AK, Hastins CA, Feusner J (2011) Hematologic supportive care for children with cancer. In: Pizzo PA, Poplack DG (eds) Principles and practice of pediatric oncology, 6th edn. Wolters Kluwer Lippinsott Williams & Wilkins, Philadelphia, pp 1152–1189

Ahmed NM, Flynn PM (2014) Fever in children with chemotherapy-induced neutropenia. In: UptoDate, Waltham, MA. http://www.uptodate.com. Accessed 23 August 2014

Alley E, Green R, Schuchter L (2002) Cutaneous toxicities of cancer therapy. Curr Opin Oncol 14:212–216

Altaf S, Enders F, Jeavons E (2013) High-BMI at diagnosis is associated with inferior survival in patients with osteosarcoma: a report from the Children's Oncology Group. Pediatr Blood Cancer 60(12):2042–2046. doi:10.1002/pbc.24580

Anghelescu DL, Oakes LL, Hankins GM (2011) Treatment of pain in children after limb-sparing surgery: and institution's 26 year experience. Pain Manag Nurs 12(2):82–94. doi:10.1016/j.pmn.2010.02.002

Baggott C, Dodd M, Kennedy C et al (2010) Changes in children's reports of symptom occurrence and severity during a course of myelosuppressive chemotherapy. J Ped Oncol Nurs 27:307–315. doi:10.1177/1043454210377619

Baggott C, Cooper B, Marina N et al (2014) Symptom assessment in pediatric oncology: how should concordance between children's and parents' reports be evaluated? Cancer Nurs 37(4):252–262. doi:10.1097/NCC.0000000000000111

Bauer J, Jurgens H, Fruhwald MC (2011) Important aspects of nutrition in children with cancer. Adv Nutr 2(2):67–77. doi:10.3945/an.110.000141

Baumann FT, Bloch W, Beulertz J (2013) Clinical exercise interventions in pediatric oncology: a systematic review. Pediatr Res 74(4):366–374. doi:10.1038/pr.2013.123

Berenson GS, Bogalusa Heart Study Group (2012) Health consequences of obesity. Pediatr Blood Cancer 58(1):117–121. doi:10.1002/pbc.23373

Bonthius D, Lee A (2013) Approach to the child with headache. Pediatric & Neonatal Lexi-Drugs Online™, Hudson. http://online.lexi.com. Accessed 30 Aug 2014

Bower JE, Crosswell AD, Slavich GM (2014) Childhood adversity and cumulative life stress: risk factors for cancer-related fatigue. Clin Psychol Sci 2(1):108–115. doi:10.1177/2167702613496243

Burgoyne LL, Billups CA, Jiron JL et al (2013) Phantom limb pain in young cancer-related amputees: recent experience at St. Jude Children's Research Hospital. Clin J Pain 28(3):222–225. doi:10.1097/AJP.0b013e318227ce7a

Burningham Z, Hashibe M, Spector L et al (2012) The epidemiology of sarcoma. Clin Sarcoma Res 2(1):2–14. doi:10.1186/2045-3329-2-14

Burris H III, Hurtig J (2010) Radiation recall with anticancer agents. Oncologist 15:1227–1237. doi:10.1634/theoncologist.2009-0090

Center for Disease Control and Prevention (2014a) About BMI for children and teens. http://www.cdc.gov/healthyweight/assessing/bmi/childrens_bmi/about_childrens_bmi.html#What%20is%20BMI%20percentile

Center for Disease Control and Prevention (2014b) Childhood obesity facts: prevalence of childhood obesity in the United States 2011–2012. http://www.cdc.gov/obesity/data/childhood.html

Chang CW, Mu PF, Jou ST et al (2013) Systematic review and meta-analysis of nonpharmacological interventions for fatigue in children and adolescents with cancer. Worldviews Evid Based Nurs 10(4):208–217. doi:10.1111/wvn.12007

Children's Oncology Group (2013) Long-term follow-up guidelines for survivors of childhood, adolescent and young adult cancer. www.survivorshipguidelines.org

Children's Oncology Group (n.d.) Hearing problems after treatment. Retrieved from http://www.childrensoncologygroup.org/index.php/sensory/hearingproblems

Collins JJ, Byrnes ME, Dunkel IJ et al (2000) The measurement of symptoms in children with cancer. J Pain Symptom Manag 19(5):363–377

Dupuis L, Boodhan S, Sung L et al (2011) Guideline for the classification of the acute emetogenic potential of antineoplastic medication in pediatric cancer patients. Pediatr Blood Cancer 57:191–198. doi:10.1002/pbc.23114

Dupuis L, Boodhan S, Holdsworth M et al (2013) Guideline for the prevention of acute nausea and vomiting due to antineoplastic medication in pediatric cancer patients. Pediatr Blood Cancer 60:1073–1082. doi:10.1002/pbc.24508

Feyer P, Maranzano E, Molassiotis A et al (2011) Radiotherapy-induced nausea and vomiting: MASCC/ESMO guideline for antiemetics in radiotherapy: update 2009. Support Care Cancer 19:S5–S14. doi:10.1007/s00520-010-0950-6

Freifeld AG, Bow EJ, Sepkowitz KA et al (2011) Clinical practice guideline for the use of antimicrobial agents in neutropenic patients with cancer: 2010 update by the infectious diseases society of America. Clin Infect Dis 52(4):e56–e93. doi:10.1093/cid/cir073

Gibson F, Auld E, Bryan G et al (2010) A systematic review of oral assessment instruments. Cancer Nurs 33(4):E1–E19. doi:10.1097/NCC.0b013e3181cb40c0

Gilchrist L (2012) Chemotherapy-induced peripheral neuropathy in pediatric cancer patients. Sem Ped Neurol 19(1):9–17. doi:10.1016/j.spen.2012.02.011

Gonzalez T (2013) Chemotherapy extravasations: prevention, identification, management, and documentation. Clin J Oncol Nurs 17(1):61–66. doi:10.1188/13.CJON.61-66

Hilliard LM, Berkow RL, Watterson J et al (1997) Retinal toxicity associated with cisplatin and etoposide in pediatric patients. Med Pediar Oncol 28(4):310–313

Hinds PS, Yang J, Gattuso JS et al (2010) Psychometric and clinical assessment of the 10-item reduced version of the Fatigue Scale-Child instrument. J Pain Symptom Manag 39(3):572–578. doi:10.1016/j.jpainsymman.2009.07.015

Hockenberry M, Kline N (2011) Nursing support of the child with cancer. In: Pizzo PA, Poplack DG (eds) Principles and practice of pediatric oncology, 6th edn. Wolters Kluwer Lippincott Williams & Wilkins, Philadelphia, pp 1295–1298

Hockenberry MJ, Hinds PS, Barrera P et al (2003) Three instruments to assess fatigue in children with cancer: the child, parent and staff perspectives. J Pain Symptom Manage 25(4):319–328

Hockenberry M, McCarthy K, Taylor O et al (2011) Managing painful procedures in children with cancer. J Pediatr Hematol Oncol 33:119–127. doi:10.1097/MPH.0b013e3181f46a65

Hockenberry MJ, Taylor OA, Pasvogel A et al (2014) The influence of oxidative stress on symptom occurrence, severity, and distress during childhood leukemia treatment. Oncol Nurs Forum 41(4):E238–E247. doi:10.1188/14.ONF.E238-E247

Hockenberry-Eaton M, Hinds P (2000) Fatigue in children and adolescents with cancer: evolution of a program. Semin Oncol Nurs 16(4):261–278

Hockenberry-Eaton M, Hinds PS, Alcoser P et al (1998) Fatigue in children and adolescents with cancer. J Ped Oncol Nurs 15(3):172–182

Hockenberry-Eaton M, Hinds P, Howard V et al (1999) Developing a conceptual model for fatigue in children. Eur J Oncol Nurs 3(1):5–11

Hogan A (2009) Implementation of an oral care protocol and its effects on oral mucositis. J Pediatr Oncol Nurs 26(3):125–135. doi:10.1177/1043454209334356

Huhmann MB, August DA (2008) Review of American Society for Parenteral and Enteral Nutrition (ASPEN) clinical guidelines for nutrition support in cancer patients: nutrition screening and assessment. Nutr Clin Pract 23:182–188. doi:10.1177/0884533608314530

Inaba H, Surprise H, Pounds S et al (2012) Effect of body mass index on the outcome of children with acute myloid leukemia. Cancer 118(23):5989–5996. doi:10.1002/cncr.27640

Jacob E (2008) Pain. In: Kline N (ed) Essentials of pediatric hematology/oncology nursing, 3rd edn. APHON, Glenview, pp 148–153

Kanellopoulos A, Hamre HM, Dahl AA et al (2013) Factors associated with poor quality of life in survivors of childhood acute lymphoblastic leukemia and lymphoma. Pediatr Blood Cancer 60(5):849–855. doi:10.1002/pbc.24375

Kennedy RM, Luhmann J, Zempsky WT (2008) Clinical implications of unmanaged needle-insertion pain and distress in children. Pediatrics 122(suppl 3):S130–S133. doi:10.1542/peds.2008-1055e

Kestler SA, LoBiondo-Wood G (2012) Review of symptom experiences in children and adolescents with cancer. Cancer Nurs 35:e31–e48. doi:10.1097/NCC.0b013e3182207a2a

Koh AY, Pizzo PA (2011) Infectious complications in pediatric cancer patients. In: Pizzo PA, Poplack DG (eds) Principles and practice of pediatric oncology, 6th edn. Wolters Kluwer Lippinsott Williams & Wilkins, Philadelphia, pp 1190–1242

Krane E, Casillas J, Zeltzer L (2011) Pain and symptom management. In: Pizzo PA, Poplack DG (eds) Principles and practice of pediatric oncology, 6th edn. Wolters Kluwer Lippincott Williams & Wilkins, Philadelphia, pp 1256–1287

Lai JS, Cella D, Kupst MJ et al (2007) Measuring fatigue for children with cancer: development and validation of the pediatric Functional Assessment of Chronic Illness Therapy-Fatigue (pedsFACIT-F). J Pediatr Hematol Oncol 29(7):471–479

Landers R, O'Hanlon-Curry J (2008) Gastrointestinal complications. In: Kline N (ed) Essentials of pediatric hematology/oncology nursing, 3rd edn. APHON, Glenview, pp 134–136

Lee M, Korner J (2009) Review of physiology, clinical manifestations, and management of hypothalamic obesity in humans. Pituitary 12(2):87–95. doi:10.1007/s11102-008-0096-4

Lehrnbecher T, Phillips R, Alexander S et al (2012) Guideline for the management of fever and neutropenia in children with cancer and/or undergoing hematopoietic stem-cell transplantation. J Clin Oncol 30(35):4427–4438. doi:10.1200/JCO.2012.42.7161

Lexicomp (2014) Pediatric & Neonatal Lexi-Drugs Online™, Hudson. http://online.lexi.com. Accessed 21 Aug 2014

Linder LA, Christian BJ (2012) Nighttime sleep characteristics of hospitalized school-age children with cancer. J Spec Pediatr Nurs 18:13–24. doi:10.1111/jspn.12005

Lustig RH (2011) Hypothalamic obesity after craniopharyngioma: mechanisms, diagnosis, and treatment. Front Endocrinol 2:60. doi:10.3389/fendo.2011.00060

Mandrell BN, Yang J, Hooke MC et al (2011) Psychometric and clinical assessment of the 13-item reduced version of the fatigue scale-adolescent instrument. J Pain Symptom Manag 28(5):287–294. doi:10.1177/1043454211418667

Marina N, Hudson MM, Jones KE et al (2013) Changes in health status among aging survivors of pediatric upper and lower extremity sarcoma: a report from the Childhood Cancer Survivor Study (CCSS). Arch Phys Med Rehabil 94(6):1062–1073. doi:10.1016/j.apmr.2013.01.013

McCarthy GM, Skillings JR (1992) Jaw and other orofacial pain in patients receiving vincristine for the treatment of cancer. Oral Surg Oral Med Oral Pathol 74(3):299–304

Meeske KA, Siegel SE, Globe DR et al (2005) Prevalence and correlates of fatigue in long-term survivors of childhood leukemia. J Clin Oncol 23(24): 5501–5510

Meeske KA, Patel SK, Palmer SN et al (2007) Factors associated with health-related quality of life in pediatric cancer survivors. Pediatr Blood Cancer 49:298–305

Montgomery K, Belongia M, Haddigan M et al (2013) Perceptions of nutrition support in pediatric oncology patients and parents. J Pediatr Oncol Nurs 30:90–98. doi:10.1177/1043454212471726

Norville R (2008) Skin changes. In: Kline N (ed) Essentials of pediatric hematology/oncology nursing, 3rd edn. APHON, Glenview, pp 142–143

Omoti AE, Omoti CE (2006) Ocular toxicity of systemic anticancer chemotherapy. Pharm Pract 4(2):55–59

Orgel E, Sposto R, Malvar J et al (2014) Impact on survival and toxicity by duration of weight extremes during treatment for pediatric acute lymphoblastic leukemia: a report from the Children's Oncology Group. J Clin Oncol 32(13):1331–1337. doi:10.1200/JCO.2013.52.6962

Orsey AD, Wakefield DB, Cloutier MM (2013) Physical activity (PA) and sleep among children and adolescents with cancer. Pediatr Blood Cancer 60(11):1908–1913. doi:10.1002/pbc.24641

Owens JA, Mindell JA (2011) Pediatric insomnia. Pediatr Clin N Am 58:555–569. doi:10.1016/j.pcl.2011.03.011

Pashankar F, Season J, McNamara J et al (2011) Acute constipation in children receiving chemotherapy for cancer. J Pediatr Hematol Oncol 33(7):e300–e303. doi:10.1097/MPH.0b013e31821a0795

Pessi M, Zilembo N, Haspinger E et al (2014) Target therapy-induced diarrhea: a review of the literature. Crit Rev Oncol Hematol 90:165–179. doi:10.1016/j.critrevonc.2013.11.008

Phillips R, Gibson F (2008) A systematic review of treatments for constipation in children and young adults undergoing cancer treatment. J Pediatr Hematol Oncol 30(11):829–830. doi:10.1097/MPH.0b013e318175898c

Phillips R, Gopaul S, Gibson F et al (2011) Antiemetic medication for prevention and treatment of chemotherapy induced nausea and vomiting in childhood. Cochrane Database Syst Rev 9(2):CD007786. doi:10.1002/14651858

Pulsipher MA (2012) Pediatric-specific guidelines for fever and neutropenia: a catalyst for improving care and focusing research. J Clin Oncol 30(35):4292–4293. doi:10.1200/JCO.2012.45.4629

Purser MJ, Johnston DL, McMillan HJ (2014) Chemotherapy-induced peripheral neuropathy among paediatric oncology patients. Can J Neurol Sci 41(4):442–447

Rehwaldt M, Wickham R, Purl S et al (2009) Self-care strategies to cope with taste changes after chemotherapy. Oncol Nurs Forum 36(2):E47–E56. doi:10.1188/09

Rodgers CC (2015) Children with cancer. In: Hockenberry M, Wilson D (eds) Wong's nursing care of infants and children, 10th edn. Elsevier, St. Louis, pp 1379–1424

Rodgers C, Young A, Hockenberry M et al (2010) The meaning of adolescents' eating experiences during bone marrow transplant recovery. J Pediatr Oncol Nurs 27(2):65–72. doi:10.1177/1043454209355984

Rodgers CC, Hooke MC, Hockenberry MJ (2013) Symptom clusters in children. Curr Opin Support Palliat Care 7(1):67–72. doi:10.1097/SPC.0b013e32835ad551

Rogers PC, Melnick SJ, Ladas E et al (2008) Children's oncology group nutrition committee. Pediatr Blood Cancer 50:447–450

Rusch R, Schulta C, Hughes L et al (2014) Evidence-based practice recommendations to prevent/manage post-lumbar puncture headaches in pediatric patients receiving intrathecal chemotherapy. J Pediatr Oncol Nurs 31(4):230–238

Ryan J (2000) Radiation somnolence syndrome. J Pediatr Oncol Nurs 17(1):50–53

Santucci G, Mack J (2007) Common gastrointestinal symptoms in pediatric palliative care: nausea, vomiting, constipation, anorexia, cachexia. Pediatr Clin N Am 54:673–689

Schulmeister L (2011) Extravasation management: clinical update. Semin Oncol Nurs 27(1):82–90. doi:10.1016/j.soncn.2010.11.010

Shaw C, Taylor L (2012) Treatment-related diarrhea in patients with cancer. Clin J Oncol Nurs 16(4):413–417. doi:10.1188/12.CJON.413-417

Sheridan D, Meckler G, Spiro D et al (2013) Diagnostic testing and treatment of pediatric headache in the emergency department. J Pediatr 163(6):1634–1637. doi:10.1016/j.jpeds.2013.07.006

Skolin I, Wahlin Y, Broman D et al (2006) Altered food intake and taste perception in children with cancer after start of chemotherapy: perspective of children, parents and nurses. Support Care Cancer 14(4):369–378

Torado B (2012) Cannabinoids in the treatment of chemotherapy-induced nausea and vomiting. J Natl Compr Canc Netw 10:487–492

Trottier E, Bailey B, Lucas N et al (2013) Diagnosis of migraine in the pediatric emergency department. Pediatr Neurol 49:40–45. doi:10.1016/j.pediatrneurol.2013.03.003

Tuca A, Jimenez-Fonseca P, Gascon P (2013) Clinical evaluation and optimal management of cancer cachexia. Clin Rev Oncol Hematol 88:625–636. doi:10.1016/j.critrevonc.2013.07.015

Ullrich N (2009) Neurologic sequelae of brain tumors in children. J Child Neurol 24(11):1446–1454. doi:10.1177/0883073809342491

Varni JW, Burwinkle TM, Katz ER et al (2002) The PedsQL in pediatric cancer: reliability and validity of the pediatric quality of life inventory generic core scales, multidimensional fatigue scale, and cancer module. Cancer 94(7):2090–2106

Vena C, Parker K, Cunningham M et al (2004) Sleep-wake disturbances in people with cancer part I: an overview of sleep, sleep regulation, and effects of disease and treatment. Oncol Nurs Forum 31(4):735–746

Viale P (2006) Chemotherapy and cutaneous toxicities: implications for oncology nurses. Semin Oncol Nurs 22(3):144–151

Webster-Gandy J, How C, Harrold K (2007) Palmar-plantar erythrodysesthesia (PPE): a literature review with commentary on experience in a cancer centre. Eur J Oncol Nurs 11:238–246

White M, Murphy AJ, Hallahan A et al (2012) Survival in overweight and underweight children undergoing hematopoietic stem cell transplantation. Eur J Clin Nutr 66(10):1120–1123. doi:10.1038/ejcn.2012.109

Withycombe JS, Post-White JE, Meza JL et al (2009) Weight patterns in children with higher risk ALL: a report from the Children's Oncology Group (COG) for CCG 1961. Pediatr Blood Cancer 53(7):1249–1254. doi:10.1002/pbc.22237

Wohlschlaeger A (2004) Prevention and treatment of mucositis: a guide for nurses. J Pediatr Oncol Nurs 21(5):281–287. doi:10.1177/1043454204265840

Woodgate R, Degner L (2003) Expectations and beliefs about children's cancer symptoms: perspective of children with cancer and their families. Oncol Nurs Forum 30:479–491

Zhang FF, Kelly MJ, Saltzman E et al (2013) Obesity in pediatric ALL survivors: a meta-analysis. Pediatrics 133(3):e704–e715. doi:10.1542/peds.2013-333

4 Assessing Family Psychosocial Risks in Pediatric Cancer

Anne E. Kazak, Stephen DiDonato, Stephanie J. Schneider, and Ahna L.H. Pai

Introduction

Although psychosocial interventions and care in pediatric cancer, based on strong scientific evidence from more than 30 years of research on youth and families, has prospered and been refined over recent decades, these findings are not consistently translated into the clinical delivery of psychosocial care for children with cancer and their families (Kazak and Noll 2015). For example, in a study of Children's Oncology Group (COG) institutions, about half of families were offered psychosocial services within the first 30 days after diagnosis. Only 9 % of institutions used empirically supported psychosocial evaluations and less than 11 % implemented empirically based treatments (Selove et al. 2012). Notably, no published data are available addressing the type or frequency of services at other points during the treatment trajectory.

There is little empirical data that documents psychosocial care and outcomes in pediatric cancer. Clinical experience and professional collaborations portray a situation in which psychosocial care is highly variable between, and even within, pediatric cancer programs. While most centers have access to some psychosocial staff, models for integrating psychosocial care in pediatric oncology programs have not been clearly articulated nor implemented consistently. Most pediatric cancer centers rely on existing psychosocial resources at a given institution and referral patterns are based on provider judgments of need. Ongoing concerns about staffing, time, and finances are pervasive.

Therefore, it is difficult to answer the basic question "What are the standards of psychosocial care in pediatric cancer?" A recent review on this point identified that, despite calls from professional organizations to screen for psychosocial distress (COC 2012; IOM 2007; Noll et al. 2013), none of the current published guidelines or stan-

A.E. Kazak, PhD, ABPP (✉)
Nemours Biomedical Research,
Nemours Center for Healthcare Delivery Science/
Alfred I. duPont Hospital for Children,
Wilmington, DE, USA
e-mail: anne.kazak@nemours.org

S. DiDonato, MS
Nemours Biomedical Research,
Center for Pediatric Traumatic Stress at the Nemours/
Alfred I. duPont Hospital for Children,
RC1 – 167, 1600 Rockland Road,
Wilmington, DE 19803, USA
e-mail: stephen.didonato@nemours.org

S.J. Schneider, MS
Nemours Biomedical Research, Nemours/
Alfred I duPont Hospital for Children,
RC1-160G, 1600 Rockland Road,
Wilmington, DE 19803, USA
e-mail: Stephanie.J.Schneider@gmail.com

A.L.H. Pai, PhD
Department of Behavioral Medicine and Clinical
Psychology, Blood Diseases Institute, Cincinnati
Children's Hospital Medical Center,
MLC 7039, Cincinnati, OH 45229-3039, USA
e-mail: ahna.pai@cchmc.org

A.N. Abrams et al. (eds.), *Pediatric Psychosocial Oncology: Textbook for Multidisciplinary Care*,
DOI 10.1007/978-3-319-21374-3_4

dards meet the comprehensive and evidenced-based criteria necessary to serve as psychosocial standards of care for pediatric cancer today (Wiener et al. 2015).

Screening to determine the level and nature of a patient and family's psychosocial status is a reasonable first step in the process of delivering care. Screening, usually for depression or distress, has become more common in adult oncology. The Commission on Cancer guidelines (COC 2012) requires distress screening but indicates that the treating institution should decide upon the method and tool for screening. Standardized and validated screening measures have preference. The COC also recommends that screening should occur at times of highest distress (i.e., at diagnosis, family meeting with oncologist to discuss treatment, transitions off treatment).

These existing recommendations for screening do not translate easily to pediatric settings. Many screening or assessment approaches are focused on the individual adult patient and are neither sufficiently broad nor inclusive of many key aspects of families and the broader social context necessary in pediatrics. In addition, there is a history of family-centered care and psychosocial support for families in pediatrics that is not typical in adult settings. Therefore, screening that corresponds to the types of services available to children and families in healthcare settings is also important.

Indeed, it is reasonable to assert that *all* families entering a pediatric healthcare setting should receive care attuned to their specific needs, including psychosocial care related to their health condition. There are distinct practice models for providing psychosocial care to children in pediatric settings. These approaches are generally aimed at treating the more severe problems identified by medical and nursing staff. For example, consultation liaison teams and referral to community providers are common approaches. However, care may be based primarily on clinical referral patterns that are not systematic but rather selective, based on individual clinical judgment and response to crisis. The availability of an "on-site" psychosocial professional integrated into the healthcare team may facilitate care to a broader range of patients and families. A population health model, looking at the needs of all patients and families and screening systematically, has the potential to overcome stigma associated with behavioral health services, change non-systematic provider-determined referral patterns, and facilitate more evidence-based and cost-effective allocation of finite resources, including more preventative care, when appropriate.

Screeners of psychosocial risk should include questions based on key research findings (e.g., factors related to adjustment over time and the need for intervention) and be administered efficiently in order to pair screening results with appropriate clinical interventions. Given the large literature on family factors that impact child functioning and well-being in both primary and tertiary healthcare settings, a contextual social ecological approach to screening offers a broad array of potential targets for intervention and provides an opportunity to appreciate the strengths as well as vulnerabilities of families (Ungar 2012).

Figure 4.1 illustrates the social ecology of child health and provides examples of how these map on to screening items. At the center are the child, the illness/condition, and the family microsystems. Family assessments/screening focuses heavily on these interrelated systems with questions about the child, family, and illness prominent. At the next level of the model are systems intimately linked to successful adaptation and child health outcomes: healthcare settings, schools, social relationships, and communities. Figure 4.1 illustrates the complex interrelationships among elements of the social ecology. The more distal macrosystem includes other influences, such as culture, laws, and social class that provide a context for a thorough conceptualization of risk and resilience. Therefore, a comprehensive screen should include quick evaluation of relevant topics of the child's social ecology and in the context of a broader systemic model in order to identify factors impacting the child's functioning and to identify and prioritize interventions.

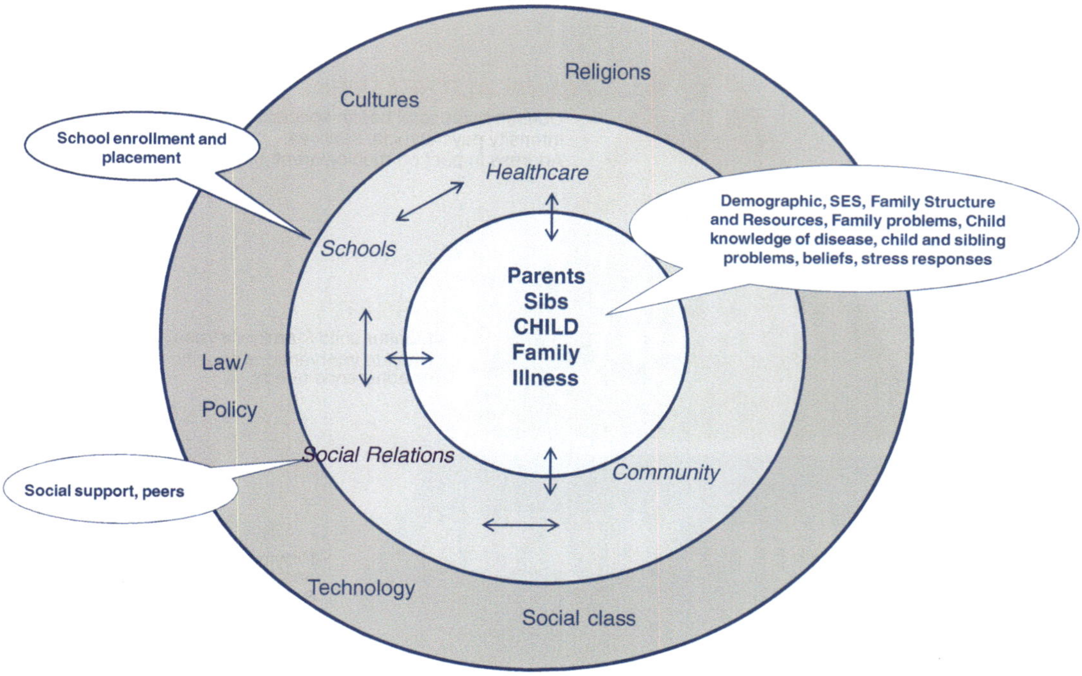

Fig. 4.1 Screening in a social ecological context

Timely screening for multifaceted family psychosocial risk is a means by which treatment needs and follow-up care for the patient and family can be identified in an effective and inclusive manner to facilitate efficient assessment and delivery of evidence-based care matched to patient and family need. In light of a recent comprehensive review of the literature on screening in pediatric cancer (Kazak et al. 2012), this chapter includes an updated search, completed in October 2014, to identify recent papers on psychosocial screening in pediatric cancer. We used the same keywords as the earlier review ("pediatric oncology" or "pediatric cancer" or "childhood cancer") AND (screen* or tool* or assess* or classify* or categorize or evaluate or "psychosocial risk" or "psychosocial need" or "psychosocial care" or at risk" or "level of risk" or "identify risk" or distress or parents) AND (NOT survivor*) and databases (PsycInfo, Cinahl, PubMed, and Health and Psychosocial Instruments Database). In addition, authors of recent papers were contacted to obtain copies of relevant presentations and prepublication work.

Models for Standardized Screening

Three primary models of risk screening were identified in a previous review (Kazak et al. 2012) – 1) the *P*ediatric *P*reventative *P*sychosocial *H*ealth *M*odel (PPPHM), 2) the Family APGAR (*A*daptability, *P*artnership, *G*rowth, *A*ffection, and *R*esolve) approach, and 3) the HEADSS (*H*ome, *E*ducation, *A*ctivities, *D*rugs, *S*exuality, and *S*uicide/Depression) framework. No additional models of psychosocial risk screening in pediatric cancer were found in the literature between 2011 and 2014.

The Pediatric Psychosocial Preventative Health Model (PPPHM; Fig. 4.2) is based on a public health framework and used to conceptualize families with varying levels of psychosocial risk along with interventions matched to risk (Kazak 2006). Each of the PPPHM levels is described below followed by a case example.

At the base of the pyramid are Universal families, who are understandably concerned or distressed about their child's health problem but who are generally resilient and able to

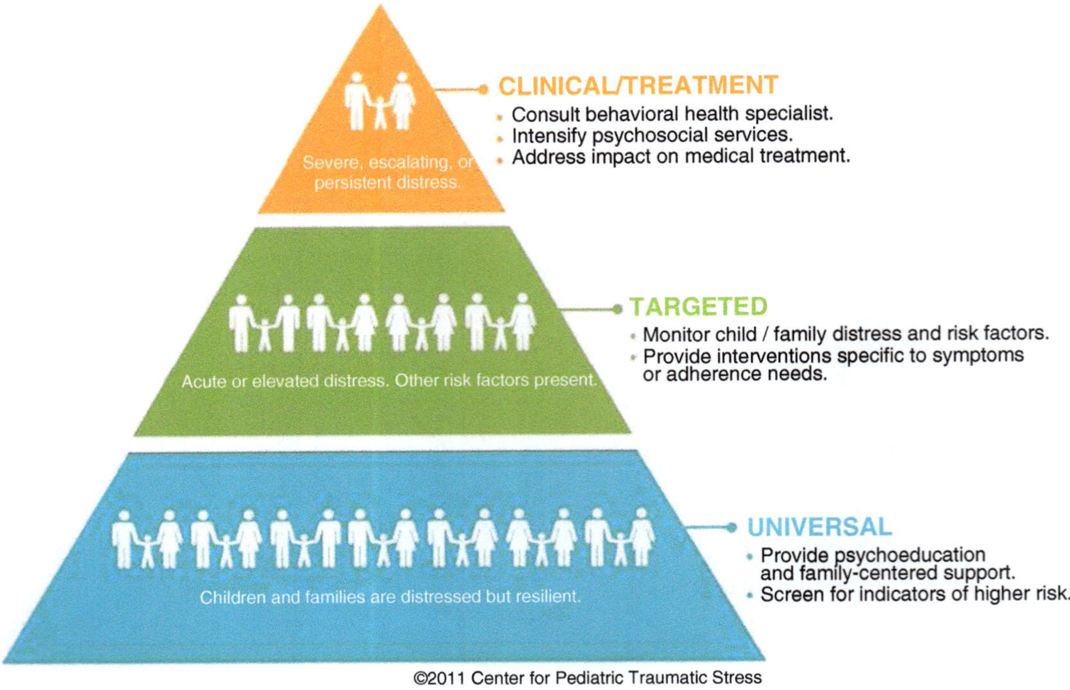

Fig. 4.2 Pediatric Psychosocial Preventative Health Model (PPPHM) (Reproduced with permission from the Center for Pediatric Traumatic Stress (CPTS) at Nemours Children's Health System © 2011. All rights reserved. The PPPHM may not be reproduced in any form for any purpose without the express written permission of CPTS. To obtain permission to use reproduce the PPPHM, contact Anne Kazak, PhD ABPP at anne.kazak@nemours.org)

cope and adapt to their child's illness and treatment.

Universal Level Case Example: Max is a 15-year-old recently diagnosed with resilient leukemia. His parents are married. They work full time outside the home but expect that their employers will afford them some flexibility over the next few months. Max has two siblings, ages 12 and 17, and a large family support system available for help. Max's parents consider him a bit of a worrier but otherwise a popular student who learns easily. His mother reports a history of frequent migraine headaches and appears sad and tired at clinic visits.

The middle tier consists of Targeted families, with preexisting concerns or difficulties that may contribute to continuing or escalating vulnerability during treatment.

Targeted Level Case Example: Aiden is a 9-year-old recently diagnosed with a rhabdomyosarcoma. His teachers have noted difficulties in attention and some challenges in learning last year and this year. His parents are executives in local businesses who separated last year and have occasional disputes about custody and child support. Both parents are present at clinic visits.

At the tip of the pyramid are Clinical families, with one or more preexisting, chronic, and complex problems and resulting greatest need for prompt and often intensive intervention.

Clinical Level Case Example: Sophia is a 5-year-old recently diagnosed with a medulloblastoma. She has three younger siblings, ages 3 and 2 years and 8 months. Her parents have many financial worries (e.g., concerns about paying phone and utility bills, rent, etc.), few people to assist them, and general apprehensiveness about treatment and its impact on their daughter and family. Sophia's parents indicate that she has several behavioral and developmental concerns (e.g., moodiness, anxiety, problems in kindergarten) and, on screening, endorses a number of behavioral concerns for at least one of the siblings. In addition, her mother has a history of anxiety and endorsed symptoms of acute stress since her daughter's diagnosis.

Using the PPPHM as a guide, treatment options vary by level. Many of the services currently provided in pediatric settings (e.g., social workers, child life specialists, chaplains, creative arts programs, family-centered care programs, financial counselors, etc.) provide a broad undergirding of care that will address many of the needs of Universal families. There are many evidence-based interventions developed that are appropriate for families at the Targeted level. These include cognitive behavioral therapy for pain and behavioral or multicomponent interventions for adherence to medical regimens (see http://www.apadivisions.org/division-54/evidence-based/). At the Clinical level, behavioral medicine teams are usually necessary to assess and provide generally more intensive interventions in addition to Universal services that families would receive. The PPPHM provides a "snapshot" of the family's risks and resilience. Screening always necessitates clinical follow-up assessment to determine a treatment plan. Continued monitoring of risk for all families is critical to capture changes in risk over time. The literature review identified eight papers that referred to the PPPHM as a model or guide for pediatric populations.

The Family APGAR (*A*daptability, *P*artnership, *G*rowth, *A*ffection, and *R*esolve) provides quantitative data on individual family member's satisfaction with their family's functioning based on the APGAR components. The items are intended to measure individual family member's perception of family functioning. The Family APGAR also allows for the integration of physician knowledge of the family and follow-up discussions with the family member to gain qualitative data of the individual family member's satisfaction and family functioning based on the quantitative APGAR data (Smilkstein 1978).

The HEADSS framework (*H*ome, *E*ducation, *A*ctivities, *D*rugs, *S*exuality, and *S*uicide/Depression) interview guide aims to engage adolescents and young adults (AYAs) in preventative healthcare throughout the course of their cancer treatment (Yeo and Sawyer 2009). Providing physicians with a developmentally appropriate guide to engage adolescents and young adults in queries of specific areas of psychosocial risk is important in building rapport and ensuring patient-centered care. Although there is limited empirical basis for the HEADSS interview, the content is consistent with general adolescent preventative care (Goldenring and Rosen 2004).

Screening Methods and Evidence-Based Tools

There are potentially many different means of conducting screening. Before discussing specific approaches and measures, the results of a listserv posting conducted as part of the Psychosocial Standards of Care Project for Childhood Cancer (PSCPCC) are noted (Kupst MJ, 2015, Personal Communication). Queries were posted in July 2013 to listservs of the Society of Pediatric Psychology (SPP) and the International Society of Pediatric Oncology (SIOP) asking what measures were used in clinical care for screening and assessment of children, adolescents, and young adults with cancer. Although not a scientific survey, the results indicated that the most frequently used screeners were the Psychosocial Assessment Tool (PAT; Pai et al. 2008), the Strengths and Difficulties Questionnaire (SDQ; Goodman 2001), the Child Behavior Checklist (CBCL; ASEBA 2015), the Distress Thermometer (DT; National Comprehensive Cancer Network® (NCCN®) 2003), the Behavior Assessment System for Children (BASC/BASC-2; Reynolds and Kamphaus 2004), and the Brief Symptom Inventory (BSI; Derogatis 2000).

Methods for Screening

One method of risk assessment is to use a battery of validated measures (e.g., well-known measures of depression, anxiety, child behavior).[1]

[1] There are many validated instruments that have been used in pediatric oncology. A review of all of them is beyond the scope of this chapter.

The advantage of these approaches is the use of established psychometrically strong instruments, usually specific to a construct (e.g., quality of life, behavior, depression) and often with clinical cutoff scores. The disadvantages are that multiple measures are often necessary to assess relevant outcomes. The number of items on these batteries can be significant and the participant burden and administration time can become longer than is feasible in a medical setting. Scoring and interpretation may also necessitate a mental health professional; adding another step can slow the communication of results and may be problematic in some settings without such staff. One of the more creative applications of this approach, measuring quality of life in the Netherlands, is KLIK, a Dutch acronym roughly translated in English as *Mapping Quality of Life in Clinical Practice*, which provides a patient and family ePROfile developed from generic and illness-related questionnaires. KLIK provides the healthcare team with direct access to patient responses, which increases communication and provider satisfaction in care (Haverman et al. 2014).

A second approach is the very brief screeners, exemplified by the Distress Thermometer (DT) and discussed below.

Another method is structured clinical interviews. Such interviews typically include standardized questions about the nature, severity, and duration of symptoms, often with the goal of determining a diagnosis. Exemplified by the HEADSS, discussed above (e.g., HEADSS 3.0; Goldenring and Rosen 2004), structured clinical interviews assess a broad range of topics in detail and facilitate rapport. Although they provide clinicians with guidance regarding which questions to ask and how to ask them, they tend to be susceptible to interviewer drift and social desirability. The standardized structured clinical interview such as HEADSS also requires trained staff and increases the burden on clinical staff, and the administration time can be problematic in healthcare settings. The structured clinical interview differs from a clinical assessment in which the clinician is asking questions about particular areas of interest but using a less formally structured protocol to do so.

Yet another approach is the use of single relatively short standardized instruments. Most focus solely on child behavior (e.g., the Pediatric Symptom Checklist) or parenting stress (e.g., the Parenting Stress Index). The Beck Youth Inventory II was found to be a feasible approach for screening depression and anxiety in adolescents in oncology treatment (Kersun et al. 2009). SCREEM-RES (*S*ocial, *C*ultural, *R*eligious, *E*conomic, *E*ducation, and *M*edical) Family Resource Survey questionnaire was developed to identify areas that families need support in order to increase the family's capacity to cope with the child's cancer (Panganiban-Corales and Medina 2011).

The Psychosocial Assessment Tool (PAT) is the only measure developed specifically for pediatric oncology, guided by research evidence and clinical experience to assess (parental report) a range of potential risks across the family's social ecology. The PAT is discussed below in more detail.

Two Empirically Supported Tools

The Distress Thermometer (DT; Fig. 4.3; NCCN® 2014) uses a graphic representation of a thermometer, generating a 1–10 unidimensional rating of how distressed the respondent has felt in the past week. The DT may also be used with a problem list of practical problems (e.g., housing, insurance), family problems (e.g., dealing with partner, children), emotional problems (e.g.., worry, sadness), spiritual and religious concerns (e.g., relating to God, loss of faith), and physical problems (e.g., pain, nausea) (NCCN 2003). The DT has been used quite extensively in adult oncology and more recently in pediatric cancer (Patel et al. 2011). Data from Patel et al. (2011) were extracted for patients and their mothers at the end of life, indicating that the DT was helpful in tracking changes at this point in treatment (Patel et al. 2011). The DT is feasible in screening for distress in children with cancer or other chronic illness and correlated with both child and parent measures of depression, anxiety, pain, and fatigue (Zadeh et al. 2014). The Distress Thermometer for Parents (DT-P) was also developed and validated for parents of children with

NCCN National Comprehensive Cancer Network®

NCCN Guidelines Version 2.2014
Distress Management

NCCN Guidelines Index
Distress Management TOC
Discussion

NCCN DISTRESS THERMOMETER

Instructions: Please circle the number (0-10) that best describes how much distress you have been experiencing in the past week including today.

Extreme distress

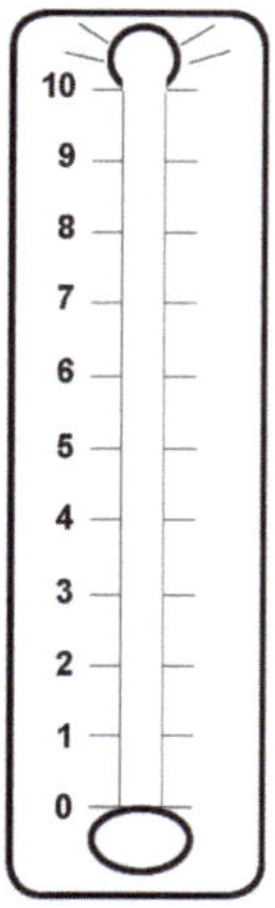

No distress

PROBLEM LIST
Please indicate if any of the following has been a problem for you in the past week including today.
Be sure to check YES or NO for each.

YES	NO	Practical Problems
❑	❑	Child care
❑	❑	Housing
❑	❑	Insurance/financial
❑	❑	Transportation
❑	❑	Work/school
❑	❑	Treatment decisions
		Family Problems
❑	❑	Dealing with children
❑	❑	Dealing with partner
❑	❑	Ability to have children
❑	❑	Family health issues
		Emotional Problems
❑	❑	Depression
❑	❑	Fears
❑	❑	Nervousness
❑	❑	Sadness
❑	❑	Worry
❑	❑	Loss of interest in usual activities
❑	❑	**Spiritual/religious concerns**

YES	NO	Physical Problems
❑	❑	Appearance
❑	❑	Bathing/dressing
❑	❑	Breathing
❑	❑	Changes in urination
❑	❑	Constipation
❑	❑	Diarrhea
❑	❑	Eating
❑	❑	Fatigue
❑	❑	Feeling Swollen
❑	❑	Fevers
❑	❑	Getting around
❑	❑	Indigestion
❑	❑	Memory/concentration
❑	❑	Mouth sores
❑	❑	Nausea
❑	❑	Nose dry/congested
❑	❑	Pain
❑	❑	Sexual
❑	❑	Skin dry/itchy
❑	❑	Sleep
❑	❑	Substance abuse
❑	❑	Tingling in hands/feet

Other Problems: ______________________________

____

 DIS-A

Fig. 4.3 NCCN® Distress Thermometer (Reproduced with permission from the NCCN Clinical Practice Guidelines in Oncology (NCCN Guidelines®) for Distress Management V.2.2014. © 2014 National Comprehensive Cancer Network, Inc. All rights reserved. The NCCN Guidelines® and illustrations herein may not be reproduced in any form for any purpose without the express written permission of the NCCN. To view the most recent and complete version of the NCCN Guidelines, go online to NCCN.org. NATIONAL COMPREHENSIVE CANCER NETWORK®, NCCN®, NCCN GUIDELINES®, and all other NCCN Content are trademarks owned by the National Comprehensive Cancer Network, Inc.)

chronic illnesses, showing associations of its 10-point Likert scale with parental distress (Haverman et al. 2013).

The advantages of the DT are brevity, simplicity, and focus on the self-reported distress of the respondent. Its simplicity allows for it to be completed by children and parents. However, a single score of one dimension (distress) may provide limited clinical information and is not highly specific in providing direction for needed intervention. The use of problem lists on the DT contributes information about areas of concern, although it adds slightly to the length, which is usually 3–5 minutes.

The Psychosocial Assessment Tool (PAT; Fig. 4.4; Pai et al. 2008), a brief (5–10 minutes administration time) screener of family psychosocial risk based on the PPPHM's trilevel of risk classification, was developed for families of children with cancer. In addition to the total score, there are seven subscales (structure/resources, family problems, social support, stress reactions, family beliefs, child problems, and sibling problems). The psychometric properties of the PAT are strong (Pai et al. 2008) and PPPHM risk classification is generally stable across 4 months (Alderfer et al. 2009). Detailed information about the history, use, and research on the PAT is detailed in a recent paper (Kazak et al. 2015). The all-literacy English and Spanish versions of the PAT (4th-grade reading level) are

PAT
PSYCHOSOCIAL ASSESSMENT TOOL

About you (person completing form):

Are you: ☐Biological Parent ☐Step-parent ☐Adoptive parent ☐Foster parent ☐Grandparent ☐Legal Guardian

Your role with the child ☐Main (daily) caregiver ☐Supporting or back-up caregiver ☐Occasional (off and on) caregiver

About the main caregiver(s) in the child's home (if you are not the main caregiver, please provide as much information, as you know):

Age of main caregiver(s) (✓all that apply): ☐Under age 21 ☐Age 21 or over ☐One is over 21 and the other is under 21

How far did you get in school? (✓one box)

☐ Started school but didn't finish ☐ Finished high school / got GED
☐ Started college or trade school ☐ Finished college or trade school
☐ Started master's or doctoral program ☐ Finished master's or doctoral program

Who can you ask to help with: (✓all boxes that apply)

	My spouse/ partner	Child's main/ other caregiver(s)	Child's Grand-parents	Other family members	Friends	People at work	Church / spiritual community	Other (list)	No One
a. Childcare / Parenting									
b. Emotional Support									

In what areas are there money problems? (✓all boxes that apply)

☐ None ☐ Phone/heat/light bills ☐ Paying rent/mortgage ☐ Buying food ☐ Car costs (upkeep /gas /insurance) ☐ Medical bills

In general, does he or she: (✓ one box for each question) →				A problem for other children at home? ☐ No other children	
	No	Some – times	Yes / Getting Help	No	Yes
a. Seem moody / change moods a lot?					
b. Seem sad or keeps to herself / himself?					
c. Have developmental problems compared to kids the same age?					

At any time during the child's illness have you. . . (circle a number for each question below)	Not at All	Some-times	Often	Very Much
a. Had unwanted memories or upsetting dreams about the child having cancer?	0	1	2	3
b. Stayed away from people, places, or things that remind you of the child's cancer?	0	1	2	3
c. Been on the lookout for signs that the cancer is getting worse or happening all over again?	0	1	2	3

As a caregiver for the child, how much do you believe. . . (✓one box for each statement below)	Not true for me	A little true for me	Mostly true for me	Very true for me
a. The doctors and nurses will know how to help				
b. My child will be in a lot of pain				
c. Our family will be closer because of this				

About the adults caring for the child... (✓one box for each question)	No	Yes
a. Has anyone had a lot of worry, fear, or anxiety at times?		
b. Have drugs or alcohol caused problems for anyone in the family?		

Fig. 4.4 Sample items from the Psychosocial Assessment Tool (PAT) (Reproduced with permission from the Center for Pediatric Traumatic Stress (CPTS) at Nemours Children's Health System © 2014–2015. All rights reserved. The PAT image above is comprised of sample items from each of the PAT subscales. The PAT image may not be reproduced in any form for any purpose without the express written permission of CPTS. To obtain permission to use or view the most recent version of the PAT, please contact CPTS at psychosocialassessmenttool@nemours.org)

being tested in a current multisite study (ACS RSG-13-015).

Recent papers support the use of a Canadian adaptation of the PAT (Barrera et al. 2014), associations between socioeconomic variables and overall risk level over a 1-year period (Karlson et al. 2013), and feasibility in survivorship care (Gilleland et al. 2013). PAT can be administered in

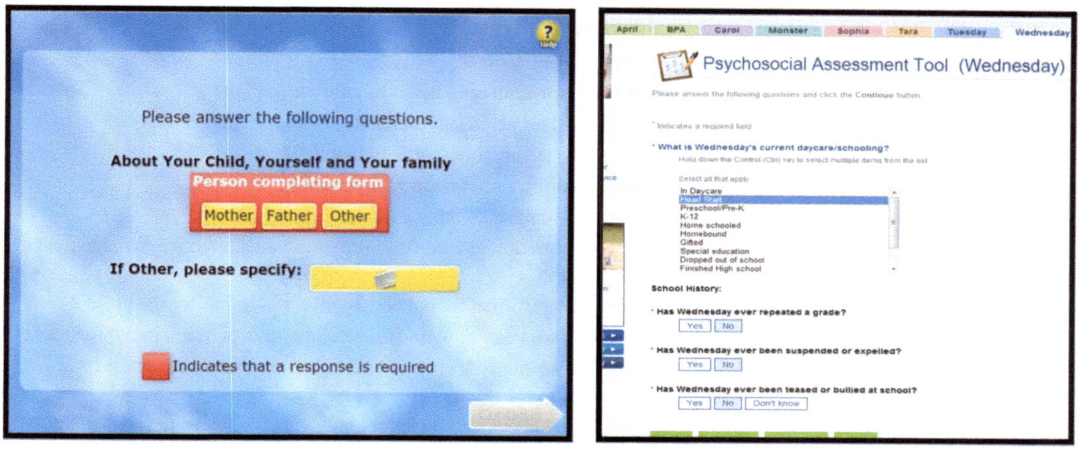

EPIC Template
Cincinnati Children's Hospital Medical Center

Patient Portal/EPIC
www.MyNemours.org

Fig. 4.5 Examples of integration into electronic health records (EPIC) at two hospitals (Reproduced with permission from Cincinnati Children's Hospital Medical Center and Nemours Children's Health System)

paper and pencil, via REDCap on a tablet computer, or using a web-based version. Interfaces with electronic health records (EHRs), specifically (EPIC; www.epic.com) at Nemours Children's Health System and Cincinnati Children's Hospital Medical Center, and in the patient/family portal at Nemours (Fig. 4.5), are available as well.

Across sites and patient groups, the distribution of patients across risk levels for the PPPHM, based on PAT scores, is reassuring in terms of the overall competence of families and also quite consistent across settings and patient populations (Kazak et al. 2015). In general, one-half to two-thirds of samples score in the Universal tier on the PAT, one-quarter to one-third in the Targeted range, and up to 15 % fall in the Clinical tier. This is generally less than anticipated by healthcare providers who fear that screening will identify a large number of previously unidentified families for whom services would have to be provided.

Implementing Psychosocial Risk Screening

Although psychosocial screening is not utilized in a consistent or systematic manner in pediatric cancer treatment programs, there are options for screening that could be implemented. For example, either the DT or the PAT could be used as a brief screener. Or other validated questionnaires could be implemented to assess more specific areas of function. Parent report measures could be augmented by inclusion of a child-report screener. For example, targeted selection of the child-report screeners could minimize the response burden on children undergoing treatment. Given the recognized importance of screening and the availability of approaches and of validated instruments, the barriers to implementation are important to address.

Integrated care rests on successful partnerships with healthcare providers and systems and care delivery models that facilitate treatment outcomes and are acceptable to patients and families. With regard to partnerships, screening is highly congruent with healthcare practice because it is quick and can be incorporated into the flow of clinical care. The brief assessment of a patient's or family's status guides treatment plans and clinical pathways. Our experience has been that physicians and nurses readily appreciate the rationale for screening and will collaborate with psychosocial staff on implementation of brief screening tools. Screening is particularly appealing when results can be readily communicated to multidisciplinary healthcare teams, patients, and families and ideally transmitted into

Table 4.1 Barriers to screening and associated strategies to overcome them

Barriers	Strategies to overcome barriers
Stigma associated with psychosocial care	Assure acceptability of screening items to families
	Make screening standard across all patients
	Provide education on comprehensive patient care
	Document patient/family satisfaction with screening
	Track items that are skipped or other evidence of concern
Need for psychosocial care not recognized	Emphasize how information gained from screening aids effective management of the child's condition
	Show the family how information collected will directly inform the child's care
	Discuss with healthcare team how information can improve care and outcomes
	Address discipline-specific concerns and facilitate coordinated support for screening
Time	Determine actual time necessary for screening
	Integrate screening into routine clinical processes
	Schedule appointments to account for time needed to complete screening
Concern about responding to needs identified	Create algorithms that match specific high-risk items with existing system resources
	Use aggregate screening data to argue for increase in psychosocial services
Impact on processes and work flow	Determine format (e.g., EHR, web) and who administers
	Create alerts for high-risk responses that require immediate action
	Identify who reviews and coordinates response
	Develop approach to provide feedback to family
	Integrate results into EHR
Sustaining screening	After processes are defined, train relevant providers to implement
	Monitor clinical pathways of care from screening to services
	Generate data to show results and further refine approaches
	Consider use of health and behavior codes to bill for screening time

EHR records for healthcare providers to consider as they treat patients and families. An example of how screening results can be communicated is shown in Fig. 4.3. Using the example of the PAT and the PPPHM, the PAT is scored quickly by computer and the overall risk level and specific high-risk responses are conveyed to the team. In this way, clinical pathways at the site can be activated immediately to match areas of risk with evidence-based treatments.

There are barriers to implementing systematic screening (Table 4.1). For example, treatment options can be limited in many, if not most, settings. That is, in many settings qualified clinicians are not perceived as available to provide care and treatment. This is a realistic concern ("should we screen if we do not have good treatment options?"). However, regardless of the size and resources of the treatment setting, problems do exist and algorithms can be created to address specific high-risk items or levels of need so that the healthcare system can predictably manage any increased burden due to issues uncovered by screening. In addition, our experiences with screening have been that fewer problems are actually found than are anticipated. And early identification of problems can facilitate earlier, less intensive, potentially more cost-effective interventions than when problems escalate and are treated later. Importantly as well, screening is a type of patient (family)-reported outcome (PRO) and also consistent with family-centered care in incorporating family input early in the treatment process. In our studies, screening tools have been acceptable to caregivers and therefore may contribute to overall positive patient experiences in healthcare settings (Table 4.2).

Table 4.2 Sample of how screening results can be communicated to treatment teams

PAT
PSYCHOSOCIAL ASSESSMENT TOOL

The family of________completed the PAT on________The items the family endorsed on the PAT are consistent with the following level of psychosocial risk and resource availability.

Overall Psychosocial Risk Level:

☐ **Low Risk:** The family reports many supportive resources and relatively low psychosocial risk (in number or severity). Any at-risk items are listed below. Recommendation: Universal interventions are recommended, including education about psychosocial impact of diagnosis / treatment, focusing on positive coping strategies and support-seeking among family members when needed.

☐ **Moderate Risk:** The family reports some supportive resources but also some psychosocial risk factors, which may impact illness adjustment or treatment adherence. Specific at-risk items are listed below. Recommendation: Further evaluation or close monitoring may be necessary. Targeted interventions are recommended, focusing on specific family problems, parent / child stress reactions, or parent beliefs that can negatively impact adjustment or adherence.

☐ **High Risk:** The family reports few supportive resources and multiple areas of difficulty that may impede illness adjustment or treatment adherence. Specific areas of difficulty are listed below. Recommendation: Clinical interventions, including mental health evaluation and more intensive family-based psychosocial services may be necessary. A team-based approach may be needed to ensure treatment adherence.

Specific areas of risk endorsed by the family: (positively scored items listed)

Family Structure / Family Resources:
Social / Family Support:
Child (Patient) Problems:
Sibling Problems:
Caregiver Problems: A caregiver in the home has experienced:
Caregiver Stress Reactions:
Caregiver beliefs that may impact treatment:
Other Notes:

Screen, Assess, Treat, Test, and Track (SATTT)

Screening is not intended to replace in-depth clinical assessment or treatment. It is the first step in a process of care delivery. A new model of *S*creen, *A*ssess, *T*reat, *T*est, and *T*rack (SATTT) has been proposed. *S*creening is a quick overview to identify families at risk (e.g., using the parent report of the DT or the PAT) and identifies "hot spots" that warrant more detailed evaluation. Therefore, screening must be followed by a more in-depth *A*ssessment/evaluation by appropriate psychosocial staff members, which then leads to implementation of the relevant evidence-based treatment. Using the subscales of the PAT as a guide, Table 4.3 provides examples of assessment topics, questions, and approaches that flow from screening. In each case, the clinician can start from an endorsed high-risk screening item to expand and understand the patient and family concerns while attending to strengths as well as challenges in each area. Standardized instruments may also be used to provide an in-depth detailed assessment. Clinical judgment and, as needed, peer and supervisory support are always

Table 4.3 Guidance for further assessment of positive screening responses

Area of risk	Topics, questions, and approaches
Family structure/family resources	Discuss, in detail, family members, those living in home, and elsewhere and role in caregiving and support
	Appraise any issues related to child custody and support
	Inquire about concrete financial concerns, employment status, transportation, etc.
Social and family support	Discuss who is available to support family throughout illness and treatment course
	Identify coping strategies used by the family
	Explore potential isolation of family or specific family members
Child (patient) problems	Ask about any child behavior items endorsed on screening
	Assess child's developmental status and any concerns
	Consider using a validated measure of child behavior, development, emotional, or social functioning to gather more detailed and normative information
	Anticipate how child and family will cope with treatment-related challenges
	Determine child's school status and identify concerns related to attendance and academic and social functioning
Sibling problems	Cover topics above
	Ask about siblings' knowledge of their brother/sister's illness/treatment and expected reactions
	Identify plans for caregiving for siblings
Caregiver problems	Obtain more information about all high-risk responses
	Consider using validated measures or structured clinical interviews to evaluate mental health concerns in detail
	Evaluate seriousness and need for referral for parents and other family members
Stress reactions	Evaluate symptoms of acute stress/traumatic stress using validated measures
	Normalize reactions and evaluate appropriateness of interventions to reduce distress and provide support
	Monitor stress reactions periodically
Family beliefs	Probe with family members about all high-risk beliefs and identify how beliefs may impact coping and interactions with the treatment team

critical in a comprehensive and accurate assessment process. It is also essential in the screening/assessment process to assure that responses that may be particularly clinically salient are addressed in a prompt and appropriate manner. While any number of items on the PAT, for example, might warrant timely clinical intervention (behavior problems, financial strains, family problems), reports of acute distress or suicidality, for example, require immediate implementation of associated clinical protocols for these concerns.

The outcome of the *T*reatment must be evaluated in a timely manner in order to determine whether to continue, discontinue, or change treatments (Test). And Tracking of psychosocial well-being over time is critical for all families, as risks can change with changes in medical treatment or with other stressors that the family may experience. Ideally, a screener should be appropriate for use at various time points in treatment and also sensitive to change over time. Both the DT and the PAT have been used at different points in care and seem applicable across the course of treatment. With a focus on current distress, the DT provides data that would be expected to reflect current events and identify elevated distress at different time points. The PAT has some subscales which are less likely to change (e.g., family structure) and others where clinically important information may reflect changes over time (e.g., child behavior, parent distress). How often screening should be repeated, which psychosocial risk factors are most associated with ongoing problems, and how screening data could be used to document clinically relevant changes are essential questions to investigate further.

There are important considerations in the refinement of screening instruments and processes for the future. Once screened, the process of SATTT should include collaboration with families. For example, families could be provided with the results of screening and participate collaboratively in subsequent care and treatment plans. The role that the child himself/herself could play in screening is another area worthy of additional consideration. Including the child's perspective is particularly important for child behavior, school issues, and adjustment to illness and treatment. Assuring that screening is responsive to the needs of families from infants through young adults is another important future consideration in screening.

Screening Within Systems of Care

While it is reasonable to think that delivering evidence-based treatments in a timely and focused manner will improve overall patient and family outcomes, this remains an area for future investigation. For example, does screening improve access to appropriate evidence-based care and patient/family satisfaction with the care received? Can we impact quality of life or other outcomes that are important to patients and families?

The PPPHM also raises interesting questions for the design of psychosocial care at a healthcare setting/system level. There is great variability in psychosocial care across medical settings, but concerns about equity in access to care, delivery of optimal interventions, and cost are common across all. Based on the PPPHM, care to families at the tip of the pyramid (Clinical) is the most expensive (e.g., psychiatric consultations, additional demands on nursing staff, physician time, patient care meetings focused on behavioral concerns, one-on-one monitoring of patients, involvement of hospital security or administration, more days in the hospital, and more clinic visits). Care at the Targeted tier is likely less intensive and less expensive and has the potential to be valuable over time, by reducing or preventing difficulties that impact healthcare (e.g., interventions related to pain, adherence to treatment, child behavior). Services at the Universal level are least expensive (e.g., social work, child life, family resources centers and programs, chaplaincy, etc.) but delivered as part of family-centered care and add value by impacting family satisfaction with care received.

The smallest number of patients (Clinical) receives the most intensive and expensive services and the largest number of patients (Universal) receives comparatively less. While clinical families must receive care to address their pressing problems, it is interesting to consider whether this scenario is optimal or whether resources could be distributed more evenly across tiers of the PPPHM and what is the perceived value in doing so. Implementation of screening would suggest that risk and services might be distributed differently, specifically with more allocation to families at the targeted tier.

Risk factors such as socioeconomic status, child difficulties, parental distress, and cultural values and beliefs may contribute to disparities by limiting engagement in care or adherence to treatment (Sato et al. 2013). Many of the areas assessed by the PAT map directly or indirectly on to areas associated with health disparities (Bhatia 2011), such as income, health insurance, knowledge, sociocultural factors, health behaviors, adherence to treatment, and health access. More effective identification of family risks can foster earlier interventions to address factors that may contribute to health disparities.

Although Electronic Health Record (EHR) systems were not designed to support psychosocial care, psychosocial risk screening can be introduced when healthcare team members endorse the concept and if screening modalities are easy to use, integrated with clinical care, and associated with improvements in care delivery. Providing screeners in user-friendly formats reduces some of the demand on the personnel responsible for conducting the screening. Tablet technology may be employed by healthcare systems to facilitate medical and psychosocial screening. And the transmission of data into the EHR has the potential to further simplify screening and facilitate integration of the results into patient records.

The Affordable Care Act mandates screening as part of preventative care without additional costs for patients. The targets for screening as described in the law, while not specifically described as psychosocial risk, include many relevant topics (e.g., developmental and behavioral concerns, obesity https://www.healthcare.gov/what-are-my-preventive-care-benefits/#part=3). We have the opportunity to assure that psychometrically strong, clinically important and family-friendly approaches are used that will not only identify risk, but guide psychosocial intervention in the pediatric oncology population.

Conclusions

Screening is the first step in assuring that the psychosocial risks and resiliencies of all families entering pediatric healthcare systems are detected early in the course of care. When linked to a conceptual model for delivering care, such as the PPPHM, clinical pathways can be developed and tested. Ideally screening is a clinical activity supported by all members of the healthcare team, including the patient and family, and can be completed in a manner that is consistent with family-centered care and appreciative of the variability in resources available across settings.

Clinical Pearls

- Screening is the first step in assuring that the psychosocial risks and resiliencies of all families entering pediatric healthcare systems are detected early in the course of care.
- Screen families early in treatment to identify and initiate interventions linked to specific patient and family risks.
- Facilitate the delivery of care to *all* families (not just those more obviously in need) by screening everyone.
- Put processes in place to complete screening systematically and to assure that results are integrated with relevant clinical information.

Appreciate that, consistent with the PPPHM, screening will necessitate immediate action for a small group of families but will promote more preventative interventions for others.

Acknowledgment The work discussed in this chapter has been supported by the National Cancer Institute (R21CA98039), St. Baldrick's Foundation, the American Cancer Society (RSG-13-015), the Substance Abuse and Mental Health Services Administration (5U79SM061255), and the Nemours Center for Healthcare Delivery Science. The PPPHM and the PAT are copyrighted and cannot be used without permission (for information, contact psychosocialassessmenttool@nemours.org). Correspondence regarding this chapter may be directed to Dr. Kazak (anne.kazak@nemours.org).

References

Achenbach System of Empirically Based Assessment (2015) The ASEBA approach www.aseba.org. Accessed 9 Apr 2015

Alderfer M, Mougianis I, Barakat L et al (2009) Family psychosocial risk, distress and service utilization in pediatric cancer: predictive validity of the Psychosocial Assessment Tool (PAT). Cancer 115:4339–4349

Barrera M, Hancock K, Rokeach A et al (2014) External validity and reliability of the Psychosocial Assessment Tool (PAT) among Canadian parents of children newly

diagnosed with cancer. Pediatr Blood Cancer 61:165–170
Bhatia S (2011) Disparities in cancer outcomes: lessons learned from children with cancer. Pediatr Blood Cancer 56:994–1002
Commission of Cancer (2012) Cancer program standards 2012: ensuring patient-centered care. American College of Surgeons, Chicago
Derogatis L (2000) Brief symptom inventory 18: administration, scoring, and procedures manual. National Computer Systems Inc., Minneapolis
Gilleland J, Reed-Knight B, Brand S et al (2013) Assessment of psychosocial functioning in survivors of pediatric cancer using the PAT2.0. Psychooncology 22:2133–2139
Goldenring J, Rosen D (2004) Getting into adolescent heads: an essential update. Contemp Pediatr 21:64–90
Goodman R (2001) Psychometric properties of the Strengths and Difficulties Questionnaire (SDQ). J Am Acad Child Adolesc Psychiatry 40:1337–1345
Haverman L, van Oers H, Limperg P et al (2013) Development and validation of the Distress Thermometer for parents of a chronically ill child. J Pediatr 163:1140–1146
Haverman L, van Oers H, Limperg P et al (2014) Implementation of electronic patient reported outcomes in pediatric daily clinical practice: the KLIK experience. Clin Prac Pediatr Psychol 2(1):50–67
Institute of Medicine (2007) Cancer care for the whole patient: meeting psychosocial health needs. The National Academies Press, Washington, DC
Karlson CW, Smith ML, Haynes S et al (2013) Risk for psychosocial problems in pediatric cancer: impact on socioeconomics. Child Health Care 42(3):231–247
Kazak A (2006) Pediatric Psychosocial Preventative Health Model (PPPHM): research, practice and collaboration in pediatric family systems medicine. Fam Syst Health 24:381–395
Kazak A, Noll R (2015) The integration of psychology in pediatric oncology research and practice: collaboration to improve care and outcomes. Am Psychol 70:146–158
Kazak A, Brier M, Alderfer M et al (2012) Review: screening for psychosocial risk in pediatric cancer. Pediatr Blood Cancer 59:822–827. PMCID: PMC3396795
Kazak A, Schneider S, DiDonato S et al (2015) Family psychosocial risk screening guided by the Pediatric Preventative Psychosocial Health Model (PPPHM) using the Psychosocial Assessment Tool (PAT). Acta Oncol 54(5):574–580
Kersun LS, Rourke MT, Mickley M et al (2009) Screening for depression and anxiety in adolescent cancer patients. J Pediat Hematol Onc 31(11): 835–839
National Comprehensive Cancer Network (2003) Distress management clinical practice guidelines. J Natl Compr Can Netw 1:344–374
Noll R, Patel SK, Embry L, COG Behavioral Sciences Committee et al (2013) Children's Oncology Group's 2013 blueprint for research: behavioral science. Pediatr Blood Cancer 60:1048–1054
Pai AL, Patino-Fernandez AM, McSherry M et al (2008) The psychosocial assessment tool (PAT2.0): psychometric properties of a screener for psychosocial distress in families of children newly diagnosed with cancer. J Pediatr Psychol 33:50–62
Panganiban-Corales AT, Medina MF (2011) Family resources study: Part 1: Family resources, family function and caregiver strain in childhood cancer. Asia Pac Fam Med 10:14
Patel S, Mullins W, Turk A et al (2011) Distress screening, rater agreement and services in pediatric oncology. Psychooncology 20:1324–1333
Reynolds CR, Kamphaus RW (2004) Manual for the behavior assessment system for children, 2nd edn. AGS Publishing, Circle Pines
Sato A, Kopel S, McQuaid E et al (2013) The home environment and family asthma management among ethnically diverse urban youth with asthma. Fam Syst Health 31:156–170
Selove R, Kroll T, Coppes M et al (2012) Psychosocial services in the first 30 days after diagnosis: results of a web-based survey of Children's Oncology Group (COG) member institutions. Pediatr Blood Cancer 58:435–440
Smilkstein G (1978) The Family APGAR: a proposal for family function test and its use by physicians. J Fam Practice 6(6):1231–1239
Ungar M (2012) The social ecology of resilience: a handbook of theory and practice. Springer, New York
Wiener L, Viola A, Koretski J et al (2015) Pediatric psycho-oncology care: standards, guidelines and consensus reports. Psychooncology 24(2):204–211. doi:10.1002/pon.3589
Yeo M, Sawyer S (2009) Psychosocial assessment for adolescents and young adults with cancer. Cancer Forum 33:18–21
Zadeh S, Wiener L, Pao M et al (2014) The use of a Distress Thermometer in a pediatric outpatient setting: evaluation, validity, acceptability and feasibility. Psychooncology 23(1):52

Coping and Adaptation in Pediatric Cancer: Current Perspectives

5

Mary Jo Kupst and Andrea Farkas Patenaude

Introduction

Ten years ago, we reviewed and summarized the literature on psychosocial aspects of pediatric cancer (Patenaude and Kupst 2005), highlighting the considerable progress made over the previous 30 years, along with the advances in cancer treatment and improved survivorship. We described the transformation in approach from keeping children in the dark about the nature of their disease and their prognosis to what is now basically taken for granted, i.e., more open communication and involvement of children and adolescents in their treatment and decision-making. The family became the unit of care. Results of behavioral studies provided interventions to help children and adolescents with procedural distress and anxiety. With the ability to conduct longitudinal studies, additional information emerged about the potential late effects that survivors faced and the need for more attention to their psychosocial and neurocognitive needs.

M.J. Kupst, PhD (✉)
Department of Pediatrics, Medical College of Wisconsin, Milwaukee, WI, USA
e-mail: mkupst@mcw.edu

A.F. Patenaude, PhD
Department of Psychosocial Oncology and Palliative Care, Dana-Farber Cancer Institute, 450 Brookline Avenue, Boston, MA 02215, USA
e-mail: andrea_patenaude@dfci.harvard.edu

Overall, studies indicated that, despite the intense stresses connected with pediatric diagnosis and treatment, most children, adolescents, and their families were able to cope and adapt adequately. However, a subset of children and families had more severe or lasting problems and required additional psychological help. It also became clear that the success of a coping effort was a complex interaction between the characteristics of the threatening situation, characteristics of the individual, the coping resources, and time; there was no one optimal way of coping in all situations. While disappointing, this realization suggested areas for further research and also clarified the continuing need for well-trained mental health professionals in the clinical setting to help evaluate how family members are coping and to provide sensitive interventions that are appropriate to the person and situation.

Recent work has increased our understanding of patient and family needs and indicated other directions for research and clinical care. Intervention research has progressed but much work remains to establish effective interventions for the full range of problems experienced by the child with cancer and their family members. While other chapters focus more thoroughly on specific psychological issues and interventions, this chapter highlights recent research findings in the area of coping and adaptation to cancer and suggests ways in which they may be clinically useful.

A.N. Abrams et al. (eds.), *Pediatric Psychosocial Oncology: Textbook for Multidisciplinary Care*,
DOI 10.1007/978-3-319-21374-3_5

What Is Coping?

Coping is universal. Life brings all kinds of stresses that must be managed in order to survive, grow, and thrive. Day-to-day living involves coping with numerous stresses and hassles. While there have been many ways to describe coping, perhaps the most comprehensive definition is that of Richard Lazarus, whose theory and research have guided much of the coping field. Coping means "cognitive and behavioral efforts to manage specific external or internal demands (and conflicts between them) that are appraised as taxing or exceeding the resources of the person" (Lazarus and Folkman 1984). Coping is essential when we are faced with a situation or condition that is both potentially stressful and meaningful. Coping is a fluid process that is a transaction between the person and the environment affected by one's age, personality, experiences, and situational demands.

Coping and Cancer

Coping in the context of cancer describes a method of integrating the cancer experience into the existing personality of the patient or family member. This requires acknowledging the threat cancer poses and the demands of cancer treatment while, at the same time, managing emotional reactions and maintaining essential aspects of the child's or family member's identity and role in the family and community.

Every cancer patient and every family member must find ways to cope with the disease, its treatment, and sequelae, each of which presents an unfamiliar set of stressful situations. From the initial difficult diagnosis discussion, to the challenges of survivorship or the heartbreak of a child's death from cancer, coping defines the interaction of the person with the cancer experience. In describing the intense emotional reactions children and families exhibit, Simms et al. (2002) referred to "clinically relevant distress" as distinguished from psychopathology, pointing out the inevitability of distress in the context of a cancer diagnosis. He noted that high-level distress in the context of a high-level threat like cancer represents an appropriate, not a pathological, response. This is true at diagnosis and also at points of potential or actual medical exacerbation, such as entry into stem cell transplantation or relapse. Sensitive experienced clinicians can distinguish appropriate reactions at such a point from reactions indicative of poor coping and unstable emotional status.

Anger is not uncommon at these times, but sometimes it is so intense and unrelenting that it signals deeper problems and requires more attention.

Case Vignette

When Chloe was referred to a new cancer center for a stem cell transplant, her mother, a lone parent, arrived in clinic and initially would not talk to staff or answer their questions. After several attempts by staff to engage her, she became visibly irritated and began pacing, swearing loudly at staff, complaining that they didn't know what they were doing. After admission, her anger did not abate, but continued, with threats of lawsuits if staff were to make any mistakes. At one point, security was called, after which her behavior was less intense. During the hospitalization, Chloe's mother slowly began to trust one nurse and one psychosocial clinician, but mostly to vent her anger about other staff (there were "good" and "bad" staff). The nurse and psychosocial clinician acknowledged her distress, but did not side with her against other staff, and encouraged her to focus more on Chloe and to work with staff to help Chloe through the hospitalization. They suggested that Chloe's mother "teach" the staff about how she helped Chloe at home. This approach helped for brief periods, but she continued to have occasional angry outbursts, though they were more contained. Staff suspected this was a preexisting pattern of behavior that went beyond a distressed response to stem cell transplantation and learned that she had a history of emotional outbursts and confrontations including similar behavior at their home hospital.

As treatment continues, stressful situations continue to present themselves and it is important to understand the specific stressors with which the person must cope, as coping depends on context. We have outlined many of the stressors that children and families have to face throughout and after treatment (Patenaude and Kupst 2011). For example, after diagnosis and in early treatment, parents must try to absorb all of the medical and treatment information they receive in order to make rapid decisions about their child's treatment. At the same time, they seek to support their child, manage their own emotions, and begin to integrate hospital demands with home, work, and family needs. Children must deal with unfamiliar, invasive, and painful procedures, side effects of treatment, and interruptions of school, peer, and social activities. They must often cope with separation from their families and friends and with adjustment to the hospital environment. Even when treatment ends, children and parents must try to balance their happiness and relief that treatment is over with the loss of the support they relied upon from treatment and staff. After so much time focusing on cancer and treatment, it is challenging to reorganize family, work, school, and social lives while maintaining optimism about future health, knowing there is the lurking possibility of recurrence or relapse.

Survivorship can mean the end of cancer, but the need to cope persists as children and parents manage the physical, neurocognitive, and/or psychosocial late effects of treatment. In some cases this involves coping with diminished cognitive functioning and changes in academic and vocational plans. Late effects may require children to cope with general medical and/or psychosocial follow-up, repeated assessments, and ongoing care for posttreatment conditions (see Chap. 15 on Survivorship).

Clinical work with children with cancer makes us aware that, in addition to the burdens and fears associated with the diagnosis of a child with cancer and the treatment and uncertainty which follow, cancer is often not the only major stressor families are experiencing. We detail here several examples of family experiences, which may further burden the coping resources of families where a child has cancer. Some relevant concurrent stressors can be serious illness in a parent themselves or in another family member (see section on the stress of hereditary cancer); chronic illness of a sibling requiring special education or home care; economic problems including work, insurance, and housing; and low levels of social support.

Family and Coping

There is no doubt that the diagnosis of a child with cancer is a life-changing event for everyone in the family. The high demands of treatment and the psychological imperative requiring a parent to be with their child through as much of the cancer experience as possible alter parents' work, home, and social lives. When there are two parents, the child's diagnosis affects their relationship as well as their relationship to their other children. We know that family conflict or lack of cohesion affects the adjustment of children and parents to cancer (Alderfer, et al. 2010; Long and Marsland 2011). Sometimes there is only a single parent or a parent who functions as a lone parent (Brown et al. 2008; Mullins et al. 2011; Wiener et al. 2013). Cancer in a child multiplies what may already be a significant care-taking burden falling on one parent. Early attention to ongoing parental and family problems is essential, given the close intercorrelation between parent and child well-being (Hile et al. 2014).

Family conflict occurs within intact families, but divorced families face special challenges when a child is diagnosed and treated for cancer. The cancer diagnosis in a child upends the familial restructuring which is often achieved only with difficulty after a divorce. Caretaking in the hospital, caring for the other children at home, and making important decisions about their ill child's care under stressful, emotional conditions often lacking in privacy put parents and stepparents into novel, often uncomfortable, juxtaposition. Being in each other's presence may itself be a stressor for divorced parents and disagreements about limit-setting, discipline, indulgence, bedtimes, and handling of the child's response to treatment medications can increase stress on parents, which is often passed on to the children in the family. Clinicians skilled in family psychotherapeutic techniques as well as in understanding the hospital climate and procedures can help strengthen coping approaches and communication between parents and between parents and staff during this difficult time. Please see Chap. 6 on Psychotherapeutic Modalities. Family-based interventions can be particularly helpful in circumstances where family relationships prior to the diagnosis were strained. Physical distance and financial issues can add to parental strain when the child is treated far from the family home. Communication technology such as texting, Skyping, sharing photos over the Internet, e-mailing, and using social media has reduced the sense of isolation experienced by both the hospitalized child and the family remaining at home.

Case Vignette

Sophie, an almost 16-year-old with osteosarcoma, was hospitalized far from home for surgery. Due to an extended hospital stay, she was going to miss her 16th birthday at home with family and friends. Her mother decorated her hospital room and brought presents and cake, but this was hardly the celebration Sophie had anticipated. Unknown to Sophie, however, her mother also had arranged two Skype video calls. One was with her father and brothers at home who had decorated the house and had a cake with candles and presents for Sophie. The other was with her friends who sang "Happy Birthday" and promised Sophie a better in-person party when she returned home. The friends also posted Instagram birthday wishes and promised to keep her updated with social happenings at school through Facebook.

Cultural Considerations

We sometimes assume homogeneity of values, meaning, and desires in patients and parents of children with cancer, but with increased diversity in our populations, it is very important to recognize and assess families for their particular views and practices related to their cultural, national, or ethnic origins. There are considerable differences in the ways people cope with cancer in different cultures. Expectations vary in how parents and their child should behave in the medical setting and what they expect from medical caregivers, especially about how and how much to tell a child about his/her disease and treatment (Gray et al. 2014). Adjustment to the hospital may be especially stressful for families who come from a distant country for the child's treatment or when the family has migrated to a new country, but are not well acculturated to their new land. Language limitations, unfamiliarity with the physical environment in and outside of the hospital, cultural disorientation, difficulty preparing familiar food for the child and other family members, and higher costs add to the family stress. Problem-solving interventions for international cancer patients who may spend prolonged periods of time in an unfamiliar cultural setting are valuable in helping them accommodate to the alterations in their environment. It should be noted albeit to a lesser extent that all families experience challenges in these areas, as the hospital environment is an unfamiliar and daunting world, demanding adaptability on the part of all whose lives become centered there. Reducing some of these practical barriers is important, but it does not treat the sadness and fear that diagnosis of cancer in a child evokes in all family members. Therapeutic support sensitive to a family's cultural perspectives should be offered to the fullest extent possible to reduce distress.

Hereditary Cancers

Hereditary cancers add additional layers of stress to the family experience. Multiple family members may concurrently be treated for cancer, are cancer survivors, or have experienced the loss of an unusual number of relatives from cancer. Identification of a cancer-predisposing mutation that affects a child's risk of developing cancer raises concern about the mutation status of the ill child's siblings. It also increases the pressures placed on parents to communicate these risks to their own siblings, cousins, parents, and other blood relatives so that other at-risk family members can have genetic testing. For those found to be mutation carriers, preventive actions or targeted screening can be undertaken to detect cancers at the earliest and most treatable point. Family communication about family history and other related matters about risk can be very difficult and add significantly to the burdens on parents. Communication between parents and children about hereditary risk has been identified by parents in high-risk cancer families as an area they find unfamiliar and one in which they would welcome help from professionals (O'Neill et al. 2015).

Relapse

Relapse or recurrence challenges the "new normal" in which families evolve in the wake of the diagnosis of a child with cancer. It reduces hope for survival and brings back fears about treatment and its effects on all aspects of the family's life. It demands a higher level of coping, not just with the personal and logistical organization required, but with the maintenance of hope in light of reduced odds for survival. It may challenge spiritual beliefs and can lead parents to question whether other doctors or hospitals might have more effective treatments. Patients, parents, siblings, and grandparents (Wakefield et al. 2014) all need support at such a juncture to help them find the strength to continue to function and to cope with what can be, at times, overwhelming fear and sometimes anger, irritation, and depression.

Coping Style and Strategies

The way people cope and the effectiveness of their coping strategies determine how well they adapt to the series of stressful situations that are part of cancer diagnosis, treatment, and survivorship. Knowing a person's typical coping style can help a clinician select optimal ways to approach children and families. Some people prefer to have a great deal of information ("monitors"), while for others a large amount of detailed information can increase anxiety ("blunters") (Miller 1995). For those who prefer the monitoring style, seeking and receiving information is a way of coping that helps them to adapt to the situation through perceived control. For those who have a blunting style, presenting an overview followed by several small increments of information may reduce anxiety. Similarly, it is often assumed that talking with others helps people cope with stress, and for some people this is true. However, others may prefer to be alone in order to process their thoughts and manage their emotions before talking with others. Knowing which way people typically cope can help in providing effective interventions. This information can also be usefully shared with the medical team to help guide their interactions with the patient and family.

It used to be that a "defensive" style was considered negative, but more recent work has tempered that belief somewhat (Phipps et al. 2006; Harper et al. 2014). In several studies, children and adolescents with cancer showed lower levels of anxiety and reported fewer psychological problems than children in the general population or those with other medical conditions. A possible explanation offered was that such reports represented denial or repression. However, a "repressive adaptational" style (Phipps et al. 2001) is not necessarily problematic and can be adaptive, especially early in the cancer experience when the volume of emotionally upsetting information received can approach unbearable levels. Finding a good fit between style or disposition to cope and the demands of the situation can enable the clinician to help improve patient or parent coping and/or to offer reassurance that the approach will not prove detrimental. Past research has helped us define successful adaptation to cancer as coping which allows the child to tolerate bad news and unpleasant treatment and to express appropriate emotions, yet to remain in reasonable interpersonal connection with others in the hospital or home setting and to continue to experience themselves as whole and cared for. For parents, coping means being able to understand the realities and implications of the medical information about diagnosis and treatment, to regulate strong emotional reactions and maintain equilibrium, and to do what is necessary to participate in care of the child and attend to other responsibilities.

The stress and coping framework suggests that when a person is presented with a stressful situation, they must determine if it represents a significant threat or stressor. If it does, the next question they need (often unconsciously) to ask is, "Can I change or affect it in some way?" This second question involves the potential use of a range of different coping strategies. Several schools of thought (see reviews by Aldridge and Roesch 2007; Skinner and Zimmer-Gembeck 2007) suggest that, in cases where something can be changed, an active, problem-focused coping "approach" can be most helpful. These would be efforts such as seeking information, problem-solving, or confronting the stressor. For a child with cancer who is going to miss school for treatment, it may mean getting information about alternative ways to keep current with schoolwork and peers. In cases where the stressor cannot be changed and the reality that cancer will mean stopping an activity such as sports may require emotion-focused coping strategies such as cognitive reappraisal or acceptance. When a situation is not changeable, a person can change how he or she thinks and feels about it and can utilize stress management techniques such as distraction, relaxation, etc., to manage the situation (see reviews by Compas et al. 2012; Vrijmoet-Wiersma et al. 2008). It is, however, always important to acknowledge that people may use many different strategies over time or even in response to the same stressor. There is no 1:1 algorithm that a particular stressor will always necessitate the use of a particular coping strategy, but rather that the circumstance and the person define the optimal approach. The solid research published in recent years by Bruce Compas and colleagues offers promise to better understand individual use of strategies in various situations, as well as development of interventions to teach or enhance coping (Compas et al. 2014).

An example of differences in coping is the way childhood cancer survivors deal with ongoing cancer activities. Some survivors become actively involved in volunteer efforts, such as camps for children with cancer, survivorship groups, fund raising for cancer-related causes, and mentoring newly diagnosed patients. It is not uncommon for survivors to pursue careers in nursing, medicine, social work, psychology, or child life and some express their desire to help others with cancer as they were helped. Others however consider their cancer experience "ancient history" as one young man put it, and they focus more on "getting on with the rest of my life." This isn't denial or repression. He freely spoke about having had cancer and his treatment, including late effects, and has kept in touch with staff and patients he met during his treatment, but his focus has shifted away from cancer. Both are ways of coping and demonstrate that individual approaches can be equally adaptive.

In our earlier review (Patenaude and Kupst 2005), we reported that many studies found most children and parents adapted remarkably well despite the intense stresses of cancer diagnosis and treatment but also that some (estimates of 20–30 %) exhibited significant or unremitting distress. More recent research supports this view, showing that a similar minority has serious problems at some time during the cancer experience (Long and Marsland 2011; Compas et al. 2012). For this group, many of the forms of intervention described in other chapters of this volume may be particularly helpful (see Chaps. 6, 8 and 9).

Developmental Aspects of Coping

As physical, cognitive, and emotional development emerges, so do ways of coping (see review by Kupst and Bingen 2006). Infants exhibit stress reactions, such as withdrawal from hurtful stimuli and stress responses, such as crying to elicit parental help. Toddlers and young children begin to show voluntary efforts and ways to better regulate their emotional reactions, including fantasy, play, and distraction. As childhood progresses, children begin to increase their ability to use voluntary control and cognitive ways of coping such as cognitive reappraisal and problem-solving. Older children and adolescents can use more cognitive strategies in problem-solving in controllable situations. They can use emotion-focused coping in uncontrollable situations, as their ability to have a future perspective increases. With maturation, coping becomes more multidimensional, complex, and flexible.

Even very young children of 3 or 4 years, however, can be helped to cope through distraction, fantasy, and play (Linn et al. 1986). Interventions with younger children are more likely to be around emotional regulation. Many of the diagnoses of childhood cancer occur when children are under 8 years of age (Bjork et al 2006). Approaches which help young children acclimate to the hospital environment, sometimes provided by activities of therapists and sometimes by mental health staff, can be very useful in containing the anxiety, fear, and sense of isolation which many children experience at diagnosis and early in their cancer treatment. Consistency of compassionate care from nursing and medical staff can also contribute to calming children in the hospital. Fantasy play including puppets (Linn 2008) in the hands of well-trained professionals can help children express the worries that are common at this stage, which can help suggest directions for further discussion and/or intervention. Surprisingly, there is relatively little published about the most ubiquitous intervention offered to children with cancer and their family members, psychotherapy or psychotherapeutic consultation. There is some European work emerging to delineate the functions of play therapy in the life of the child with cancer (Pitillas 2014).

As school and peer relationships are crucial for school-age children, where possible, continuation of schoolwork should be fostered through ongoing communication with teachers and educators, sometimes including visual connections to the classroom via the Internet and return to school as early as possible. Contact with peers should be maintained in person, if possible, or if not, children can keep in touch through notes, phone calls, the Internet, or Skype. School-age children can benefit from interactions with other children with cancer (if they and parents desire it), as well as a combination of child psychotherapy and play activities. Similarly, adolescents benefit from academic and peer support, as well as environments and activities appropriate to their developmental level, including web-based resources and psychotherapy for relevant stresses. If they were actively involved in sports or extracurricular activities such as music or theater, they should be encouraged to continue their participation even if it is limited by treatment or disease impact.

Other Variables Related to Coping with Cancer

Factors found to be related to coping include time since diagnosis, duration of treatment, late effects resulting from diagnoses and treatment involving the CNS, previous functioning and family functioning, and socioeconomic resources. Coping and adjustment are, of course, also closely connected (Patenaude and Kupst 2005). Later work has also noted the role of early psychological functioning, past traumatic events, family functioning, and emotional resources (Rodriguez et al. 2012; Vrijmoet-Wiersma, et al. 2008).

Time since diagnosis has been recognized as an important factor, with reductions in distress typically, but not always, occurring with additional time to cope and to adjust to the routines of a changed reality. Those who were able to cope early in the cancer experience tended to cope more effectively throughout the experience. Studies have supported that coping and psychological functioning early in treatment are predictive of later functioning (Aldridge and Roesch 2007; Klassen et al. 2011). This is why it is especially important to see children and families soon after diagnosis to assess how they are coping and to determine a strategy to help them adapt.

Assessment

The need for early and repeated assessment of the coping and adjustment of children and families affected by pediatric cancer has been increasingly recognized as the basis of good clinical care over the challenging period of treatment, in the years of survivorship, in the circumstance of recurrence, and at the end of life (Wiener et al. 2015). Measures developed in the 1980s and 1990s continue to be widely utilized in assessment of actual coping behavior (Patenaude and Kupst 2015) and newer measures have been developed. Some common coping measures include the Ways of Coping Questionnaire (Folkman and Lazarus 1988) for adolescents and adults, the Kidcope (Spirito et al. 1988) for children over 7 years of age and adolescents, and the Responses to Stress Questionnaire (Connor-Smith et al. 2000) for adolescents. More generally, measurement development in recent years has focused on the development of new tools to assess psychological functioning of children with cancer and their families. Established and promising new measures of psychosocial outcomes including adjustment, distress, anxiety, and depression can be used to assess the efficacy of coping as well.

Until recently, attempts to assess psychological outcomes in children with cancer involved lengthy batteries of neurocognitive and psychosocial tests. While these are reliable and valid tests in common use in clinical psychology, they also are labor-intensive, take hours to administer and score, and are costly. The Children's Oncology Group Behavioral Sciences Committee developed a relatively brief screening battery. The Neuropsychological, Social, Emotional, and Behavioral Outcomes in Children with Cancer (ALTE07C1) (Embry et al. 2012), a battery of standardized neurocognitive and psychosocial measures, is currently for use in a clinical research context, but is increasingly seen as having clinical value as a first step to determine which children with cancer are in need of additional cognitive or psychological assessment and intervention.

PROMIS and NIH Toolbox Resources

There are many traditional measures of psychosocial functioning that continue to be used in pediatric cancer. Recently, two large-scale projects, the Patient Reported Outcomes Measurement Information System (PROMIS) and the NIH Toolbox for Neurological and Behavioral Function, have developed brief measures of psychological functioning, including stress and coping, that can be used across the life span (including measures for children and parent proxy (Forrest et al. JPP 2012; Salsman et al. 2013; Kupst et al. 2015), have good psychometric properties, and are free of charge. They are largely intended for use in clinical research but can be valuable measures for psychologists and other trained clinicians as well. The Psychosocial Assessment Tool (PAT) has sparked international research to assess the value and limitations of its predictive utility for child, parent, and family functioning (Kazak et al. 2011). See Chap. 4, Assessment, for more details about the PAT. Initial use of the PAT provides a standardized measure of psychosocial risk and can help clinicians to determine the level, intensity, and nature of psychosocial intervention that is particularly needed immediately following a child's cancer diagnosis. This can be especially valuable in clinical settings with limited resources. The PAT is a useful adjunct to, but not, however, a replacement for a diagnostic interview with the child and his/her parents near the point of diagnosis, during which the initial steps toward relationship building can take root. An important part of that clinical interview is a determination of the nature and success of past coping strategies and assessment of the most pressing current issues affecting the family members. For example, a recent study showed that shortly after diagnosis, it was the role disturbances, not concern about the medical treatment, which were most upsetting to children with cancer (Rodriguez et al. 2012). Children especially needed help coping with their inability to go to school, play sports, or have typical peer interactions, as these losses were the most upsetting aspects of the early treatment experience.

The diagnosis and treatment of cancer can be particularly difficult for children and adolescents who have been actively involved in sports. Physical activity is often their primary and most effective way to cope with stress.

Case Vignette

Justin, a 12-year-old boy who was a star pitcher for his baseball team was diagnosed with ALL. He became quite depressed when he was told he would not be able to play baseball for the season. When questioned, Justin said that missing games and feeling like he was letting his team down made him more upset than having cancer. He was also worried that he would *never* be able to play again. Additionally, his involvement in sports had helped him deal with family stresses. Recognizing the important role baseball had been playing in Justin's life, his psychosocial provider and medical team found a way for him to remain connected to his team that was medically feasible. Justin spoke with his coach who reassured him he had a place on the team and made him a "player-coach." His coach videotaped practices and games and asked Justin for input on team members' performances. His coach also gave him a medically approved workout routine to help him keep in shape and reminded him of his ultimate return to the lineup. After induction therapy, Justin was able to attend home games and sat on the bench continuing in his role as a "player-coach." The following spring he was able to return to playing with his team.

Justin was fortunate. In some cases, especially those involving permanent loss of limb or function, children are not able to continue in sports which have sustained them in the past. After amputation or other "career-stopping" surgeries, they must develop other ways to deal with stress and may need help from psychosocial clinicians to find new activities that can be rewarding or stress reducing. Some choose an alternative type of physical activity, while others may turn to music, writing, making videos, increased concentration on school or work, or developing new social groups. The social support from other patients is often helpful because others who have gone through similar situations can discuss what they did to cope with these significant losses.

Trauma and Resilience in Pediatric Cancer

There are currently several models to explain the psychological impact of pediatric cancer. One model views the experience of cancer as a trauma, where children and families are at risk for posttraumatic stress responses. Research has been done to assess whether children and parents have posttraumatic stress disorder (Bruce 2006). While most do not meet diagnostic criteria for the disorder, some could be said to have posttraumatic stress symptoms (PTSS). However, the prevalence of PTSS was relatively low in children undergoing cancer treatment and only moderately higher in parents and survivors (Alderfer et al. 2010). Data from these studies indicated that, even with significant trauma, most did not have PTSD or PTSS and, in fact, many experienced posttraumatic growth (Picoraro et al. 2014).

What has emerged is a model that shows that many children and families are resilient, in spite of the frightening, sometimes overwhelming traumatic situations they experience in the context of the child's diagnosis and treatment for pediatric cancer and in spite of intense distress they experience in responses to these situations, (see reviews by Noll and Kupst 2007; Phipps et al. 2014; Wechsler and Sanchez-Iglesias 2013; Harper et al. 2014). Haase's (2014) Resilience in illness model stresses the importance of coping as a protective factor and this research has provided the basis for interventions to promote coping and resilience.

Interventions: Helping Children and Families Cope with Cancer

Coping is often viewed, if effective, as a way to achieve better adjustment or adaptation. The questions of (a) "What, in particular, is most important to cope with at a particular time in treatment?" and (b) "What are the available personal and environmental resources?" must be answered to determine what the most effective intervention will be. In most cases, multiple levels of intervention are needed over time, as the stressors are typically environmental, physical, and psychosocial. Unfortunately many different factors can influence an individual child's or parent's response to an intervention, so even with knowledge of a problem area, knowledge of particular individual or family strengths or weaknesses (Scholten et al. 2015), and access to an established intervention, the desired relief is not always achieved. Cultural, educational, cognitive, attentional, and physical factors can complicate the utility of a particular intervention at a point in treatment or afterward and can sometimes be barriers to the success of the intervention. The expertise and experience of mental health clinicians are often called upon to view the composite family situation and to assess the strengths of the family members as well as to understand the particular stressors of the clinic or ward environment in relation to the current coping of the child and close relatives.

While they may not be designated as "coping" interventions per se, a number of interventions have been designed to help optimize coping for members of families of children with cancer. For example, cognitive-behavioral therapy (CBT) has been found to be effective in reducing anxiety and distress, and most current interventions include some components of CBT. See Chap. 6 on Psychotherapeutic modalities for details. Problem-solving skills training (Sahler et al. 2005) has been found to be helpful in teaching mothers of children with cancer how to reduce negative emotions and anxiety, using the role of active, problem-focused coping. Similarly, helping parents develop coping strategies, such as acceptance and cognitive reappraisal, can be helpful in dealing with uncontrollable aspects of the cancer experience (Rodriguez et al. 2012). Other interventions have involved attempts to help parents cope with their child's cancer diagnosis, (Kazak et al. 2007; Mullins, et al. 2012), as well as completion of treatment (Wakefield, et al. 2011). In addition, there are several approaches to help terminally ill adolescent patients cope with fears and make end of life plans (Zadeh et al. 2014) and help parents and families with reactions to bereavement (Donovan et al. 2015).

Technology promises to make longitudinal assessment of children's coping and quality of life easier in coming decades. A study in the Netherlands showed that a program of home-based, electronic child self-report of quality of life in which data is provided before clinic visits to the medical providers resulted in greater discussion of psychosocial topics within the patient visit (Engelen et al. 2012). Such interventions may especially help more reticent children share information with providers; may remove the burden from either patient, provider, or parent to ensure psychosocial factors well-being is discussed (a necessary preliminary to intervention); and can actually save physician time.

Summary

Coping represents a universal phenomenon which all parents and patients engage in when a child is diagnosed with and treated for cancer. We continue to learn more about coping and to enhance our theoretical understanding about the ways in which personal, medical, and environmental factors affect coping and, subsequently, affect the success of interventions to improve psychosocial outcomes and reduce distress. The skill of psychosocial clinicians continues to be essential in assessing coping strategies in individual patients and families. This clinical expertise is also important in the selection and administration of effective interventions that take into account relevant factors exerting major influences on coping in the child's and family's experience.

Clinical Pearls

- The diagnosis of a child with cancer is a life-changing event for everyone in the family; it may not be the only major stressor families are experiencing.
- Successful adaptation to cancer involves coping which allows the child to tolerate bad news and unpleasant treatment and to express appropriate emotions while remaining in reasonable interpersonal connection with others in the hospital or home setting and continuing to experience themselves as whole and cared for.
- For parents, coping means being able to understand the realities and implications of the medical information about diagnosis and treatment they have been given, to regulate strong emotional reactions and maintain equilibrium and to do what is necessary to participate in the care of the child and to attend to other essential responsibilities.
- A clinical diagnostic interview early in treatment can determine the nature and success of past coping strategies and assessment of the most pressing issues currently affecting the family.
- The skill of psychosocial clinicians is essential in observing coping strategies in individual patients and families and in selecting and administering effective developmentally and culturally appropriate interventions.

References

Alderfer MA, Long KA, Lown A, Marsland AL, Ostrowski NL, Hock JM, Ewing LJ (2010) Psychological adjustment of siblings of children with cancer: a systematic review. Psychooncology 19:789–805

Aldridge AA, Roesch SC (2007) Coping and adjustment in children with cancer: a meta-analytic study. J Behav Med 30:115–129

Bjork M, Nordstrom B, Hallstrom I (2006) Needs of young children with cancer during their initial hospitalization: an observational study. J Pediatr Oncol Nurs 23:210–219

Brown RT, Wiener L, Kupst MJ, Brennan T, Behrman R, Compas BE, David Elkin T, Fairclough DL, Friebert S, Katz E, Kazak AE, Madan-Swain A, Mansfield N, Mullins LL, Noll R, Patenaude AF, Phipps S, Sahler OJ, Sourkes B, Zeltzer L (2008) Single parents of children with chronic illness: an understudied phenomenon. J Pediatr Psychol 33:408–421

Bruce M (2006) A systematic and conceptual review of posttraumatic stress in childhood cancer survivors and their parents. Clin Psychol Rev 26:233–256

Compas BE, Jaser SS, Dunn MJ, Rodriguez EM (2012) Coping with chronic illness in childhood and adolescence. Annu Rev Clin Psychol 8:455–480

Compas BE, Desjardins L, Vannatta K, Young-Saleme TY, Rodriguez EM, Dunn M, Bemis H, Snyder S, Gerhardt CA (2014) Children and adolescents coping with cancer: self- and parent report of coping and anxiety/depression. Health Psychol 33:853–861

Connor-Smith JK, Compas BE, Wadsworth ME, Thomsen AH, Saltzman H (2000) Responses to stress in adolescence: measurement of coping and involuntary responses to stress. J Consult Clin Psychol 68:976–992

Donovan LA, Wakefield CE, Russell V, Cohn RJ (2015) Hospital-based bereavement services following the death of a child: a mixed study review. Palliat Med 29:193–210

Embry L, Annett RD, Kunin-Batson A, Patel SK, Sands S, Reaman G, Noll RB (2012) Implementation of multi-site neurocognitive assessments within a pediatric cooperative group: can it be done? Pediatr Blood Cancer 59:536–539

Engelen V, van Zweiten M, Koopman H, Detmar S, Caron H, Egeler M, Kaspers GJ, Grootenhuis M (2012) The influence of patient reported outcomes on the discussion of psychosocial issues in children with cancer. Pediatr Blood Cancer 59:161–166

Folkman S, Lazarus RS (1988) Ways of coping questionnaire. Consulting Psychologists Presss, Palo Alto

Forrest CB, Bevans KB, Tucker C, Riley AW, Ravens-Sieberer U, Gardner W, Pajer K (2012) The patient-reported outcomes measurement system (PROMIS©) for children and youth: application to pediatric psychology. J Pediatr Psychol 37:614–621

Gray WN, Szulczewski LJ, Reagan SMP, Williams JA, Pai AH (2014) Cultural influences in pediatric cancer: from diagnosis through care/end of life. J Pediatr Oncol Nurs 31:252–271

Haase JE, Kintern EK, Monhan PO, Robb SL (2014) The resilience in illness model, part 1: an exploratory evaluation in adolescents and young adults with cancer. Cancer Nurs 34:E1–E12

Harper FWK, Goodlett BD, Trentacosta CJ, Albrecht TL, Taub JW, Phipps S, Penner LA (2014) Temperment, personality, and quality of life in pediatric cancer patients. J Pediatr Psychol 39:459–468

Hile S, Erickson SJ, Agee B, Annett RD (2014) Parental stress predicts functional outcome in pediatric cancer survivors. Psychooncology 23:1157–1164

Kazak AE, Rourke MT, Alderfer MA, Pai A, Reilly AF, Meadows AT (2007) Evidence-based assessment, intervention and psychosocial care in pediatric oncology: a blueprint for comprehensive services across treatment. J Pediatr Psychol 32:1099–1110

Kazak AE, Barakat LP, Ditaranto S, Biros D, Hwang WT, Beele D, Kersun L, Alderfer MA, Mougianis I, Hocking MC, Reilly A (2011) Screening for psychosocial risk at pediatric cancer diagnosis: the psychosocial assessment tool. J Pediatr Hematol Oncol 33:289–294

Klassen AF, Anthony SJ, Khan A, Sung IL, Klassen R (2011) Identifying determinants of quality of life of children with cancer and childhood cancer survivors: a systematic review. Support Care Cancer 19:1275–1287

Kupst MJ, Bingen K (2006) Stress and coping in the pediatric cancer experience. In: Brown RT (ed) Comprehensive handbook of childhood cancer and sickle cell disease: a biopsychosocial approach. Oxford University Press, New York, pp 35–52

Kupst MJ, Butt Z, Stoney C, Salsman J, Griffith J, Folkman S, Cella D (2015) Assessment of stress and self-efficacy for the NIH toolbox for neurological and behavioral functioning. Anxiety Stress Coping 23: 531–544

Lazarus RS, Folkman S (1984) Stress, appraisal and coping. Springer, New York

Linn S (2008) The case for make-believe: saving play in a commercialized world. The New Press, New York

Linn S, Beardslee W, Patenaude AF (1986) Puppet therapy with pediatric bone marrow transplant patients. J Pediatr Psychol 11:37–46

Long KA, Marsland AL (2011) Family adjustment to childhood cancer: a systematic review. Clin Child Fam Psychol Rev 14:57–88

Miller SM (1995) Monitoring versus blunting styles of coping with cancer influence the information patients want and need about their disease. Implications for cancer screening and management. Cancer 76:167–177

Mullins LL, Wolfe-Christensen C, Chaney JM, Elkin TD, Wiener L, Hullmann SE, Fedele DA, Junghans A (2011) The relationship between single-parent status and parenting capacities in mothers of youth with chronic health conditions: the mediating role of income. J Pediatr Psychol 36:249–257

Mullins LL, Fedele DA, Chaffin M, Hullman SE, Kenny C, Eddington AR, Phipps S, McNall-Knapp RY (2012) A clinic-based inter-disciplinary intervention for mothers of children newly diagnosed with cancer. J Pediatr Psychol 37:1104–1115

Noll RB, Kupst MJ (2007) Commentary: the psychological impact of pediatric cancer hardiness, the exception or the rule? J Pediatr Psychol 32:1089–1098

O'Neill SC, Mays D, Patenaude AF, Garber JE, DeMarco TA, Peshkin BN, Schneider KA, Tercyak KP (2015) Women's concerns about the emotional impact of awareness of heritable breast cancer risk and its implications for their children. J Community Genet 6:55–62

Patenaude AF, Kupst MJ (2005) Psychosocial functioning in pediatric cancer. J Pediatr Psychol 30:9–27

Patenaude AF, Kupst MJ (2011) Coping in pediatric cancer. In: Wiener L, Pao M, Kazak AE, Kupst MJ, Patenaude AF, Holland JC (eds) Quick reference for pediatric oncology clinicians: psychiatric and psychological dimensions of pediatric cancer symptom management. APOS Press, Charlottesville

Patenaude AF, Kupst MJ (2015) Coping in pediatric cancer. In: Wiener L, Pao M, Kazak AE, Kupst MJ, Patenaude AF, Arceci R (eds) Quick reference for pediatric oncology clinicans: psychiatric and psychological dimensions of pediatric cancer symptom management, 2nd edn. Oxford Press, New York

Phipps S, Steele RG, Hall K, Leigh L (2001) Repressive adaptation in children with cancer: a replication and extension. Health Psychol 20:445–451

Phipps S, Larsen L, Long A, Rai SN (2006) Adaptive style and symptoms of posttraumatic stress in children with cancer and their parents. J Pediatr Psychol 31:296–309

Phipps S, Klosky J, Long A, Hudson MM, Huang Q, Zhang H, Noll RB (2014) Posttraumatic stress and psychological growth in children with cancer: has the traumatic impact of cancer been overestimated? J Clin Oncol 32:641–646

Picoraro JA, Womer JW, Kazak AE, Feudtner C (2014) Post-traumatic growth in parents and pediatric patients. J Palliat Med 17:209–218

Pitillas C (2014) A theoretical model involving four different uses of play therapy within Pediatric Psycho-Oncology. Paper presented at the International Psycho-Oncology Society Annual Meeting, Lisbon, 22 Oct 2014

Rodriguez EM, Dunn M, Zuckerman T, Vannatta K, Gerhardt CA, Compas BE (2012) Cancer-related sources of stress for children with cancer and their parents. J Pediatr Psychol 37:185–197

Sahler OJ, Fairclough DL, Phipps S, Mulhern R, Dolgin MJ, Noll RB, Katz ER, Varni JW, Copeland DR, Butler RW (2005) Using problem-solving skills training to reduce negative affectivity in mothers of children with newly diagnosed cancer: report of a multisite randomized trial. J Consult Clin Psychol 73:272–283

Salsman JM, Butt Z, Pilkonis PA, Cyranowski JM, Zill N, Hendrie HC, Kupst MJ, Kelly MA, Bode RK, Choi SW, Lai JS, Griffith JW, Stoney CM, Brouwers P, Knox SS, Cella D (2013) Emotion assessment using the NIH toolbox. Neurology 80:S76–S86

Scholten L, Willemen AM, Napoleone E, Maurice-Stam H, Last BF, van Dijk-Lokkart EM, Zandbelt N, Ensink E, Grootenhuis MA, Schuengel C (2015) Moderators of the efficacy of a psychosocial group intervention for children with chronic illness and their parents. J Pediatr Psychol 40:214–227

Simms S, Kazak AE, Golomb V, Goldwein J, Bunin N (2002) Cognitive, behavioral, and social outcome in survivors of childhood stem cell transplantation. J Pediatr Hematol Oncol 2:115–119

Skinner EA, Zimmer-Gembeck MJ (2007) The development of coping. Annu Rev Psychol 58:119–144

Spirito A, Stark LJ, Williams C (1988) Development of a brief checklist to assess coping in pediatric patients. J Pediatr Psychol 13:555–574

Vrijmoet-Wiersma CMJ, van Klink JMM, Kolk AM, Koopman HM, Ball LM, Egeler M (2008) Assessment of parental psychological stress in pediatric cancer: a review. J Pediatr Psychol 33:694–706

Wakefield CE, McLoone JK, Bulow P, Lenthen K, Cohn RJ (2011) Parental adjustment to the completion of their child's cancer treatment. Pediatr Blood Cancer 56:524–531

Wakefield CE, Drew D, Ellis SJ, Doolan EL, McLoone JK, Cohn RJ (2014) Grandparents of children with cancer: a controlled study of distress support and barriers to care. Psychooncology 23(8):855–861

Wechsler AM, Sanchez-Iglesias I (2013) Psychological assessment of children with cancer as compared with healthy children: a meta-analysis. Eur J Cancer Care (Engl) 22:314–325

Wiener L, Pao M, Battles H, Zadeh S, Patenaude AF, Madan-Swain A, Friebert S, Elkin D, Kupst MJ (2013) Socio-environmental factors associated with lone parenting of chronically ill children. Child Health Care 42:264.280

Wiener L, Viola A, Koretski J, Perper ED, Patenaude AF (2015) Pediatric psycho-oncology care: standards, guidelines and consensus reports. Psychooncology 24:204–211

Zadeh S, Pao M, Wiener L (2014) Opening end-of-life discussions: how to introduce voicing my CHOiCES™, an advance care planning guide for adolescents and young adults. Palliat Support Care 13:1–9

6 Psychotherapeutic Modalities for Children with Cancer and Their Families

Larry L. Mullins, Alayna P. Tackett, and Kristina I. Suorsa

Introduction

Monumental changes have taken place in the field of pediatric cancer in the past three to four decades (Brown 2006) through dramatically improved and innovative treatments and improved survival rates with a greater focus on long-term survivorship and quality of life. Increasingly, efforts have been extended to better understand the short- and long-term adjustment of children with cancer and their families and, consequently, the means by which this adjustment may be facilitated by psychosocial interventions. With this in mind, the goal of this chapter is to highlight current psychotherapeutic modalities utilized in the treatment of youth with cancer and their families, including those with empirical support as well as those that are considered promising or have demonstrated support with other populations experiencing similar difficulties (e.g., heightened stress, depression, anxiety). Our focus will be on practical applications, with the goal of this chapter being a resource for clinicians working with children with cancer and their families. Although this chapter will be arranged by specific therapeutic modalities, it should be taken into account that some of the work reviewed will describe interventions that are by design multimodal and multifaceted in nature. For an overview of the modalities described in this chapter, potential target symptoms and populations, and challenges to implementation, see Table 6.1.

L.L. Mullins, PhD (✉) • A.P. Tackett, MS
K.I. Suorsa, MS
Department of Psychology,
Oklahoma State University,
116 N. Murray Stillwater,
Stillwater, OK 74078, USA
e-mail: Larry.Mullins@okstate.edu; alayna.tackett@okstate.edu; suorsa@okstate.edu

Individual Therapy for Adolescents and Parents

Although we know very little about the actual practice patterns of clinicians in pediatric cancer centers, it is safe to say that individual psychotherapy broadly defined (e.g., supportive, nondirective, or eclectic) is a commonly delivered treatment modality for both parents as well as adolescents. This individual therapy probably takes many forms, depending upon the unique presentation of each individual, but it most often takes the form of crisis intervention (especially in the days and weeks following the initial diagnosis) or supportive psychotherapy, also referred to as Rogerian client-centered therapy (Rogers 1959). Key considerations in providing individual therapy would include (1) the development of a strong therapeutic alliance with the parent and adolescent and the establishment of trust; (2) "normalization" of the symptoms, fears, and

A.N. Abrams et al. (eds.), *Pediatric Psychosocial Oncology: Textbook for Multidisciplinary Care*,
DOI 10.1007/978-3-319-21374-3_6

Table 6.1 Therapeutic approaches

	Key aspects	Symptom focus	Population	Challenges[a]
Traditional individual therapy	Tailored to individual needs, psychoeducation, crisis intervention, supportive psychotherapy, normalization of symptoms, and coping strategies	Premorbid psychiatric condition or adjustment difficulties	Adolescents and parents	Adolescent resistance/ reluctance to participate. Multitude of modalities exist – previous experiences may influence interest to participate/seek services
Family and marital therapy cognitive behavioral therapies (CBT)	Tailored to family needs and may include medical family therapy, supportive care, family crisis intervention psychoeducation, encouraging expression of emotion, identifying automatic thoughts, thought logging, behavioral activation, relaxation strategies, and assertiveness and communication skills	Family conflict, family role relationships, marital conflict Maladaptive thoughts, feelings, and behaviors	Families and couples Children, parents, siblings	Resistance to discussing family problems and marital conflict. May require additional visits to clinicians Developmental level can be a barrier to engaging in the cognitive aspects of CBT, possible cultural and language barriers
Problem-solving therapy	Provide strategies to engage in effective problem-solving	Difficulties in making decisions and challenged in problem-solving	Parents and families	Best paired within a multimodal approach, difficult to implement just PST
Structured parent and family interventions	Psychoeducation, enhancing communication skills, problem-solving skills, Adversity-Belief-Consequence framework, self-talk, and reframing child's diagnosis and related concerns	Parent adjustment, coping, stress, and general psychological functioning	Parents and families	Scheduling sessions with families due to more time-consuming nature of treatment interventions
Play therapy	Play activities	Emotional difficulties	Younger children and siblings	Obtaining parent involvement and limited empirically supported evidence for efficacy of treatment
Art therapy	Drawing	Emotional difficulties and communication	Children and siblings	Obtaining parent involvement and limited empirically supported evidence for efficacy of treatment
Social skills training	Psychoeducation, modeling, and practice	Social skills	Children	Frequently provided as a group intervention which can be difficult to provide in more rural settings

Table 6.1 (continued)

	Key aspects	Symptom focus	Population	Challenges[a]
Adherence to medical regimens	Psychoeducation, assess and overcome adherence barriers, and monitoring regimen	Nonadherence to medical regimen	Children, adolescents, young adults, caregivers	Monitoring adherence can be difficult due to the high cost of the devices. Some families have a difficult time navigating the use of these devices. Frequency of clinic appointments may limit opportunity to get blood assay levels and/or electronic downloaded of the adherence data device. Barriers to care (e.g., costs, transportation, access to care/information) can limit caregivers' ability to provide the appropriate resources for children/adolescents
Health promotion interventions	Psychoeducation, behavioral plans, problem-solving, assessing barriers, and coping skills	Health-risk behaviors (e.g., dietary choices, smoking cessation, and patient knowledge surrounding illness information)	Children and parents	Unwillingness to engage in behavior change and limited knowledge regarding the importance of certain health behaviors
Bibliotherapy	Psychoeducation, self-management, and coping skills	Anxiety related to procedures and treatments, uncertainty of cancer diagnosis and symptoms, and coping with distress	Children, parents, and siblings	May potentially confuse the patient or parent if material is too complex or arouses additional anxiety
Acceptance and commitment therapy	Engaging in acceptance, cognitive diffusion, being in the present moment, viewing the self as context, identifying and working towards the individuals' values, and committing actions	Psychological flexibility, acceptance of symptoms and diagnosis	Children and parents	Limited training opportunities and limited research support within pediatric cancer[b]
Mindfulness	Psychoeducation, focusing awareness, meditation, and nonjudgment	Anxiety and rumination	Children and parents	Ensuring mindfulness activities are age-appropriate and limited research support within pediatric cancer[b]

(continued)

Table 6.1 (continued)

	Key aspects	Symptom focus	Population	Challenges[a]
Trauma-focused cognitive behavioral therapy	Psychoeducation, relaxation strategies, development of trauma narrative, repeated exposure to trauma narrative, and identifying and challenging maladaptive thoughts	Relieving PTSS related to cancer-specific procedures	Children and siblings	Limited research support within pediatric cancer[b]

PTSS posttraumatic stress symptoms

Note

[a]Common concerns across all treatment modalities include developing a therapeutic alliance with children and families, completing homework, and overcoming barriers to treatment

[b]As these emerging therapies become more prominent in the extant literature, it is likely that additional challenges specific to these treatment modalities will be identified and suggestions for management provided

concerns that characterize the cancer experience; (3) provision of resources and assessing the specific needs for the family, such as support groups, liaisons to other parents who are further past the initial diagnosis and who are in a good position to provide valuable insights; and (4) provision of coping strategies for dealing with negative emotions and the crisis at hand.

Many parents and adolescents diagnosed with cancer are individuals who could best be characterized as, "psychologically healthy" prior to the child's diagnosis. For these individuals, the diagnosis is a major stressor to which, with time and appropriate support as described throughout this chapter, they will adjust. However, it is sometimes the case that a parent or adolescent presents with a challenging premorbid psychiatric condition. A small but significant subset of parents and adolescents will evidence a serious mental health problem that comes to the attention of the treatment team at some point after the diagnosis. These psychological difficulties can range from serious problems with drug and alcohol dependence to major mental illness such as bipolar disorder or obsessive-compulsive disorder. In each of these situations, the clinician must be prepared to either provide direct individual therapy services to the individual or refer to another mental health professional that can provide appropriate services.

Not surprisingly, in working with adolescents with cancer, a number of other unique challenges emerge in providing traditional individual therapy. Establishing trust is essential in developing a therapeutic relationship and can be quite challenging with adolescents. In adolescents, the "typical themes" of the desire for increased independence and autonomy, the importance of peer relationships, and the emotional upheaval that can become magnified at the time of diagnosis and throughout the course of treatment usually emerge. The many physical changes that may occur including hair loss, fatigue, weight changes, and cushingoid facies can also contribute to increased distress and sense of "being different." While some adolescents report that their friends lavish them with support, others find that they become estranged from their old friends. With these issues in mind, it is essential that clinicians do a careful, thorough assessment of the concerns of each adolescent and develop an appropriate treatment plan that addresses these issues.

Family and Marital Therapy Approaches

In the context of pediatric cancer, it is clear that the need often exists for supportive, crisis-oriented interventions to help the family as a whole or to help parents with issues in their marriage. This is particularly true in light of the many role changes and challenges to cohesiveness that can occur within the family system. Family and marital therapy interventions can often prove helpful in these situations and can help restore homeostasis and reduce stress and conflict (see Chap. 9 for additional information on families of youth with cancer).

Family and marital therapy interventions of this type tend to be flexible and often do not necessarily follow an explicit protocol or manual. McDaniel and colleagues (McDaniel et al. 2002; Ruddy and McDaniel 2013) have written extensively about this approach, referring to it as medical family therapy (MFT). Using a biopsychosocial systems perspective (i.e., there are no psychosocial problems without biological features, and there are no biomedical problems without psychosocial features), MFT is designed to engage the patient and family and to actively collaborate between the family and the interdisciplinary team (Tyndall et al. 2012). In an effort to help families attenuate distress, the fundamental goals for this therapy are as follows:

1. Help the family identify which aspects of the disease are controllable.
2. Work to help families find sources of social support and avoid isolation. In this manner, the therapist attempts to encourage the family to not let the illness dominate their lives.
3. Help the family set new routines while continuing to meet the needs of others in the family, such as siblings.
4. Help the family to manage communication about the illness, particularly as it concerns balancing the amount of information given to the child about their illness and insuring that secrets about the disease are not being kept.
5. Help the family actively collaborate with the multidisciplinary team.

Specific to marriage, the stress of pediatric cancer clearly has the potential to take a toll, particularly if a marriage was fragile prior to the diagnosis. Financial pressures, time spent apart due to hospitalizations, changing role relationships, and disrupted family routines can result in a loss of closeness and intimacy as well as direct conflict. In some case, couples may seek help directly from the existing support team. Other couples may be reluctant, however, to bring up marital concerns with the medical team, and therefore, it is important for personnel to be able to refer to marriage and family therapists in the community who are mindful of the themes that parents of youth with cancer face.

Traditional family therapy and marital therapy approaches clearly have a role in the context of pediatric cancer. MFT has been widely discussed in the health psychology literature and has been utilized extensively. Unfortunately, there are few studies that have evaluated its effectiveness in the context of pediatric chronic illness, specifically cancer, or adaptations that focus specifically on marriage and support for parents. Campbell (2003) has suggested that forms of MFT indeed have potential benefits for youth with cancer, asthma, cystic fibrosis, and cardiac disease. MFT and adaptations thereof that involve systemic interventions should continue to be evaluated as frontline interventions for families of youth with cancer.

Cognitive Behavioral Approaches

Cognitive behavioral therapies (CBT) constitute a family of therapeutic interventions that have been applied to a wide variety of presenting problems with both adult and child populations. The fundamental basis or premise for the majority of CBT approaches is that cognitive factors, including cognitive schemas, belief systems, cognitive distortions, and dysfunctional or maladaptive beliefs, serve to predispose and or maintain various types of psychological distress. It is argued that targeting and altering these maladaptive cognitions or beliefs can alleviate distress. CBT also includes some interventions that may appear less "cognitive" and more behavioral, including behavioral activation (Kanter et al. 2010) and exposure techniques. CBT approaches have been applied to depressive disorders, anxiety disorders, general distress, sleep disorders, and somatoform disorders, among many others in literally hundreds of studies, and the evidence base for the efficacy of these interventions is considerable. CBT has targeted distress associated with medical conditions in adults and children, as well as in pediatric cancer populations.

In the 1990s, Hoekstra-Weebers et al. published one of the first studies examining CBT in parents of children newly diagnosed with cancer (Hoekstra-Weebers, et al. 1998). Cognitive behavioral strategies employed in the study included the encouragement of emotional expression, identification of distorted automatic thoughts, use of problem-focused coping skills, discussion of psychosocial impact on the family, and training in assertiveness and communication skills. Importantly, the intervention was tailored to meet the expressed needs of the parents and also took into account the developmental level of their child. Compared to standard care (which did include provision of psychosocial services from a social worker), few differences in outcomes were found. This may have been a function of the overall lack of intensity of the intervention or lengthy time periods between intervention sessions. Importantly, it may have also been the result of high-quality services delivered to the standard care group. However, it did appear that the intervention was both feasible and acceptable to the families and set the stage for future structured/semistructured psychosocial interventions.

Streisand and colleagues (2000) also piloted a brief (one 90-min session) stress management intervention using cognitive behavioral techniques with a small sample of parents of children undergoing bone marrow transplant (Streisand et al. 2000). This intervention included an educational component, the teaching of relaxation skills, and communication skills, augmented by handouts that reviewed the components of the program as well as a tape player and headset for them to practice their relaxation skills. Although no differences were found between the treatment and control group, the results did indicate that parents in the intervention group successfully learned and subsequently employed these strategies in their efforts to manage stress.

More recently, efforts have been made to pilot and test the potential effectiveness of CBT in conjunction with other therapies. Seitz and colleagues (2014) developed an Internet-based intervention called "Onco-STEP" for cancer survivors who are off treatment (Seitz et al. 2014). Based in part on Pennebaker's expressive writing disclosure task, this intervention consists of 10 writing sessions that involve standard text messages and instructions. "Onco-STEP" includes two essential treatment modules, one of which involves helping the individual reprocess traumatic experiences associated with their cancer experience and the second module focusing on developing coping skills for dealing with remaining fears related to their cancer. Although this was only a single arm study, the authors did find significant decreases in self-reported anxiety, posttraumatic symptoms, depressive symptoms, and fears of relapse. Notwithstanding the small sample size and control group, this work demonstrates the promise of CBT interventions delivered through electronic means and certainly warrants replication (see Chap. 20 eHealth).

Importantly, children undergoing treatment for cancer and survivors of childhood cancer have been identified as being particularly at risk for anxiety and somatic concerns. The Coping Cat is a well-established manualized cognitive behavioral treatment that assists children ages 10–17 years in (Kendall 1994; Kendall 2000; Kendall et al. 2005):

1. Identifying feelings and physical reactions to anxiety
2. Understanding and restructuring maladaptive cognitions and beliefs surrounding anxiety-provoking situations
3. Learning to develop a coping plan for situations and determining the most effective coping actions
4. Learning how to evaluate and alter coping strategies as needed

Techniques presented to children throughout each training session include modeling real-life situations, role-playing, relaxation training, and contingent reinforcement. In addition, therapists use social reinforcement to encourage and reward the child, who is then encouraged to verbally reinforce their own successful coping. The Coping Cat is comprised of 16 sessions; the first eight sessions are training sessions in which each of the basic concepts is introduced individually and then practiced and reinforced (Kendall 1994; Kendall 2000). During the second set of eight sessions, the child practices the new skills in both imaginary and real-life situations varying from low stress/low anxiety to high stress/high anxiety situations, depending on their needs (Kendall 1994; Kendall 2000). Although there are currently no published studies available in the literature using the Coping Cat specifically with pediatric cancer patients, the strong empirical support for this approach in reducing anxiety in youth would argue for its use, particularly with youth who are experiencing significant symptoms of anxiety.

Similar to the strategies of the Coping Cat, a program targeting coping with cancer featuring a stuffed toy named "Cellie" was developed by psychologists at The Children's Hospital of Philadelphia for children aged 6–12 years (Marsac et al. 2012). The Coping Kit includes "Cellie," cancer coping cards, and a book for caregivers. The cancer Coping Cards, found hidden inside "Cellie's" zippered mouth, provide children with strategies to deal with numerous cancer-related stressors, ranging from medical procedures and hospital visits to feelings of anxiety, distress, and uncertainty (Marsac et al. 2012). The "Cellie Cancer Coping Kit" is flexible and can be used in a number of settings including the home, clinic, and/or hospital (see http://www.chop.edu/health-resources/cellie-cancer-coping-kit-prezi#; Marsac et al. 2012). "Cellie" can also help families begin discussions surrounding difficult topics including care, treatment decisions, and managing hospital stays via the deck of Coping Cards. Once a problem has been identified, the child or caregiver finds the relevant Coping Card and takes the card(s) along wherever they go by placing and zipping them into "Cellie's" mouth. In addition to providing support, "Cellie" also comes with a caregiver book that offers advice for dealing with common cancer-related challenges caregivers often face, such as caring for siblings and working with the medical team (Marsac et al. 2012). The acceptability and efficacy of "Cellie" has been examined in families who have a child diagnosed with cancer, and all parents reported that Cellie was an engaging, helpful, and easy-to-use coping tool they would recommend to other parents of children with cancer (Marsac et al. 2012). Children reported using the "Cellie" Kit for multiple reasons, including it being a playtime activity as well as a way to express difficult topics surrounding their treatment and care.

Another unique intervention that employs a cognitive element is the game "Shop Talk" (Wiener et al. 2011). "ShopTalk" is a therapeutic game with versions in Spanish and English, designed for children ages 7–16 diagnosed with cancer. It also can be used with children and youth who have been diagnosed with other types of serious medical illness (Wiener et al. 2011). "ShopTalk" can be used in individual or group therapy sessions to assist in starting conversations about difficult emotional issues related to the child or adolescent's medical illness and the impact their illness has in various situations (e.g., school, home, peer relations). During the game, "ShopTalk" players visit ten different "shops" around the board, choosing one of six "gifts" from each store to place in their individual shopping bag when they choose to answer the question. One example of a "shop" that is visited during the game is a pet store called "Unconditional Love," that provides a series of questions pertaining to aspects of the child's life that are accepting, supportive, and helpful in addition to assessing for fears of rejection and/or abandonment. Another shop visited during game play is a sports store called "Balls in Your Court," which provides a series of questions examining different social scenarios that can occur throughout the course of treatment and then specific ways to handle these situations. "ShopTalk" is an effective tool in identifying a multitude of psychological adjustment issues, such as family relationships, sadness, peer relationships, and self-esteem (Wiener et al. 2011). Two additional versions of "ShopTalk" are now available. A sibling version can be obtained through (http://www.alexslemonade.org/campaign/supersibs) and a version for children whose parents have cancer is available through the National Cancer Institute (http://pediatrics.cancer.gov/scientific_programs/psychosocial/educational.asp)

Cognitive behavioral interventions have become a mainstay treatment for many psychological disorders, including the distress associated with a diagnosis of pediatric cancer. Although studies evaluating the impact of CBT have not always shown significant improvement in symptoms above and beyond standard care, it is worth noting that there have actually been very few studies that have attempted to deliver CBT as a standalone, intensive intervention. The existing studies involved very brief interventions and used personnel with limited training in use of these techniques. Indeed, it may also be that these studies included a significant number of individuals who evidenced relatively low levels of depression and anxiety, both of which are traditional targets of CBT interventions. Thus, CBT may be best suited for individuals with higher levels of distress.

As will be seen later in this chapter, some clinicians have integrated CBT techniques with other modalities (e.g., family therapy, communication training) and have witnessed stronger findings. Indeed, a strength of CBT is the ease in which it can be integrated into other psychotherapeutic approaches (e.g., family therapy, mindfulness training, acceptance and commitment therapy), as well as its strong empirical underpinnings. For more information on CBT and its implementation, see *Cognitive Behavior Therapy: Core Principles for Practice* (O'Donohue and Fisher 2012), *General Principles and Empirically Supported Techniques of Cognitive Behavior Therapy* (O'Donohue and Fisher 2009), as well as *The Case Formulation Approach to Cognitive Behavior Therapy: Guides to Individualized Evidence Based Treatment* by Jacqueline Persons (Persons 2012).

Case Vignette

Paul, a 16-year-old adolescent with non-Hodgkin Lymphoma, approached a physician's assistant (PA) during a regular clinic visit 3 months after his diagnosis and asked if he could get a prescription for his "nerves." After asking a few follow-up questions about his specific complaints and history, the PA referred him to the mental health clinician for additional assessment and possible treatment. Apparently, Paul had experienced a number of significant stressors in the year prior to his diagnosis, including the loss of his grandmother from breast cancer, feelings of separation from his friends, and anxiety surrounding his performance in school. To Paul, his diagnosis was "the last straw." He reported increased sadness and irritability, avoidance of activities that typically brought him pleasure, significant weight gain, and sleep problems. He agreed with the clinician to try short-term cognitive behavior therapy to address what appeared to be a major depressive disorder. The counselor began by having Paul self-monitor his mood and thoughts via the 3-column technique (situation-thought-feeling relationships) as a means of identifying his cognitive beliefs and schemas. Over the first few sessions, it appeared that he was harboring rather significant negative beliefs related to his self-worth ("I am useless unless I am valedictorian," "I am a loser now because I don't have as many friends as I had before I got sick") as well as to his future ("bad things are going to continue to pile up in my life and I'll never get past them"). Paul's counselor helped him to begin to understand how his cognitions and beliefs contributed to his depressed mood, and slowly he was asked to assess the validity of these beliefs though Socratic questioning. Cognitive coping strategies were shared with Paul such that he could address his cognitive distortions on his own ("what evidence do I have that other bad things are actually going to happen or that I can't cope with them?"). In addition, Paul was asked to increase the frequency of his activities, particularly those activities that he had previously enjoyed. Over the course of 10–12 sessions, Paul reported decreasing depressive symptoms and improvement in mood.

Problem-Solving Therapy

Problem-solving therapy (PST), a well-established model of intervention, has considerable empirical support for a wide range of psychosocial issues. Originally, this therapeutic modality was developed to help clients solve "real-life" problems and was not necessarily targeted at psychopathology per se. Problem-solving therapy involves teaching the client a very broad, general strategy that is designed to address any given problem situation and involves the following steps: (1) teach the patient to identify and clearly define the problem, (2) establish all available strategies that will address or solve the problem, (3) evaluate the specific pros and cons of each possible solution to the problem, (4) select a solution and take action, (5) evaluate the effectiveness of that action, and (6) determine whether another option or course of action is needed in order to effectively solve the problem (Nezu et al. 2013) (Table 6.2).

Problem-solving therapy has received considerable attention as an effective treatment for parents of youth with pediatric cancer. In a programmatic series of studies, Sahler and colleagues (2002, 2005) and Varni and colleagues (1999) evaluated the effectiveness of PST with mothers of children newly diagnosed with cancer. The problem-solving intervention utilized was called "Bright IDEAS." The term "bright" was meant to convey a sense of optimism to the parents as they approached the problem-solving process. The acronym *IDEA* refers to:

1. *I*dentify the problem.
2. *D*etermine the options available.
3. *E*valuate the options and choose the best possible solution.
4. *A*ct on the solution.
5. *S*ee if the solution worked, thus mirroring the problem-solving process outlined above.

Eight one hour therapy sessions were conducted in either the clinic or hospital setting, so that parents need not travel back to the hospital for additional meeting times. Parent worksheets facilitated the problem-solving process, and homework tasks were included as part of the intervention to help parents continue to practice problem-solving skills outside of the clinic and hospital setting.

Table 6.2 Example steps in problem-solving therapy

1. Identify and clearly define the problem	"I have no childcare options for my healthy child when I have to take my child with cancer to the clinic for their outpatient visits"
2. Establish all available strategies that will address or solve the problem	"Check with the social worker at the hospital to see what options might be available at the hospital itself" "Look in the yellow pages for affordable childcare options" "Check with my friends at church to see who might be available"
3. Evaluate the specific pros and cons of each possible solution to the problem	"Checking with the social worker would be easy and I would know very quickly if there are such services. But my child would be with folks they don't know well" "The yellow pages would have lots and lots of options, but I'd have to call around, investigate their safety, and it would be expensive" "Checking with the church would be easy and affordable, and my child would be with someone they know. Having someone who can be flexible in their schedule is the biggest challenge"
4. Select a solution and take action	"I think I'm going to call the church and see if they can help. I'm going to call tomorrow"
5. Evaluate the effectiveness of that action,	"The church has agreed that they are going to send out an immediate message to all members and have assured me that they will identify a group of individuals who can watch my child in my home on the days that I have to go to the hospital"
6. Determine whether another option or course of action is needed in order to effectively solve the problem	"No other solution is necessary. A list of members was established and volunteers were scheduled to help for the next 4 clinic visits"

Importantly, this study found considerable support for its efficacy in reducing what has been referred to as "negative affectivity" (e.g., anxiety, depression, and posttraumatic stress symptoms) as well as improvement in overall problem-solving skills. Additionally, this intervention was particularly effective for younger, single mothers, as well as for Hispanic mothers. PST has also been incorporated into other multimodal treatments in the context of pediatric cancer. Sahler et al. (2013) later compared the "Bright IDEAS" problem-solving intervention to a more active treatment (nondirective supportive therapy) and concluded that PST is not only effective in reducing symptoms of distress but also in eliciting improvements that continue over time. These positive long-term changes are most likely due to the acquisition of active coping skills.

Problem-solving therapy appears to have great promise in the pediatric cancer setting. Such an approach is very easily taught to both older children and parents, is cost-effective in terms of the number of sessions needed to teach these skills, can be delivered in virtually any setting by a number of modalities (e.g., outpatient clinic, hospital room, by phone or Skype), and is acceptable to diverse populations (Nezu et al. 2013). PST is also a strategy that can be readily incorporated with other cognitive behavioral intervention tools. Law et al. (2014) recently concluded in their meta-analysis that PST is one of the few interventions with considerable demonstrated research support as an effective treatment for parents of children with a medical condition. An excellent resource for clinicians on problem-solving therapy is "Problem-Solving Therapy: A Treatment Manual" by Arthur and Christine Nezu et al. (2013).

Structured Parent and Family Interventions

In light of the fact that cancer affects the entire family, structured interventions have been developed to broaden the focus of psychological support to encompass the parent and the family system of the child with a diagnosis of cancer. These interventions are structured to provide education and psychological skills, which are typically provided within a CBT framework.

Mullins and colleagues (2012) developed an interdisciplinary intervention to provide support for mothers of children with newly diagnosed pediatric cancer (i.e., within 6–12 weeks following the initial diagnosis), which was tested as part of a randomized controlled trial. This intervention focused on illness uncertainty as a mechanism for reducing parental stress. Six modules were developed as part of the standardized intervention, including (1) understanding the nature of uncertainty in the context of pediatric cancer, (2) enhancing communication with medical staff, (3) training in cognitive coping skills (i.e., CBT), (4) problem-solving training, (5) learning how to garner social support, and (6) consolidating all of these skills (Mullins et al. 2012). Sessions were led in clinic by a psychologist, followed by a nurse interventionist contacting mothers by phone to provide additional support and reinforcement related to each module topic. The intervention was designed to allow mothers to meet with the psychologist on odd weeks and receive follow-up care from the nurse interventionist on even weeks.

Mothers reported high levels of satisfaction with the overall protocol and with each individual intervention session. For all measures of distress, consistent significant effects or trends in favor of the intervention were found. Such results suggest that the intervention can reduce maternal psychological distress, posttraumatic stress symptoms, and burden. It was also interesting to note that several mothers in the treatment as usual group showed *worsening* scores over time, a pattern not observed in mothers in the intervention group. One possible interpretation is that the intervention served a preventive or buffering function for those mothers who were at risk for worsening symptoms over time.

Other structured parent and family interventions have similarly been developed. "The Surviving Cancer Competently: An Intervention Program (SCCIP)" was a pilot study designed by Kazak and colleagues (1999). SCCIP is a 1-day, 4-session intervention that incorporates both

CBT strategies and family therapy in order to reduce symptoms of distress and posttraumatic stress. During the intervention, families meet all together and in four separate groups. These four groups include (1) the child with the cancer diagnosis, (2) siblings, (3) mothers, and (4) fathers. Families received psychoeducation, practiced self-talk and reframing, and discussed beliefs about cancer.

The SCCIP study was later adapted to the Surviving Cancer Competently Intervention Program – Newly Diagnosed (SCCIP-ND; Kazak et al. 2005). This protocol was developed for caregivers of newly diagnosed cancer patients. This specific intervention consists of 3-sessions lasting 45 min each conducted during the first month after the child's cancer diagnosis. During Session 1, the goal is to develop a collaborative relationship with caregivers and introduce an A-B-C framework for identifying concerns about cancer-related difficulties or concerns and examining thoughts, feelings, behaviors, and relationships. Session 2 provides psychoeducation, modeling, and practice for caregivers to change their maladaptive thoughts in order to produce different behaviors. Specifically, these cognitive strategies examine the relationship between thoughts or beliefs and behaviors that result in negative consequences for the family. Caregivers are given tools to be able to identify maladaptive thoughts and then identify new beliefs that address: (1) accepting events related to their child's illness that cannot be controlled, (2) turning their attention on events that can be controlled, (3) bringing their attention and efforts towards utilizing and maximizing their strengths, and (4) focusing on positives. The third session is aimed at encouraging caregivers to nurture the growth of their family beyond the cancer diagnosis. Tools the psychologist provided in order to accomplish this included "The Family Survival Roadmap" and "Putting Cancer in Its Place." The Family Survival Roadmap is a visual map that caregivers utilize to plan a course of action for themselves and their family as they maneuver through the cancer diagnosis and plan for resuming a more typical course in light of the uncertainty their child's illness may cause. Putting Cancer in Its Place helps caregivers to incorporate their child's cancer diagnosis into the family structure while also providing boundaries so the diagnosis does not take over all aspects of family life. Studies suggest that the SCCIP-ND is both useful to families and that caregivers in the intervention group show reduced posttraumatic stress. Importantly, the Intervention Manual for SCCIP-ND is available at https://www.healthcaretoolbox.org/images/pdf/sccipnd_info.pdf.

Case Study Tracy, a 25-year-old single mom, requested psychological services through the Pediatric Hematology/Oncology Clinic in order to help her cope with her daughter Melissa's new diagnosis of leukemia. During the initial session, which was conducted in clinic following Melissa's appointment to see her physician, Tracy and the clinical psychologist, Dr. Smith, first discussed Tracy's concerns and goals for therapy. Tracy reported that she felt completely overwhelmed by Melissa's diagnosis; had stopped going to work because she was so nervous about Melissa's care, even though Tracy's mother typically watched Melissa during the day while she went to work; and was not sleeping well. Tracy completed several measures to assess her current mood, including the Beck Depression Inventory and the Beck Anxiety Inventory, the results of which placed her in the moderate range of clinical depression and anxiety. Tracy indicated that she would like to gain skills to better manage her stress surrounding Melissa's leukemia diagnosis and treatment.

The following week, Tracy again saw Dr. Smith after Melissa's appointment in the Pediatric Hematology/Oncology Clinic. During this session, Dr. Smith provided psychoeducation about the Adversity-Belief-Consequence (A-B-C) framework to identify concerns about Melissa's cancer diagnosis and examine the impact of subsequent thoughts, feelings, behaviors, and relationships, as in:

1. *A*dversity: Tracy identified Melissa's leukemia diagnosis as a significant *A*dversity for her and worrying about Melissa's health had taken over most of her thoughts.

2. *B*elief: Tracy was also able to identify the *B*elief that if she was not there to care for Melissa, something bad would happen and Melissa would likely get sicker.
3. *C*onsequence: As a *C*onsequence, Tracy had not gone to work in 3 weeks; she was spending most of her time worrying about Melissa and was sleeping only 3 to 5 hours per night. Dr. Smith and Tracy worked together to reframe Tracy's concerns related to her daughter's diagnosis. For example, Tracy was able to change her belief that her going to work would affect Melissa's health in light of the fact that her mother was a wonderful caregiver and completely competent to take care of Melissa during the day.

The following week, Tracy indicated that she had started back to work, beginning with a 2-day trial. Due to this success, Tracy felt she could continue to attend work on more regular basis. Tracy also stated that she thought therapy had been helpful but no longer needed services. Dr. Smith reiterated the importance of the A-B-C framework and encouraged Tracy to follow-up with her if she needed support in the future.

Play Therapy with Children

Play therapy as a modality for treating children's emotional difficulties has been in existence for almost a century, with reports of its use going back to the early 1900s. Play therapy was specifically designed for younger children whose capacity for abstract thought has yet to be developed. In this regard, play is utilized as a substitute for verbal expression; it is argued that through their play activities, children can express negative emotions, achieve conflict resolution, and ultimately a resolution of symptoms and psychological distress. Many forms of play therapy exist including filial, patient-centered, ecosystemic, prescriptive, and sand therapy. A thorough review of all of these modalities is beyond the scope of this chapter (see Bratton and colleagues 2005 for an excellent overview and meta-analysis of play therapy outcomes). Although not formally studied, it is safe to say that play therapy can be utilized for children with cancer, particularly those whose capacity for verbal expression and learning of coping skills may be limited.

Although there has been some debate about the effectiveness of play therapy in general, Bratton et al.'s (2005) results suggest that play therapy can result in positive and significant outcomes, particularly if parents are involved in the play therapy training. Philips (2010) argues that some of the best evidence for play therapy comes from work with children with health conditions, including those who are facing needle sticks and medical procedures.

In the medical setting, play therapy has been utilized to ease children's fears and help them adjust to stressful and challenging situations. Providing puzzles, pictures, or other fun activities can help children ease into a therapeutic atmosphere. These approaches can be combined with other modalities (e.g., relaxation training, cognitive coping strategies) to facilitate child adjustment.

Art Therapy with Children

For many years, art therapy has been used consistently with children who experience both acute and chronic medical conditions (Prager 1995), such as pediatric cancer (Coucil 1993; Sourkes 1991). Specifically, art therapy is the use of drawing to allow an individual to communicate about or explore a particular situation they are experiencing. Having a child with a pediatric cancer diagnosis engage in art therapy allows them to express their feelings related to their illness and treatments. Additionally, it can be useful in developing a therapeutic alliance and sense of support for the child. This practice has been linked to improvements in the patient's sense of self and quality of life (Madden et al. 2010). Sourkes (1991) used structured art therapy techniques with pediatric cancer patients and their siblings in order to facilitate the expression of emotions. Techniques used included (1) mandalas, (2) the change-in-family drawing, and (3) and scariest drawing. While the child is engaged in drawing, the therapist asks specific questions related to the subject of the drawing. In examining the mandala of a 12-year-old boy, Sourkes stated that "a black triangle indicates endlessness, a yellow one has gratefulness for being alive, pink for hating the feeling of having no control, and mauve for invasion of his privacy which is part of hospital life" (Chester 1998 p. 1). Art therapy with pediatric cancer patients can be used in both individual and group settings. Additionally, this technique can be used in conjunction with other treatments, such as cognitive behavioral therapy.

Social Support Groups

Support groups have a long history in the context of pediatric cancer as well as other health conditions, including those developed for the child with cancer, parents, and siblings. Support groups are based on the fundamental principle that social support buffers the impact of highly stressful life events, for which there is considerable scientific evidence. The setting for scheduling support groups is flexible, but typically they take place in the hospital, clinics, in the community setting, or online. While some are highly structured and consist of a series of informative lectures about coping with cancer followed by open discussion, others are much less formal and primarily revolve around allowing members to voice their individual concerns with facilitation from a group leader. Some support groups are led by trained professionals with a mental health background, while others are led by parents or survivors or a combination of both.

In an effort to evaluate the needs of adolescent cancer survivors, Cassano and colleagues (2008) described a number of themes that emerged for youth who were involved in a support group. The importance of being able to speak to other youth with the same experience, share inspirational messages, and have fun as a normal teenager were common threads of conversation. Other topics that have been the focus of discussion in teen support groups include the responses of healthy peers to the diagnosis of cancer, reintegration into school, dealing with medical staff, improving communication between teenagers and parents, inclusion in medical decision-making, and positive communication between the physician and the teenager (Orr et al. 1984; Palmer et al. 2000). The importance of having support groups for siblings of youth with cancer has also been underscored, with efforts made to help siblings reduce their own anxiety and fear about the cancer experience (Houtzager et al. 2001). Additionally, support groups have been effective for parents of children with pediatric cancer (Foreman et al. 2005).

For both parents and children, the American Childhood Cancer Organization (ACCO) provides links to online support groups, email support groups, and listserves meant to connect children, parents, and siblings to other individuals experiencing similar difficulties. The online support group resources can be found at https://www.inspire.com/groups/american-childhood-cancer-organization/. It is also recommended that families be encouraged to ask their oncology provider what support groups are available in the hospital and in their community.

Support groups are a long-standing tradition in the care of youth with cancer and their families. They appear to be widely available to families, and resources typically can be found in pediatric cancer centers, in the community, through professional foundations, and electronically.

Social Skills Training

Pediatric cancer survivors, specifically those diagnosed with brain or central nervous system (CNS) tumors, can potentially experience significant deficits in social functioning. Problems with social interactions in these youth have been noted throughout the literature across self, parent, and teacher reports. It has been hypothesized that social deficits are related to concomitant declines in executive functioning (Wolf et al. 2013). Due to these deficits, interventions have been developed in order to provide support and encourage the strengthening of social interactions for children and adolescents with pediatric cancer. Social skills interventions involve providing children with tools to better maneuver their social interactions. Gaining these skills is achieved through (1) psychoeducation, (2) modeling, and (3) practice.

Social skills interventions have been created to help children with a new diagnosis of pediatric cancer reintegrate into the classroom (Varni et al. 1993). Children engaged in social cognitive problem-solving, assertiveness training, and ways to manage teasing and name-calling. Specific to problem-solving, children as young as 5 years old were taught to approach problems as if they are solvable, outline the importance of identifying specific problems, identify antecedents of the problem, brainstorm potential solutions, and plan solutions and assess outcomes. Children were provided with information about asserting their concerns, wishes, and thoughts to their parents, teachers, medical staff, and peers. Furthermore, assertive, passive, and aggressive behavior was defined. Children were also given skills for managing teasing and name-calling due to changes in their appearance from cancer.

More recently, Schulte and colleagues (2014) developed an 8-week social skills group intervention with pediatric brain tumor survivors. The intervention was developed to enhance skills related to (1) making friends, (2) cooperation, (3) dealing with bullies, (4) resolving conflicts, (5) empathy, and (6) assertiveness. Psychoeducation, modeling, and practice were interwoven with activities that helped participants practice intervention skills. The introduction of social skills and practice took place during the first 6 sessions of the intervention. Session 7 focused on reviewing all skills learned in the previous sessions, and the final session enabled children to practice their skills and share what they had learned throughout the study with their families. Children in the control group experienced significant increases in social problems from pre- to post-intervention per parent report, compared to children in the intervention group, whose social problem levels remained stable. Additionally, children in the intervention group reported a significant improvement in social functioning, compared to the control group who experienced no change.

Social skills training can be an integral aspect of providing psychosocial support for children with a diagnosis of pediatric cancer and their families. The negative cognitive outcomes associated with a cancer diagnosis and treatments as well as the social isolation that comes from missing school due to treatment speak to the importance of social skills training in this population.

Adherence to Medical Regimens

Adherence to medical regimens has been a major focus for improving pediatric outcomes for over 30 years. Adherence has been defined as "the extent to which a person's behavior (in terms of taking medications, following diets, or executing lifestyle changes) coincides with medical or health advice" (Haynes 1979). Adherence rates vary tremendously depending on specific disease factors (e.g., severity, length of illness, etc.), complexity of the treatment regimen (e.g., number of medications, varying times per day medication is required, intravenous versus oral ingestion), and the method of monitoring adherence (e.g., pill count, daily diary, electronic monitoring). In general, across studies and disease groups in which adherence rates have been extensively assessed, estimates for adherence in children and adolescents are typically below 50 % (Rapoff 2010; La Greca and Bearman 2003). Specific to cancer, Kondryn and colleagues (2011) reviewed the literature on treatment nonadherence to oral medications in adolescents and young adults (AYA) and found that there are only four studies focusing on nonadherence with rates ranging from 27 to 63 %. The cost of this nonadherence is extremely serious for the individual. Failure to adhere to medication regimens can result in drug resistance, unexpected adverse medical events (e.g., negative drug reactions), increased rates of relapse, as well as morbidity and mortality and can lead to unnecessary increased dosages or discontinuation of a medication due to the belief that it is ineffective for the individual (Bhatia et al. 2012; DiMatteo et al. 2002). Therefore, it is clear that nonadherence is a significant but understudied problem among pediatric cancer patients.

Patients with behavioral or emotional problems are less likely to adhere to regimens for cancer, diabetes, and renal disease (Rapoff 2010). Additionally, ambiguity within the family context of who is in charge or has primary responsibility of monitoring regimen tasks (e.g., making sure the medication was taken and completing refills) also tends to be associated with lower adherence (Rapoff 2010). Specifically related to effective treatments, behavioral interventions and multicomponent interventions with a treatment focus on the individual, family, and broader community within which the family operates have been identified as the most effective in improving treatment adherence (Butow et al. 2010). Adherence in younger children may also be affected by inability to or aversion to swallowing pills. Strategies for pill swallowing are described in Chap. 13, Stem Cell Transplantation.

In one approach to remedying nonadherence in AYAs, AYAs were given a mini-PC computer that contained either the intervention game ("Re-Mission") and/or the commercial game (i.e., "Indiana Jones and the Emperor's Tomb") and were asked to play the game(s) for at least 1 hour per week during the 3-month study period (Kato et al. 2008). "Re-Mission" (HopeLab 2015) addresses issues of cancer treatment and care for teenagers and young adults. The game includes missions such as destroying cancer cells and managing common treatment-related effects (e.g., bacterial infections, nausea, constipation) by using chemotherapy, antibiotics, and stool softeners as ammunition. Players are also encouraged to use relaxation techniques to reduce stress, and eat healthy foods to gain energy. During any point in the game, neither the Nano-Bot nor any of the virtual patients "die." If players fail to complete a mission or level at any point in the game, then the Nano-Bot powers down and players are given the opportunity to try the mission again. Players must complete missions successfully prior to moving to the next level. Importantly, Kato et al. (2008) found that individuals who played the game evidenced improved levels of adherence to treatment protocols, increased self-efficacy, and higher levels of cancer-related knowledge compared to those that did not.

Currently, "Re-Mission 2" has open access to six games, "Nano-Bot's Revenge," "Stem Cell Defender," "Nano Dropbot," "Leukemia," "Feeding Frenzy," and "Special Op" online (http://www.re-mission2.org), which allows players to engage in different tactics to defend the body against mutant cells. It also provides access to information regarding research supporting the game platform and resources for families to become engaged in "Re-Mission 2." This is one example of an innovative intervention that incorporates multiple approaches to the management of treatment adherence in the context of pediatric cancer.

A significant gap in the literature still exists for proven interventions to improve adherence in adolescents and young adults undergoing treatment for cancer (Butow et al. 2010). Numerous pediatric cancer researchers (e.g., La Greca and Schuman 1995; Gray et al. 2014; McGrady et al. 2014; Pai and Drotar 2010) have suggested general approaches to the management of treatment adherence as interventions that primarily emphasize (1) learning new skills and behaviors specific to adherence, (2) providing supervision and/or feedback, (3) providing incentives for improved treatment adherence, (4) enhancing family support and/or problem-solving, and (5) offering conventional psychiatric treatment. Pediatric interventions that include a multitude of these modules are likely to be most beneficial in assisting the patient and their family with adherence issues. For example, interventions may need to include one-on-one psychoeducation instruction surrounding specific disease management techniques, medical education (e.g., knowledge of medication side effects), problem-solving techniques, and adherence feedback (e.g., medical bioassay levels and/or MEMsCaps®), coupled with nurse consultation in order to be maximally effective. With the advent of new technology (e.g., Medication Even Monitoring System® (MEMSCap®; © 2002, 2003, 2005 by AARDEX® Ltd., Untermüli 6, CH-6302 Zug); Maya Pill Dispenser (MedMinder™ © 2014); MedFolio Pillbox (©

MedFolio 2014)), adherence to medical regimens has become an integral part of many interventions within the context of pediatric cancer treatment. Each of these technological devices provides the clinician, patient, and/or family members the ability to track adherence, set phone, text message, and/or email reminders to take medication. These devices can be excellent resources for providing additional assistance to children and families having significant difficulties with adherence to medication.

Health Promotion Interventions

Similar to adherence interventions, which focus on a multitude of constructs (e.g., behavior, cognitive functioning, psychosocial functioning) to improve outcomes, health promotion interventions target modifiable behaviors such as dietary choices, smoking cessation, and patient knowledge surrounding illness information. Health-risk behaviors, such as smoking, drug use, sun exposure, and sedentary lifestyles can place individuals at risk for maladaptive psychosocial and physical outcomes (Hudson and Findlay 2006). Pediatric cancer and subsequent treatments can place patients at even greater risk for morbidity secondary to engaging in the same risky behaviors as their peers without cancer (Hudson et al. 1997; Mertens et al. 2002). Several interventions to motivate the practice of health behaviors have been a focus of childhood cancer research (Nathan et al. 2009); however, little is currently known regarding the use of health promotion behaviors to optimize health status and decrease cancer-related health effects (Hudson and Findlay 2006) in children who have undergone pediatric cancer treatment.

One area of health promotion literature examines the importance of physical activity. In the adult literature, research on exercise interventions during cancer treatment is well established (Knols et al. 2005), yet very few studies exist in children. Despite methodological limitations and small sample sizes, existing evidence strongly suggests that exercise is not only safe and feasible during cancer treatment, but that it can also improve physical functioning, quality of life, and potentially cognitive functioning (Knols et al. 2005; Schmitz et al. 2005).

A recent study involving pediatric patients with a malignant bone tumor investigated the effects of individualized exercise interventions versus a control condition during their inpatient stays (Winter et al. 2013). Due to varying degrees in exercise history and disease severity, exercise plans were tailored individually to each participant to include different exercise elements such as strength, endurance, coordination, and flexibility exercises as well as games and relaxation training. Overall, the physical activity intervention group increased in overall physical activity, yet differences decreased after the cessation of the intervention. While no durable significant differences were observed, this is an important intervention program which gives pediatric cancer patients individualized exercise knowledge and education about healthy activity levels.

What have sometimes been referred to as "psychoeducational" interventions are another type of health promotion intervention that can be implemented by pediatric healthcare providers. This approach addresses informational transactions, discussions of problem-solving techniques and/or concerns surrounding the individual/illness/family, and use of coping skills training and psychosocial support. While this was briefly discussed in the adherence section regarding knowledge of medication and disease prognosis, the role of psychoeducational interventions in facilitating adaptation to chronic disease has received growing recognition, especially with the development of patients and families advocating for greater involvement in their own care (please see Chap. 24 for additional information on Advocacy).

According to the systematic review of informational interventions designed to influence knowledge among pediatric cancer patients, the development of health-related knowledge in children is best accompanied by information transfer methods that are highly interactive and individualized (Bradlyn et al. 2003), such as interactive multimedia formats. Lastly, an online interactive website including webisodes and chat rooms, created by HopeLabs and the StarLight Children's

Foundation, called *Coping With Chemo*, is another resource for children and families (http://chemo.starlight.org/). Webisodes include information about the diagnosis, telling your friends you have cancer and making decisions about your treatment.

Other psychoeducational interventions have focused on reduction of secondhand smoke exposure among children with cancer. Secondhand smoke exposure is carcinogenic and can lead to significant health consequences such as respiratory illness, ear infections, and reduced pulmonary functioning (United States Department of Health & Human Services 2006). This is particularly worrisome for children who are diagnosed with cancer as it may increase vulnerability to health risks associated with their diagnosis (Tyc et al. 2013). A recent innovative intervention attempted to decrease secondhand smoke exposure in children undergoing active cancer treatment. This intervention involved three individual, face-to-face, biweekly 1 hour sessions followed by three 25-minute telephone sessions with parents with the goals of reducing children's exposure to tobacco smoke, increasing parental self-monitoring of smoking around the child, and problem-solving barriers to smoking around the child and social reinforcement for success (Tyc et al. 2013). Overall, the intervention was successful in significantly reducing parent-reported child secondhand smoke exposure. While no significant changes in cotinine levels were observed, overall parents reported a willingness to participate. While Tyc and colleagues (2013) provided a significant first step in assessing secondhand smoke in children with pediatric cancer, more studies are needed to assess interventions for secondhand smoke exposure.

It is essential that effective interventions are implemented and embedded within multidisciplinary care in addition to including a multitude of formats (e.g., electronic, web-based) in order to maximize positive health outcomes for children, adolescents, and their parents. These interventions will also need to take into account different learning styles (e.g., auditory versus visual, desire for written materials versus electronic modalities) and take into account developmental levels.

Case Vignette

Gus, a 14-year-old male who was diagnosed with acute lymphoblastic leukemia (ALL), was referred to the psychologist due to staff concern about his nonadherence with his medical regimen, which was interfering with his recovery and ability to attend school. Gus was withdrawn, depressed and anxious about medical complications, and felt little control over his treatment and disease. The psychologist arranged an initial care conference that included Gus, a social worker, the primary nurse coordinator, nutritionist, and the psychologist.

The team began by trying to increase Gus' sense of control by informing him about painful procedures at least 3 days in advance and choosing which days of the week he preferred to receive his chemotherapy. The team also worked to improve Gus' activity in support groups, provided him additional knowledge of his illness via interactive forums (i.e., video games and interactive videos), and implemented electronic monitoring with text messaging reminders sent to both Gus and his parents to improve adherence.

While the team worked with Gus, it became clear that Gus' parents experienced significant conflict surrounding his care and would often yell at each other during clinic visits. His parents were seen together for one session to negotiate who would bring Gus to clinic visits and to identify communication difficulties. To address Gus' exposure to his father's secondhand smoke, the psychologist implemented a behavioral smoking cessation intervention (e.g., nicotine replacement therapy products) for Gus' father. After two months, Gus' parents were successful in decreasing Gus' exposure to secondhand smoke, as measured by oral cotinine levels and exhaled carbon monoxide. In addition, Gus increased his school attendance, improved his adherence with his treatment regimen, and became more social in school activities.

Bibliotherapy

From a formal perspective, bibliotherapy has been defined as the "use of written materials to gain understanding and engage in problem-solving" (Goddard 2011). Bibliotherapy can be particularly useful in settings where engaging in a therapeutic treatment protocol that requires multiple sessions would simply not be feasible (e.g., with families living in rural setting; Elgar and McGrath 2003). Bibliotherapy has four components, including:

1. Identification
2. Selection
3. Presentation
4. Follow-up (Pardeck 1992)

Identification involves working with the family and patient to pinpoint their specific psychosocial needs. The process of selection consists of selecting materials that coincide with the family and patients identified needs. Presentation involves the clinician giving the selected information to the patient in a manner that is appropriate to their specific developmental level. Finally, follow-up involves the clinician checking in with the patient to ensure they understood the information given, offer the opportunity for the patient to explain the information they found helpful, and address or elaborate on any questions. Pardeck (1992) suggests that bibliotherapy with patients is a process whereby the clinician is involved directly with the patient during therapy, as opposed to the patient reading materials on their own without the presence of the clinician. Additionally, bibliotherapy can be used in sessions with the clinician and patient as a means of modeling of skills and generating discussion.

Bibliotherapy and multimedia such as film and short stories have a long history of clinical utilization in the pediatric context. Numerous books are available for both parents and children whose lives have been affected by pediatric cancer (see Chap. 25 for additonal resources). These books include those written for parents that cover material relevant to diagnosis and treatment (see Nancy Keene's series of books on a variety of topics specific to pediatric cancer) to books that specifically help children cope with negative feelings and fears. Many resources for parents can be found on the Internet.

As mentioned previously, bibliotherapy has been widely used to provide psychoeducational support for pediatric cancer patients, but rarely has it been investigated from a research perspective (Schneider et al. 2013). Schneider and colleagues (2013) completed a bibliotherapy intervention with 21 pediatric cancer patients. A social worker read *Nikki's Day at Chemo*, a book developed for the study to facilitate discussions of coping strategies, emotions, diagnosis, and treatment, to the cancer patient and then asked pointed questions in order to assess the child's understanding of the book. The child was asked how the story might be applicable to their own cancer diagnosis and treatment, using specific examples from the book to prompt the child. The discussion of the use of the tools provided in the book typically lasted about 15 minutes. They found that it helped to improve interpersonal functioning and was also rated as a satisfying activity by both patients and families. There was also an improvement in intrapersonal functioning several months post-intervention compared to pre-intervention. Bibliotherapy has also been suggested as a useful tool for psychologists, educators, physicians, other healthcare providers (Elgar and McGrath 2003) and school counselors when working specifically with pediatric cancer patients (Karayanni and Spitzer 1984). Bibliotherapy can be a helpful tool in providing support when used within the context of a larger treatment protocol (see Chap. 25).

Emerging New Therapies

Acceptance and commitment therapy (ACT), mindfulness, and trauma-focused cognitive behavioral therapy (TF-CBT) are three relatively new therapeutic approaches that may be used within the pediatric cancer population. The main focus of ACT is to increase psychological flexibility by engaging in acceptance, cognitive defusion, practicing being in the present moment, viewing the self as context, identifying and working towards the individual's values, and committing actions (Hayes et al. 2006). Mindfulness is the "awareness that emerges through paying attention, purposefully and nonjudgmentally, to the unfolding of experience moment to moment, including one's thoughts, feelings, and body sensations" (Jones et al. 2013). TF-CBT within pediatric cancer is aimed at alleviating posttraumatic stress symptoms resulting from disease-related procedures in order to elicit improvements in quality of life and psychosocial adjustment.

There is limited research examining the effectiveness of ACT within a pediatric cancer population. Masuda and colleagues (2010) developed a protocol of eight 60-minute family sessions within the context of sickle-cell disease. Sessions were broken into 3 sections. The first section, lasting 5–10 minutes, involved the patient and family discussing the patient's activities throughout the week and any medical concerns the patient or family had. The second section, about 30–40 minutes long, was comprised of utilizing ACT tools to address the concerns of the patient and family. These included acceptance, values clarification, and mindfulness. The final section, lasting 10–15 minutes, was geared towards having the patient and family develop specific values-based goals for the coming week. Additionally, Burke and colleagues (2014) developed the Take a Breath Intervention for parents of children with life-threatening conditions (i.e., parents of youth with cancer or cardiac disease). This intervention involved five 90-minute sessions. During these group sessions, parents participated in the use of metaphors, experiential exercises, and self-reflection, all elements of ACT. Parents also worked to identify personal values and then utilized those values to help enhance problem-solving skills. From pre- to post-intervention, parents reportedly experienced decreases in posttraumatic stress symptoms and impact of illness scores and increases in psychological flexibility and mindfulness. Parents also reported an improvement in access to emotional resources.

Mindfulness involves both elements of psychoeducation and practice. Patients practice observing their external surroundings and internal thoughts and sensations as ever changing while refraining from identifying with or reacting to these stimuli (Jones et al. 2013). Mindfulness also typically involves setting an intention. This is typically related to showing compassion and kindness towards the self and others. It has been suggested in the literature that using these skills will help pediatric cancer patients shift their cognitive focus from uncertain future-oriented thoughts to focusing on the present moment through a nonjudgmental lens. Lagor and colleagues (2013) developed a mindfulness-based intervention for children with various chronic illnesses. There were six group sessions that provided psychoeducation through interactive exercises and metaphors and practice. Sessions towards the beginning of the intervention focused on making patients aware of their environment. An example of this would be mindful touching, where patients were asked to describe a mystery object that was in a paper bag using nonjudgmental words. Sessions towards the end of the intervention focused on patients practicing mindfulness of their internal experiences. These sessions were aimed at using visual imagery and playful curiosity in order to practice mindfulness. An example of visual imagery was being mindful of thoughts by sorting them into boxes (Lagor et al. 2013).

Although there is no data on the use of TF-CBT in pediatric cancer, a review completed by Nenova and colleagues (2013) found that with adult cancer patients, cognitive behavioral strategies can alleviate cancer-related posttraumatic stress symptoms (PTSS). Results from the adult literature suggest that cognitive behavioral strategies may be effective in reducing PTSS, but more research is needed to better understand the implication of trauma-focused interventions within pediatric cancer samples. As with all psychotherapeutic modalities, there can be barriers that arise in providing TF-CBT effectively. These include, but are not limited to, the developmental and cognitive level of the child, resistance to homework, and cultural considerations. Therefore, it is important for the clinician to consider these potential barriers when engaging in treatment.

ACT, mindfulness, and TF-CBT are emerging therapies that have the potential to be clinically useful tools when working with children with chronic illness. Within the pediatric cancer population, additional research needs to be done before we can understand the implications of these interventions within this population; however, preliminary work thus far seems promising.

Case Study *Background*

Brock, a 5-year-old boy, was referred for psychotherapy by his pediatric oncologist and multidisciplinary team following his recent diagnosis of acute lymphoblastic leukemia (ALL). Brock had been diagnosed at a regional hospital in a rural part of the state and had been medically evacuated to the pediatric cancer center in a university teaching hospital approximately 160 miles from his home. Ten weeks into his treatment protocol, he began to show signs of withdrawal and sadness. Notably, his mother had also begun to show signs of depression, isolating herself from the other parents, asking minimal questions to the medical team, and experiencing significant weight loss.

The treatment team noticed that the vast majority of hospitalizations and outpatient visits involved only Brock and his mother; rarely did visits occur with Brock's father and two siblings. Brock's mother was found sobbing in the bathroom one morning, stating that she was completely overwhelmed by everything that she had to deal with. She also stated concerns about the uncertainty surrounding Brock's illness, including his long-term prognosis and possibility of late effects, stating "even if he does survive, what will his future be like?" She noted that the family was excessively burdened by the increased financial and logistical demands (e.g., travel to the hospital, childcare for their other children, and management of business needs) and that her husband felt compelled to work even harder in order to keep them financially afloat. Although Brock's paternal grandmother was able to provide some childcare, his dad had considerable new responsibilities being the primary care provider for Brock's siblings managing two other small children on a daily basis.

Intervention

In a meeting with the pediatric oncology psychologist, Brock's mother revealed her own history of episodic depressive episodes, triggered by major stressors in her life, for which she had successfully sought treatment through a local mental health provider. The psychologist proposed conducting weekly family sessions that would coincide with Brock's treatment, and Brock's father would call in if he were unable to attend.

During the subsequent three sessions, a number of potential problem areas were identified using a medical family therapy approach. Both parents underscored how difficult communication between them had been, in part due to the physical distance between home and hospital and also due to their desire not to stress each other further. Apparently, both individuals were "conflict-avoidant," and the diagnosis of cancer had further accentuated that pattern. In addition, both acknowledged the considerable uncertainty they felt. On the one hand, they acknowledged the good prognosis their son had and their trust in the treatment team, and yet they were both experiencing the "what if" phenomenon, (i.e., "what if he doesn't respond to chemotherapy," "what if his port gets infected"?). They both voiced their concerns for Brock's siblings as well, believing that they were "short-changing them" and worried in particular that Brock's older brother would be resentful about the attention Brock was receiving and the additional chores that he was being asked to assume. The therapist attempted to "normalize" yet legitimize their concerns while offering support and continuing to develop the therapeutic relationship. She also reframed their conflict-avoidant style intended to protect one another as potentially causing detriment in the long run.

In later sessions, it appeared that both parents were experiencing a sense of relief and a new commitment to maintaining communication. Brock's father was reassured that they could discuss these issues without his wife plunging further into depression. In order to further support the mother's coping with her depressive symptoms, the therapist implemented CBT approaches such as having her monitor symptoms through a daily thought diary and increasing social interactions, which had been helpful to her in the past.

A *problem-solving approach* (PST) was taken to address the family's financial concerns, including (1) checking with his insurance coverage to determine what treatment is covered, (2) consulting with a financial advisor to further determine their actual financial status and the long-term impact on his business, and (3) consulting with the social worker at the hospital to see if funds were available to support them. Through each of these efforts, they were able to determine their financial needs, and while not a specific goal of therapy, a number of fundraisers were held in their home community.

Additional visits were conducted with Brock to assess his level of distress. Not unlike many 5-year-old boys, his preference was to talk about toys and his favorite superheroes. Although Brock initially appeared somewhat sad, his mood slowly lifted as he talked about his various interests. When the therapist asked him in the third meeting what he worried about the most, he very quickly said "my mom" and changed the topic. The therapist continued to keep the topic "light" over the next few sessions while continuing to meet with his mother and father. As the mother's mood lifted, so did Brock's, indicating that his "depression" was in large part a reflection of his mother's challenges in coping.

When the family was seen 10 weeks later, the therapist reviewed their progress. Brock's parents were concerned about his reintegration into the school environment and the questions his friends may have about his treatment and health status. Fortunately, the treatment center had a well-established school reintegration tool kit they had developed, with an array of informational pamphlets and handouts for teachers and schoolmates. A release was obtained and the reintegration coordinator contacted the school, offering to visit with the staff and students. The parents also agreed to schedule a meeting with Brock's teacher, principal, and special education director to discuss these issues further.

Approximately 6 months into Brock's treatment, his parents described being "in a much better place," both individually and as a couple. They reported that although they still experienced uncertainty and knew that their son had a lot of treatment remaining, they felt they had the skills to manage their fears. They did not think they needed more sessions with the therapist, but wanted to make sure they could "touch base" should the need arise. Additionally, the therapist spoke with Brock's treatment team to obtain their perspective on the family's adjustment and ensure that the family was coping more effectively and was appropriately engaged in oncology treatment.

This case study illustrates a multicomponent cognitive behavior therapy and problem-solving therapy (PST) approach in the context of a family systems intervention. Such a case demonstrates the integration of empirically supported strategies but in the context of a flexibly instituted family systems framework. In this treatment approach, the therapist took care to (1) assess the family dynamics, including their strengths and weaknesses prior to the diagnosis of cancer, role definitions, and role shifts that had occurred; (2) clearly assess how the family defined their greatest stressors/challenges, including how they were coping with uncertainty; (3) establish multiple therapeutic plans at different systems levels (e.g., parent, child, sibling, medical team) for enhancing their coping; (4) subsequently implement the plan; and (5) evaluate its effectiveness. Care was taken throughout the course of treatment to establish and maintain the therapeutic alliance, assess for cultural issues, integrate procedures/resources with the multidisciplinary team, and assess for barriers. A basic assumption at all times was that *all families seek to do the very best they can under extraordinary circumstances* and that the role of the therapist is to facilitate the process of coping while hopefully mitigating maladaptive responses.

Future Directions

A wide array of approaches and techniques have been utilized to address the needs of children with cancer and their families. These range from broad and general strategies aimed at alleviating family distress to very specific and targeted therapies aimed at reducing pain or enhancing adherence or exercise. Clinicians now have the ability to employ various interventions depending on the needs of a given family.

In light of the current state of intervention science, where do we need to go from here? First, it appears that while a wide range of psychotherapeutic modalities are available, many of these modalities would benefit from continued empirical scrutiny. Some of the interventions that have been employed to date actually have limited support from a research perspective in children with cancer (e.g., CBT, Coping Cat) compared to treatment as usual. Although randomized clinical trials are time-consuming and expensive, it remains important to find ways to document "best practices" if we are to provide the best possible care to our families. Additionally, although a number of emerging therapies have been identified as effective with adult cancer patients (e.g., ACT, mindfulness, and TF-CBT), the utility of these interventions should be explored within pediatric cancer in order to provide patients with cutting-edge empirically supported psychological treatments.

Second, it is clear that the movement towards electronic dissemination of interventions has great potential for utilization in pediatric cancer centers around the country (see Chap. 20). Families can already access an immense amount of information online, including coping resources, support groups, and education about treatment, side effects, and new developments in the field. Such interventions may be particularly helpful for those families who live in rural areas or who have limited resources to travel for additional psychotherapeutic services. This technology is already available, and both patient and parent can track cognitive (e.g., thoughts and beliefs), emotional (e.g., depressive and anxiety symptoms), and physical variables (e.g., activity levels and exercise) electronically with relative ease and low expense. Although there are issues of confidentiality to contend with, technology such as Skype allows for real time face-to-face intervention from virtually any location (including around the world). Such technology may be the primary means by which we can enhance the delivery of services to families whose lives are often fragmented by the diagnosis of cancer.

Clinical Pearls

- Resiliency is the norm! However, there are those subsets of families that need support and who are at risk for various types of psychological distress (e.g., anxiety, depression). Each family should be approached through a unique lens to provide the appropriate and necessary psychological assistance.
- Use a multidisciplinary team approach to benefit the family. Such a team can provide resources, assist with care management decisions, and implement interventions in several settings (e.g., hospital, home, school), which will help to improve psychosocial functioning.
- When you have worked with one family with a child with cancer, you have worked with one family with a child with cancer. Do not assume they are all the same and will fit neatly into a single conceptual framework.
- The best predictor of child adjustment is parent adjustment. All psychotherapeutic endeavors should attempt to involve the parents and the entire family system in some form or fashion.
- We cannot provide all resources to all parents, but with careful assessment, we can address their most pressing needs.
- Craft interventions to the needs and desires of the families. Some families may want to problem solve and share openly with other families; other families may want to be listened to and desire privacy. Continual assessment of the family needs over time is important, as needs may well change over the trajectory of survivorship.

References

AARDEX® Ltd. (© 2002, 2003, 2005). MEMsCap® MEMs® 6 Medication event monitoring system. Retrieved from http://www.aardexgroup.com/upload/pdf/mems6_trackcap_datasheet.pdf

Bhatia S, Landier W, Shangguan M et al (2012) Nonadherence to oral mercaptopurine and risk of relapse in Hispanic and non-Hispanic white children with acute lymphoblastic leukemia: a report from the Children's oncology group. J Clin Oncol 30:2094–2101

Bradlyn AS, Beale IL, Kato PM (2003) Psychoeducational interventions with pediatric cancer patients: part I. Patient information and knowledge. J Child Fam Stud 12:257–277. doi:10.1023/A:1023983609702

Bratton SC, Dee R, Rhine T et al (2005) The efficacy of play therapy with children: a meta-analytic review of treatment outcomes. Prof Psychol Res Pract 36:376–390

Brown RT (2006) Introduction: why the need for a comprehensive handbook on pediatric psychosocial oncology/hematology. In: Brown RT (ed) Comprehensive handbook of childhood cancer and sickle cell disease: a biopsychosocial approach. Oxford University Press, Oxford

Burke K, Muscara F, McCarthy M et al (2014) Adapting acceptance and commitment therapy for parents of children with life-threatening illness: pilot study. Fam Syst Health 32:122–127. doi:10.1037/fsh0000012

Butow P, Palmer S, Pai A et al (2010) Review of adherence-related issues in adolescents and young adults with cancer. J Clin Oncol 28:4800–4809. doi:10.1200/JCO.2009.22.2802

Campbell TL (2003) The effectiveness of family interventions for physical disorders. J Marital Fam Ther 29:263–281. doi:10.1111/j.1752-0606.2003.tb01204.x

Cassano J, Nagel K, O'Mara L (2008) Talking with others who "just know": perceptions of adolescents with cancer who participate in a teen group. J Pediatr Oncol Nurs 25:193–199. doi:10.1177/1043454208319972

Chester B (1998) The privilege of working with children faced with death. Retrieved from http://reporter-archive.mcgill.ca/Rep/r3015/sourkes.html

Coucil T (1993) Art therapy with pediatric cancer patients: helping normal children cope with abnormal circumstances. Art The 10:78–87

Dimatteo MR, Giordani PJ, Lepper HS et al (2002) Patient adherence and medical treatment outcomes: a meta-analysis. Med Care 40:794–811. doi:10.1037/0278-6133.23.2.207

Elgar FJ, McGrath PJ (2003) Self-administered psychosocial treatments for children and families. J Clin Psychol 59:321–339. doi:10.1002/jclp.10132

Foreman T, Willis L, Goodenough B (2005) Hospital-based support groups for parents of seriously unwell children: an example from pediatric oncology in Australia. Social Work Groups J Commun Clin Pract 28:3–21. doi:10.1300/J009v28n02_02

Goddard AT (2011) Children's books for use in bibliotherapy. J Pediatr Health Care 25:57–61, doi:http://dx.doi.org/10.1016/j.pedhc.2010.08.006

Gray WN, Szulczewski LJ, Regan SMP et al (2014) Cultural influences in pediatric cancer from diagnosis to cure/end of life. J Pediatr Oncol Nurs 31:252–271. doi:10.1177/1043454214529022

Hayes SC, Luoma JB, Bond FW et al (2006) Acceptance and commitment therapy: model, processes and outcomes. Behav Res Ther 44:1–25, doi:http://dx.doi.org/10.1016/j.brat.2005.06.006

Haynes RB (1979) Introduction. In: Haynes RB, Taylor DW, Sackett DL (eds) Compliance in health care. Johns Hopkins University Press, Baltimore

Hoekstra-Weebers JEHM, Heuvel F, Jaspers JPC et al (1998) Brief report: an intervention program for parents of pediatric cancer patients: a randomized controlled trial. J Pediatr Psychol 23:207–214. doi:10.1093/jpepsy/23.3.207

HopeLab (2015) Innovative solutions: re-mission™. Retrieved from http://www.hopelab.org/innovative-solutions/re-mission/

Houtzager BA, Grootenhuis MA, Last BF (2001) Support groups for siblings of pediatric oncology patients: Impact on anxiety. Psychooncology 10:315–324

Hudson MM, Findlay S (2006) Health-risk behaviors and health promotion in adolescent and young adult cancer survivors. Cancer 107:1695–1701. doi:10.1002/cncr.22103

Hudson MM, Jones D, Boyett J et al (1997) Late mortality of long-term survivors of childhood cancer. J Clin Oncol 15:2205–2213

Jones P, Blunda M, Biegel G et al (2013) Can mindfulness-based interventions help adolescents with cancer? Psychooncology 22:2148–2151. doi:10.1002/pon.3251

Kanter JW, Manos RC, Bowe WM et al (2010) What is behavioral activation?: a review of the empirical literature. Clin Psychol Rev 30:608–620

Karayanni M, Spitzer A (1984) The role of the school counselor in the rehabilitation of children with cancer. Int J Adv Couns 7:209–215. doi:10.1007/BF00116193

Kato PM, Cole SW, Bradlyn AS et al (2008) A video game improves behavioral outcomes in adolescents and young adults with cancer: a randomized trial. Pediatrics 122:e305–e317. doi:10.1542/peds.2007-3134

Kazak AE, Simms S, Barakat L et al (1999) Surviving cancer competently intervention program (SCCIP): a cognitive-behavioral and family therapy intervention for adolescent survivors of childhood cancer and their families. Fam Process 38:175–191. doi:10.1111/j.1545-5300.1999.00176.x

Kazak AE, Simms S, Alderfer MA et al (2005) Feasibility and preliminary outcomes from a pilot study of a brief psychological intervention for families of children newly diagnosed with cancer. J Pediatr Psychol 30:644–655. doi:10.1093/jpepsy/jsi051

Kendall PC (1994) Treating anxiety disorders in children: results of a randomized clinical trial. J Consult Clin Psychol 62:100–110

Kendall PC (2000) Coping cat workbook. Workbook Publishing, Ardmore

Kendall PC, Robin JA, Hedtke K et al (2005) Considering CBT with anxious youth? Think exposures. J Cogn Behav Pract 12:136–150

Knols R, Aaronson NK, Uebelhart D et al (2005) Physical exercise in cancer patients during and after medical treatment: a systematic review of randomized and controlled clinical trials. J Clin Oncol 23:3830–3842. doi:10.1200/JCO.2005.02.148

Kondryn HJ, Edmondson CL, Hill J et al (2011) Treatment non-adherence in teenage and young adult patients with cancer. Lancet Oncol 12:100–108. doi:10.1016/S1470-2045(10)70069-3

La Greca AM, Bearman KJ (2003) Adherence to pediatric regimens. In: Roberts MC (ed) Handbook of pediatric psychology. Guilford Press, New York, pp 119–140

La Greca AM, Schuman W (1995) Adherence to prescribed medication regimens. In: Roberts MC (ed) Handbook of pediatric psychology. Guilford Press, New York

Lagor AF, Williams DJ, Lerner JB et al (2013) Lessons learned from a mindfulness-based intervention with chronically ill youth. Clin Pract Pediatr Psychol 1:146–158. doi:10.1037/cpp0000015

Law EF, Fisher E, Fales J et al (2014) Systematic review and meta-analysis of parent and family-based interventions for children and adolescents with chronic medical conditions. J Pediatr Psychol 39:866–886. doi:10.1093/jpepsy/

Madden JR, Mowry P, Gao D et al (2010) Creative arts therapy improves quality of life for pediatric brain tumor patients receiving outpatient chemotherapy. J Pediatr Oncol Nurs 27:133–145

Marsac ML, Hildenbrand AK, Clawson K et al (2012) Acceptability and feasibility of family use of the cellie cancer coping kit. Support Care Cancer 20:3315–3324. doi:10.1007/s00520-012-1475-y

Masuda A, Cohen LL, Wicksell RK et al (2010) A case study: acceptance and commitment therapy for pediatric sickle cell disease. J Pediatr Psychol 36:398–409

McDaniel SH, Belar CD, Schroeder C et al (2002) A training curriculum for professional psychologists in primary care. Prof Psychol 33:65. doi:10.1037/0735-7028.33.1.65

McGrady ME, Williams SN, Davies SM et al (2014) Adherence to outpatient oral medication regimens in adolescent hematopoietic stem cell transplant recipients. Eur J Oncol Nurs 18:140–144

MedFolio© (2014) MedFolio© Pillbox. Retrieved from http://www.medfoliopillbox.com/product/medfolio-pillbox/

MedMinder™ © (2014) Maya medical alert and pill dispenser. Retrieved from http://www.medminder.com/pill-dispensers/maya-medical-alert-and-pill-dispenser

Mertens AC, Yasui Y, Liu Y et al (2002) Pulmonary complications in survivors of childhood and adolescent cancer. Cancer 95:2431–2441. doi:10.1093/jnci/djp148

Mullins LL, Fedele DA, Chaffin M et al (2012) A clinic-based interdisciplinary intervention for mothers of children newly diagnosed with cancer: a pilot study. J Pediatr Psychol 37:1104–1115. doi:10.1093/jpepsy/jss093

Nathan PC, Ford JS, Henderson TO et al (2009) Health behaviors, medical care, and interventions to promote healthy living in the Childhood Cancer Survivor Study cohort. J Clin Oncol 27:2363–2373. doi:10.1200/JCO.2008.21.1441

Nenova M, Morris L, Paul L et al (2013) Psychosocial interventions with cognitive-behavioral components for the treatment of cancer-related traumatic stress symptoms: a review of randomized controlled trials. J Cogn Psychother 27:258–284. doi:10.1891/0889-8391.27.3.258

Nezu AM, Nezu CM, D'Zurrilla T (2013) Problem-solving therapy: a treatment manual. Springer Publishing, New York

O'Donohue WT, Fisher JE (2009) General principles and empirically supported techniques of cognitive behavior therapy. Springer Publishing, New York

O'Donohue WT, Fisher JE (2012) The Core Principles of Cognitive Behavior Therapy. Cognitive Behavior Therapy: Core Principles for Practice, John Wiley and Sons, Inc., Hoboken p1–12

Orr DP, Hoffman MA, Bennetts G (1984) Adolescents with cancer report their psychosocial needs. J Psychosoc Oncol 2:47–59

Pai AL, Drotar D (2010) Treatment adherence impact: the systematic assessment and quantification of the impact of treatment adherence on pediatric medical and psychological outcomes. J Pediatr Psychol 35:383–393

Palmer L, Erickson S, Shaffer T et al (2000) Themes arising in group therapy for adolescents with cancer and their parents. Int J Rehabil Health 5:43–54. doi:10.1023/A:1012959119398

Pardeck JT (1992) Bibliotherapy and cancer patients. Fam Ther 19:223–232

Persons JB (2012) The case formulation approach to cognitive-behavior therapy (guides to individualized evidence-based treatment). Guilford Press, New York

Philips RD (2010) How firm is our foundation? Current play therapy research. Int J Play Ther 19:13–25

Prager A (1995) Pediatric art therapy: strategies and applications. Art Ther 12:32–38

Rapoff MA (2010) Adherence to pediatric medical regimens. Springer Press, New York. doi:10.1007/978-1-4419-0570-3_2

Rogers C (1959) A theory of therapy, personality, and interpersonal relationships, as developed in the client-centered framework. In: Koch S (ed) Psychology: a study of a science. McGraw Hill, New York

Ruddy NB, McDaniel SH (2013) Medical family therapy in the age of health care reform. Couple Fam Psychol 2:179, doi:http://dx.doi.org/10.1377/hlthaff.28.5.1253

Sahler OJZ, Varni JW, Fairclough DL et al (2002) Problem-solving skills training for mothers of children with newly diagnosed cancer: a randomized trial. J Dev Behav Pediatr 23:77–86. doi:10.1097/00004703-200204000-00003

Sahler OJZ, Fairclough DL, Phipps S et al (2005) Using problem-solving skills training to reduce negative affectivity in mothers of children with newly diagnosed cancer: report of a multisite randomized trial. J Consult Clin Psychol 73:272. doi:10.1200/JCO.2011.39.1870

Sahler OJZ, Dolgin MJ, Phipps S et al (2013) Specificity of problem-solving skills training in mothers of children newly diagnosed with cancer: results of a multisite randomized clinical trial. J Clin Oncol 31:1329–1335. doi:10.1200/JCO.2011.39.1870

Schmitz KH, Holtzman J, Courneya KS et al (2005) Controlled physical activity trials in cancer survivors: a systematic review and meta-analysis. Cancer Epidemiol Biomarkers Prev 14:1588–1595. doi:10.1158/1055-9965

Schneider NM, Peterson M, Gathercoal KA et al (2013) The effect of bibliotherapy on anxiety in children with cancer. Int J Child Health Hum Dev 6:337–345. doi:10.3322/caac.20006

Schulte F, Bartels U, Barrera M (2014) A pilot study evaluating the efficacy of a group social skills program for survivors of childhood central nervous system tumors using a comparison group and teacher reports. Psychooncology 23:597–600, doi:http://dx.doi.org.argo.library.okstate.edu/10.1002/pon.3472

Seitz DCM, Knaevelsrud C, Duran G et al (2014) Efficacy of an internet-based cognitive-behavioral intervention for long-term survivors of pediatric cancer: a pilot study. Support Care Cancer 22(8):2075–2083. doi:10.1007/s00520-014-2193-4

Sourkes BM (1991) Truth to life: art therapy with pediatric oncology patients and their siblings. J Pediatr Oncol 9:81–96, doi:http://dx.doi.org/10.1300/J077v09n02_06

Streisand R, Rodrigue JR, Houck C et al (2000) Brief report: parents of children undergoing bone marrow transplantation: documenting stress and piloting a psychological intervention program. J Pediatr Psychol 25:331–337. doi:10.1093/jpepsy/25.5.331

Tyc VL, Huang Q, Nicholson J et al (2013) Intervention to reduce secondhand smoke exposure among children with cancer: a controlled trial. Psychooncology 22:1104–1111. doi:10.1002/pon.3117

Tyndall LE, Hodgson JL, Lamson AL et al (2012) Medical family therapy: charting a course in competencies. Contemp Fam Ther 34:171–186. doi:10.1037/1091-7527. 22.2.245

US Department of Health and Human Services (2006) The health consequences of involuntary exposure to tobacco smoke: a report of the surgeon general. US Department of Health and Human Services, Centers for Disease Control and Prevention, Coordinating Center for Health Promotion, National Center for Chronic Disease Prevention and Health Promotion, Office of Smoking and Health, Atlanta

Varni JW, Katz ER, Colegrove R et al (1993) The impact of social skills training on the adjustment of children with newly diagnosed cancer. J Pediatr Psychol 18:751–767. doi:10.1093/jpepsy/18.6.751

Varni JW, Sahler OJ, Katz ER et al (1999) Maternal problem-solving therapy in pediatric cancer. J Psychosoc Oncol 16:41–71. doi:10.1300/J077v16n03_0

Wiener L, Battles H, Mamalian C et al (2011) Shop Talk: a pilot study of the feasibility and utility of a therapeutic board game for youth living with cancer. Support Care Cancer 19:1049–1054. doi:10.1007/s00520-011-1130-z

Winter CC, Müller C, Hardes J et al (2013) The effect of individualized exercise interventions during treatment in pediatric patients with a malignant bone tumor. Support Care Cancer 21:1629–1636. doi:10.1007/s00520-012-1707-1

Wolf KR, Walsh KS, Reynolds NC et al (2013) Executive functions and social skills in survivors of pediatric brain tumor. Child Neuropsychol 19:370–384, doi:http://dx.doi.org.argo.library.okstate.edu/10.1080/09297049.2012.669470http://dx.doi.org.argo.library.okstate.edu/10.1080/09297049.2012.669470

7 Preparation, Education, and Procedural Support in Pediatric Cancer

Caroline H. Armington, Heather E. Peach, and Stephanie Hopkinson

Introduction

Considering the rigorous treatment involved with a cancer diagnosis and the stress it inflicts on pediatric patients, defining best practices to enhance emotional and psychosocial well-being has become vital. One area where best practices are needed is procedural support. Built on the premise of providing honest, accurate, and developmentally appropriate information to children with cancer, procedural support includes education about the diagnosis, preparation for tests and procedures, and supportive interventions to enhance coping of the patient and family throughout the course of oncology treatment.

Childhood cancer treatment often includes repetitive, invasive, painful, and anxiety-producing procedures. As research has revealed, with increased anxiety comes the increased perception of pain and the occurrence of chemotherapy side effects (DuHamel et al. 1999). Inadequately addressed pediatric pain can lead to "conditioned anxiety" (Slifer et al. 2011), pain intolerance, and increased distress and anxiety during subsequent procedures leading to long-term negative neurological, emotional, and health outcomes (Cramton and Gruchala 2012; Taddio et al. 2010). Pain memories of children receiving cancer therapy (Kennedy et al. 2008) can lead to fear of future procedures (Corwin et al. 2012). Therefore, creating the best possible first experience for children by minimizing procedure-related anxiety and pain through the use of procedural support techniques is crucial for children who will face a long road of treatment and repeated procedures.

C.H. Armington, MS, CCLS
H.E. Peach, MS, CCLS (✉)
Division of Pediatric Hematology and Oncology, MassGeneral Hospital for Children, Yawkey 8B, 55 Fruit Street, Boston, MA 02114, USA
e-mail: charmington@mgh.harvard.edu; hpeach@mgh.harvard.edu

S. Hopkinson, MA CCLS
Child Life Services, Development and Continuing Education, Allied Health, Sidra Medical and Research Center, 26999, Doha, Qatar
e-mail: shopkinson@sidra.org
http://www.sidra.org

Education and Preparation

The first step to providing procedural support for children and their families is the implementation of developmentally appropriate education about the diagnosis and procedural preparation. Uncertainty, fear, anxiety, and pain are closely intertwined for many patients with medical conditions. In a 2010 study examining fear of the hospital, Salmela et al. found that 91 % of preschoolers ages four to six expressed fear of at least one element of the hospital or medical treatment with 48 % reporting over seven fears.

A.N. Abrams et al. (eds.), *Pediatric Psychosocial Oncology: Textbook for Multidisciplinary Care*,
DOI 10.1007/978-3-319-21374-3_7

Based on their cognitive development, young children may struggle to cope with medical experiences that are perceived as threatening (Salmela et al. 2010). However providing applicable interventions can reduce medically related anxiety and distress not only for preschoolers but also for children of all ages. Increased general anxiety, eating problems (Salmela et al. 2010), aggression, separation anxiety, sleep disturbances, and behavioral changes (Gaynard et al. 1990) are potential short- and long-term detrimental effects of hospitalization for which practical supportive interventions have become a critical element of caring for children with cancer. In addition to age and cognitive development, it is important to consider the child's premorbid temperament and coping style, previous healthcare experiences, diagnosis, and family dynamics (Koller 2007).

Diagnosis Education: Interventions and Tools

Providing children with information about their illness and medical care at the beginning of their cancer treatment can help to frame the purpose of subsequent procedures, increase understanding, address misconceptions, and open the door for continued communication. Information should be culturally sensitive, accurate, honest, and developmentally appropriate and provided in a child- and family-focused, nonthreatening environment (Mahan 2005; Sobo and Kurtin 2007). Education generally begins by describing how a healthy body functions and then transitions into explaining what is happening in the body when a child has cancer. Various teaching tools, including dolls, books, visuals, and interactive activities, can assist the psychosocial clinician and provide learning opportunities that are tailored to the specific diagnosis of the patient.

Teaching Dolls

Common diagnosis education materials include dolls such as MediKin™ teaching aids. These dolls offer a wide variety of accessories that can be adapted for multiple oncology diagnoses including leukemia, brain, and bone tumors. Since children typically receive a PORT-A-CATH® (port) or central line soon after their diagnosis, the MediKins™ can also be a helpful tool to illustrate where the lines will be placed and how they feel through the "skin" of the doll. For many children, having the opportunity to ask questions about the doll and being able to touch and feel the port, for example, before it is surgically placed, is very empowering. Dolls can serve as a meaningful tool to increase understanding and familiarity not only during diagnosis education but also for procedural preparation.

Diagnosis and Emotion-Themed Reading and Visual Materials

Child friendly books can provide an overview of what children and families can expect while demystifying potentially threatening terms such as "cancer" or "oncology." Helpful explanations of treatment and coping tools can be found in books such as *Chemo, Craziness & Comfort: My book about childhood cancer* and *Healing Images for Children: Teaching Relaxation and Guided Imagery to Children Facing Cancer and Other Serious Illnesses* which serve as useful guides for parents and children. At this early stage in forming a relationship of trust and in an effort to encourage self-expression, books with general themes of identifying and sharing feelings can also be helpful. Some examples include: *How Are You Peeling? Foods with Moods*, *It's Okay to Be Different*, and *Moody Cow Meditates*. For additional suggestions see Chap. 6 regarding bibliotherapy and Chap. 25 for resources. Visual materials such as diagrams or interactive iPad applications ("My Incredible Body" for 9–11-year-olds or "3D Anatomy Lite" for 12–18-year-olds) can assist older school-age patients and adolescents learn about how the body works and launch further discussion regarding diagnosis and treatment.

Interactive Educational Activities

Interactive, hands-on activities can also help children explore the fundamentals of how the body works in relation to their diagnosis. The opportunities for creativity are endless and interventions will vary depending on the child's specific diagnosis and development. One example is a "blood workshop" to help patients diagnosed

Table 7.1 Blood workshop

Ingredients and descriptions
Plasma (*corn syrup*): makes our body's blood, like a workshop
Red blood cells (*dry kidney beans or red hot candies*): give our bodies energy
White blood cells (*dry navy beans or white jellybeans*): keep us healthy
Platelets (*rice or white sprinkles*): help our bodies heal
Leukemia cells "blasts" (*mini marshmallows or white hard candies*): fill up the blood workshop of children who have leukemia
Instructions
1. Fill 2 specimen cups with plasma and explain that these are like the body's blood workshops
2. In one of the cups, make "healthy blood" by inviting the patient to add the red and white blood cells and platelets while you explain the role of each
3. In the second cup, make "unhealthy blood" by inviting the patient to fill this cup nearly all the way with the leukemia cells while explaining that when someone has leukemia, the body's blood workshop makes too many of these cells so that there is no room for the healthy parts of the blood to be made. The child can then add 2 or 3 of the red and white cells and platelets
4. Compare the two cups and explain that the job of the medicine "chemotherapy" is to take the leukemia cells out of the body's blood workshop to make room for healthy blood to be made

with leukemia understand what is happening in their body (Table 7.1). This activity makes the abstract and confusing medical terminology more tangible and easier to visualize. It also gives clinicians the opportunity to explain the purpose of treatment. Other options include beading programs, such as "My Story in Beads" and "Legacy Beads", which offer children an opportunity to document and honor their cancer journey by stringing together beads specific for each aspect of their treatment. Journaling is oftentimes a component of beading journey programs and allows the patients or parents to record treatment facts and/or their feelings about the process.

Role of Child Life Specialists

As described throughout this chapter, children benefit from diagnosis education and procedural preparation and support, which can be provided by various members of the pediatric oncology team. Child life specialists are specifically trained and certified to assist children by optimizing their growth and development, decreasing their anxiety, and fostering positive coping skills through the use of play, education, and art. Child life specialists strive to positively impact how children with cancer manage their medical journey by helping them process potentially traumatic healthcare experiences. Through consultations and interventions, child life specialists address the impact of a cancer diagnosis on children and families and utilize the tools discussed in this chapter to support self-expression, learning, and optimal coping.

Procedural Preparation: Interventions and Tools

The American Pain Society and American Academy of Pediatrics state that one of the keys to managing pain and distress is preparation (Cramton and Gruchala 2012). In turn, preparation can reduce the perception of pain particularly in perioperative settings (Fincher et al. 2012). Therefore, once clinicians have established a relationship of trust and an understanding of treatment goals, procedural preparation becomes the next integral piece to providing continued support. Detailed procedural preparation sessions are most effective for children over 2 years of age (Schechter et al. 2007) and include education about procedure duration, sequence of events, role of the child and caregiver, and sensory information (what the child will see, hear, smell, taste, and feel) (DeMaso and Snell 2013; Mahan 2005). Common procedures that patients may face include surgery, bone marrow aspirations (BMA), lumbar punctures (LP), port accesses, dressing changes, MRIs, CT scans, IVs, and IM injections. The tools psychosocial clinicians implement should be tailored to the developmental needs of the child and may vary in detail depending on the child's learning and coping style, purpose of the procedure, and time frame of the intervention.

Considering the timing for procedural preparation, it is important to allow enough time for information processing while not causing increased anxiety to build (Cramton and Gruchala 2012; Schechter et al. 2007). Generally speaking, procedural preparation should take place earlier for adolescents and closer to the time of the procedure for younger children and always in collaboration with parents to tailor the timing of preparation to the individual needs of the child.

Preparation Books

Preparation books, including those printed, electronic, or on an iPad, can also help to describe the steps of upcoming procedures and encourage dialogue about any concerns or questions that a child may have. Younger children may feel less threatened by illustrated images or photos of a stuffed animal undergoing the procedure, while older children may respond better to photos of a child their own age. To ensure comprehension and to minimize potential misconceptions, it is helpful to ask patients to share their questions, to repeat the steps of the procedure, and to identify their role in the process, for example, to hold their arm as still as a statue. In addition to understanding a child's learning style, coping strategies must also be assessed and understood as a continuum as a child may respond differently to various stressors over time (Kuttner 1996). See Chap. 5 on coping for details. Children who utilize a problem-oriented coping strategy would be more likely to participate in preparations where they generate their own questions; whereas, children with an emotion-oriented coping style may call upon denial tactics or silence (Salmela et al. 2010; Li et al. 2011a). While research suggests that problem-focused coping tends to be more effective for patients, it is important to utilize interventions that reflect each child's needs, comfort level, and ability to engage in the intervention.

Medical Play

In addition to creating pleasure and joy, play can assist children as they prepare for and reenact stressful or threatening medical experiences. Children who engaged in a therapeutic play intervention prior to day surgery demonstrated decreased anxiety scores and emotional behaviors both pre- and postoperatively (Li et al. 2011b). Medical play is a powerful tool that can help children process their treatment journey prior to and following procedures. The goal of medical play is to increase communication, self-expression, preparation, familiarization, and reflection in a developmentally appropriate manner. Medical play provides opportunities for children to practice the steps of a procedure on a doll (role rehearsal/role reversal); engage with symbolic, real, or play medical equipment (medical fantasy play); use medically themed games or puzzles (indirect medical play); or manipulate medical supplies through expressive painting, sculpting, or collage (medical art) (Goldberger 1984). By facilitating educational opportunities in a supervised, nonthreatening environment, psychosocial clinicians can help to reduce the child's fears surrounding their treatment.

Examples of medical play dolls include blank muslin dolls that children can personalize or teaching dolls that are specifically designed for children with cancer. These include Gabe's Chemo Duck Program™ and Shadow Buddies™ which teach children about ports or central lines. With guided supervision, children can practice port accesses or lab draws on their dolls using play or real medical equipment to increase familiarity and empowerment.

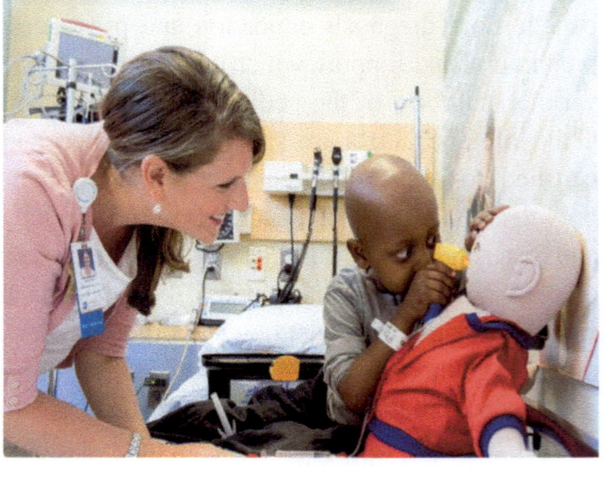

Case Vignette
Chris, a 4-year-old boy with ALL, always arrived to the outpatient hematology and oncology unit with his doll named Annie. At the onset of his diagnosis, the child life specialist had inserted some tubing into Annie that replicated Chris' port. While initially observing the child life specialist with some trepidation, Chris began to actively participate in the steps of "accessing" Annie's port in subsequent sessions. As he gained mastery over this procedure, these medical play opportunities translated into Chris becoming more comfortable when his own port was accessed.

In addition to these medical play materials, Cuzzocrea et al. (2013) found that significant reductions in anxiety can occur following preparation using puppets and storytelling, involving exploratory opportunities with relevant medical equipment, and having a supportive adult present during procedures to remind children of their practiced coping techniques. Preparation, in addition to the use of distraction tools, was most effective in increasing adherence and reducing anxiety compared to distraction alone (Cuzzocrea et al. 2013). Role play and preparation techniques have also been found to increase understanding of what to expect during procedures, reduce fear in younger children, reduce anxiety in older children, and increase overall satisfaction (Hatava et al. 2000).

Providing the opportunity to practice coping strategies through developmentally appropriate procedural education prior to surgery has been shown to minimize the child's and family's anxiety as well as increase coping ability (Fein et al. 2012). Such interventions can also foster trust, reduce uncertainty, correct misconceptions, enhance self-efficacy, and decrease distress (DeMaso and Snell 2013) while increasing coping, understanding, medical adherence, and a sense of control for the child and parent (Schechter et al. 2007; Pattillo and Itano 2001). Diagnosis education and procedural preparation tools help psychosocial clinicians collaborate with children and families to develop a coping plan for the procedure and may involve some of the techniques reviewed in the following section.

Procedural Support: Non-Pharmacological Interventions and Tools

Procedural support works best when both pharmacological and non-pharmacological interventions are utilized when appropriate (Cuzzocrea et al. 2013). The primary purpose of non-pharmacological procedural support interventions is to increase the child's coping ability and sense of control while reducing fear, distress, and pain (Wente 2013). Non-pharmacological strategies may even reduce the overall need for opioid use when effective pain management is achieved (Ahmed et al. 2014). Establishing optimal procedural support includes listening to the child and parents about what has been helpful in the past and introducing supplementary coping tools that build upon what is familiar. More on pain management can be found in Chap. 3.

Environmental Considerations

Creating a calm, child-friendly, engaging environment is essential for anxiety reduction (Fein et al. 2012). Hospital design and its impact on patients exceed the scope of this chapter; however, environmental adjustments can make a tremendous difference. For example, the child's inpatient hospital room should be maintained as a safe haven as much as possible and treatment rooms should be used for invasive procedures (DeMaso and Snell 2013). Removing excess stimuli can help to create a relaxing environment regardless of the procedure taking place in a treatment, exam, or infusion room. When possible, dimming bright lights (Baxter 2013), playing music of the patient's choice, speaking softly, and limiting speakers (Pasero and Smith 1997) establish a setting of comfort. Reducing the number of healthcare providers in the room by implementing the ONE VOICE™ approach includes assigning one person to provide verbal instruction to

Table 7.2 Procedural communication and language considerations

Helpful	Not helpful
• Simple, honest, concrete explanations of procedures • Talk with a child before touching him and speak with firm but warm confidence • Use soft language such as "pressure," "tight squeeze," or "uncomfortable." For example, "some children say that they can feel pressure, you can tell me how it feels for you" • Offer choices only when possible and give directions in the positive: "You will need to keep your body very still, but you can choose something to hold" • Implement a practiced coping plan • Redirect with humor or nonprocedural talk • Recognize a child's specific behavior during procedure, for example, "You held your arm very still"	• Confusing medical jargon: "CAT scan" (cats), IV (ivy plants), shot (guns, punishment), or dressing change (removing clothing) • Apologizing and allowing children to delay procedures. Examples include: "I'm sorry" or "You'll be OK" • Threatening language like "burn," "cut," or "hurt." Examples include: "we are giving you a shot and this may hurt" • Unrealistic choices, criticism, threatening punishment, and negative instructions. For example, "you're such a big boy, you didn't cry last time" or "don't move!" • Lack of a discussed coping plan or strategy • Excess clinician and/or caregiver side conversations during procedure or talking as if child is not present • Generalizing comments about the child such as "You're such a brave patient" that can lead to shame or a seemingly unattainable expectation

the child during the procedure (Baxter 2013), thus avoiding an otherwise chaotic scene. While limiting the number of clinicians is important, encouraging parental presence once parents have been coached on coping techniques and their role can provide increased security for the child in addition to a comfort item such as a stuffed animal from home (Cramton and Gruchala 2012).

Communication and Language

Honesty before and during interventions will help build trust between the clinician and patient (DeMaso and Snell 2013). Telling children "it won't hurt" does not decrease pain perception and erodes the trust between the patient and clinician if discomfort is felt. Table 7.2 provides communication and language considerations that have been found to both increase and decrease children's ability to cope with procedures. In general, terms of reassurance, apologies, and criticisms (Cramton and Gruchala 2012) have been shown to increase distress during procedures, while positive encouragement and validation (Leahy et al. 2008) can help to decrease stress. Additionally, humor can facilitate coping as well as physical, emotional, and spiritual healing by reducing tension and stress while supporting the immune system and increasing control, relaxation, and the release of endorphins (Pattillo and Itano 2001).

Positioning

During a procedure, the experience of fear, lack of control, or a sense of helplessness can be impacted by the child's physical position. Research supports that the supine position causes greater distress to children and parents. Coached and practiced comfort holding techniques can therefore offer more choice, control, and security for the child (Taddio et al. 2010). "Lying supine is the most vulnerable position for humans, particularly when physically restrained with a papoose board or by adults" (Baxter 2013); whereas, sitting upright, having the opportunity to watch the procedure, and being held by a parent can increase a sense of empowerment and safety. The Comfort Measures model developed by Stephens et al. (1999) starts by welcoming parents to be present during the procedure but not forcing parents to do so if they are not comfortable. To enhance coping, the team involved in a procedure should review procedural positioning choices and each person's role so that the child and parent have comfortable physical contact, and the clinician has necessary access and room to perform the medical intervention. A study by Sparks et al. (2007) found that seated parental holding decreased anticipatory stress, recovery time, and distress pre-, during, and post-IV placement and increased comfort and parental satisfaction. Additional benefits of this positioning included fewer staff required to safely hold a child still and a reduction in the time it took

Table 7.3 Cognitive-behavioral procedural distraction and relaxation interventions

Infant: birth–1 year	• Maternal nursing or sweetened solutions on a pacifier • Gently stroking a baby's face or rubbing their back • Singing softly or playing soothing music • Having comfort item (blanket or stuffed animal)
Toddler: 1–3 years	• Blowing bubbles or pinwheels • Shaking rattles, watching light up toys • Reading books that make noise or pop up • Playing peek-a-boo
Preschool: 3–5 years	• Playing with interactive toys (matchbox cars, trains, dolls, or puppets) • Storytelling and singing • Blowing bubbles or pinwheels • Reading books
School-age: 6–12 years	• Holding a parent or clinician's hand • Reading books, toys, counting games, or I Spy games • Breathing exercises: bubble blowing, party blowers, or controlled/conscious breathing such as imagining blowing up a balloon or blowing out birthday candles • Using your imagination to "travel" to a favorite or calming place
Adolescent: 13–18 years	• Practicing coping techniques in advance • Utilizing relaxation, breathing, guided imagery, or progressive muscle relaxation • Squeezing a stress ball or parent's hand • Listening to calming or favorite music

for IV placement (Sparks et al. 2007). Certainly, considerations of safety for the patient, parent, and clinician must always be taken into account.

Distraction

Children who have experienced extreme distress in previous procedures typically respond similarly in later procedures. With the intention of alleviating distress and increasing children's ability to cope (Heden et al. 2009), distraction redirects attention away from the pain-inflicting stressor and positively influences their reactions to future procedures (McCarthy et al. 2010). Benefits of distraction for children with chronic conditions include improving cooperation and reducing self-reported pain (Slifer et al. 2011). Distraction is commonly utilized during needlesticks (Sadeghi et al. 2013) and may also be extremely helpful during other repeated procedures such as dressing changes in pediatric oncology treatment.

Distraction interventions can be considered *active* when patients are fully engaged during the procedure and are using multiple senses such as breathing exercises, interactive toys, and guided imagery or *passive* when the child remains focused on a stimulus such as reading, watching a movie, or listening to music (Sadeghi et al. 2013; Koller and Goldman 2012). For example, children distracted by interactive electronic tablets during IM injections and port accesses reported significantly less distress the second time the procedure took place compared to those who did not have the intervention (Dahlquist et al. 2002). Distraction can also influence perceived pain perception. In a prospective, randomized controlled study of 123 children, 96 % of the children in the experimental group using Flippits® cards as distraction during venipuncture reported less pain than their previous experience without the cards (Inal and Kelleci 2012).

For some children active distraction can be more effective as it is multisensory; however, passive distraction can benefit children who may have difficulty engaging in a complex activity while undergoing a procedure. Similar to the other interventions described in the chapter, distraction techniques should be tailored to the individual child and the procedure involved (Koller and Goldman 2012; Sadeghi et al. 2013). Table 7.3 reviews cognitive-behavioral procedural distraction and relaxation interventions that empower children by giving them a defined role and the tools to help themselves during a procedure.

Children with cancer can gain a greater sense of control when given a choice of specific distraction interventions to help them through a procedure.

Lazarus and Folkman's (1984) theory on cognitive appraisal, stress, and coping links one's sense of control over a threatening source to one's assessment of that threat. Accordingly, children who have more control over their procedures and environment experience decreased perceived threat appraisal and distress (Li et al. 2011b). For children who like to be actively involved, they might cope best by participating in removing their dressing, counting, or watching the port access (Pasero and Smith 1997); whereas, for information-avoiders, watching the procedure may increase their level of distress and looking away would be more applicable (Walworth 2005). While research indicates that children who like to be actively involved experience better patient outcomes (DeMaso and Snell 2013), careful assessment of each child's unique coping abilities during the time of the intervention is necessary in order to develop a personalized coping plan.

Relaxation

Teaching and implementing relaxation techniques provide another option for procedural support. An essential element of "relaxation training" includes deep breathing exercises which bring awareness to the breath (DeMaso and Snell 2013). Breathing exercises can be a powerful tool to help children practice for repeated port accesses and dressing changes. Children's yoga taught by certified practitioners can also assist children in gaining a sense of empowerment, control, relaxation, mindfulness, confidence, and self-esteem.

Case Vignette

Amy, a 7-year-old girl with rhabdomyosarcoma, participated in a weekly yoga class for children with cancer taught by the child life specialist. She learned a number of breathing techniques and chose the "snake breath," breathing in deeply and steadily releasing the breath with a hissing sound, to help her relax prior to and during her weekly port accessing. Throughout the course of her year-long treatment, she used the "snake breath" as her primary coping tool during her many procedures.

In addition to controlled breathing, progressive muscle relaxation is another empowering intervention that can promote a sense of calm and tension release. This requires complete concentration and involves the flexing and relaxation of isolated muscle groups (DeMaso and Snell 2013). Engaging the natural creativity of children through relaxation and imagery techniques may also be very beneficial. Guided imagery and visualization actively engage children in vividly reconstructing a place that brings a sense of comfort and happiness or even alters the pain perception and sensation (Kuttner 1996), for example, shrinking a "boulder" of pain down to a "pebble."

Visualization is an important tool that encourages relaxation and sleep and even decreases the need for medications and restraining measures by increasing endorphins and lowering blood pressure (Hoffart and Keene 1998). For pediatric patients in particular, visualization harnesses their imaginations, helps them to develop a sense of inner strength and confidence, and reduces anxiety, thus making this a helpful support for children with cancer (Hoffart and Keene 1998). For example, during a guided imagery session, a clinician can work with the patient to determine a setting to which he would like to travel, such as the beach. This "visit" to the beach should include all of the sensory experiences in order to fully engage the child's imagination and shift the focus from the stress of the procedure to a relaxed and calm state.

"The Magic Glove" is an example of a hypnotic pain management technique used to control anticipatory anxiety. It involves having the child concentrate and imagine the magic glove protecting the child's hand and creating an analgesic response to pain stimuli. This technique is generally most successful among 3–12-year-olds (Kuttner 2013). Procedural support techniques can offer children the opportunity to gain self-confidence and feel empowered as they learn coping strategies which may also be utilized for stressors beyond their medical treatment. The more often a tool such as progressive muscle relaxation or visual imagery is used, the more quickly the child is likely to experience benefits (Kuttner 1996). Therefore it is important to introduce such resources early on and repeatedly in a child's treatment.

Family-Centered Procedural Preparation and Support

The family plays an integral role during procedural support interventions as the core source of comfort for the child. Parental presence has been found to be the most common benefiting factor for preschoolers while they are in the hospital (Salmela et al. 2010). According to Ross and Ross (1984), 99 % of children ages five to twelve (n=994) stated that having their parents present would have helped them the most during their procedure regardless of the level of reported pain involved.

When parents are empowered and well informed of the procedure, coping tools, and their role, their own anxiety decreases and they are better able to support and reduce the anxiety felt by their child (Fein et al. 2012; Fincher et al. 2012). Parental presence and involvement during behavioral interventions have been found to decrease procedural-related distress and impact how the child reacts to painful procedures (McCarthy et al. 2010). Since calm parental presence is most beneficial to children (DeMaso and Snell 2013; Yip et al. 2009), it is important to increase parental understanding and decrease their procedure-related stress as well. However, parents who do not feel comfortable being present should be respected for their decision and not forced to participate (Fincher et al. 2012) as they can still provide comfort and support to their child in many other meaningful ways both prior to and following medical procedures.

Procedure Processing and Reflection

Following each stage of intervention, be it diagnosis education, procedural preparation, or procedural support, the clinician should engage the child to make sure that there are no misunderstandings and correct misconceptions. Regardless of the tool(s) used, post-procedural review with the child to determine the accuracy of the preparation and to make any notable changes for future treatment is important (DeMaso and Snell 2013). It is useful to ask the child what the experience was like. For example, questions such as "Was it what you expected?," "Were there any surprises?," and "Was the distraction you chose helpful?" can empower children to reflect on the procedure and their coping strategy. These conversations bring the process of preparation and support full circle and ensure that the interventions were beneficial in reducing distress. By obtaining feedback, clinicians are able to validate children's feelings and assure them that their needs were heard and that they will remain involved in their care. As children may receive active treatment for 2–3 years, and follow-up well beyond, revisiting coping strategies as they progress through treatment is important to make sure that with growth and development, any questions or adaptations to coping techniques are addressed.

Conclusion

Throughout the cancer trajectory, children will face multiple invasive procedures. By involving children in a procedural plan, psychosocial clinicians empower patients in their care and decrease their stress. Diagnosis education, procedural preparation, and procedural support are crucial elements in caring for children with cancer. While the American Academy of Pediatrics recommends the incorporation of child life specialists or other psychosocial team members trained in non-pharmacological strategies for reducing anxiety and perceived pain in children (Fein et al. 2012), supportive interventions can also be implemented by other members of the multidisciplinary team. As each child is unique, psychosocial clinicians, parents, and children should collaborate to create an individual care plan that enhances development, optimal coping skills, and ultimately mastery of procedures throughout cancer treatment.

Clinical Pearls

- Diagnosis education, preparation, and supportive interventions are key elements of procedural support.
- Children, parents, and psychosocial clinicians should work together to create a procedural support plan that reflects each child's unique needs to maximize optimal coping and mastery.
- Providing children with information about their illness and medical care at the beginning of their cancer treatment can help to frame the purpose of subsequent procedures, increase understanding, address misconceptions, and open the door for continued communication.
- Education and preparation should include accurate, honest, and developmentally appropriate information given within a culturally sensitive, child- and family-focused nonthreatening environment.

  Considerations for non-pharmacological procedural interventions should include distraction, relaxation, environment, positioning, and communication/language to help children cope throughout their cancer treatment.

Additional Resources

Suggested Book Resources

3 months to 3 years:

This Is my Hair. Parr, T (2011). Little, Brown Books for Young Readers, New York, NY.

3 to 7 years:

It's Okay to Be Different. Parr, T (2001). Little, Brown Books for Young Readers, New York, NY.

Feelings. Parr, T (2009). Little, Brown Books for Young Readers, New York, NY.

4 to 8 years:

How Are You Peeling? Foods with Moods. Play with Your Food. Freeymann, S., and Elffers, J. (2004). LLC. Scholastic, New York, NY.

Visiting Feelings. Rubenstein, L (2002). Magination Press. American Psychological Association, Washington, DC.

Moody Cow Meditates. MacLean,K.L (2009). Wisdom Publications MA. Somerville, MA.

Websites

Medkin Teaching Aids: https://legacyproductsinc.com/

Cloth Dolls: http://www.mefinefoundation.org/what-we-do/striving-for-more/cancer-support-programs/medical-play-dolls/

Shadow Buddies Foundation: http://www.shadowbuddies.org/product/port-a-cath-buddy/

Gabe's Chemo Duck: http://chemoduck.org/for-kids/meet-chemo-duck/

ONE VOICE: http://www.onevoice4kids.com/

Legacy Beads: http://www.stjude.org/legacy-beads

Educational Apps

My Incredible Body-Guide to learn about the human body for children (age 4+ but designed for 9–11)

The Human Body by Tinybop (ages 6–8)

Visual Anatomy Lite (12+)

3D Anatomy Lite (12+)

References

Ahmed M, Modak S, Sequeira S (2014) Acute pain relief after Mantram meditation in children with neuroblastoma undergoing anti-GD2 monoclonal antibody therapy. J Pediatr Hematol Oncol 36(2):152–155

Baxter A (2013) Common office procedures and analgesia considerations. Pediatr Clin North Am 60:1163–1183

Corwin DJ, Kessler DO, Auerbach M et al (2012) An intervention to improve pain management in the pediatric emergency department. Pediatr Emerg Care 28(6):524–8

Cramton RE, Gruchala NE (2012) Managing procedural pain in pediatric patients. Curr Opin Pediatr 24(4):530–538

Cuzzocrea F, Gugliandolo MC, Larcan R et al (2013) A psychological preoperative program: effects on anxi-

ety and cooperative behaviors. Paediatr Anaesth 23(2):139–43
Dahlquist LM, Pendley JS, Landthrip DS et al (2002) Distraction intervention for preschoolers undergoing intramuscular injections and subcutaneous port access. Health Psychol 21(1):94–99
DeMaso DR, Snell C (2013) Promoting coping in children facing pediatric surgery. Semin Pediatr Surg 22(3):134–138
DuHamel KN, Redd WH, Vickberg SM (1999) Behavioral interventions in the diagnosis, treatment and rehabilitation of children with cancer. Acta Oncol 38(6):719–34
Fein J, Zempsky W, Cravero J (2012) Relief of pain and anxiety in pediatric patients in emergency medical systems. Pediatrics 130(5):1391–1405
Fincher W et al (2012) The effectiveness of a standardized preoperative preparation in reducing child and parent anxiety: a single-blind randomized controlled trial. J Clin Nurs 21:946–955
Gaynard L, Wolfer J, Goldberger J et al (1990) Psychosocial care of children in hospitals: A clinical practice manual. Association for the Care of. Children's Health, Bethesda
Goldberger J (1984) The use of toys with hospitalized children. Child Environ Q 1(3):56–62
Hatava P, Olsson G, Lagerkranser M (2000) Preoperative psychosocial preparation for children undergoing ENT operations: A comparison of two methods. Paediatr Anesthesiol 10:477–486
Heden L, VON Essen L, Ljungman G (2009) Randomized interventions for needle procedures in children with cancer. Eur J Cancer Care 18(4):358–63
Hoffart MB, Keene E (1998) Body-mind-spirit: the benefits of visualization. Am J Nurs 98(12):44–47
Inal S, Kelleci M (2012) Distracting children during blood draw: Looking through distraction cards is effective in pain relief of children during blood draw. Int J Nurs Pract 18:210–219
Kennedy R, Luhmann J, Zempsky W (2008) Clinical implications of unmanaged needle-insertion pain and distress in children. Pediatrics 122:130–133
Koller D (2007) Child life council evidence-based practice statement preparing children and adolescents for medical procedures. Child Life Council. Available http://www.childlife.org. Accessed 24 Oct 2014
Koller D, Goldman R (2012) Distraction techniques for children undergoing procedures: a critical review of pediatric research. J Pediatr Nurs 27:652–681
Kuttner L (1996) A child in pain. Hartley & Marks Publishers, Seattle, Washington
Kuttner L (2013) The magic glove: a hypnotic pain management technique. Available http://pediatric-pain.ca/wp-content/uploads/2013/04/The_Magic_Glove12.pdf. Accessed 3 Apr 2015
Lazarus R, Folkman S (1984) Stress, appraisal, and coping. Springer, New York
Leahy S, Kennedy R, Hesselgrave J et al (2008) On the front lines: lessons learned in implementing multidisciplinary peripheral venous access pain-management programs in pediatric hospitals. Pediatrics 122(3):161–170
Li W, Chung J, Ho E et al (2011a) Coping strategies used by children hospitalized with cancer: an exploratory study. Psychooncology 20(9):969–76
Li W, Chung J, Ho E (2011b) The effectiveness of therapeutic play, using virtual reality computer games, in promoting the psychological well-being of children hospitalized with cancer. J Clin Nurs 20(15–16): 2135–43
Mahan CC (2005) Preparing children for health-care encounters. In: Rollins J, Bolig R, Mahan CC (eds) Meeting children's psychosocial needs across the health-care continuum. PRO-ED, Austin, Texas, pp 43–75
McCarthy AM, Kleiber C, Hanrahan K et al (2010) Factors explaining children's responses to intravenous needle insertions. Nurs Res 59(6):407–416
Pasero CL, Smith NK (1997) Pain control: nondrug measures for painful procedures. Am J Nurs 97(8):18–20
Pattillo CGS, Itano J (2001) Laughter is the best medicine. Am J Nurs 101(4):40–43
Ross D, Ross S (1984) Childhood pain: the school-aged child's viewpoint. Pain 20:179–191
Sadeghi T, Mohammadi N, Shamshiri M et al (2013) Effect of distraction on children's pain during intravenous catheter insertion. J Spec Pediatr Nurs 18(2):109–114
Salmela M, Salanterä S, Aronen E (2010) Child-reported hospital fears in 4 to 6-year-old children. Pediatr Nurs 35(5):1222–1231
Schechter NL, Zempsky WT, Cohen LL et al (2007) Pain reduction during pediatric immunizations: Evidence-based review and recommendations. Pediatrics 119(5):1184–1198
Slifer KJ, Hankinson JC, Zettler MA et al (2011) Distraction, exposure therapy, counterconditioning, and topical anesthetic for acute pain management during needle sticks in children with intellectual and developmental disabilities. Clin Pediatr 50(8):688–697
Sobo E, Kurtin P (eds) (2007) Optimizing care for young children with special health care needs: knowledge and strategies for navigating the system. Brookes Publishing, Baltimore
Sparks L, Setlik J, Luhman J (2007) Parental holding and positioning to decrease IV distress in young children: a randomized controlled trial. J Pediatr Nurs 22(6):440–447
Stephens B, Barkey M, Hall H (1999) Techniques to comfort children during stressful procedures. Adv Mind Body Med 15(1):49–60
Taddio A, Appleton M, Bortolussi R et al (2010) Reducing the pain of childhood vaccination: an evidence-based clinical practice guideline. CMAJ 182(18):843–855
Walworth DD (2005) Procedural-support music therapy in the healthcare setting: a cost-effectiveness analysis. J Pediatr Nurs 20(4):276–284
Wente S (2013) Nonpharmacologic pediatric pain management in emergency departments: a systematic review of the literature. J Emerg Nurs 39(2):140–150
Yip P, Middleton P, Cyna AM et al (2009) Non-pharmacological interventions for assisting the induction of anaesthesia in children. Cochrane Database Syst Rev. doi:10.1002/14651858.CD006447

Psychiatric Issues in Pediatric Oncology: Diagnosis and Management

8

Julia Kearney, Abraham S. Bartell, and Maryland Pao

Psychiatric Issues in Pediatric Oncology: Diagnosis and Management

The presentation of intense distress of patients, parents, and others on the pediatric cancer unit remains all too common. From uncertainty and worry to suffering, grief, and loss, the emotional reality of the life-threatening and life-limiting nature of the disease is ever present. An essential skill of the psycho-oncologist (and any oncologist) is "normalization" of negative emotions and behaviors, in other words, reassuring an individual that their sadness, anxiety, fear, sense of helplessness, and possibly guilt are normal responses to a profoundly challenging experience. It can therefore be a subtle matter to determine the presence of psychopathology in people presenting in distressing situations. How much sadness or distress is "normal," when does it cross into a disorder, what behaviors are "understandable," when is mental illness present, and how do we explain it to someone who is in such a situation? This chapter addresses these questions and specific treatment recommendations when a psychiatric disorder is suspected in the pediatric oncology patient, with support from available literature and clinical experience.

J. Kearney, MD (✉) • A.S. Bartell, MD
Departments of Pediatrics and Psychiatry & Behavioral Sciences, Memorial Sloan Kettering, 641 Lexington Avenue, 7th Floor, New York, NY 10022, USA
e-mail: kearneyj@mskcc.org; bartella@mskcc.org

M. Pao, MD
Office of the Clinical Director, National Institute of Mental Health (NIMH), 10 Center Drive 10/6-5340, Bethesda, MD 20892-1276, USA
e-mail: paom@mail.nih.gov

The Consultation-Liaison Child and Adolescent Psychiatrist in Pediatric Oncology

The pediatric consultation-liaison (C/L) psychiatrist, also referred to as pediatric psychosomatic specialist in some hospitals, is a child and adolescent psychiatrist with an expertise through specific experience and/or training in the psychiatric care of children and adolescents with medical illness (such as in triple board and/or psychosomatic medicine fellowship training programs). Many models of C/L psychiatry exist, but recent focus is on the development of integrated behavioral health programs embedded physically in pediatric centers, with a focus on collaborative multidisciplinary care and provider continuity (Talmi and Fazio 2012; AAP. National Center for Medical Home Implementation 2015). At a minimum, pediatric oncology programs should develop relationships with C/L child psychiatry services within their center to provide access to

A.N. Abrams et al. (eds.), *Pediatric Psychosocial Oncology: Textbook for Multidisciplinary Care*, DOI 10.1007/978-3-319-21374-3_8

psychiatric consultation when needed. Close collaboration and mutual support between C/L child psychiatrists and pediatric oncologists, nurses, social workers, psychologists, child life, and other psychosocial clinicians is the essence of this work, from introduction of the psychiatric consultant to biopsychosocial evaluation, workup, and treatment planning.

Diagnostic Considerations

For accurate treatment formulation and clear communication with patients, families, and medical teams, it is important to be able to diagnose primary and secondary psychiatric syndromes, often in the context of complicated physical and emotional symptom burden. Psychiatric disorders may be present prior to a diagnosis of cancer (e.g., ADHD, separation anxiety disorder), precipitated by the stress of disease or treatment (e.g., reactive depression or disease related anxiety in a vulnerable patient with a family history of anxiety and mood disorders), directly caused by the disease or treatment (steroid-related psychosis or postsurgical posterior fossa syndrome), or completely coincidental to cancer (development of bipolar disorder or schizophrenia). Evaluation starts by collecting a comprehensive history of present illness from multiple sources (patient, caregiver, and hospital staff familiar with the patient). It is critical to get baseline information of the patient's development and prior psychological, emotional, and academic functioning. Discussion of family history is key for recognition of genetic predisposition for hereditary mental illnesses, mood disorders and anxiety. The child psychiatrist consultant should be familiar with cancer treatments and supportive medications, their expected courses, side effects, and treatment road maps to help with diagnosis, treatment planning, and anticipatory guidance with families. Regular examination of medication regimens and laboratory trends is essential.

Many psychiatric diagnoses are the same in children with or without cancer and must remain on the mind of the clinician: e.g., ADHD, oppositional defiant disorder (ODD), panic attacks, separation anxiety, and selective mutism. Some diagnoses, however, have particular presentations in the psycho-oncology setting and those will be discussed specifically here.

Family Functioning and Mental Illness

The impact of parent functioning on child adjustment, coping, and functioning should not be underestimated in the general pediatric psychosocial assessment and specifically in pediatric psycho-oncology (Rosenberg et al. 2014; Pai et al. 2007) (see Chap. 9, Family Interventions). The consultant should take this opportunity to screen parents for mental illness, an important part of a holistic assessment, as parent distress and impairment is common and may affect a child's coping with cancer. Parent assessment is important for understanding a child's presentation. Evidence suggests that identification and treatment of parent psychopathology, or other systemic interventions (e.g., provision of alternate caregivers for respite, etc.) to buffer the effects of parents' symptoms on children, may result in more rapid and complete resolution of psychiatric symptoms of children, with less potential for side effects of psychopharmacologic intervention (Waters et al. 2009)

Psychopharmacology for Medically Ill Children

Psychotropic medication can be safe and effective even in the medically complex pediatric oncology population. Estimates show that psychotropic medications are used in 6 % of the general pediatric population and at likely double that rate in the pediatric cancer population (Zito et al. 2003; Pao et al. 2006) The process of Federal Drug Administration approval for use of drugs in children is based on limited available evidence from specific pediatric psychopharmacologic studies (Kearns and Hawley 2014). While child psychiatrists prefer to use psychotropic medications "on-label" for their pediatric patients; it is not uncommon that certain medications are used "off-label" when no other treatment is available or when the usual treatments are contraindicated. This practice is guided by evidence for the use of these medications in adults but not yet approved in pediatrics or FDA approval for use in pediatrics but for different disorders or symptoms than the labeling indicates.

The threshold to consider medication treatment of psychiatric symptoms is reached when symptoms interrupt or disrupt necessary medical treatment (e.g., through nonadherence, inability to communicate with or assess the patient), present safety concerns (e.g., agitation while connected to intravenous infusions or with severe thrombocytopenia), or cause the patient significant suffering. The choice of which medication to recommend follows the framework of *applied clinical therapeutics*, which is the consideration of all evidence and experience about the patient, the disease, and the medication, integrated and applied to clinical decision making. Considerations within this framework may include:

- Pharmacokinetics: *the study of the biological fate of external substances or medication administered from the moment of administration to complete elimination from the body.*
  - Routes of administration may be limited by developmental stage, nausea, gastrointestinal (GI) disease, or toxicity (e.g., impaired oral absorption in patients with severe diarrhea and transdermal formulations contraindicated with severe skin rashes).
  - Distribution can be affected by height, weight, nutritional state, and fluid balance.
  - Hepatic cytochrome p450 interactions of multiple drug regimens can profoundly affect metabolism.
  - Excretion affected by liver, GI, and renal function.
- Pharmacodynamics: *the study of a drug's biochemical and physiological effects on the body including mechanisms of action and the dose–response relationship.*
  - Drug–disease-state interactions (e.g., hypotensive effects of drugs in patients with low blood pressure; possible suppressive effects on bone marrow in patients with hematologic illness)
  - Consideration of potential serotonin syndrome and neuroleptic malignant syndrome in differential diagnosis of vital sign abnormalities
- Pharmacogenomics (or pharmacogenetics): the study of the role of genetic variations in drug response by correlating gene expression or single-nucleotide polymorphisms with drug absorption, distribution, metabolism, and elimination, as well as drug receptor target effects. *Pharmacogenetics* focuses on single drug–gene interactions, while *pharmacogenomics* encompasses a more genome-wide association approach, incorporating genomics and proteomics to consider the effects of multiple genes on drug response.
  - Patients with particular *p450 polymorphisms* are prone to nonresponse, overresponse, or increased toxicity due to individual metabolism. Genetic testing can predict this in some cases and dosing can be adjusted (Drug-Gene Alerts — Mayo Clinic Center for Individualized Medicine, 2014).
  - *Family history* of response to drugs may imply similar inherited pharmacogenomics, even if testing is not available to show this empirically.

Psychiatric Treatment Planning in the Medical Setting

The final recommendation for treatment with a psychotropic medication should take into consideration practical issues such as the availability of the medication, cost, route of administration and dosage forms, dosage range, flexibility of dosing, interactions with other medications, and other special characteristics of the medication. Consultants should collaborate by problem-solving with medical teams, families, and patients for devising and implementing successful drug treatment regimens.

Informed consent for psychotropic medication should include discussion of treatment options and alternatives, risks, and benefits of the treatment, known adverse effects, dosing scheme ("How much?"), duration and timing of treatment ("How long?"), and legal and ethical considerations including off-label use and black box warnings.

Inherent to successful psychiatric treatment in the pediatric medical setting is the establishment of a four-way relationship of collaboration and open communication between the patient, parent, medical team, and psychiatric consultant. The medical team may need support and education about the consultant's formulation of the patient and their symptoms and the medical provider's own countertransference. This is traditionally considered the "liaison" aspect of the C/L work. Ideally, psychoeducation in the context of collaborative relationships will help manage all parties' expectations of the treatment effects: what symptoms will and won't respond to medications, what is an expected timeline for response to medication, and what is the role of adjunctive therapies in addition to medications. The team can then reinforce the psychiatric treatment plan as part of the patient's overall care, and the patient and parent are able to feel supported with consistent, psychologically informed care.

Psychiatric Disorders and Symptoms in Pediatric Psycho-oncology

Complex Symptom Management: Distinguishing Psychological from Medical Symptoms

Few patients with cancer present with psychosomatic syndromes that meet full diagnostic criteria, such as functional neurological symptom disorder (formerly known as conversion disorder in DSM-IV). Much more common, however, is the request to determine whether a patient has a psychological cause of unexplained or difficult to manage physical symptoms (e.g., pain, nausea/vomiting, headache, fatigue, etc.) that seem out of proportion to known pathophysiology. The interaction between psychological stressors and physical symptoms of disease is thought to account for the increased rates of anxiety disorders in young patients with medical illness (Pao and Bosk 2011). Patients with poor coping, lack of psychosocial supports, or lack of age appropriate explanations for their symptoms may be particularly at risk for this type of presentation. School-age children (or older children with behavioral and emotional regression) may present with developmentally typical somatic symptoms (such as headaches and stomachaches) as a manifestation of anxiety. A full psychiatric evaluation and review of the medical record, patterns and triggers of the physical symptoms, workup for alternate causes of the symptoms, and success of treatments attempted is warranted. Evaluation of the child's explanation of the symptoms and understanding of their own illness can uncover fears and misconceptions that may feed anxiety around a particular symptom. An understanding of the parent (or caregiver)–child relationship is helpful in determining whether parents can distinguish pain from anxiety, behavioral distress, or manipulation, in their child. For an accurate assessment, the consultant may need to confront the defensiveness that can result from a patient thinking a psychiatrist has been called because the medical team believes the symptoms (pain, nausea, etc.) are "all in my head," exaggerated, or manufactured. An up-front explanation of the mind–body connection, anxiety components of pain or nausea, and reassurance that the mental health evaluation is not an attempt to discredit the patient but to help them improve the teams' understanding and ability to treat their symptoms can help form an alliance with the patient and their family.

If anxiety or depression is present, treatment is warranted regardless of whether the psychological symptoms "cause," worsen, or are a reaction to the physical symptoms, and it is not necessary to insist the patient believes or admits to the diagnostic formulation to proceed with an evidence-based therapy. Even without realizing the full impact of their emotional distress on their physical well-being, many patients and families benefit from medical play, cognitive behavioral techniques, and motivational interviewing to reduce fear of the physical symptoms, improve communication with medical staff, clarify medical assessment, and improve patient functioning. Family psychoeducation and support can modify family response to symptoms and reduce the unwitting reinforcement of the child's symptom with undue anxiety and attention.

Depression

Case Vignette

Nick, a 9-year-old boy, with a strong family history of mood disorders in mother, presented 3 months post-diagnosis of high-risk acute lymphocytic leukemia (HR-ALL) with severe anorexia, lethargy, and marked anhedonia persisting through a recovery period in his chemotherapy schedule, where he had not received treatment for over 2 weeks. Medical complications were ruled out and psychiatric consultation was sought. He had demonstrated irritable mood and loss of energy during steroid courses in induction and consolidation, but post-steroids the irritable mood had given way to a flat affect, helpless behaviors, and periods of crying. A G-tube was placed for nutritional repletion and support. This had stabilized his weight loss but he did not gain weight and his appetite and energy did not improve. On interview with the child psychiatrist, he reported feeling guilty for the trouble he was causing his mother since he got sick and only having interest in doing things he could no longer do like riding his bike. He asked if he would die from his cancer and shared that he thought he would, but denied wanting to die. Over the following 10 days, he and his mom were seen three times for assessment and initiation of therapy. However, he did not engage in the therapy and did not show any improvement. ***Diagnosis***: major depressive episode. ***Recommendations***: He was started on sertraline 12.5 mg daily and titrated to 50 mg daily over the course of the following month (an off-label use of a commonly used SSRI that is only FDA approved in children ages 6–17 for OCD). ***Outcome***: He had an excellent response to the medication and nutritional repletion and was able to participate in multiple integrative medicine and psychosocial supportive therapies at the center. His appetite, mood, energy, and interest improved to baseline level and he again demonstrated a mischievous wit and fascination with war-themed video games and films. He was maintained on sertraline for 2 years until 6 months post-leukemia therapy when he tolerated a slow taper off the medication.

While studies have shown that it is common for pediatric cancer patients and their families to experience intense transient distress around the diagnosis of cancer, and at other vulnerable points in the treatment trajectory, most demonstrate resilience in the face of this distress and do not meet criteria for psychopathology (Stuber 2012). A recent Children's Oncology Group (COG) prospective study of a homogeneous group of 159 children with standard risk acute lymphoblastic leukemia (SR-ALL) showed that children in this population do have a higher than expected risk for anxiety (25 %) and depression (21 %) at 1 month post-diagnosis and the risk of depression persists up to 1 year post-diagnosis, particularly in children who are Hispanic and whose families are poorly functioning (Myers et al. 2014). Similar studies are needed to investigate the risks for other oncology patient populations, who may have additional disease and treatment-related risk factors such as poorer prognosis, higher symptom burden, and cranial radiation or other CNS-related effects.

Recognition of depression is an important clinical issue. At the time of cancer diagnosis, initial adjustment difficulties with depressed or anxious mood may commonly appear due to the idea of having cancer and the rapid drastic life changes that follow. However, the acceptance (by inexperienced or nonpsychiatric staff or families) "that everyone who has cancer is depressed" or that depression is "appropriate" or normal can be misleading and allow impairing anxiety and depression to be underdiagnosed and undertreated in this population (Ruland et al. 2009; Kersun et al. 2009). Depression may develop as a patient's vulnerability (due to a strong positive family history of psychiatric disorder or the child's own previous psychiatric history) (Rosenstein et al. 2014) becomes exacerbated by the biological and psychological stresses of cancer and treatment. As cancer treatment duration continues, patients who become clinically depressed may have difficulty coping and be less adherent with their cancer treatment which can then create a downward spiral and lead to worsening depressive symptoms (Patenaude and Kupst 2005). In survivorship, children who have significant and severe late side effects also tend to have poorer self-esteem and be more depressed (Institute of Medicine (US) and National Research Council (US) and National Cancer Policy Board 2003).

Even for experienced clinicians, it can be challenging to determine if a child with cancer has major depression given the number of overlapping somatic symptoms such as changes in sleep, appetite, level of energy or fatigue, and concentration. These concomitant neurovegetative symptoms and the mental symptoms of lassitude and apathy mimic symptoms of depression when a patient is neutropenic in the same way some animal models demonstrate cytokine-induced "sickness behaviors" (Cleeland et al. 2003). There are suggestions that a subtype of depression may be related to inflammatory pathways which could prove particularly relevant in cancer patients (Raison and Miller 2011). Clinicians working with children with cancer may need to focus on the more cognitive aspects of depression such as anhedonia, guilt, poor self-esteem, or feeling like a burden on others to distinguish more syndromic major depression. It is important to diagnose depression as it can affect quality of life and treatment adherence in patients with childhood cancer (Kersun et al. 2009).

Suicidal Ideation

If the oncologic disease progresses with relapses and treatment failures, it can sometimes be difficult to understand what a child means if they articulate "feeling tired of fighting." These passive thoughts about dying or "giving up" may be realistic and not a sign of intention for self-harm, but are frightening to the patient, family, and staff. Clinicians need to gently probe for active suicidal ideation in the setting of depression, but often clinicians are afraid to ask for fear of upsetting the child or "putting ideas in their head." The myth of iatrogenic suicidal ideation by asking children about suicide during an assessment has been refuted in a randomized controlled clinical trial (RCT) (Gould et al. 2005).

In adult patients at end of life, the "desire for hastened death" has been associated with demoralization syndrome and is more prevalent in patients with poorly controlled physical symptoms, inadequately treated depression and anxiety, and reduced social functioning and support (Robinson et al. 2014). While this has not been studied in children or adolescents, it is essential that pediatric clinicians obtain a comfort level and skill in discussing death and dying with parents and then with pediatric patients themselves. Prudent management of suicidality in pediatric cancer patients is to aggressively address all modifiable symptoms while ensuring the patient's safety (see Chap. 14 on palliative care). As dual-diagnosis medical–psychiatric inpatient units are rare, the inpatient pediatric oncology ward with 1:1 companion for suicide precautions may sometimes be the safest location, medically and psychiatrically, for treatment of a suicidal pediatric oncology patient.

Finally, adult survivors of childhood cancers are at increased risk for suicidal ideation related to cancer diagnosis as well as posttreatment mental and physical health problems, even many years after completion of therapy and therefore should be monitored in outpatient settings into adulthood (Recklitis et al. 2010).

Anxiety

Case Vignette

Leah, a 7-year-old girl with stage IV neuroblastoma, presents for evaluation and treatment of anxiety in the context of antibody therapy. She has no evidence of active disease after five cycles of high-dose chemotherapy, surgical resection of primary abdominal tumor, and radiation to two small sites of bony metastases. She has undergone two prior cycles of the anti-GD2 antibody therapy, which she found very difficult to tolerate as it caused abdominal and back pain during infusion. She understands the disease and the purpose of the antibody very well and she and her parents benefited from working with child life and dance therapy to learn coping and relaxation techniques to use during treatment. On the way to the medical center for another week long course of antibody therapy, she develops stomach pain and nausea, which she says comes from "thinking about the medicine." On arrival to clinic, she is retching and unable to take her oral premedications. Parents report she is a mildly anxious child at baseline, with no history of psychiatric treatment, but report she had self-limited separation anxiety at the start of school and nightmares for 1 month after the death of grandfather last year. However, they report that over the past month, between the cycles of antibody, she has been playful, social, and interactive at home, with improving physical status after her intensive therapies. She says she is looking forward to going to school again when they return home after this cycle of antibody. ***Diagnosis***: Adjustment disorder with anxiety. ***Recommendations***: Child psychiatry recommends a trial of lorazepam 0.5 mg orally on the mornings prior to her clinic visits for the rest of this cycle and the next cycle. ***Outcome***: The next morning, after the first dose, she tolerates antibody therapy much better with minimal opiate medication for pain. By the fifth cycle, 2 months later, she only needs a single dose of lorazepam on the way to clinic the first day of treatment and copes well with treatment the rest of the week.

Anxiety symptoms are common in medically ill children, often manifesting as irritability, anticipatory anxiety for procedures, sleep disturbance, behavioral regression, and unexplained physical symptoms (Pao and Bosk 2011). Prevalence of anxiety disorders in medically ill children and adolescent age ranges from 7 to 40 % in studies, compared to approximately 13 % in the general population of children and adolescents (Lavigne and Faier-Routman 1992). In the COG study discussed above, children with SR-ALL had a higher rate of anxiety disorders at 1 month post-diagnosis but this normalized at 6 months and 12 months (Myers et al. 2014). Diagnosis of an anxiety disorder in a child or adolescent with cancer must take into account a patient's understanding of and adjustment to the illness and treatment, possible contribution of cancer and directed therapies producing anxiety symptoms (e.g., corticosteroids, thyroid abnormalities), and family coping and adjustment. Adjustment to illness is related more to psychosocial than medical factors, such as parental adjustment, socioeconomic status, social support, and intelligence, and psychotherapeutic interventions can be targeted at these factors. Psychoeducation and psychotherapeutic techniques (primarily cognitive behavioral therapy) have been developed around pediatric medical traumatic stress and coping and resiliency frameworks and form the mainstay of evidence-based universal and targeted psychosocial supports and preventive services which pediatric cancer centers should provide as standard of care (see Chap. 6 Psychotherapeutic Modalities) (Kazak et al. 2012; Pao and Wiener 2011).

When anxiety symptoms have not responded to usual psychotherapeutic interventions or disrupt a child's medical treatment (e.g., nonadherence with treatment or assessment), normal routines (e.g., prolonged sleep disruption or inability to separate from parent), or family functioning (e.g., child requires so much attention from parents that siblings are starting to manifest adverse symptoms as well), medication management of anxiety may be appropriate. Medication selection is guided by applied clinical therapeutics and one or more drugs may be appropriate, depending on the evidence base for specific disorders, FDA approval for children, need for short- or long-term management, and comorbid medical symptoms and treatments. Family history of childhood anxiety may be relevant to the decision to medicate a child for anxiety (e.g., initiation of selective serotonin reuptake inhibitor (SSRI)) as it may indicate underlying vulnerability to anxiety across many situations and triggers and beyond a particular period of acute stress. SSRIs, selective norepinephrine reuptake inhibitors (SNRIs), benzodiazepines, and antipsychotics are included in detailed clinical cases, the Medication section discussion, and tables in this chapter. Buspirone has not been found efficacious in the management of pediatric anxiety disorders (Strawn et al. 2012).

Posttraumatic Disorders and Symptoms

The diagnosis of pediatric medical traumatic stress (posttraumatic effects of a medical illness or related event) may be appropriate if a child or adolescent identifies cancer or aspects of their cancer treatment to be extremely traumatic. The previously held thought that PTSD occurs with high prevalence (20–30 %) in patients and family members (Stuber 2012; Bruce 2006) has been refuted recently with a matched-peer controlled study by Phipps et al., who found no higher rates of PTSD than the general population, at around 0.4 % (current, lifetime prevalence was 2.8 %.) (Phipps et al. 2014). This difference has been attributed to research methodologies used, in particular use of screening instruments (vs. diagnostic interview), focusing effects of mentioning cancer as a traumatic event prior to assessment of symptoms, and lack of the use of normal controls. It will be important that this single center study be reproduced. Diagnosis of medical PTSD should follow DSM-5 criteria, and consideration of prior traumas (not just assuming cancer is the "Criterion A event") is important. If PTSD is diagnosed, pharmacologic support for control of symptoms (anxiety, insomnia, hyperactivity/hypervigilance) and comorbid psychiatric disorders is the appropriate approach. Due to the theory that patients with PTSD have overactive adrenergic systems, anti-adrenergic medications (guanfacine, clonidine) have theoretical value and have shown some benefits in subsets of patients, but more research is needed (Strawn et al. 2010; Dowben et al. 2011). In adults, prazosin, another alpha-adrenergic blocker, has shown promise in reducing nightmares in trials with civilians and combat veterans with PTSD (Green 2014). Atypical antipsychotics and mood stabilizers also have limited benefits depending on symptoms presented and functional impairment.

Delirium

Case Vignette

Psychiatry team is called to see Matthew, a 14-year-old boy with aplastic anemia, in remission 4 months post-stem cell transplant admitted with Epstein–Barr Virus (EBV) related lymphoma of multiple sites including chest and neck, to assess "anxiety." He has a history of recent airway obstruction which caused significant anxiety and is aware of his guarded prognosis and reliance on experimental anti-EBV T-cell therapy. Over the course of his 2-week admission, he has received liberal doses of hydromorphone and lorazepam to treat pain, nausea, and anxiety. Medication review reveals he is also receiving corticosteroids, multiple antifungals, and antibiotics. He had fevers a day prior to consult, but is afebrile when seen. On exam, patient is a pleasant, knowledgeable, anxious adolescent who is unable to fully participate in conversations as he nods, off in the middle of sentences due to sedation. When he awakens he asks to be reoriented "Where was I?" He apologizes for his inability to focus. He reports there have been some "misunderstandings" about his medication use with staff, and he feels persecuted as a "drug seeker." He worries that people in the hallway are talking about him. He complains of very poor sleep at night but inability to

Table 8.1 Delirium in children with cancer

DSM-5	
Acute-onset, fluctuating, usually reversible, change in mental status	
Disturbance in attention and awareness	
Change in at least one domain of cognition (e.g., memory, orientation, language, perceptual disturbances)	
Symptoms in infants and children (hypoactive, hyperactive, or both)	
Disoriented (both)	Refractory agitation (hyperactive)
Inattentive (both)	Requiring escalating doses of sedation (hyperactive)
Disorganized sleep (both)	Pulling lines and tubes (hyperactive)
Sparse or delayed responses (hypoactive)	Withdrawal, flat affect (hypoactive)
Oversleepy (hypoactive)	
Screening tools	*Ages for use*
Pediatric Anesthesia Emergence Delirium (PAED) (Sikich and Lerman 2004)	Over 18 months old
Pediatric Confusion Assessment Method (pCAM) (Smith et al. 2011)	Over 5 years old
Preschool Confusion Assessment Method (ps-CAM)	2–5 years old (pending publication)
Cornell Assessment of Pediatric Delirium (CAPD) (Traube et al. 2014)	From newborn and up (0–21 year)
Etiologies	
Common	*Less common*
Anesthetics (except dexmedetomidine)	Biological therapy (antibody or cell therapies)
Antihistamines	Catatonia
Benzodiazepines (intoxication or withdrawal)	CNS vascular event (hemorrhagic or embolic)
CNS disease	Ifosfamide/other chemotherapy toxicities
Infection (systemic or localized)	NMDA receptor encephalitis
Metabolic/electrolyte derangements	Other paraneoplastic encephalitis
Opiates (intoxication or withdrawal)	Opsoclonus-myoclonus
Scopolamine/anticholinergics	Posterior reversible encephalopathy syndrome (PRES) (Kushner et al. 2013)
Seizure	Severe vitamin deficiencies (or rapid repletion in refeeding)
Steroids (intoxication or withdrawal)	
Behavioral/environmental interventions	
Use familiar toys, music, and caregivers	Diurnal cycle preservation
Primary nursing care	Encourage awake in day, sleep in night
Frequent reorientation	Cluster nursing care to reduce unnecessary awakenings
Nonconfrontation of delusions/hallucinations	Timing of sedating medications
Encourage oral hydration	Early mobilization/encouragement of physical therapy
Reduction in stimulation	

stay awake during the day. ***Diagnosis***: Delirium – multifactorial, secondary to recent fever, polypharmacy, exacerbated by poor sleep. ***Recommendations***: Child psychiatry recommended that team decrease the use of lorazepam and add olanzapine 2.5 mg at night to help manage his delirium as well as improve his sleep and alleviate nausea and anxiety. It was also recommended that he be reoriented frequently, cluster night nursing care to preserve sleep, and encourage oral intake, mobility, and physical therapy during the day. ***Outcome***: Patient showed significant improvement over the course of the ensuing 24 hours. Olanzapine greatly improved sleep and nausea and was continued in lieu of lorazepam for several weeks. Parents demonstrated improved insight and early recognition of future episodes of subthreshhold delirium which were quickly reversed. Patient engaged in ongoing psychotherapy for anxiety related to his illness.

Delirium is an acute brain dysfunction related to systemic illness, affecting 10–30 % of critically ill children in pediatric intensive care units (PICU). It carries significant risk for prolonged hospital and PICU stays and is associated in adults with increased mortality and prolonged neurocognitive sequelae. Diagnosis in children, like adults, follows DSM-5 criteria (Table 8.1) and may present as hyperactive, hypoactive, or mixed type. Research on pediatric delirium has increased in recent years with new screening and diagnostic tools and treatment algorithms (Smith et al. 2009; Creten et al. 2011; Silver et al. 2014). Pediatric clinicians must consider the differential presentation of delirium through a developmental lens. Consensus is emerging that with careful consideration of a child's baseline development and functioning in each symptom domain of delirium, it is possible to diagnose delirium from infancy and even in the context of developmental delay (Table 8.1) (Turkel et al. 2013; Silver et al. 2014). Coordination of care with family caregivers and inpatient nurses is critical to understand fluctuating mental status in delirious children.

The differential diagnosis of delirium may include undertreatment of pain or other physical symptoms, emotional distress (depression vs. hypoactive delirium), tantrums, and traumatic symptoms (Creten et al. 2011; Turkel et al. 2006). Once identified, clinicians should first seek to reverse delirium by treating underlying medical etiologies and/or removing offending "deliriogenic" medications (Table 8.1). Medical workup of the newly identified delirious patient should include blood and urine cultures, physical exam, and routine laboratories. Other workup will depend on the specific symptoms and history of each patient. In immunocompromised patients, a high index of suspicion for infection should be present.

In pediatric oncology, the most common causes of delirium include: opiates (intoxication and withdrawal), anesthesia, benzodiazepines, antihistamines, steroids, and infection. In the case of opiates, changing to another opiate ("rotation") may relieve symptoms as patients may be more sensitive to side effects of a particular drug and more tolerant of another. While most general anesthetics may be a risk factor, there is evidence that use of dexmedetomidine, during surgical procedures or for sedation in the PICU, may be protective against delirium (Dahmani et al. 2014).

Interventions for Delirium

The consulting psychiatrist can recommend a change in sedatives or anesthesia, after which dosing and management would be at the discretion of the intensivist or anesthesiologist. In addition to addressing underlying medical etiologies, staff can implement environmental changes that assist with comforting, reorienting, and promoting normal sleep for delirious patients. While environmental or sensory disruptions alone will not cause delirium, a calm and non-threatening environment helps reduce distress and agitation in the disoriented patient and should be a goal for all hospitalized patients. When possible, clustering of nursing care (to reduce interruptions at night and preserve sleep), frequent reorientation of the patient, preservation of day/night cues (e.g., lights on in the day, off at night), early mobilization even in the PICU, and encouraging oral hydration can all improve sleep quality and reduce disorientation and agitation in delirious and at-risk patients (Silver et al. 2014).

While addressing these factors, if symptom management is required for reasons of safety or distress (e.g., the child is pulling lines and tubes, hallucinating, or frightened), the off-label use of low-dose atypical antipsychotics is the recommended intervention in adults and children (Turkel and Hanft 2014). Use of atypical antipsychotics has been found to be safe in low doses and often allows for reduced use of other sedatives, which may be causing delirium and normalization of sleep/wake cycle. As sleep disruption is now understood to be a critical mechanism and core symptom of delirium, it is not surprising that studies are investigating use of melatonin to reset (or prevent disruption of) circadian rhythm in patients at risk or already experiencing delirium. Melatonin and melatonin agonist studies in adults, which have been small, have found they are well tolerated with modest benefit in prevention but not resolution of delirium. As melatonin is known to be safe and helpful in multiple types of pediatric sleep disorders, it is reasonable to consider its use in targeted cases of sleep disruption (Turkel and Hanft 2014; Chakraborti et al. 2014; Özcan and Dönmez 2014).

Since antihistamines and benzodiazepines are routinely used in daily pediatric oncology care, it is common to see children who have "paradoxical" reactions and become agitated, enraged, hyperactive, disinhibited or present with the full syndrome of delirium. In general, antihistamines and benzodiazepines should be avoided for children with a history of paradoxical reactions; however, sometimes these medications are unavoidable (e.g., blood transfusions requiring premedication with antihistamines) and concomitant use of a low-dose atypical antipsychotic may be needed to offset these adverse effects. Antipsychotics and other dopaminergic drugs like metoclopramide can induce extrapyramidal symptoms (EPS) (e.g., oculogyric crisis, torticollis) or akathisia (a type of psychomotor agitation, often described as "ants in pants" or a "restless leg" type of feeling all over the body). A careful history about the timing of medications and the development of symptoms can help differentiate these types of symptoms in a patient who may have an evolving delirium in the context of polypharmacy, which is very common. Further discussion of doses and scheduling follows in the Medications section.

Withdrawal Syndromes

Some patients with cancer experience chronic symptoms such as pain, nausea, and anxiety, which may necessitate long-term administration of habit-forming medications such as opiates or benzodiazepines. This can occur in an inpatient setting (e.g., during a prolonged critical illness or stem cell transplant) or with chronic comorbidities (e.g., avascular necrosis of joints related to corticosteroids, phantom limb pain, persistent nausea) of cancer therapy as an outpatient. Acute or subacute changes in a patient's clinical status (for better or worse) may result in the rapid reduction of these medications and cause opiate or benzodiazepine withdrawal symptoms if a patient had developed physiological dependence to the drug. It is common for these sorts of dose changes, made 2–3 days prior to presentation of withdrawal symptoms, to be overlooked when a patient's medical problems are complex, acute, and fluctuating. Therefore, careful review of the medications dispensed over the course of the symptoms is important.

While the classic syndrome of opiate withdrawal includes hypertension, tachycardia, vomiting, diarrhea, and diaphoresis, milder symptoms experienced by patients still on some dose of opiate often appear psychiatric in nature, including dysphoria, anxiety, emotional lability, tremulousness, fatigue, myalgias, and nausea. With the recognition of withdrawal, these symptoms can be easily treated and reversed. For patients on a short course of opiate therapy (less than 14 days), the World Health Organization (WHO) guidelines recommend discontinuation by a taper which decreases the original dose by 10–20 % every 8 hours, gradually increasing the time interval. However, for patients on opiates for longer periods, dose reduction should not exceed *10–20 % per week* and management should include a measurement of withdrawal symptoms using a standard scoring system (World Health Organization 2012). The treatment of cancer-related and treatment-related pain in children is covered in Chap. 3 and in the WHO Guidelines on the Pharmacological Treatment of Persisting Pain in Children with Medical Illnesses.

Benzodiazepine withdrawal can present similarly, with symptoms of nausea, agitation, anxiety, tremulousness, myalgia, tachycardia, and hypertension. Benzodiazepine withdrawal, like alcohol withdrawal, can cause dangerous hypertension and seizures and should be considered in any new onset seizure in a medically complex patient who has recent exposure to benzodiazepines. As with opiates, tapers in chronic users should be slow and based on prevention of objective signs of withdrawal (like the Withdrawal Assessment Tool (WAT-1) or the Sophia Observation Withdrawal Scale). Research in the area of monitoring and guidelines for tapering of sedation and other uses of opiates and benzodiazepines in pediatrics is urgently needed (Poh et al. 2014; Galinkin et al. 2014; Ista et al. 2013).

Other Iatrogenic Symptoms

Case Vignette

Lucy, a 3-year-old girl with acute myelogenous leukemia (AML), who receives steroids for 1 week each month, has been exhibiting worsening irritability over the 7-day course of steroids each cycle. Her pediatric oncologist requests child psychiatry consultation to assess her mood and behavior. Parents report escalating outbursts to rageful tantrums in which she is inconsolable, irrational, screaming, and throwing herself on the floor for up to 90 minutes regardless of any intervention by parents. Parents note that despite offering her whatever she wants she doesn't stop until she "cries herself to sleep." She also has started threatening to pull out her central line when agitated. Her sleep is erratic, waking during the night crying and hungry. The symptoms escalate over the week and finally dissipate 2–3 days after steroids are stopped. ***Diagnosis***: Substance (corticosteroid)-induced mood disorder. ***Recommendation***: Start risperidone at 0.25 mg at bedtime and titrate up to 0.25 mg in AM and 0.5 mg at bedtime during steroid courses only. ***Outcome***: The patient responded well with better sleep at night and fewer, self-limited tantrums lasting less than 5 minutes with consolable irritability. Mother reports patient still has personality changes the week on steroids, but they are much more manageable. The patient's appetite is ravenous during the day due to the additive effects of steroids and risperidone, but with safety concerns and sleep both greatly improved, her mother feels this is acceptable.

Many cancer treatments cause iatrogenic psychiatric symptoms. Administration of corticosteroids, which is commonly used for the treatment of ALL and lymphoma, causes varying degrees of irritability, mood lability, impulsivity, lethargy and/or insomnia (Ularntinon et al. 2010). These changes can be intense but are usually limited to the duration of the treatment. Psychoeducation may be sufficient in supporting a patient and family through their course of corticosteoids, but if significant impairment is present, a short-acting agent like risperidone can be extremely helpful in reducing impairment and distress. If chronic steroid use is needed for graft versus host disease (GVHD) or other illnesses, frank clinical depression or anxiety disorders may develop which warrant other targeted therapies.

Another medication that warrants close monitoring of psychiatric symptoms is isotretinoin (Accutane), most commonly used for severe cystic acne, but due to its effect on inhibition of tumorigenesis, it has also been used in regimens treating neuroblastoma, medulloblastoma, and other skin and brain cancers. Prescription of isotretinoin in the United States can only occur if patient is registered and monitored on an FDA-administered website due to its side effects of severe teratogenicity, blood dyscrasias, and psychiatric effects, which include depression and mood lability and, rarely, suicidal ideation or completed suicide. It is often well tolerated. If needed, atypical antipsychotics can be useful for offsetting any mild to moderate psychiatric effects, but the presentation of severe psychiatric symptoms warrants reevaluating the risks and benefits of the treatment.

Interferon alpha (IFN-alpha), an immunotherapy used for treatment of metastatic melanoma, hepatitis B and C, giant cell tumors, and rarely other disorders, carries significant side effects including flu-like symptoms, fatigue, anorexia, and neuropsychiatric symptoms like depression, mania, and psychosis. It is generally better tolerated in children than adults but symptoms, if present, often respond well to targeted therapy with antidepressant, antimanic, or antipsychotic medication.

Neurocognitive Impairment

The evaluation and management of neurocognitive adverse effects of cancer illness and therapy in children and adolescents are discussed in

Chap. 10. As part of a differential diagnosis during psychiatric evaluation, neurocognitive symptoms may include impairment of any domain of cognition, in particular, memory, attention, processing speeds, and visual motor integration (Castellino et al. 2014). A patient with acquired neurocognitive impairment may present to psychiatric evaluation with secondary anxiety or frustration with daily tasks (e.g., due to reduced ability to attend or process information), amotivation, or underachievement in academics. For the assessment of inattention and other cognitive symptoms after cancer treatments, an ADHD framework is insufficient, as many at-risk patients will not meet diagnostic criteria (Kahalley et al. 2011). Of note, depression, anxiety, and PTSD can also have cognitive symptoms like attention impairment and should be ruled out. Neuropsychological testing is an essential part of evaluation and treatment planning for patients with these types of symptoms. Some patients with attentional issues due to ADHD or acquired cognitive deficits may benefit from stimulant therapy to improve performance on focused tasks (Pao et al. 2006). In pediatric cancer survivors who received CNS directed therapy (ALL with cranial radiation and brain tumors), response to methylphenidate (MPH) is less robust (45 %) than in the ADHD population (75 %) . A history of preexisting inattention/ADHD is the best predictor of response. Given that the safety and tolerability are favorable, and similar to the ADHD population, and nearly half will have a response, Conklin et al. recommend a trial of methylphenidate with a slow titration and close monitoring of treatment response and side effects (Conklin et al. 2014). See Table 8.5, Stimulants, for specific medication information.

Medications

Antidepressants (Table 8.2)

Retrospective reviews of antidepressant use in pediatric oncology patients have been conducted (Pao et al. 2006; Portteus et al. 2006; Kersun and Elia 2007; Phipps et al. 2012). In most centers, pediatric oncologists prescribe antidepressants, but fewer than 10 % of the oncologists report specifically assessing for suicidal ideation despite the institution of a black box warning on use of selective serotonin reuptake inhibitors (SSRIs) in adolescents (Phipps et al. 2012). Consultation with a child psychiatrist by the pediatric oncology medical team is encouraged for the selection and monitoring of psychotropic medications for pediatric oncology patients. There are no randomized controlled trials (RCTs) in children with cancer and depression using antidepressants including SSRIs, the current antidepressant treatment of choice in children and adolescents (Valluri et al. 2012). In the United States, only fluoxetine and escitalopram have pediatric Food and Drug Administration (FDA) indications for depression (see Table 8.2 Antidepressants). Two small open-label trials of antidepressants have been reported in children with cancer (DeJong and Fombonne 2007; Gothelf et al. 2005).

Other medications used in the treatment of depression include mirtazapine and stimulants. Mirtazapine is a noradrenergic and specific serotonin agent that is a partial 5HT-3 receptor antagonist. Its use off-label has become more popular as it is sedating, causes weight gain, has antiemetic properties, and has few significant drug interactions, but it is not FDA approved for use in children. Children and adolescents who cannot tolerate antidepressants may, assuming cardiac stability, benefit from a trial of stimulants for depression and apathy. Tricyclic antidepressants do not have demonstrated efficacy for depression in children but may be useful for headache prophylaxis or enuresis (Daly and Wilens 1998). It is important to note they can be dangerously cardiotoxic in overdose and have anticholinergic side effects (e.g., dry mouth, sedation) at therapeutic doses.

Primary considerations in antidepressant selection include drug-drug interactions and side effect profiles. Practitioners must be aware that some antibiotics commonly used in resistant infections such as linezolid, a weak monoamine oxidase inhibitor, have a small but documented risk of leading to serotonin syndrome when

Table 8.2 Preparations and dosages of antidepressant medications in children

Medication	Prescribing information (Starting dose – general range) Routes of administration	FDA indication in children	Psycho-oncology uses and specific notes
Selective serotonin reuptake inhibitors (SSRIs)			Depression Anxiety Caution with linezolid (MAOI) Note p450 interactions Black box warning
Citalopram (Celexa®) Escitalopram (Lexapro®)	5–40 mg/day, increase by 5–10 mg/day PO[a] 5–20 mg/day Increase by 5–10 mg/day PO[a]	No 12 years and older for depression	Few drug-drug interactions; EKG changes above 40 mg Few drug–drug interactions
Fluoxetine (Prozac®)	5–60 mg/day Increase by 5–10 mg/day PO[a]	8 years and older for depression; 7 years and older for OCD	Long half-life, p450 issues
Fluvoxamine (Luvox®)	25–200 mg/day, increase by 25 mg/day Max 300 mg PO	8 years and older for OCD	Sedation, dry mouth, tachycardia
Paroxetine (Paxil®)	5–20 mg/day, increase by 5 mg/day PO	No	Prohibited in Europe under 18, short half-life, increased rate of discontinuation symptoms
Sertraline (Zoloft®)	12.5–150 mg/day, Increase by 12.5–25 mg/day Max 200 mg PO[a]	Yes, 6 years and older for OCD	
Other antidepressants			
Bupropion (Wellbutrin®)	37.5–300 mg/day, increase by 37.5–50 mg/day Max 450 mg PO	No	Depression Anxiety ADHD (3rd line) Decreases seizure threshold
Duloxetine (Cymbalta®)	20–60 mg/day, increase by 10–20 mg/day Max 120 mg PO	7 years or older for generalized anxiety disorder	Depression Anxiety Pain
Mirtazapine (Remeron®)	7.5–45 mg/day, increase by 7.5–15 mg/day Max 45 mg PO[b]	No	Depression Anxiety Boosts appetite (weight gain), antiemetic, helps sleep (sedation) at lower doses
Venlafaxine (Effexor®)	18.75–300 mg/day, increase by 18.75–37.5 mg/day Max 375 mg PO	No	Depression Anxiety Pain Monitor blood pressure (hypertension) and heart rate (tachycardia)

PO per os/by mouth, *IM* intramuscular, *IV* intravenous
[a]Liquid form available
[b]Oral disintegrating tablet available http://www.micromedexsolutions.com/accessed 1/19/2015

Table 8.3 Preparations and dosages of antipsychotic medications in children

Medication	Prescribing information (Starting dose – general range) Maximum dose allowed Routes of administration	FDA indication in children	Psycho-oncology uses and specific notes
Atypical antipsychotics			*Need to monitor QT intervals*
Aripiprazole (Abilify®)	2 mg–15 mg/day, increase by 5 mg/day Max 30 mg PO[a, b], IM	6–17 years agitation in autism; 10 years or older in bipolar I; 6–18 years in Tourette's; 13–17 years in schizophrenia	Delirium (hypoactive, adults primarily); long half-life
Olanzapine (Zyprexa®, Zydis®)	2.5–10 mg/day, increase by 2.5–5 mg/day Max 20 mg PO[b], IM	13–17 years bipolar I acute, schizophrenia; depressed bipolar I with fluoxetine 10–17 years	Delirium Nausea Steroid-related mood problems
Quetiapine (Seroquel®)	12.5–50 mg/day, increase by 12.5–25 mg/day Max 600–800 mg PO	10–17 years bipolar mania; 13–17 years acute schizophrenia	Delirium Agitation Used in low doses (<200 mg/day)
Risperidone (Risperdal®, Risperdal Consta®, Risperidone M-Tab®)	0.25–3 mg/day, increase 0.25–0.5 mg/day Max 6 mg/day PO[a, b], IM	5 years or older irritability in autism; 10 year or older bipolar I; 13 years or older schizophrenia	Delirium Agitation Steroid-related mood problems
Typical antipsychotics			*Need to monitor QT intervals*
Chlorpromazine (Thorazine®)	0.25 mg/lb body weight – 50 mg (Titrate by weight) PO, IM	6 months to 12 years for nausea and vomiting; severe problem behavior; 1–12 years tetanus	Delirium Hiccups Agitation; highly sedating
Haloperidol (Haldol®)	0.25–5 mg/day PO, IM, IV	3 years or older Tourette's, hyperactive or severe behavioral problems, schizophrenia	Delirium Agitation

PO per os/by mouth, *IM* intramuscular, *IV* intravenous
[a]Liquid form available
[b]Oral disintegrating tablet available http://www.micromedexsolutions.com/accessed 1/19/2015

combined with SSRI use. Serotonin syndrome is characterized by change in mental status, autonomic instability, and neuromuscular abnormalities and can be lethal if not identified and treated by discontinuation of the SSRI and providing autonomic support. Clinicians may have to decide to discontinue either linezolid or SSRI in situations in which both medications are present. Similarly, when patients must undergo prolonged periods of no intake by mouth during transplant or postoperatively, a clinical decision as to the severity of the depression may warrant continuation of the antidepressant via liquid form or per nasogastric tube.

Antipsychotics (Table 8.3)

Off-label use of antipsychotics, particularly atypical antipsychotics, may be beneficial for symptom management for children with cancer in several clinical scenarios. As discussed above in the section on pediatric delirium, atypical antipsychotics are the recommended treatment for symptoms of agitation or distress in delirious infants and children. Their use in this setting may reduce exposure to other offending agents causing delirium, decrease time the patient is delirious, decrease traumatic disorientation and distress, and reduce length of stay in the PICU and hospital. Quetiapine and risperidone have been most commonly cited. Dose ranges have been anecdotally reported (Turkel and Hanft 2014; Silver et al. 2010) (Table 8.3), but studies are needed to determine the safest and most efficacious dosing regimens in medically ill children. In situations where a child is unable to take oral medications, low-dose intravenous haloperidol may be used.

For children with disabling corticosteroid-related mood and behavioral changes, medication treatment may be warranted. Risperidone has been widely used for this complaint, because it is generally well tolerated and rapidly effective (in the first 1–2 days of administration) and has a safety record (and FDA approval) in children with autism down to age 5 years. In this setting, risperidone is prescribed during steroid courses only and can be discontinued between cycles of treatment (Ularntinon et al. 2010). Children with irritability, impulsivity, or mood swings due to CNS insults, like brain tumors or posterior reversible encephalopathy syndrome (PRES), can also benefit from risperidone or other low-dose antipsychotic (Pangilinan et al. 2010).

Olanzapine was found to be effective against chemotherapy-induced nausea in adults in the early 1990s. It has been found most useful for delayed nausea and works with moderate and highly emetogenic chemotherapy regimens (Wang et al. 2014). It is hypothesized that its efficacy for this symptom can be attributed to its activity at multiple types of nausea-related receptors (dopamine, serotonin, antihistamine, etc.). Similarly, it is known to stimulate appetite and cause weight gain, a side effect which may be beneficial in the medically anorexic population. A meta-analysis examining 47 studies for safety of olanzapine use in children under 13 years showed it was well tolerated with 15 % EKG changes and 9 % extrapyramidal symptoms, thus setting the stage for further trials examining its use in this population (Flank et al. 2014).

In general, the side effects of weight gain, appetite stimulation, and sedation can be secondary benefits for many pediatric oncology patients, and during the short-term symptomatic use of these drugs, metabolic side effects are not usually seen. Monitoring of EKG is important in hospitalized children on antipsychotics as illness, electrolyte abnormalities, and polypharmacy may predispose these children to prolongation of QTc interval (corrected QT interval, a measurement of the interval between Q wave and T wave on EKG tracing, representing electrical depolarization and repolarization of the ventricles, corrected for normal changes in relation to the patients current heart rate.) QTc prolongation, usually defined by QTc>500 ms, is a congenital or acquired change in electrophysiologic function of the heart and is a risk factor for a potentially fatal cardiac arrhythmia, known as torsade de pointes. Discontinuation of causative drugs may be warranted. Cardiology consultation can be valuable in situations where medications are critical for patient management. It is important that serum levels of magnesium, potassium, and calcium, which affect heart function, are repleted if deficient in this context. In general terms, atypical antipsychotics prolong QTc less than typical antipsychotics, with olanzapine and aripiprazole having the least QTc prolongation overall. Further studies are needed into the absolute and relative risks of QTc prolongation and link to risk for torsades de pointes (Hasnain et al. 2014).

Benzodiazepines (Table 8.4)

The use of benzodiazepines in oncology is ubiquitous mostly in the context of nausea and anxiety management but also for sleep, muscle relaxation in musculoskeletal pain, and sedation for procedures or long-term critical illness. Pediatric oncology clinicians are comfortable using this class of medications, particularly lorazepam and diazepam for symptom management of nausea, anxiety, and sleep and midazolam for sedation and usually follow dosing in the Harriet Lane, Micromedex, or other pediatric guides. The child and adolescent psychiatrist consultant may be involved in complex symptom management where balancing the benefits of these medications with their side effects can be delicate. Benzodiazepines may cause sedation, confusion, respiratory depression, delirium, and, particularly in young, developmentally delayed

Table 8.4 Preparations and dosages of benzodiazepine medications in children

Medication	Prescribing information (Starting dose – general range) Maximum dose Routes of administration	Approximate equivalence	Route of administration	Onset of action	Psycho-oncology uses and specific notes
Clonazepam (Klonopin®)	0.25–3 mg/day 0.01 mg/kg/24 h ÷ q8 h, increase by 0.25–0.5 mg/day	0.25 mg	PO[a]	Slow	Anxiety REM-sleep disorders
Diazepam (Valium®)	2–10 mg/day IV: 0.04–0.25 mg/kg, increase by 1–2 mg/day PO: 0.12–0.8 mg/kg/day	5 mg PO, PR 2.5 mg IV	PO, IV, IM, PR	Intermediate	Anxiety Muscle relaxation
Lorazepam (Ativan®)	0.5–6 mg/day, increase by 0.25–0.5 mg/day	0.5 mg PO, IV	PO, IV	Rapid	Nausea/vomiting Anxiety Catatonia
Midazolam (Versed®)	0.025–0.05 mg/kg IV Max 0.4 mg/kg 0.25–1 mg/kg PO Max 20 mg	2.5 mg IV	PO[b], IV, IM	Rapid	Procedural sedation

PO per os/by mouth, *IM* intramuscular, *IV* intravenous, *PR* per rectum
[a]Oral disintegrating tablet available http://www.micromedexsolutions.com/accessed 1/19/2015
[b]Liquid form available

or neurologically impaired children, "paradoxical reactions." Tolerance, dependence, and withdrawal are important to monitor and can be avoided with careful medication tapers. The primarily hepatic metabolism of lorazepam makes it a safe choice in renal impairment. It is also well tolerated in hepatic failure and can be given in a continuous drip for palliative sedation. Short-acting alprazolam, while highly effective for acute situational anxiety, has a limited role in treatment of most oncology patients whose "triggers" are often frequent and repeated. The repeated use of short-acting benzodiazepines can lead to marked, undesired swings in emotional and physiological withdrawal symptoms due to additive effects of onset/offset of action of the drug and the underlying anxiety. In patients requiring continuous coverage of symptoms with benzodiazepines, longer acting agents such as clonazepam may be desirable and (as with opiates) cross tapering of the drugs can be safely accomplished with careful attention to published benzodiazepine equivalency references (and in Table 8.4) and close supervision of the patient (Watson 2009). Weaning schedules and careful monitoring for withdrawal are discussed above. Clonazepam is also helpful for generalized anxiety and is an adjunctive management of anxiety components of pain or while waiting for antidepressant onset of action.

The effects of chronic benzodiazepine exposure, as well as other anesthetic and sedative exposure, in the developing brain are not well understood, but animal studies in mice and in vitro models have raised concern about neurotoxicity. Research is ongoing to identify cellular mechanisms of action and developmental windows of vulnerability to these toxic effects in humans (Mintz et al. 2012).

Mood Stabilizers

The presence of a family or personal history of bipolar disorder or a manic reaction to steroids or antidepressants could necessitate the need for a mood stabilizer in patients with cancer. During cancer treatment, however, the choice of mood stabilizers is particularly limited. Most antiepileptic drugs usually used for mood stabilization are to be avoided due to hepatic p450 enzyme interactions affecting chemotherapy metabolism and hematologic side effects. Valproate and valproic acid have been shown to have some antitumor properties, but even so are usually avoided in oncology patients because of metabolic interactions, blood dyscrasias, and hepatotoxicity. Lamotrigine has antidepressant and mood-stabilizing properties, although research is ongoing regarding its role in bipolar spectrum disorders; its practical use, which requires slow titrations for starting and discontinuing to avoid triggering Stevens–Johnson syndrome, may be difficult to maintain through some cancer treatment regimens. Levetiracetam is a commonly recommended antiepileptic for seizure prophylaxis and control in pediatric oncology because it has limited p450 interactions, but does not have strong mood-stabilizing properties and can have significant behavioral side effects (Ruggiero et al. 2010). Lithium requires close management of fluid and electrolytes to avoid nephrotoxicity and may cause leukocytosis, electrocardiographic changes, and thyroid toxicity. Atypical antipsychotics are a well-tolerated option for mood stabilization in cancer patients.

Stimulants (Table 8.5)

The use of stimulants in pediatric oncology is surprisingly low, compared to the general pediatric population, according to a review of psychotropic prescribing in pediatric oncology (Pao et al. 2006). Many families stop stimulant medication for a child previously diagnosed with ADHD when the child is not attending school and/or on treatment for pediatric cancer, but if

Table 8.5 Preparations and dosages of stimulant medications in children

Medication	Prescribing information (Starting dose – general range) Maximum dose allowed Routes of administration	FDA indication in children	Psycho-oncology uses and specific notes
Stimulants			*Monitor weight loss, decreased growth, insomnia, tachycardia, hypertension, headaches, irritability, tics*
Dextroamphetamine/ mixed amphetamine salts (immediate release) Dexedrine	2.5 mg orally once or twice daily (am and noon); increase by 2.5 mg/day at 1-week intervals to optimum response Max 40 mg/day PO[a]	3 to 16 years immediate release for ADHD; 6 to 16 years sustained release for ADHD, narcolepsy	Poor attention and concentration ADHD Depressed mood with fatigue
Methylphenidate Ritalin (immediate release)	2.5–5 mg orally twice daily (am and noon); dose adjustments of 2.5–5 to 10 mg at weekly intervals Max dose 60 mg/day PO[a, b] patch	6 to 17 years for ADHD	Poor attention and concentration ADHD Depressed mood with fatigue
Modafanil Provigil®	50–100 mg orally to start for at least 1–3 days, then titrate up as needed, typical dose 100–200 mg Max dose 400 mg PO	Over 16 years for narcolepsy, obstructive sleep apnea	Depression with fatigue, adjunct

ADHD attention deficit hyperactivity disorder, *PO* per os/by mouth
[a]Liquid form available
[b]Oral chewable tablet available http://www.micromedexsolutions.com/accessed 1/26/2015

they present with behavioral or emotional issues during cancer treatment, it may be warranted to restart. These medications may be useful for symptom management of opiate-related sedation, radiation-related somnolence syndrome, or adjunctive treatment of depression, although they have been largely disproven to be of benefit in cancer-related fatigue in randomized controlled trials in adults (Ruddy et al. 2014). Anorexia and insomnia may be treatment-limiting side effects of stimulants in this population.

As mentioned above, the use of stimulants in pediatric cancer survivors with inattention and other cognitive complaints is a subject of ongoing research. Studies show a trial of methylphenidate (MPH) is warranted if stimulants are not medically contraindicated, for ALL patients and brain tumor patients who are struggling with executive functioning. Gains were seen on objective measures of attention, teacher report of academic and social skills, and parent reports of academic and executive functioning (turning in assignments, planning ahead, etc.) While response rates did not approach those of the ADHD population, 45 % of children with these complaints did benefit and tolerated the medication well (Conklin, et al. 2014). Over the first year of treatment with MPH, pediatric cancer survivors do experience small but significant deceleration in body mass index (BMI) and weight but not height (Jasper et al. 2009).

Other Psychotropic Medications and Dietary Supplements

The α-2 agonists clonidine and guanfacine are used frequently for adjunctive treatment of ADHD, particularly for hyperactivity, aggression, and insomnia symptoms and comorbid tic disorders. Patients should be monitored for hypotension, bradycardia, and somnolence (Hirota et al. 2014). Clonidine has also been explored as a treatment for PTSD, thought to modulate adrenergic system dysregulation; however this is yet to be proven in randomized controlled trials (RCTs). Along with guanfacine, it may also be useful for management of steroid-induced insomnia and dysregulation as an alternative medication to children in whom benzodiazepines or antipsychotics are contraindicated or poorly tolerated (such as those with CNS insults or developmental delays.) (Pangilinan et al. 2010)

The dietary supplements omega fatty acids (n3FAs) and melatonin warrant a brief discussion because of their low side effect profile, evidence base of possible psychiatric benefits in certain subpopulations, and common use in community samples. N3FA supplementation, found deficient in most Western diets low in fish and nut intake, is postulated to reverse a potentially proinflammatory state and prevent or reverse certain cardiovascular and psychiatric disorders. Studies have focused on the n3Fas EPA and DHA, derived from fish oil, but remain mixed as to their efficacy in treatment of unipolar depression and bipolar disorder in adults. Side effects are minor GI upset, possible rapid cycling in bipolar disorder, and hypothetical risk of bleeding in combination with other thrombolytic medications (aspirin or warfarin) or illness states. Herbal supplements, including n3FAs should be avoided during chemotherapy as potential interactions are largely unstudied but have implications in treatment efficacy (Mischoulon and Freeman 2013; Omega-3 | Memorial Sloan Kettering Cancer Center 2014). Melatonin, not a medication but a natural supplement, has proven efficacy and safety in a myriad of pediatric sleep disorders; however, it has not been tested in pediatric cancer patients (Carter et al. 2014; Özcan and Dönmez 2014). Pediatric starting doses range from 1 to 3 mg but much higher doses have been reported safe. As it is a non-prescription supplement, it is unregulated by the FDA and care must be taken that patients (or hospital pharmacies) choose reputable brands to purchase (see Integrative therapies Chap. 16) .

Conclusions

The diagnosis and management of psychiatric problems can greatly enhance the care of the pediatric oncology patient, from significantly improving quality of life and reducing suffering to managing psychiatric comorbidities that allow for life-saving or life-prolonging oncology treatment to continue. Psychotropic medications are an important treatment modality in the psycho-oncologists' "toolbox" and should be prescribed in the context of comprehensive, multimodal, multidisciplinary care. Evidence-based psychotherapies delivered by trained mental health clinicians, directed at specific psychiatric disorders, and symptoms should be sought for children with cancer and their families throughout the disease trajectory. Consultation psychiatrists may work in many practice settings, but whether functioning as a medication consultant or multidisciplinary team leader, it is the physician's responsibility to provide a comprehensive, holistic approach in assessment, diagnosis, and treatment planning for the child with cancer and their family.

Clinical Pearls

Collaboration and open communication between the patient, parent, medical team and psychiatric consultant is essential for successful psychiatric treatment in the pediatric medical setting. A proactive explanation of the mind-body connection, the contribution of anxiety to pain or nausea, and reassurance that the mental health evaluation is intended to improve the teams' understanding and ability to treat their symptoms, can help form an alliance with the patient and their family.Psychotropic medication in the medically complex pediatric oncology population can be a safe and effective tool to provide relief of psychological/psychiatric symptoms and facilitate oncologic treatment. Clinicians working with children with cancer may need to focus on the more affective aspects of depression (vs. the neurovegetative symptoms) such as anhedonia and hopelessness to diagnose major depression and distinguish it from the effects of illness and treatment. Depression in the context of cancer can affect quality of life and treatment adherence.Standardized screening tools and patient education materials for pediatric delirium should be used to engage nurses and parents in identifying delirium in children of all ages. Delirium risk factors can be minimized, and environmental and pharmacologic interventions can improve mental status.

References

AAP. National Center for Medical Home Implementation (2015). http://www.medicalhomeinfo.org. Accessed 25 Jan

Bruce M (2006) A systematic and conceptual review of posttraumatic stress in childhood cancer survivors and their parents. Clin Psychol Rev 26(3):233–256. doi:10.1016/j.cpr.2005.10.002

Carter KA, Hathaway NE, Lettieri CF (2014) Common sleep disorders in children. Am Fam Physician 89(5):368–377

Castellino SM, Ullrich NJ, Whelen MJ, Lange BJ (2014) Developing interventions for cancer-related cognitive dysfunction in childhood cancer survivors. J Natl Cancer Inst 106(8). doi:10.1093/jnci/dju186

Chakraborti D, Tampi DJ, Tampi RR (2014) Melatonin and melatonin agonist for delirium in the elderly patients. Am J Alzheimers Dis Other Demen. doi:10.1177/1533317514539379

Cleeland CS, Bennett GJ, Dantzer R, Dougherty PM, Dunn AJ, Meyers CA, Miller AH et al (2003) Are the symptoms of cancer and cancer treatment due to a shared biologic mechanism? a cytokine-immunologic model of cancer symptoms. Cancer 97(11):2919–2925. doi:10.1002/cncr.11382

Conklin HM, Reddick WE, Khan RB (2014) Comment on Smithson et al.'s review of stimulant medication usage to improve neurocognitive and learning outcomes in childhood brain tumour survivors. Eur J Cancer 50(8):1566–1568. doi:10.1016/j.ejca.2014.01.032

Creten C, Van Der Zwaan S, Blankespoor RJ, Leroy PL, Schieveld JN (2011) Pediatric delirium in the pediatric intensive care unit: a systematic review and an update on key issues and research questions. Minerva Anestesiol 77(11):1099–1107

Dahmani S, Delivet H, Hilly J (2014) Emergence delirium in children: an update. Curr Opin Anaesthesiol 27(3):309–315. doi:10.1097/ACO.0000000000000076

Daly JM, Wilens T (1998) The Use of tricyclic antidepressants in children and adolescents. Pediatr Clin North Am 45(5):1123–1135

DeJong M, Fombonne E (2007) Citalopram to treat depression in pediatric oncology. J Child Adolesc

Psychopharmacol 17(3):371–377. doi:10.1089/cap.2006.0076

Dowben JS, Grant JS, Keltner NL (2011) Clonidine: diverse Use in pharmacologic management: biological perspectives. Perspect Psychiatr Care 47(2):105–108. doi:10.1111/j.1744-6163.2011.00302.x

Drug-Gene Alerts — Mayo Clinic Center for Individualized Medicine (2014). http://mayoresearch.mayo.edu/center-for-individualized-medicine/drug-gene-alerts.asp. Accessed 25 Nov

Flank J, Sung L, Dvorak CC, Spettigue W, Lee Dupuis L (2014) The safety of olanzapine in young children: a systematic review and meta-analysis. Drug Saf. doi:10.1007/s40264-014-0219-y

Galinkin J, Koh JL, Committee on drugs, and Section on Anesthesiology and Pain Medicine (2014) Recognition and management of iatrogenically induced opioid dependence and withdrawal in children. Pediatrics 133(1):152–155. doi:10.1542/peds.2013-3398

Gothelf D, Rubinstein M, Shemesh E, Miller O, Farbstein I, Klein A, Weizman A, Apter A, Yaniv I (2005) Pilot study: fluvoxamine treatment for depression and anxiety disorders in children and adolescents with cancer. J Am Acad Child Adolesc Psychiatry 44(12):1258–1262. doi:10.1097/01.chi.0000181042.29208.eb

Gould MS, Marrocco FA, Kleinman M, Thomas JG, Mostkoff K, Cote J, Davies M (2005) Evaluating iatrogenic risk of youth suicide screening programs: a randomized controlled trial. JAMA 293(13):1635–1643. doi:10.1001/jama.293.13.1635

Green B (2014) Prazosin in the treatment of PTSD. J Psychiatr Pract 20(4):253–259. doi:10.1097/01.pra.0000452561.98286.1e

Hasnain M, Victor W, Vieweg R (2014) QTc interval prolongation and torsade de pointes associated with second-generation antipsychotics and antidepressants: a comprehensive review. CNS Drugs 28(10):887–920. doi:10.1007/s40263-014-0196-9

Hirota T, Schwartz S, Correll CU (2014) Alpha-2 agonists for attention-deficit/hyperactivity disorder in youth: a systematic review and meta-analysis of monotherapy and add-on trials to stimulant therapy. J Am Acad Child Adolesc Psychiatry 53(2):153–173. doi:10.1016/j.jaac.2013.11.009

Institute of Medicine (US) and National Research Council (US) National Cancer Policy Board; Hewitt M, Weiner SL, Simone JV (eds) (2003) Childhood cancer survivorship: improving care and quality of life. National Academies Press (US), Washington (DC). http://www.ncbi.nlm.nih.gov/books/NBK221742/

Ista E, de Hoog M, Tibboel D, Duivenvoorden HJ, van Dijk M (2013) Psychometric evaluation of the Sophia observation withdrawal symptoms scale in critically ill children. Pediatr Crit Care Med 14(8):761–769. doi:10.1097/PCC.0b013e31829f5be1

Jasper BW, Conklin HM, Joanne L, Brannon Morris E, Howard SC, Shengjie W, Xiong X, Shelso J, Khan RB (2009) Growth effects of methylphenidate among childhood cancer survivors: a 12-month case-matched open-label study. Pediatr Blood Cancer 52(1):39–43. doi:10.1002/pbc.21770

Kahalley LS, Conklin HM, Tyc VL, Wilson SJ, Hinds PS, Shengjie W, Xiong X, Hudson MM (2011) ADHD and secondary ADHD criteria fail to identify many at-risk survivors of pediatric ALL and brain tumor. Pediatr Blood Cancer 57(1):110–118. doi:10.1002/pbc.22998

Kazak AE, Brier M, Alderfer MA, Reilly A, Parker SF, Rogerwick S, Ditaranto S, Barakat LP (2012) Screening for psychosocial risk in pediatric cancer. Pediatr Blood Cancer 59(5):822–827. doi:10.1002/pbc.24166

Kearns MA, Hawley KM (2014) Predictors of polypharmacy and off-label prescribing of psychotropic medications: a national survey of child and adolescent psychiatrists. J Psychiatr Pract 20(6):438–447. doi:10.1097/01.pra.0000456592.20622.45

Kersun LS, Elia J (2007) Depressive symptoms and SSRI Use in pediatric oncology patients. Pediatr Blood Cancer 49(7):881–887. doi:10.1002/pbc.21208

Kersun LS, Rourke MT, Mickley M, Kazak AE (2009) Screening for depression and anxiety in adolescent cancer patients. J Pediatr Hematol Oncol 31(11):835–839. doi:10.1097/MPH.0b013e3181b8704c

Kushner BH, Modak S, Basu EM, Roberts SS, Kramer K, Cheung NK (2013) Posterior reversible encephalopathy syndrome in neuroblastoma patients receiving anti-GD2 3F8 monoclonal antibody. Cancer 119(15):2789– 2795. doi: 10.1002/cncr.28137

Lavigne JV, Faier-Routman J (1992) Psychological adjustment to pediatric physical disorders: a meta-analytic review. J Pediatr Psychol 17(2):133–157

Mintz CD, Wagner M, Loepke AW (2012) Preclinical research into the effects of anesthetics on the developing brain: promises and pitfalls. J Neurosurg Anesthesiol 24(4):362–367. doi:10.1097/ANA.0b013e31826a0495

Mischoulon D, Freeman MP (2013) Omega-3 fatty acids in psychiatry. Psychiatr Clin N Am 36(1):15–23. doi:10.1016/j.psc.2012.12.002

Myers RM, Balsamo L, Xiaomin L, Devidas M, Hunger SP, Carroll WL, Winick NJ, Maloney KW, Kadan-Lottick NS (2014) A prospective study of anxiety, depression, and behavioral changes in the first year after a diagnosis of childhood acute lymphoblastic leukemia: a report from the Children's Oncology Group. Cancer 120(9):1417–1425. doi:10.1002/cncr.28578

Omega-3 | Memorial Sloan Kettering Cancer Center (2014). http://www.mskcc.org/cancer-care/herb/omega-3. Accessed 2 Nov

Özcan Ö, Dönmez YE (2014) Melatonin treatment for childhood sleep terror. J Child Adolesc Psychopharmacol 24(9):528–529. doi:10.1089/cap.2014.0061

Pai ALH, Greenley RN, Lewandowski A, Drotar D, Youngstrom E, Peterson CC (2007) A meta-analytic review of the influence of pediatric cancer on parent and family functioning. J Fam Psychol 21(3):407–415. doi:10.1037/0893-3200.21.3.407

Pangilinan PH, Giacoletti-Argento A, Shellhaas R, Hurvitz EA, Hornyak JE (2010) Neuropharmacology in pediatric brain injury: a review. PM R 2(12):1127–1140. doi:10.1016/j.pmrj.2010.07.007

Pao M, Bosk A (2011) Anxiety in medically ill children/adolescents. Depress Anxiety 28(1):40–49. doi:10.1002/da.20727

Pao M, Wiener L (2011) Psychological symptoms. In: Wolfe J, Hinds PS, Sourkes BM (eds) Textbook of interdisciplinary pediatric palliative care. Elsevier/Saunders, Philadelphia

Pao M, Ballard ED, Rosenstein DL, Wiener L, Wayne AS (2006) Psychotropic medication use in pediatric patients with cancer. Arch Pediatr Adolesc Med 160(8):818–822. doi:10.1001/archpedi.160.8.818

Patenaude AF, Kupst MJ (2005) Psychosocial functioning in pediatric cancer. J Pediatr Psychol 30(1):9–27

Phipps S, Buckholdt KE, Fernandez L, Wiener L, Kupst MJ, Madan-Swain A, Mullins L et al (2012) Pediatric oncologists' practices of prescribing selective serotonin reuptake inhibitors (SSRIs) for children and adolescents with cancer: a multi-site study. Pediatr Blood Cancer 58(2):210–215. doi:10.1002/pbc.22788

Phipps S, Klosky JL, Long A, Hudson MM, Huang Q, Zhang H, Noll RB (2014) Posttraumatic stress and psychological growth in children with cancer: has the traumatic impact of cancer been overestimated? J Clin Oncol 32(7):641–646. doi:10.1200/JCO.2013.49.8212

Poh YN, Poh PF, Buang SNH, Lee JH (2014) Sedation guidelines, protocols, and algorithms in PICUs: a systematic review. Pediatr Crit Care Med 15(9):885–892. doi:10.1097/PCC.0000000000000255

Portteus A, Ahmad N, Tobey D, Leavey P (2006) The prevalence and use of antidepressant medication in pediatric cancer patients. J Child Adolesc Psychopharmacol 16(4):467–473. doi:10.1089/cap.2006.16.467

Raison CL, Miller AH (2011) Is depression an inflammatory disorder? Curr Psychiatry Rep 13:467–475

Recklitis CJ, Diller LR, Li X, Najita J, Robison LL, Zeltzer L (2010) Suicide ideation in adult survivors of childhood cancer: a report from the Childhood Cancer Survivor Study. J Clin Oncol 28(4):655–661. doi:10.1200/JCO.2009.22.8635

Robinson S, Kissane DW, Brooker J, Burney S (2014) A systematic review of the demoralization syndrome in individuals with progressive disease and cancer: a decade of research. J Pain Symptom Manage. doi:10.1016/j.jpainsymman.2014.07.008

Rosenberg AR, Wolfe J, Bradford MC, Shaffer ML, Yi-Frazier JP, Randall Curtis J, Syrjala KL, Scott Baker K (2014) Resilience and psychosocial outcomes in parents of children with cancer. Pediatr Blood Cancer 61(3):552–557. doi:10.1002/pbc.24854

Rosenstein DR, Elswick DE, Fleisch S, Maryland P (2014) Psychopharmacologic management in oncology. In: Jame A, Gulley JL, Allegra CJ (eds) Bethesda handbook of clinical oncology, 4th edn. Wolters Kluwer/Lippincott Williams & Wilkins Health, Philadelphia

Ruddy KJ, Barton D, Loprinzi CL (2014) Laying to rest psychostimulants for cancer-related fatigue? J Clin Oncol 32(18):1865–1867. doi:10.1200/JCO.2014.55.8353

Ruggiero A, Rizzo D, Mastrangelo S, Battaglia D, Attinà G, Riccardi R (2010) Interactions between antiepileptic and chemotherapeutic drugs in children with brain tumors: is it time to change treatment? Pediatr Blood Cancer 54(2):193–198. doi:10.1002/pbc.22276

Ruland CM, Hamilton GA, Schjødt-Osmo B (2009) The complexity of symptoms and problems experienced in children with cancer: a review of the literature. J Pain Symptom Manage 37(3):403–418. doi:10.1016/j.jpainsymman.2008.03.009

Sikich N, Lerman J (2004) Development and psychometric evaluation of the pediatric anesthesia emergence delirium scale. Anesthesiology 100(5):1138–1145. PMID: 15114210

Silver GH, Kearney JA, Kutko MC, Bartell AS (2010) Infant delirium in pediatric critical care settings. Am J Psychiatry 167(10):1172–1177

Silver G, Kearney J, Traube C, Hertzig M (2014) Delirium screening anchored in child development: the Cornell assessment for pediatric delirium. Palliat Support Care. doi:10.1017/S1478951514000947

Smith HA, Fuchs DC, Pandharipande PP, Barr FE, Ely EW (2009) Delirium: an emerging frontier in the management of critically ill children. Crit Care Clin 25(3):593–614, x

Smith HA, Boyd J, Fuchs DC, Melvin K, Berry P, Shintani A, Eden SK, Terrell MK, Boswell T, Wolfram K, Sopfe J, Barr FE, Pandharipande PP, Ely EW (2011) Diagnosing delirium in critically ill children: Validity and reliability of the Pediatric Confusion Assessment Method for the Intensive Care Unit. Crit Care Med 39(1):150–157. doi: 10.1097/CCM.0b013e3181feb489

Strawn JR, Keeshin BR, DelBello MP, Geracioti TD, Putnam FW (2010) Psychopharmacologic treatment of posttraumatic stress disorder in children and adolescents: a review. J Clin Psychiatry 71(7):932–941. doi:10.4088/JCP.09r05446blu

Strawn JR, Sakolsky DJ, Rynn MA (2012) Psychopharmacologic treatment of children and adolescents with anxiety disorders. Child Adolesc Psychiatr Clin N Am 21(3):527–539. doi:10.1016/j.chc.2012.05.003

Stuber M (2012) Psychiatry impact of childhood cancer. In: Pediatric psycho-oncology psychosocial aspects and clinical interventions. Wiley-Blackwell, Chichester, pp 43–51

Talmi A, Fazio E (2012) Commentary: promoting health and well-being in pediatric primary care settings: using health and behavior codes at routine well-child visits. J Pediatr Psychol 37(5):496–502. doi:10.1093/jpepsy/jss047

Traube C, Silver G, Kearney J, Patel A, Atkinson TM, Yoon MJ, Halpert S, Augenstein J, Sickles LE, Li C, Greenwald B (2014) Cornell Assessment of Pediatric Delirium: a valid, rapid, observational tool for screening delirium in the PICU. Crit Care Med 42(3):656–663. doi: 10.1097/CCM.0b013e3182a66b76

Turkel SB, Hanft A (2014) The pharmacologic management of delirium in children and adolescents. Paediatr Drugs 16(4):267–274. doi:10.1007/s40272-014-0078-0

Turkel SB, Trzepacz PT, Tavare CJ (2006) Comparing symptoms of delirium in adults and children. Psychosomatics 47(4):320–324

Turkel SB, Jacobson JR, Jane Tavaré C (2013) The diagnosis and management of delirium in infancy. J Child Adolesc Psychopharmacol 23(5):352–356. doi:10.1089/cap.2013.0001

Ularntinon S, Tzuang D, Dahl G, Shaw RJ (2010) Concurrent treatment of steroid-related mood and psychotic symptoms with risperidone. Pediatrics 125(5):e1241–e1245. doi:10.1542/peds.2009-1815

Valluri S, Zito JM, Pao M, Ballard ED, Safer DJ, Korelitz JJ, Mattison DR, Wayne AS (2012) Antidepressant treatment of medicaid-insured youth with a cancer diagnosis: antidepressant treatment of medicaid-insured youth with cancer. J Pharm Health Serv Res 3(2):109–114. doi:10.1111/j.1759-8893.2011.00069.x

Wang X-f, Feng Y, Chen Y, Gao BL, Han B-h (2014) A meta-analysis of olanzapine for the prevention of chemotherapy-induced nausea and vomiting. Sci Rep 4:4813. doi:10.1038/srep04813

Waters AM, Ford LA, Wharton TA, Cobham VE (2009) Cognitive-behavioural therapy for young children with anxiety disorders: comparison of a child+parent condition versus a parent only condition. Behav Res Ther 47(8):654–662. doi:10.1016/j.brat.2009.04.008

Watson M, Lucas C, Hoy A, Wells J (2009) Psychiatric symptoms in palliative care In: Watson MS (ed) Oxford handbook of palliative care, 2nd edn. Oxford handbooks. Oxford University Press, Oxford/New York, p 507–523

World Health Organization (2012) WHO guidelines on pharmacological treatment of persisting pain in children with medical illnesses. World Health Organization, Geneva. http://whqlibdoc.who.int/publications/2012/9789241548120_Guidelines.pdf

Zito JM, Safer DJ, DosReis S, Gardner JF, Magder L, Soeken K, Boles M, Lynch F, Riddle MA (2003) Psychotropic practice patterns for youth: a 10-year perspective. Arch Pediatr Adolesc Med 157(1):17–25

The Impact of Pediatric Cancer on the Family

9

Cynthia A. Gerhardt, Christina G. Salley, and Vicky Lehmann

Case Vignette

"I didn't hear anything after the doctor told us Jason had cancer. My mind went blank. We were terrified." During an initial consult with their psychosocial provider, Jennifer and Tom described the moment they found out their 5-year-old son, Jason, had acute lymphoblastic leukemia (ALL), and they shared their concerns about what the next few years of treatment would mean for their family. Although the oncologist explained that Jason had a good chance of cure, they worried about his future and felt overwhelmed by all the medical information they were given. Managing intense treatment demands while continuing to work and care for Jason's sisters seemed impossible. The psychosocial provider first reassured Jennifer and Tom that their worries were very normal and then helped them to problem solve these early challenges. Rallying support to assist with immediate needs was an important, practical step. The psychosocial provider also assessed their understanding of Jason's situation and discussed how to appropriately share this information with him and his 8- and 13-year-old sisters. These strategies relieved some of Jennifer and Tom's anxiety in the first days after diagnosis and allowed the family to find a routine that now included cancer, but worked effectively for them.

Even under the best circumstances, when the likelihood of cure is good, families experience considerable stress and disruption when a child is diagnosed with cancer. In addition to adjusting to the initial shock of the diagnosis and making difficult treatment decisions, families must cope with the demands of treatment, changes in family routines, financial costs, chal-

C.A. Gerhardt, PhD (✉) • V. Lehmann, PhD
Department of Pediatrics and Psychology,
The Ohio State University, 700 Children's Drive, Rm. JW4992, Columbus, OH 43201-2696, USA

Center for Biobehavioral Health,
The Research Institute at Nationwide Children's Hospital, 700 Children's Drive, Columbus, OH 43201-2696, USA
e-mail: cynthia.gerhardt@nationwidechildrens.org; Vicky.Lehmann@nationwidechildrens.org

C.G. Salley, PhD
Department of Psychiatry & Behavioral Sciences, Memorial Sloan Kettering Cancer Center, 641 Lexington Avenue, 7th Floor, New York, NY 10022, USA
e-mail: salleyc@mskcc.org

A.N. Abrams et al. (eds.), *Pediatric Psychosocial Oncology: Textbook for Multidisciplinary Care*, DOI 10.1007/978-3-319-21374-3_9

lenging conversations with healthcare providers and other family members, and the lingering possibility of relapse or death (Rodriguez et al. 2012). Disruption in normative activities, such as school and extracurricular functions, is common for patients and siblings during treatment (Katz and Madan-Swain 2006; Alderfer et al. 2010). In survivorship, a significant proportion of families must also deal with the child's late effects and ongoing healthcare needs. When treatment is unsuccessful, parents and siblings are faced with the overwhelming task of managing end-of-life decisions, their personal grief, and adjusting to life without the child. Thus, the diagnosis of cancer in childhood has significant and enduring implications for the psychosocial well-being of the entire family.

We begin this chapter by highlighting theoretical models that guide research and supportive care of families of children with cancer. Research on the psychosocial outcomes of parents and siblings, including aspects of family functioning, is summarized across the continuum during diagnosis and treatment, survivorship, and/or end of life. A particular focus is on innovative work that illustrates the transaction of family factors and processes that contribute to outcomes for individual family members. Although limited research has evaluated clinical trials to improve psychosocial outcomes for these families, we highlight this work when possible. Attention is focused on implications for the psychosocial assessment and ongoing care of the family. Finally, directions for future research are summarized.

Theoretical Perspectives

Family systems and socioecological models emphasize that the stress of childhood cancer affects all members of the family, as individuals make adjustments to accommodate the illness and treatment in the family system (Alderfer and Kazak 2006). Bronfenbrenner (1977) proposed that an individual is nested centrally within an expanding set of rings or systems that reflect more proximal (e.g., family, school/work) to distal spheres of influence (e.g., society, culture; see Fig. 9.1). These systems have reciprocal effects on each other and the individual. Thus, a family system model considers a child's diagnosis of cancer within the context of a family that has preexisting patterns of relationships and interactions. This climate, or the common values, rules, and beliefs within the family, provides a framework for how parents and children respond to one another with respect to the challenges presented throughout treatment and afterward. For example, family environment influences how openly the family talks about the diagnosis, shares emotion and affect, and collaborates in decision making. Family members are interdependent, such that an individual's adjustment is influenced not only by intrinsic characteristics but also by the significant others in his or her life. In other words, family functioning may set the stage for how individual family members will manage cancer-related stress as a system.

Because the needs of families of children with cancer are ongoing and complex, research and clinical care is optimized when also considered within a life-span developmental perspective. As a growing number of childhood cancer survivors mature into adults, we have gained a better understanding of the evolving and lasting influence of cancer on the developing individual and family. This approach requires sensitivity to the dynamic nature of the child and family's illness experience over time (Wong et al. 2010; Kazak 2001). Transitions between developmental periods are important, as major changes in social roles and contexts can alter the course of physical and psychosocial well-being for both children and adults. For example, a child's age or the timing of diagnosis and treatment are important as they can imply different risks for psychosocial problems and provision of appropriate supportive care. Young children with cancer may have young parents who are less financially stable or new to the demands of caring for multiple, small children in the home, further compounding the strain of the cancer experience. Other parents may have different challenges, such as the cost of college tuition for older children or managing the care of elderly parents, in addition to the ill child's

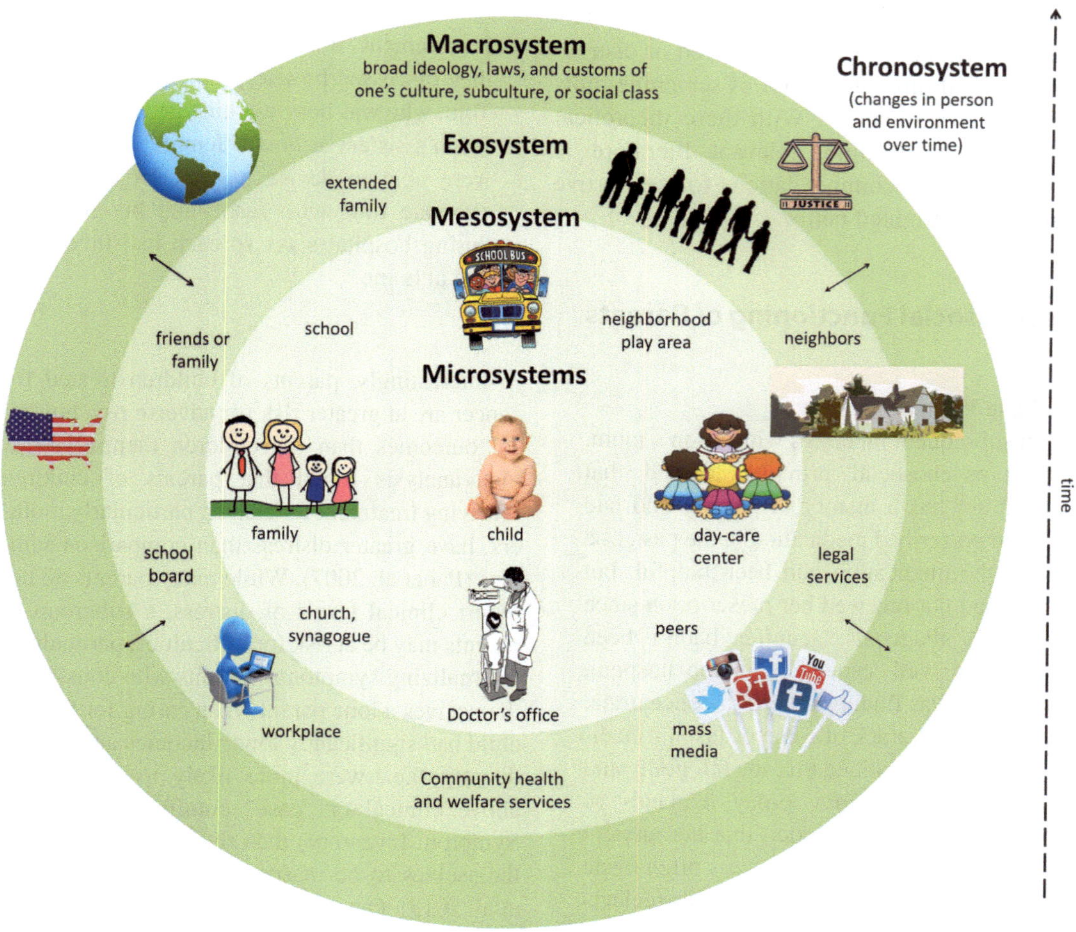

Fig. 9.1 Ecological systems theory

care. There is also evidence that childhood cancer can affect the patient's transition between developmental periods after diagnosis, including the attainment of socially valued milestones (e.g., graduation, employment) (Stam et al. 2006). Thus, a delay or failure to achieve these milestones can have lasting implications for the family system based on the child's ultimate level of independence.

Disability/stress models suggest that a variety of risk and protective factors contribute to the development of psychopathology or negative outcomes in response to adversity (Wallander and Varni 1992; Lazarus and Folkman 1984). For example, medical or disease factors, intrapersonal traits, and socioecological and environmental factors are proposed to interact over time to influence an individual's trajectory of adjustment. Many families of children with cancer exhibit resilience after initial treatment and have few lasting negative effects. However, some families or individuals struggle to adapt to a child's diagnosis and treatment for cancer and may have long-term difficulties even after treatment is completed. Researchers continue to examine the interplay of factors that contribute to variation in outcomes for families over time. The Pediatric Psychosocial Preventative Health Model (PPPHM) may provide practical guidance on how to triage services based on a family's risk profile (Kazak 2006). Please see Chap. 4 on assessment for details. This model proposes a three-tiered approach to matching the level of psychosocial intervention (i.e., universal, clinical, or targeted) with the level of family need or distress as identified through the use of screening tools or clinical assessment. With these theoretical perspectives in mind, relevant literature is reviewed and recommendations for supportive care are highlighted below.

Psychosocial Functioning of Parents

Case Vignette

In subsequent meetings with Jason's mom, the psychosocial provider learned that Jennifer has a history of anxiety and had been prescribed medication in the past. She felt the medication had been helpful, but she had not renewed her prescription since Jason's diagnosis. Jennifer hadn't been sleeping well, especially in the hospital, and she was finding it hard to concentrate. She had lost track of some of Jason's medications and confided that she felt guilty and stressed by the day-to-day demands of care. The nurses reported that her anxiety during Jason's mediport access often made it difficult to keep him calm. "I just feel terrible that he has to go through this. It breaks my heart. I worry about everything." Near the end of the session, Jennifer also shared that she had befriended another family on the unit whose child relapsed a few days earlier. Witnessing this family's pain was a stark reminder of the precarious situation that her family faced, despite her best attempts to reassure herself that Jason would be fine. The psychosocial provider discussed the importance of self-care and helped coordinate Jennifer's treatment with her primary care provider. They discussed cognitive–behavioral strategies to manage her worries and to establish better sleep hygiene. The psychosocial provider also taught Jennifer how to distract Jason and coordinated sessions with the medical team and child life professionals to facilitate her involvement in his procedures. Finally, they discussed how to problem solve with Tom, who was busy working and caring for Jason's sisters at home. Jennifer and Tom were able to devise a workable plan to alternate time with Jason and his sisters during hospital stays so each had time to rest at home.

Interestingly, parents of children treated for cancer are at greater risk for adverse psychological outcomes than the children themselves. A meta-analysis found that parents of children receiving treatment for cancer, particularly mothers, have greater distress than comparison samples (Pai et al. 2007). While many parents do not report clinical levels of distress, a subgroup of parents may be at risk for difficulties, particularly internalizing symptoms. Parents who considered themselves a lone parent when caring for their ill child had significantly lower incomes and greater distress (i.e., were more likely to score at or above clinical or "case" cutoffs on the Brief Symptom Inventory) than those who considered themselves to be married or partnered (Wiener et al. 2013). Other work suggests single mothers, and those with fewer socioeconomic resources, may be at the highest risk for internalizing symptoms and benefit the most from clinical assistance (Dolgin et al. 2007). Parent distress tends to be higher near diagnosis and during treatment but usually declines over time. However, the end of treatment may be a period of psychosocial risk, as fears of recurrence can surface for parents (Wakefield et al. 2011). Oftentimes, long-term adjustment is conceptualized in terms of posttraumatic responses to the stress of the child's cancer diagnosis, painful procedures, and threat to life. Elevations in posttraumatic stress symptoms have been reported for up to 54 % of parents at some time during or after their child's cancer treatment (Bruce 2006; Kazak et al. 2005). Concurrent stressors due to the child's limitations in functioning and resultant caregiver strain can also be a potent or proximal predictor of distress for parents of survivors.

Little research has focused on the experience of parents near the end of their child's life. Caring for a seriously ill child can have deleterious effects on parental quality of life, mood, sleep, and fatigue, with fear of the child's death and physical symptoms as frequent concerns (Klassen et al. 2008; Theunissen et al. 2007). As a child approaches the end of life, these stressors can be magnified. About half of parents of children with advanced cancer have been found to have high rates of distress (Rosenberg et al. 2013). These outcomes may be worse for parents of children with poorer health status, more intense treatment, less time since diagnosis, and more economic hardship (Klassen et al. 2008; Rosenberg et al. 2013). In fact, parents whose children have a "difficult death" or unrelieved pain, anxiety, and sleep disruption may report more internalizing symptoms and poorer quality of life 4–9 years after the death (Kreicbergs et al. 2005; Jalmsell et al. 2010). A systematic review indicates that bereaved parents are at risk for depression, anxiety, prolonged grief, and poor quality of life (Rosenberg et al. 2012). They routinely score worse on most scales of adjustment, especially internalizing problems, relative to norms and controls. Compared to other types of loss, parental grief is also more severe with a greater risk for complicated or prolonged grief reactions, particularly among mothers (Lannen et al. 2008; Lichtenthal et al. in press). However, over time, some parents can also recognize personal growth and positive outcomes, such as greater compassion and closer relationships, in response to a child's illness and/or death (Gilmer et al. 2012).

Psychosocial Functioning of Siblings

Case Vignette

Following reports from Jennifer and Tom, the psychosocial provider met with their family to address concerns about behavioral issues and declining school performance for Jason's oldest sister, Janet. Janet reluctantly disclosed that she felt bad for Jason, but she also wanted to be a normal teenager and hang out with her friends. Since Jason was diagnosed, she had received two Ds on her report card and had taken on more chores at home, often caring for her younger sister in the mornings and evenings when her dad was at work. "I don't really get to see my friends that much. Jason's at the hospital a lot, and I don't really know what's going on. Mom used to take me shopping and come to my things at school, but now she's always tired or dealing with other stuff. Everything's just different now." The psychosocial provider discovered that Jason's sisters didn't visit him when he was in the hospital, and their parents hadn't talked much about his illness since the initial diagnosis. Janet had gotten bits of information while overhearing her parents on the phone, but she was afraid to ask questions because she didn't want to upset them. The psychosocial provider worked with the family to improve communication and to address Janet's academic and social concerns with the school counselor. Jennifer and Tom updated the girls on Jason's treatment and reassured them that it was okay to ask questions. They also made plans to reinstate family movie night on Friday evenings, even when Jason was in the hospital, and scheduled occasional one-on-one time with the girls to regain a sense of normalcy.

Nearly 80 % of U.S. children grow up with a brother or sister in the home (U.S. Census Bureau 2008), underscoring the importance of sibling dynamics as part of the family system. In fact, U.S. children are now more likely to grow up with a sibling than with a father (U.S. Census Bureau 2008). Siblings share many experiences, resulting in a unique and powerful bond that is often lifelong (McHale et al. 2006). They are attachment figures that can serve as teachers, friends, comforters, protectors, competitors, and antagonists. Siblings are role models for behavior and can exert both positive (e.g., social competence, academic engagement) and negative influences (e.g., substance use, delinquency) on one another. Furthermore, managing sibling relationships, particularly conflict, is one of the top child-rearing challenges for parents (Feinberg et al. 2012). Thus, sibling relationships are a key component of family functioning and child development. When cancer disrupts this relationship and the home environment, it may have significant implications for sibling well-being.

Much of the research on siblings of children with cancer is qualitative in nature (Vermaes et al. 2012). As parents are involved in the care of the ill child, siblings may experience additional demands at home (von Essen and Enskar 2003). Because they often do not want to further burden parents, they may be left to manage their worries and fears alone. Perception of parental differential treatment (PDT) is a family dynamic that occurs naturally in families (Feinberg et al. 2012), but may be exacerbated in the case of childhood cancer. Comparison with the ill child is common, and siblings may feel jealous, resentful, or neglected at times (Wilkins and Woodgate 2005). In many cases, there are several years of treatment during which much of the family's attention and resources are directed toward the patient. Older children may be caregivers for both healthy and ill siblings and can assume other adult roles in the home (Gaab et al. 2014). Challenges to maintaining normalcy and to engaging in typical developmental activities have been reported. Siblings report that they would like to visit the hospital more often and be involved in conversations about the ill child. However, there may be challenges to providing information about the ill child and to communicating openly about the impact of the illness on siblings (Patterson et al. 2011; von Essen and Enskar 2003). These unique stressors, coupled with parents who are less available or distressed due to the child's illness, leave siblings of children with cancer at risk for acute and long-term psychosocial difficulties.

A meta-analysis found siblings of children with chronic illness are at risk for multiple difficulties (Vermaes et al. 2012). Recent reviews focused specifically on siblings of children with cancer suggest a subset experience symptoms of anxiety, depression, posttraumatic stress, reduced quality of life and lower healthcare utilization, and disruption to academic and social functioning (Alderfer et al. 2010; Wilkins and Woodgate 2005). Several factors, such as age, gender, premorbid distress, coping, and family functioning, may be associated with sibling outcomes (Houtzager et al. 2004; Long et al. 2013). Furthermore, parents report that psychosocial support for siblings is inadequate (Ballard 2004; Patterson et al. 2011). In a large-scale survey of professionals from three pediatric oncology organizations, only 25 % reported providing psychosocial services to siblings (Wiener et al. 2012).

Most difficulties for siblings dissipate over the first year after diagnosis, but there is evidence that they may resurface or worsen in response to declines in the ill child's health or death. In the few studies using standardized measures, bereaved siblings have been noted to have lower social competence and more internalizing and externalizing problems relative to norms or controls within 2 years of the death (McCown and Davies 1995; Rosenberg et al. 2015). Self-concept may decline (Eilegard et al. 2013), and bereaved siblings who are younger or male can also exhibit difficulties in peer relationships relative to classmates (Gerhardt et al. 2012). Grief symptoms, such as sadness, sleep disruption, and inattention, can resurface years later as children mature and reflect on the loss from a different perspective (Sveen et al. 2014). However, bereaved siblings can also demonstrate positive growth, such as having a better outlook on life, being kinder, and more tolerant of others (Foster et al. 2012).

Couple and Marital Relationships

Case Vignette

As Jason's treatment progressed, Jennifer and Tom reported that they felt like they were living parallel lives, often passing each other during the changing of shifts while caring for the children. Although they had been happily married for 15 years, they admitted to having more arguments lately. Some of this had spilled over to irritability toward the children as well. "We've always had a good relationship, but it's hard to find time to really talk. Jennifer used to be the one I'd go to when things were bothering me, but she's got enough on her plate. We both do!" The psychosocial provider helped the couple find ways to reconnect and find private time so they could share each other's fears and hopes during Jason's treatment. They discussed other outlets for stress and sources of support. Both realized the importance of resolving their conflicts without involving the children when possible. A focus on Jason's transition to maintenance therapy, which would be less demanding, allowed them to see some relief on the horizon.

Parents of children with cancer may perceive increased marital distress and strain, especially soon after diagnosis (Long and Marsland 2011; Grootenhuis and Last 1997). A meta-analysis found significantly higher marital distress in parents of children with cancer at diagnosis compared to parents of healthy children, but not after 1-year postdiagnosis (Pai et al. 2007). Newer studies corroborate earlier research (Wijnberg-Williams et al. 2015). Effects on marital satisfaction vary and may follow one of three patterns, reflecting increasing, decreasing, or stable satisfaction over the course of treatment. Strengthened marital relationships are most likely to be found among parents long after childhood cancer treatment. Hence, time since diagnosis, as well as the strength of the relationship before cancer onset, may impact marital satisfaction. Although cancer can strain marital or couple relationships, parents of children with cancer do not appear more likely to divorce over the long term, even in the case of bereaved couples (Schwab 1998; Syse et al. 2009).

Parents often feel that their marriage is put on hold as they devote time to their sick children while juggling other daily life tasks (e.g., household chores, work, or caring for other children) (Long and Marsland 2011). As a result, parents feel communication, shared decision making, and closeness decrease, while loneliness increases (Bjork et al. 2005). The greatest source for conflict may be differences in the way each parent copes with the child's disease. Holding back emotions in order to protect the other seems most detrimental and contributes to a loss of intimacy. Although partner's behaviors can be a source of stress and conflict, parents can also serve as a great source of support for each other. However, the type of support can vary between practical support (e.g. household tasks, taking care of other children) and emotional support. Recent work has shown interesting patterns of coping among couples of children with cancer, such that mothers' use of secondary control strategies involving cognitive reappraisal, positive thinking, acceptance, and distraction may have a compensatory effect against fathers' use of disengagement coping (e.g., avoidance, wishful thinking) in predicting both mother and father distress (Compas et al. 2015).

Family Environment and Parent–Child Relationships

While many individual and family factors can contribute to the development of psychopathology more generally, often proximal factors (e.g., parental depression, family conflict) are the most common contributors to a child's risk in the context of cancer (Robinson et al. 2007; Drotar 1997). This mirrors the developmental literature indicating the two primary factors that buffer the impact of stress on children are often intelligence and having a warm and consistent caregiver (Masten 2001). For example, both parental depression and anxiety have been associated with greater distress in children (Garber and Cole 2010), and similar patterns have been identified in families of children with cancer.

Transmission of distress between family members may be accounted for or modified by family environment. For example, Varni and colleagues (1996) found that in families of children newly diagnosed with cancer, cohesion and expressiveness were associated with fewer child internalizing problems. In general, children in families high in conflict are more prone to difficulties, while children in a positive family environment are more likely to adjust well to the stress of a chronic illness or cancer (Drotar 1997; Long and Marsland 2011). There is some evidence that mothers of children with cancer report more family conflict relative to control mothers (Pai et al. 2007), but there is variability across families, and other aspects of family functioning may be preserved (Long and Marsland 2011).

With respect to parenting, there are mixed reports with some evidence that parenting stress is elevated during treatment and among mothers of brain tumor survivors (Long and Marsland 2011), but others find no group differences. Parenting stress has been related to greater emotional, behavioral, and social difficulties among children with cancer, while perceived vulnerability may contribute to emotional difficulties (Colletti et al. 2008). Parents may be more concerned, overindulgent, and lenient than parents of children without cancer (Long et al. 2014), but it is important to note that most studies focus on the ill child as opposed to siblings. In a seminal article on sibling adjustment within 2 years of a child's cancer diagnosis (Long et al. 2013), more family functioning problems, higher parent psychological control, and lower parent acceptance were associated with sibling distress. Family functioning contributed the most variance to sibling distress, but support was also found for a cumulative risk model with a higher overall risk score also contributing to distress.

Families also undergo significant change after a child's death. One study reported higher family cohesion among bereaved families than controls (Davies 1988), but others suggest less cohesion and increased parental strain (Martinson et al. 1994; West et al. 1991). Parents may be consumed by grief and "overlook" surviving children, or they may be closer and overprotective (Lehman et al. 1989; Gilmer et al. 2012). Bereaved parents have reported more parenting stress than controls (Lehman et al. 1989), and bereaved siblings have reported less communication, availability, and support from their parents (Foster et al. 2012).

Recommendations for Supportive Care

Providing supportive care that is sensitive to the context of the family system is important throughout cancer treatment, survivorship, and/or end of life. Comprehensive standards for psychosocial care in pediatric psycho-oncology are currently under development and are family focused, including recommendations for the care of ill children, parents, and siblings (Wiener et al. 2015). Multidisciplinary psychosocial services that include family access to chaplains, child life specialists, school intervention, social work, psychologists, and psychiatrists are ideal. However, resources are limited, and the availability of clinical services varies both between and within centers. Recommendations for multidisciplinary care of families of children with cancer include assistance with the practical and financial burdens of treatment; communication and shared decision making between the family and healthcare providers; routine screening for family risk and protective factors that may contribute to overall adjustment; and cognitive–behavioral strategies to facilitate adaptation (Wiener et al. 2015). However, flexibility in location and modality of care is important, as contact with family members may be restricted due to hospital visitation policies or for practical reasons. This is especially true after a child's death. Obtaining parent proxy report or telephone contact with parents or siblings may be necessary. Referrals to existing resources within the community or online also may be helpful.

Regular screening for family psychosocial challenges and the assessment of strengths and available resources can more accurately inform the allocation of services depending on family risk and needs. Referrals should be made for evidence-based treatments to reduce psychological problems when warranted (Pai et al. 2006;

Kazak 2006). Novel studies have shown promise in reducing parent distress, such as Problem-Solving Skills Training (PSST) in mothers of children near diagnosis (Sahler et al. 2005, 2013) and cognitive–behavioral strategies to reduce PTSS in fathers of survivors (Kazak et al. 2004). Interventions to address sibling needs and difficulties vary, but most often sibling support groups or camps have been described in the literature (Carpenter et al. 1990; Houtzager et al. 2001; Sidhu et al. 2006). A recent cognitive–behavioral intervention has shown success at reducing distress in children with cancer by targeting maternal distress near diagnosis (Fedele et al. 2013). Overall, there is a relative lack of randomized controlled trials targeting parents and siblings relative to children with cancer, necessitating a reliance on evidence-based strategies derived from work with other populations.

Communication is an ongoing issue in the supportive care of families. Parents may struggle with how and what to share with children throughout the illness and treatment. Children should be provided with information in a developmentally appropriate manner throughout the course of the illness and end of life if applicable. In some cases, siblings are called upon to serve as a donor for stem cell transplant. These siblings represent a special circumstance in which communication, informed consent, and potential for distress should be evaluated and addressed (Macleod et al. 2003; Packman et al. 2004; Wiener et al. 2008). Siblings should receive education about tests and procedures as well as information about the potential for success and/or failure of the transplant. See Chap. 13 on Stem Cell Transplant for additional details.

Psychosocial providers should also assess the long-term needs and concerns of families during survivorship. This is an important time for preparing a diagnosis and treatment summary and providing education to the family regarding the need for follow-up. This includes determining the ongoing role of family members in the survivor's care, screening for distress (e.g., PTSS, depression, risk behaviors), and facilitating transitions to adult providers. Natural transitions in life roles and developmental contexts (e.g., child moving away from home, parent returning to work) will likely affect the family's financial stability, health insurance coverage, and access to care. The ability to provide ongoing support to survivors and their families, such as educational accommodations or vocational rehabilitation, may help optimize the family's success with long-term adaptation to the child's diagnosis and potential late effects.

Supportive care is also critically important at end of life. Although siblings report a desire to be involved and informed when their brother or sister is dying (Nolbris and Helstrom 2005; Steele et al. 2013), parents may not feel fully informed or have an accurate understanding of the child's prognosis (Wolfe et al. 2000; Kohler et al. 2011). Attention should focus on these difficult conversations; assessing family beliefs about death and previous losses; helping parents talk about death with the ill child and siblings; giving the child a chance to ask questions and express themselves through developmentally appropriate means (e.g., journal, artwork); allowing the family to share feelings for one another; and preparing them to say goodbye. Some children may wish to give gifts or will belongings to loved ones, participate in funeral planning, and make special requests for after their death (Foster et al. 2009). These discussions, while difficult, have the potential to promote healing, provide closure, and minimize guilt and regrets for family members after the death.

Research suggests that bereaved individuals underutilize services, and support groups may be seen as stigmatizing or unhelpful (Levy and Derby 1992; Cherlin et al. 2007; Lichtenthal et al. 2015). Grief is often described as an intensely personal experience, so interventions tailored to individual or family needs may be more acceptable and effective. The family's reluctance to return to the hospital after a child's death and limitations in the availability of bereavement services are often a challenge for providing continuity of care. Thus, community-based referrals or telemedicine approaches may be more feasible for bereaved families. Several meta-analyses of grief interventions have come to variable conclusions about efficacy, with the largest improvements found for individuals with more severe or complicated courses (Larson and

Hoyt 2007; Jordan and Neimeyer 2003; Neimeyer 2000; Currier et al. 2007; Rosner et al. 2010; Allumbaugh and Hoyt 1999). Thus, current recommendations suggest services focus on those bereaved individuals who experience the highest levels of symptoms.

Directions for Future Research

While we are gaining more knowledge about the impact of cancer and its treatment on families, there is more to learn. A growing body of research has focused on outcomes of children with cancer and parents. However, less attention has focused specifically on siblings. Much of our knowledge of psychosocial outcomes in families comes from research during survivorship. Few studies have followed a large cohort of families prospectively from diagnosis into long-term survivorship to gain an in-depth assessment of predictors and processes related to psychosocial outcomes. Researchers must understand the explanatory factors that account for variation in outcomes over time as well as how development differs from typical families who have not experienced cancer.

Other methodological points for research include the need for multiple informants and mixed method approaches that move beyond paper and pencil measures. Assessments such as lab-based tasks, "real-world" observations, qualitative interviews, and biological measures (e.g., actigraphy, psychoneuroimmunology) will enhance the quality of our science. Most importantly, research that can inform the development and evaluation of interventions to prevent difficulties and promote psychosocial resilience is paramount. These interventions will be most effective if they can capitalize on innovative technologies or approaches that allow for wider dissemination and easy access to underserved populations.

Summary

We now expect that most children diagnosed with cancer will live long and full, happy lives. Thus, considering the long-term implications of the cancer experience within the family system will help ensure the provision of appropriate supportive care and optimize outcomes for the entire family. Targeting services to subgroups at risk for distress, such as mothers near diagnosis or bereaved families, is recommended. Ongoing research that is methodologically rigorous will advance our understanding of issues relevant to families of children with cancer and inform evidence-based care. With these goals in mind, we can ensure that families affected by childhood cancer are provided with the best care to promote resilience throughout the illness, treatment, and long term.

Clinical Pearls

- Cancer has a widespread impact on the entire family system. Ongoing assessment and triaging of services for parents and siblings are important.
- The impact of cancer on family interactions and relationships can evolve as the demands of the illness and treatment change. These family factors play a critical role in the well-being of children and are important targets for intervention.
- Consideration of child development is paramount to understanding the influence of cancer on the family and providing appropriate supportive care.
- Interventions that incorporate evidence-based techniques to improve individual coping strategies and family interactions are recommended for families identified to be at risk for difficulties.

References

Alderfer MA, Kazak AE (2006) Family issues when a child is on treatment for cancer. In: BROWN RT (ed) Comprehensive handbook of childhood cancer and sickle cell disease: a biopsychosocial approach. Oxford University Press, New York

Alderfer MA, Long KA, Lown EA et al (2010) Psychosocial adjustment of siblings of children with cancer: a systematic review. Psychooncology 19: 789–805

Allumbaugh DL, Hoyt WT (1999) Effectiveness of grief therapy: a meta-analysis. J Couns Psychol 46:370–380
Ballard KL (2004) Meeting the needs of siblings of children with cancer. Pediatr Nurs 30:394–401
Bjork M, Wiebe T, Hallstrom I (2005) Striving to survive: families' lived experiences when a child is diagnosed with cancer. J Pediatr Oncol Nurs 22:265–275
Bronfenbrenner U (1977) Toward an experimental ecology of human development. Am Psychol 32:513–531
Bruce M (2006) A systematic and conceptual review of posttraumatic stress in childhood cancer survivors and their parents. Clin Psychol Rev 26:233–256
Carpenter PJ, Sahler OJ, Davis MS (1990) Use of a camp setting to provide medical information to siblings of pediatric cancer patients. J Cancer Educ 5:21–26
Cherlin EJ, Barry CL, Prigerson HG et al (2007) Bereavement services for family caregivers: how often used, why, and why not. J Palliat Med 10:148–158
Colletti CJM, Wolfe-Christiansen C, Carpentier MY et al (2008) The relationship of parental overprotection, perceived vulnerability, and parenting stress to behavioral, emotional, and social adjustment in children with cancer. Pediatr Blood Cancer 51:269–274
Compas BE, Bemis H, Gerhardt CA et al. (2015) Mothers and fathers coping with their child's cancer: Individual and interpersonal processes and symptoms of depression. Health Psychol (in press)
Currier JM, Holland JM, Neimeyer RA (2007) The effectiveness of bereavement interventions with children: a meta-analytic review of controlled outcome research. J Clin Child Adolesc Psychol 36:253–259
Davies B (1988) The family environment in bereaved families and its relationship to surviving sibling behavior. Child Health Care 17:22–31
Dolgin MJ, Phipps S, Fairclough DL et al (2007) Trajectories of adjustment in mothers of children with newly diagnosed cancer: a natural history investigation. J Pediatr Psychol 32:771–782
Drotar D (1997) Relating parent and family functioning to the psychological adjustment of children with chronic health conditions: what have we learned? What do we need to know? J Pediatr Psychol 22:149–165
Eilegard A, Steineck G, Nyberg T et al (2013) Psychological health in siblings who lost a brother or sister to cancer 2 to 9 years earlier. Psychooncology 22:683–691
Fedele DA, Hullman SE, Chaffin M et al (2013) Impact of a parent-based interdisciplinary intervention for mothers on adjustment of children newly diagnosed with cancer. J Pediatr Psychol 38:531–540
Feinberg ME, Solmeyer AR, Mchale SM (2012) The third rail of family systems: sibling relationships, mental and behavioral health, and preventive intervention in children and adolescence. Clin Child Fam Psychol Rev 15:43–57
Foster TL, Gilmer MJ, Davies B et al (2009) Bereaved parents' and siblings' reports of legacies created by children with cancer. J Pediatr Oncol Nurs 26:369–376
Foster TL, Gilmer MJ, Vannatta K et al (2012) Changes in siblings after the death of a child from cancer. Cancer Nurs 35:347–354
Gaab EM, Owens GR, Macleod RD (2014) Siblings caring for and about pediatric palliative care patients. J Palliat Med 17:62–7
Garber J, Cole DA (2010) Intergenerational transmission of depression: a launch and grow model of change across adolescence. Dev Psychopathol 22:819–830
Gerhardt CA, Fairclough DL, Grossenbacher JC et al (2012) Peer relationships of bereaved siblings and comparison classmates after a child's death from cancer. J Pediatr Psychol 37:209–219
Gilmer MJ, Foster TL, Vannatta K et al (2012) Changes in parents after the death of a child from cancer. J Pain Symptom Manage 44:572–582
Grootenhuis MA, Last BF (1997) Adjustment and coping by parents of children with cancer: a review of the literature. Support Care Cancer 5:466–484
Houtzager BA, Grootenhuis MA, Last BF (2001) Supportive groups for siblings of pediatric oncology patients: impact on anxiety. Psychooncology 10:315–324
Houtzager BA, Oort FJ, Hoekstra-Weebers JEHM et al (2004) Coping and family functioning predict longitudinal psychological adaptation of siblings of childhood cancer patients. J Pediatr Psychol 29:591–605
Jalmsell L, Kreicbergs U, Onelov E et al (2010) Anxiety is contagious – symptoms of anxiety in the terminally ill child affect long-term psychological wellbeing in bereaved parents. Pediatr Blood Cancer 54:751–757
Jordan JR, Neimeyer RA (2003) Does grief counseling work? Death Stud 27:765–786
Katz ER, Madan-Swain A (2006) Maximizing school, academic, and social outcomes in children and adolescents with cancer. In: BROWN RT (ed) Comprehensive handbook of childhood cancer and sickle cell disease: a biopsychosocial approach. Oxford University Press, New York
Kazak AE (2001) Comprehensive care for children with cancer and their families: a social ecological framework guiding research, practice, and policy. Children's Services: Soc Policy Res Prac 4:217–233
Kazak AE (2006) Pediatric Psychosocial Preventative Health Model (PPPHM): Research, practice, and collaboration in pediatric family systems medicine. Fam Syst Health 24:381–395
Kazak AE, Alderfer MA, Streisand R et al (2004) Treatment of posttraumatic stress symptoms in adolescent survivors of childhood cancer and their families: a randomized clinical trial. J Fam Psychol 18:493–504
Kazak AE, Boeving CA, Alderfer MA et al (2005) Posttraumatic stress symptoms during treatment in parents of children with cancer. J Clin Oncol 23:7405–7410
Klassen AF, Klassen R, Dix D et al (2008) Impact of caring for a child with cancer on parents' health-related quality of life. J Clin Oncol 26:1–6
Kohler BA, Ward E, Mccarthy BJ et al (2011) Annual report to the nation on the status of cancer, 1975–2007, featuring tumors of the brain and other nervous system. J Natl Cancer Inst 103:714–736

Kreicbergs U, Valdimarsdottir U, Onelov E et al (2005) Care-related distress: a nationwide study of parents who lost their child to cancer. J Clin Oncol 23:9162–9171

Lannen PK, Wolfe J, Prigerson HG et al (2008) Unresolved grief in a national sample of bereaved parents: impaired mental and physical health 4 to 9 years later. J Clin Oncol 26:5870–5876

Larson DG, Hoyt WT (2007) What has become of grief counseling? An evaluation of the empirical foundations of the new pessimism. Prof Psychol Res Prac 38:347–355

Lazarus RS, Folkman S (1984) Stress, appraisal, and coping. Springer, New York

Lehman DR, Lang ER, Wortman CB et al (1989) Long-term effects of sudden bereavement: marital and parent–child relationships and children's reactions. J Fam Psychol 2:344–367

Levy LH, Derby JF (1992) Bereavement support groups: who joins; who does not; and why. Am J Community Psychol 20:649–662

Lichtenthal WG, Corner GW, Sweeney CR et al. Mental health services for parents who lost a child to cancer: if we build them, will they come? J Clin Oncol Published online before printJune 1, 2015, doi:10.1200/JCO.2014.59.0406

Long KA, Marsland AL (2011) Family adjustment to childhood cancer: a systematic review. Clin Child Fam Psychol Rev 14:57–88

Long KA, Marsland AL, Alderfer MA (2013) Cumulative family risk predicts sibling adjustment to childhood cancer. Cancer 119:2503–2510

Long KA, Keeley L, Reiter-Purtill J et al (2014) Child-rearing in the context of childhood cancer: perspectives of parents and professionals. Pediatr Blood Cancer 61:326–332

Macleod KD, Whitsett SF, Mash EJ et al (2003) Pediatric sibling donors of successful and unsuccessful hematopoietic stem cell transplants (HSCT): a qualitative study of their psychosocial experience. J Pediatr Psychol 28:223–231

Martinson IM, Mcclowry SG, Davies B et al (1994) Changes over time: a study of family bereavement following childhood cancer. J Palliat Care 10:19–25

Masten AS (2001) Ordinary magic. Resilience processes in development. Am Psychol 56:227–238

Mccown DE, Davies B (1995) Patterns of grief in young children following the death of a sibling. Death Stud 19:41–53

Mchale SM, Kim JY, Whiteman SD (2006) Sibling relationships in childhood and adolescence. In: Noller P, Feeney JA (eds) Close relationships: functions, forms, and processes. Psychology Press, New York

Neimeyer RA (2000) Searching for the meaning of meaning: grief therapy and the process of reconstruction. Death Stud 24:541–558

Nolbris M, Helstrom AL (2005) Siblings' needs and issues when a brother or sister dies of cancer. J Pediatr Oncol Nurs 22:227–233

Packman W, Gong K, Vanzutphen K et al (2004) Psychosocial adjustment of adolescent siblings of hematopoietic stem cell transplant patients. J Pediatr Oncol Nurs 21:233–248

Pai ALH, Drotar D, Zebracki K et al (2006) A meta-analysis of the effects of psychological interventions in pediatric oncology on outcomes of psychological distress and adjustment. J Pediatr Psychol 31:978–988

Pai ALH, Lewandowski A, Youngstrom E et al (2007) A meta-analytic review of the influence of pediatric cancer on parent and family functioning. J Fam Psychol 21:407–415

Patterson P, Millar B, Visser A (2011) The development of an instrument to assess the unmet needs of young people who have a sibling with cancer: piloting the Sibling Cancer Needs Instrument (SCNI). J Pediatr Oncol Nurs 28:16–26

Robinson KE, Gerhardt CA, Vannatta K et al (2007) Parent and family factors associated with child adjustment to pediatric cancer. J Pediatr Psychol 32:400–410

Rodriguez EM, Dunn MJ, Zuckerman T et al (2012) Cancer-related sources of stress for children with cancer and their parents. J Pediatr Psychol 37:185–197

Rosenberg AR, Baker KS, Syrjala K et al (2012) Systematic review of psychosocial morbidities among bereaved parents of children with cancer. Pediatr Blood Cancer 58:503–512

Rosenberg AR, Dussel V, Kang T et al (2013) Psychological distress in parents of children with advanced cancer. JAMA Pediatr 167:537–543

Rosenberg AR, Postier A, Osenga K et al (2015) Long-term psychosocial outcomes among bereaved siblings of children with cancer. J Pain Symptom Manage 49:55–65

Rosner R, Kruse J, Hagl M (2010) A meta-analysis of interventions for bereaved children and adolescents. Death Stud 34:99–136

Sahler OJ, Fairclough DL, Phipps S et al (2005) Using problem-solving skills training to reduce negative affectivity in mothers of children with newly diagnosed cancer: report of a multisite randomized trial. J Consult Clin Psychol 73:272–283

Sahler OJ, Dolgin MJ, Phipps S et al (2013) Specificity of problem solving skills training in mothers of children newly diagnosed with cancer: results of a multisite randomized clinical trial. J Clin Oncol 31:1329–1335

Schwab R (1996) Gender differences in parental grief. Death Stud 20:103–113

Schwab R (1998) A child's death and divorce: dispelling the myth. Death Stud 22:445–468

Sidhu R, Passmore A, Baker D (2006) The effectiveness of a peer support camp for siblings of children with cancer. Pediatr Blood Cancer 47:580–588

Stam H, Hartman EE, Deurloo JA et al (2006) Young adult patients with a history of pediatric disease: impact on course of life and transition into adulthood. J Adolesc Health 39:4–13

Steele AC, Kaal J, Thompson AL et al (2013) Bereaved parents and siblings offer advice to healthcare providers and researchers after a child's death from cancer. J Pediatr Hematol Oncol 35:253–259

Sveen J, Eilegard A, Steineck G et al (2014) The still grieve: a nationwide follow-up of young adults 2–9 years after losing a sibling to cancer. Psychooncology 23:658–664

Syse A, Loge JH, Lyngstad TH (2009) Does childhood cancer affect parental divorce rates? A population-based study. J Clin Oncol 10:872–877

Theunissen JM, Hoogerbrugge PM, Van Achterberg T et al (2007) Symptoms in the palliative phase of children with cancer. Pediatr Blood and Cancer 49:160–165

U.S. Census Bureau (2008) American Community Survey [Online]. Available: http://factfinder.census.gov/servlet/STTable?_bm=yand-qr_name=ACS_2008_1YR_G00_S0101and-geo_id=01000US&-ds_name=ACS_2008_1YR_G00_&-_lang=en&-redoLog=false&-state=st. Accessed 25 June 2010

Varni JW, Katz ER, Colegrove R et al (1996) Family functioning predictors of adjustment in children with newly diagnosed cancer: a prospective analysis. J Child Psychol Psychiatry 37:321–328

Vermaes IPR, Van Susante AMJ, Van Bakel HJA (2012) Psychological functioning of siblings in families of children with chronic health conditions: a meta-analysis. J Pediatr Psychol 37:166–184

Von Essen L, Enskar K (2003) Important aspects of care and assistance for siblings of children treated for cancer. Cancer Nurs 26:203–210

Wakefield CE, Mcloone JK, Butow P et al (2011) Parental adjustment to the completion of their child's cancer treatment. Pediatr Blood and Cancer 56:524–531

Wallander J, Varni JW (1992) Adjustment in children with chronic physical disorders: programmatic research on a disability-stress-coping model. In: Lagreca A, Siegel L, Wallander J, Walker C (eds) Stress and coping in child health. Guilford Press, New York

West SG, Sandler I, Pillow DR et al (1991) The use of structural equation modeling in generative research: toward the design of a preventive intervention for bereaved children. Am J Community Psychol 19:459–480

Wiener L, Steffen-Smith E, Battles H et al (2008) Sibling stem cell donor experiences at a single institution. Psychooncology 17:394–307

Wiener L, Oppenheim D, Breyer J et al (2012) A worldview of the professional experiences and training needs of pediatric psycho-oncologists. Psychooncology 21:944–953

Wiener L, Pao M, Zadeh S et al (2013) Socio-environmental factors associated with lone parenting chronically ill children. Child Health Care 42:264–280

Wiener L, Viola A, Koretski J et al (2015) Pediatric psycho-oncology care: standards, guidelines and consensus reports. Psychooncology 24:204–211

Wijnberg-Williams BJ, Van De Wiel HBM, Kamps W et al (2015) Effects of communication styles on marital satisfaction and distress of parents of pediatric cancer patients: a prospective longitudinal study. Psychooncology 24:106–112

Wilkins KL, Woodgate RL (2005) A review of qualitative research on the childhood cancer experience from the perspective of siblings: the need to give them a voice. J Pediatr Oncol Nurs 22:305–319

Wolfe J, Klar N, Grier HE et al (2000) Understanding of prognosis among parents of children who died of cancer: impact on treatment goals and integration of palliative care. JAMA 284:2469–2475

Wong TM, Branje SJ, Vandervalk IE et al (2010) The role of siblings in identity development in adolescence and emerging adulthood. J Adolesc 33:673–682

Neurocognitive Late Effects in Children with Cancer

10

Sunita K. Patel, Fiona Schulte, Natalie C. Kelly, and Amii C. Steele

Introduction

Families of children recently diagnosed with cancer may experience disruptions across multiple domains in their normal daily life and routine. Disruption in the child's cognitive and educational development during treatment for cancer has the potential to adversely impact quality of life well into the child's future. Fortunately, most children with cancer are able to successfully resume their premorbid cognitive and educational trajectories once their acute medical symptoms have resolved and their physical health has stabilized following completion of their cancer treatments.

However, there are subgroups of survivors who remain at risk for prolonged disruption as well as the development of new deficits in the years following completion of cancer therapies. Primarily, these are patients who have survived cancers involving the central nervous system (CNS) or who have received cancer therapy that can damage the developing brain, placing them at risk of developing long-term neurocognitive and behavioral sequelae. Survivors of acute lymphoblastic leukemia (ALL) and brain tumors, the two most common malignancies of childhood, are especially susceptible to these negative outcomes. Other groups that are relatively less studied but thought to be at risk due to the therapies received include patients who undergo stem cell transplantation, survivors of acute myelocytic leukemia (AML), and non-Hodgkin lymphoma (NHL), as some of these patients may receive intrathecal chemotherapy and/or total body irradiation depending on their disease status.

Research over the past three decades has helped us to identify some of the biological, clinical, and patient-related risk factors associated with neurocognitive impairment and has increased our understanding of the types of neurocognitive late effects that may be experienced

S.K. Patel, PhD (✉)
Departments of Population Sciences and Supportive Care Medicine, City of Hope Medical Center, Duarte, CA 91010, USA
e-mail: spatel@coh.org

N.C. Kelly, PhD, ABPP
Department of Supportive Care Medicine, City of Hope Medical Center, Duarte, CA 91010, USA
e-mail: nkelly@coh.org

F. Schulte, PhD, R Psych.
Departments of Oncology and Paediatrics, University of Calgary, Calgary, AB, Canada

Haematology, Oncology and Transplant Program, Alberta Children's Hospital, 2888 Shaganappi Trail NW, Calgary, AB, Canada
e-mail: fiona.schulte@albertahealthservices.ca

A.C. Steele, PhD
Department of Pediatric Hematology, Oncology, and BMT, Levine Children's Hospital at Carolinas Medical Center, 1001 Blythe Blvd, Medical Center Plaza, Suite 601, Charlotte, NC 28203, USA
e-mail: Amii.Steele@carolinas.org

A.N. Abrams et al. (eds.), *Pediatric Psychosocial Oncology: Textbook for Multidisciplinary Care*, DOI 10.1007/978-3-319-21374-3_10

by childhood cancer survivors. More recently, these lines of research have led us to begin to evaluate potential prevention and intervention approaches to address these problems in the subpopulations most at risk. In this chapter, we present information on the disease, treatment, and patient-related factors relevant in understanding neurocognitive outcomes in high-risk survivors of childhood cancer. We also provide information on common areas of neurocognitive dysfunction, general considerations and clinical practice in the neuropsychological evaluation of children with cancer, and an overview of research investigating a variety of interventions and approaches to prevent or reduce neurocognitive dysfunction.

Disease and Treatment-Related Risk Factors

Children with Brain Tumors

Approximately 70 % of pediatric brain tumors are classified as malignant, typically requiring aggressive, CNS-directed therapy consisting of surgery, radiation, and chemotherapy, either alone or in some combination. Cranial radiation was the cornerstone of pediatric brain tumor therapy for many years and has contributed to a 5-year survival rate of about 66 % overall and 70–80 % for medulloblastoma (Imbach et al. 2006). Radiation therapy involves the delivery of high-intensity radiation beams to tumor sites and is most effective in tumors that are aggressive and have rapid cell division. Radiation therapy for CNS tumors may be delivered to the entire brain, to the entire brain and spinal axis, or to a focal area of the brain. In many cases, whole brain radiation is combined with an increased dose boost to the site of the tumor and sometimes to the area surrounding the tumor (e.g., the posterior fossa). However, as long-term survival was achieved, radiation to the brain was quickly identified as a major reason for the emergence of long-term neurocognitive deficits, ranging from declines in global intelligence to reduced functioning in specific neurocognitive processes (Packer et al. 1987). Cranial radiation is also associated with other late effects, such as neuroendocrine abnormalities and fatigue, which may further exacerbate lowered neurocognitive functioning (Schwartz et al. 2000).

Because of these adverse late effects, there are ongoing efforts to alter the intensity of treatment provided to children with CNS tumors. Specifically, protocols have attempted a more targeted approach where children with a relatively lower risk clinical profile (i.e., less aggressive disease) receive a reduced dose of radiation therapy, and radiation is substituted with chemotherapeutic agents for very young children (Baron et al. 2013). In contemporary treatment protocols for children with brain tumors, patients classified as high risk based on clinical characteristics continue to receive higher dose of cranial radiation while the dose to average-risk patients is lower. Recent prospective, longitudinal follow-up of children with medulloblastoma clearly shows a substantial difference in neurocognitive decline between children who received 23.4Gy of craniospinal irradiation compared to those who received 36–39.6Gy, with poorer outcomes in high-risk patients (Palmer et al. 2013).

Children with brain tumors frequently have a number of disease- and treatment-related factors which can adversely impact their neurocognitive functioning. These factors include the location and infiltration of the tumor in the brain, the presence or absence of hydrocephalus, and the postsurgical complications which may occur, such as posterior fossa syndrome. The most common neurosurgical complications are bleeding, which can result in hemiparesis, speech impairment, visual deficits, and a variety of motor and sensory impairments (Packer et al. 1987). While there typically is some recovery of functioning after an acute neurosurgical event due to brain plasticity, long-term disability may also occur.

Neurocognitive outcomes in children with brain tumors may also be further impacted by possible neurotoxicity due to chemotherapy. The chemotherapy agents most commonly used in the high-dose regimen for childhood brain tumors include cisplatin, cyclophosphamide, etoposide, methotrexate, thiotepa, carboplatin, and topotecan. The effects of chemotherapy in children treated without radiation has not been well studied yet; however, preliminary findings suggest brain injury occurs even without cranial radiation, possibly due to a combination of tumor, surgery, and chemotherapy effects (Nelson et al. 2014).

Children with Leukemia

Acute lymphoblastic leukemia (ALL) is the most common childhood cancer and is the most frequently cited example of success following the advances in cancer treatment for children, with cure rates today of 80 % without relapse at 7–10 years after diagnosis (Imbach et al. 2006). However, earlier treatment regimens involving aggressive therapies that resulted in the improved survival rates were found to often occur at the expense of significant late effects in health outcomes, especially neurocognitive functioning.

As in the case of pediatric CNS tumor patients, there has been considerable literature documenting the adverse impact of cranial radiation therapy (CRT) on the cognitive outcomes of patients diagnosed with ALL. CRT is currently employed as a treatment procedure for ALL patients considered at high risk for relapse within the CNS (Moleski 2000). However, there appears to be a threshold of radiation intensity at which cognitive deficits are seen in patients with ALL, with evolving consensus that there are minimal cognitive late effects observed in most children who receive 1800 cGy or less, as their performances on cognitive tests are comparable to the normal population (Waber et al. 2007). Further, there is emerging evidence that proton radiation therapy may be associated with fewer cognitive deficits compared to traditional photon radiation therapy and this is an ongoing area of investigation in the effort to reduce risk for neurocognitive dysfunction (Pulsifer et al. 2010).

Given the known deleterious effects of CRT on neurocognitive function, CNS-directed chemotherapy has largely replaced CRT for patients diagnosed with ALL. Methotrexate (MTX), an antifolate, is an important component of all therapies for ALL. It is administered intrathecally to prevent leukemic involvement of the CNS and on a weekly oral schedule for 2–3 years as a component of virtually all maintenance therapies. MTX is also given intravenously, although the dose and schedule of infusion vary across treatment protocols and may include leucovorin rescue. There is ongoing research within the Children's Oncology Group to evaluate the cognitive and behavioral effects associated with these newer, potentially less neurotoxic treatment approaches (Noll et al. 2013). Results from these prospective, longitudinal studies will be helpful as the current published literature is mixed with respect to neurocognitive outcomes in ALL patients treated without radiation and only chemotherapy ranging from no effect of MTX to others identifying deficits in a wide range of neurocognitive processes (Buizer et al. 2009; Peterson et al. 2008). For the most part, findings suggest that IQ remains relatively intact; however, there may be subtle deficits in more specific neurocognitive functions, particularly attention and executive functioning processes (Buizer et al. 2009), as well as processing speed (Kahalley et al. 2013). Processing speed deficits can be particularly challenging, because children/teenagers have the cognitive capacity to do their work but are unable to complete it in a timely manner and this can lead to significant frustration and demoralization. There are no empirically validated treatments for slow processing speed.

More recently, Conklin and colleagues (2012) examined outcomes from the St. Jude Total Therapy Study XV which follows a protocol for induction therapy of intrathecal MTX for 13–25 treatments depending on risk status of the disease, as well as high-dose MTX given intravenously every other week for four cycles. The authors reported that while the ALL group was at significantly greater risk for sustained attention difficulties compared to a normative sample, no significant differences emerged for measures of intellectual functioning, academic skills, or memory (Conklin et al. 2012).

Discrepancies in findings about the impact of MTX on the cognitive outcomes of patients diagnosed with ALL may be related to the differences in the samples included in each study or may also reflect differences in the time since treatment. Time since treatment is an important predictor of neurocognitive outcomes, as longer time since treatment is more consistently associated with impaired performance on neurocognitive assessment, as well as self-reports of poor cognitive and psychosocial functioning (Krull et al. 2013b). Although the mechanism by which neurotoxic chemotherapies such as MTX work on cognition is not entirely clear, there is some evidence of reduced cerebral white matter in the brain, in a similar fashion to CRT (Reddick et al. 2005).

Other CNS-directed systemic agents that have been used in the treatment of ALL include corticosteroid therapy. The type of steroid used (i.e., dexamethasone vs. prednisone) has not been found to have clinically meaningful differences on the cognition of ALL patients (Warris et al. 2014). However, it is difficult to assess the impact of these treatments alone since they are typically administered concurrently with MTX. Nevertheless, future research investigating the effect of CNS-directed systemic therapies on cognition, including corticosteroid therapy and high-dose MTX, is needed.

Hematopoietic Stem Cell Transplant

The research related to the cognitive outcomes of ALL patients who receive hematopoietic stem cell transplant (HSCT) is generally inconclusive. Some reports indicate no effect on cognition (Phipps et al. 2008), yet there is some evidence to suggest increased use of special education services in long-term survivors and decreased language skills relative to controls (Sanders et al. 2010). One retrospective study identified that children transplanted at a younger age and treated with CRT were found to have increased cognitive deficits (Smedler et al. 1990). In the largest, prospective, longitudinal study of children who underwent transplantation, Phipps et al. (2008) concluded that there may be some risk among those who received CRT but determined that this risk was not clinically significant. The difficulty in generating conclusive statements about the cognitive outcomes for HSCT patients is that many of these patients approach the transplant already immersed in intensive treatments and therefore, baseline assessments of functioning pre-transplant may not be an accurate reflection of premorbid function.

Lymphoma

Survivors of childhood cancers other than brain tumors and leukemia may also experience some neurocognitive late effects as a consequence of their cancer treatment. Similar to ALL, treatment for non-Hodgkin lymphoma (NHL) also involves intrathecal chemotherapies and survivors may have increased risk for neurocognitive deficits, especially if treated at a young age and with cranial radiation (von Der Weid 2008). Because of the biological and therapeutic similarities between ALL and NHL, many researchers have examined impact in these patients as a single group, and thus, there is relatively limited knowledge about neurocognitive outcomes in survivors of NHL. Self-reports of neurocognitive functioning from the Childhood Cancer Survivorship Study (CCSS) found that 13–21 % of adult survivors of childhood, non-CNS cancers had impairment on various aspects of executive functioning, when compared to a sibling cohort. In this sample, 9–18 % of NHL survivors placed in the impaired range on various executive function scales. Impaired executive functioning was also associated with lack of employment in this study (Kadan-Lottick et al. 2010). A recent publication documented significantly lower objective neurocognitive performance among long-term survivors of childhood Hodgkin lymphoma (HL) relative to national age-adjusted norms, as well as leukoencephalopathy in 53 % of the survivors (Krull et al. 2012). These results were attributed to delayed effects of cardiac and pulmonary toxicities from mantle field radiation; however, the study design did not permit examination in patients treated with chemotherapy only.

Neuroblastoma

Another compelling finding from the CCSS study is that hearing difficulty was associated with an increased risk in self-reported neurocognitive dysfunction (i.e., task efficiency, organization, and emotional regulation; Kadan-Lottick et al. 2010). The association between hearing and academic performance has also been established in otherwise healthy children but is only starting to gain recognition among childhood cancer survivors. Gurney et al. (2007) studied 137 survivors of neuroblastoma and found that hearing loss was associated with learning problems and worse school functioning. Hearing loss is associated with chemotherapy such as cisplatin used to treat other malignancies; but interestingly with children with neuroblastoma, their neurocognitive deficits appear to be directly related to their hearing loss as opposed to other CNS-directed therapies.

Other Malignant Tumors of Childhood

Generally, survivors with soft tissue sarcoma, Ewing tumor, or Wilms tumor had self-reported neurocognitive functioning scores that were similar to or better than when compared with a sibling cohort (Kadan-Lottick et al. 2010). Survivors of osteosarcoma who receive IV methotrexate reported slightly poorer scores in task efficiency and emotional regulation when compared to siblings. It is unclear whether this difference is solely due to the effects of IV methotrexate or other aspects of their disease and treatment. Kadan-Lottick et al. (2010) reported that survivors who endorsed emotional distress, including anxiety and depression, were at elevated risk for impaired task efficiency, organization, memory, and emotional regulation.

Mechanisms of Neurocognitive Damage

Neurocognitive dysfunction secondary to CRT or chemotherapy results predominantly from cortical and subcortical white matter damage, with demyelination and glial cell destruction. Quantitative MRI studies in brain tumor patients have shown that the volume of normal-appearing white matter declines over time from the start of CRT and that this correlates with decreases in IQ. Additionally, CRT may disrupt the microvascular system supplying blood to the brain, resulting in calcification of fiber tracts and restriction of oxygen supply to portions of the brain (Kun 1997). Initially, radiation therapy was thought to cause acute, irreversible injury to normal tissues at the cellular level, leading to irreparable insults to organ function that remained stable over time. Currently, it is increasingly speculated that although radiation injures neurons, it is the response of multiple cell types to the radiation injury that creates chronic processes leading to progressive damage that continues over time (Wong and Van Der Kogel 2004).

Patient-Related Risk Factors for Neurocognitive Impairments

Neurocognitive late effects typically emerge within approximately 2 years following treatment completion. However, the degree of neurobehavioral deficit differs in magnitude based on a number of disease, treatment, and individual factors. Intensity of treatments and the age of the child at diagnosis and treatment are moderating factors, with younger age and higher treatment intensity associated with worse cognitive and behavioral outcomes. The interval between age at diagnosis and at time of cognitive assessment is also an important predictor with more severe deficits observed with longer time since treatment for some patient groups. At the same time, decline is also thought to eventually stabilize and may not be a linear process (Nathan et al. 2007).

The potential for adverse treatment-related neurocognitive impact appears to be associated with the degree of brain maturation at the time of therapy, with younger children being at great risk. Children with brain tumors who receive high-dose CRT prior to age four are at the greatest risk for severe, global neurocognitive deficits. For these survivors, graduation from high school outside of a specialized educational program is rare, and many are unlikely to be able to live independently as adults (Packer et al. 1987). However, for the majority of affected childhood cancer survivors, cognitive difficulties are to a less severe degree and affect discrete areas of cognition rather than having global impact. Many of these survivors are presumed to be able to compensate for specific cognitive weaknesses by employing targeted learning interventions, by utilizing environmental supports, and by relying on areas of relative strength. Gender of the child and extent of resources (i.e., quality health care, optimal school and tutoring services, parent involvement, etc.) available to the child and family are additional predictors speculated as contributing to long-term outcomes but are not yet well studied (Patel et al. 2014a). Further, individual variation in neurocognitive outcomes following diagnosis and treatment for cancer may also be a result of genetic predispositions, such as polymorphisms in genes that modulate response to therapy or predispositions that influence response to physiologic stress and CNS integrity (Krull et al. 2013a). A list of the aforementioned factors that are thought to influence the nature and extent of neurocognitive impact experienced by children with cancer is presented below. See Box 10.1.

Box 10.1 Factors Contributing to Neurocognitive Outcome

Disease/treatment factors
Cranial radiation
Presence and location of a brain tumor
Surgical resection of a brain tumor
Chemotherapies known to be associated with neurotoxicity (neurocognitive, neuropathy, hearing loss, etc.) Methotrexate Vincristine Carboplatin/cisplatin
Type and severity of cancer (e.g., brain tumor, leukemia, etc.)
Modality and dose intensity (IV, IO, IT) Drug combinations such as with or without corticosteroids, leucovorin, cytarabine, asparaginase, etc.
Individual factors
Time since diagnosis/age at assessment
Age of child at disease onset
Gender
Pre-diagnosis functioning/precancer trajectory
Environmental factors (e.g., quality of school resources)
Genetic predisposition
Family functioning

Profile of Cognitive Impairment in Childhood Cancer Survivors

Common areas of dysfunction observed in survivors with a history of CRT and/or intrathecal chemotherapy include attention/concentration skills, processing speed, memory, visual-motor integration, and executive functions (e.g., planning and organizational skills, etc.) (Buizer et al. 2009; Robinson et al. 2010). Such abilities represent "core" mental processes by which children learn, store, organize and integrate, and effectively apply new knowledge and skills. In particular, changes in the underlying basic processes of attention and memory are associated with a lowered acquisition rate of new knowledge and skills relative to same age peers and, over time, impact the survivor's IQ and academic achievement (Palmer et al. 2001). Dysfunction in attention/concentration, processing speed, and executive function skills appear to be consistently reported in studies focused on neurocognitive impact in childhood cancer survivors and warrant special attention as they can initially be easily misinterpreted as volitional nonadherence by caregivers. See Box 10.2 for common manifestations in the child's daily life.

Box 10.2 Manifestations of Neurocognitive Dysfunction in Daily Life

Attention

- Trouble sustaining focus on a task over long periods of time and may lack awareness of these episodes of disrupted attention.
- Inattention may be overlooked or even mistaken for deliberate noncompliance.
- A tendency to miss bits of information when somebody is talking, especially if there is a lot of noise or commotion nearby.
  - May lead to inability to follow directions or understanding complex concepts.
- Careless errors, incomplete homework assignments, and inconsistent performance.

- May appear to have poor memory for things like schoolwork, but good memory for more personal things that are of greater interest.
- Negative social impact since kids do not notice when they are making mistakes, or doing or saying something wrong, but peers may notice.

Processing Speed
- Needs more time to finish tasks or to respond to a question
- Trouble keeping pace with the flow of instructions, demonstrations, and explanations

Working Memory
- Trouble attending to many different things or aspects of a problem at the same time
- Limitation on the ability to mentally "hold" information, instructions, or ideas in mind temporarily while performing other mental operations

Planning and Organizing Skills
- Trouble breaking down large projects into steps and figuring out the order in which to start
- Difficulty organizing time, as they do not know how much time to allow themselves to complete an assignment or job

Quality of Life Outcomes in Survivors with Neurocognitive Impairments

The impact of neurocognitive late effects on survivors of pediatric cancer is widespread and adult survivors of childhood cancer have been found to experience long-standing economic, psychological, and social consequences (Zebrack et al. 2004). Specifically, these survivors are more likely than their siblings to require special education services, less likely to attend college, and less likely to live independently as adults (Gurney et al. 2009). In addition, survivors of childhood cancer are at increased risk of unemployment compared to their siblings and are more likely to never marry (Gurney et al. 2009). See chapter 15 (survivorship) for more details.

Survivors of pediatric cancer, and particularly those with neurocognitive late effects, experience deficits in social adjustment (Schulte and Barrera 2010). Social adjustment has been defined as the extent to which individuals are achieving socially appropriate goals (Cavell 1990). These deficits worsen with time, affecting survivors' quality of life (Schulte and Barrera 2010). Research examining the relationship between neurocognitive processes and social adjustment is scarce in pediatric brain tumor survivors and has been identified as a gap in the literature. Typically, these constructs have been investigated independently. However, cognitive processes would be expected to have pervasive effects on a child's perception and interpretation of social situations and behavioral responses in social interactions. For example, children with cognitive-executive deficits may have difficulty thinking about multiple social perspectives or response options when determining how to respond to social stimuli. A link between attention dysfunction and social outcomes in survivors of childhood cancer has been reported (Moyer et al. 2012; Patel et al. 2007).

Considerations in Neuropsychological Evaluation of Children with Cancer

The field of pediatric neuropsychology has developed significantly over the years and the practice currently involves work with children and families in varied clinical settings, including children with cancer. In addition to the general qualifications for neuropsychology, providers who wish to practice in a pediatric oncology setting are encouraged to specifically pursue training opportunities under the direct supervision of a licensed neuropsychologist experienced in the area.

From a research perspective, neurocognitive and behavioral assessments are valuable to conduct in conjunction with contemporary pediatric cancer therapies to examine differences between treatments which, in cases of similar medical outcomes, may ultimately determine treatment preference. From a clinical perspective, monitoring of neuropsychological functioning in children at risk for neurocognitive impairments is valuable to provide the medical team and the child's family with information relevant to the child's health status, particularly with respect to the emergence of late effects across time. Importantly, information from comprehensive assessments can be used to identify any delayed sequelae and to develop a plan of care for remediation of cognitive impairments. Results from the initial neuropsychological assessment are particularly helpful in guiding the course, timing, and plan of action for the child's transition back to academic and social environments. Subsequent assessments are helpful in tracking developmental progress, or lack of, in neuropsychological functioning. Results may also assist the family and medical team in understanding "problematic" behaviors. For example, identification of attention or memory problems may explain child's "nonadherence" in remembering to take medications or identify emerging problems that may impact daily living skills, such as effectively managing time to complete school assignments or activities of daily living. Ongoing monitoring of the child's neuropsychological functioning is also helpful to keep the family and medical team informed of changes across time, such as the emergence of new deficits or worsening of previously identified dysfunction.

Timing of Assessments

In general, a baseline neuropsychological evaluation is recommended following completion of primary treatments and after acute symptoms have resolved. Typically, this coincides with the child's transition back to the school environment. The Children's Oncology Task Force on Neurocognitive/Behavioral Complications after Childhood Cancer provided an expansion on the Children's Oncology Group's (COG) Long-Term Follow-Up Guidelines that offer direction on the timing of neuropsychological evaluation in pediatric cancer populations. According to these guidelines, survivors of childhood cancer should receive a baseline evaluation as they enter long-term follow-up (approximately 1–2 years post treatment), should be monitored annually for educational and vocational progress in the long-term survivorship follow-up program, and should be referred for periodic comprehensive neuropsychological reevaluations as clinically indicated (www.survivorshipguidelines.org). Typically, it is appropriate to reevaluate the patient during educational milestones and developmental transitional points (e.g., elementary to middle school, middle school to high school, and high school to college, etc.) and always when there are concerns of worsening functioning (Nathan et al. 2007). Unfortunately, not all centers have survivorship programs or staffing to provide repeated neuropsychological evaluations. Further, difficulties in securing insurance reimbursement for the neuropsychological evaluations, if done, can pose an operational barrier in providing an optimal level of care.

As described previously, children with brain tumors and ALL are at greatest risk for cognitive impairment, but the recommendation for regular monitoring of educational and vocational progress extends to children of any cancer diagnosis or treatment history. Prolonged school absences are common in children undergoing treatment for cancer which can negatively impact the child's ability to maintain pace academically; therefore, monitoring of learning and school-related difficulties would be appropriate in these cases as well. Neuropsychological evaluations can be helpful for children in this group as well, particularly for those who are struggling at school. Please see Chap. 11 (education) for more details.

General Clinical Practices in Neuropsychological Evaluation

One of the initial steps in neuropsychological assessment is a thorough review of records, which requires sifting through all the layers of information contained in medical records which may or may not be fully relevant to the case at hand. A review of neuroimaging reports (e.g., MRI, CT scans, etc.) is helpful in formulating the approach to neuropsychological evaluation, particularly in patients with brain tumor or CNS complications, given that the particular type of neuroanatomical involvement influences decisions about the battery of tests to administer. Further, in pediatric oncology specifically, it is important to gather records about the onset and associated history of the particular cancer diagnosis, as clinical-, disease-, and treatment-related factors are known to confer varying degrees of risk for cognitive and behavioral dysfunction. Also, information regarding the patient's specific treatment protocol is crucial in helping to attribute the various etiologies for any impairments that are identified as a result of the neuropsychological evaluation. In pediatric assessments, review of school records is essential to understand the patient's educational exposure and to correlate any academic and behavioral difficulties with neuropsychological performances. This process may include requesting previous educational plan documentation (e.g., Individualized Education Program), progress reports, report cards, or documentation from other providers in the school setting (e.g., school psychologist).

The clinical interview is another key aspect of neuropsychological assessment and the detailed information obtained using this procedure frequently facilitates conceptualization and hypothesis generation with respect to the child's struggles and how they manifest in daily functioning. The interview process frequently provides nuanced information regarding the severity, duration, or frequency of cognitive and behavioral symptoms that is typically not available in medical records. Incorporating details from collateral interview of parents, caregivers, teachers, other providers (e.g., therapists), etc., is also essential toward a comprehensive understanding of the child's struggles and how these are manifested in daily life. By the end of the clinical interview, the interviewer has gathered and clarified details regarding the patient's history across various domains (e.g., medical, developmental, family, psychosocial, educational, psychiatric, etc.).

Following the clinical interview, the pediatric neuropsychologist finalizes the specific tests to administer related to the neurocognitive functions of interest. When a comprehensive assessment is indicated, evaluation typically includes the following cognitive domains: academic achievement, attention/concentration, working memory, processing speed, language/verbal reasoning, verbal and visual learning and memory, executive functioning, daily behavioral and adaptive functioning, sensory, and gross and/or fine motor skills. As previously mentioned, particular domains known to be at risk for impairment in pediatric oncology populations should be the focus including global intellectual functioning, attention, executive functioning, processing speed, and nonverbal/visuospatial reasoning. Aspects of the neurological examination may also be administered based on the patient's level of direct neuroanatomical involvement or sensory presentation (e.g., visual field defect secondary to tumor resection). In addition to cognitive functioning, neuropsychologists evaluate psychological, behavioral, adaptive, and personality characteristics of their patients as well as how they integrate with the patient's neurocognitive presentation. Although generally less common in pediatric cancer populations, symptom validity testing may also be employed to provide information regarding the examinee's level of motivation or effort during the testing process (AACN 2007).

Screening Approaches

Comprehensive neuropsychological evaluations for patients at high risk for neuropsychological impairments following cancer diagnosis and treatment are the gold standard but may not always be feasible given the practical challenges that arise in the current health-care setting. As noted earlier, comprehensive neuropsychological evaluations can be quite costly and are not always covered by insurance. In addition, full assessments can take a long time (e.g., 5 or more hours), and this is not always practical for families or within the time constraints of the clinic setting. Additionally, there may not be sufficient staffing to provide timely services to all children at high risk. In contrast, routine screening could become a fiscally responsible strategy used to target patients who are in need of more comprehensive evaluation (Krull et al. 2008b). Neurocognitive screening may range from a detailed interview to assess the child's school, social, and learning development to administration of brief, standardized neurocognitive measures, depending on the child's risk level. Given this context, a number of screening approaches are being evaluated (Embry et al. 2012; Krull et al. 2008a).

Regardless of whether a comprehensive or brief neurocognitive screening approach is used, test administration, scoring, and interpretation of test data are often considered the "core" components of a neuropsychological assessment and each has its standards and competencies characteristic of the process. However, with each step, it is important to consider not just the *test scores* but the larger context that provides the framework for the quantitative "data." For example, in an adolescent patient preparing for their senior year, what effect could recent news of relapse have had on the testing results? The patient could potentially become depressed and these symptoms might influence how scores from some or all of the neurocognitive tests are interpreted.

Feedback

There is evidence that parents of children with cancer have a strong interest and need for information about the impact of treatment on their child's neurocognitive functioning, both during treatment and in the years following its completion. Therefore, feedback and discussion of findings from the neuropsychological evaluation with the family are very important and frequently are dynamic processes (Trask et al. 2009). Feedback with patients and their parents in a pediatric oncology setting is typically provided in a separate face-to face session after the testing is complete, allowing clinicians to be in dialogue with parents about the assessment and recommendations.

Feedback from neuropsychological testing may at times take on a therapeutic tone during which the neuropsychologist aligns with the family in communicating the results. Feedback itself is more than simply reporting the patient's test scores and implications of the findings, and it should also be a comprehensive clinical interaction that helps a family or patient understand their child or themselves perhaps from a new perspective. The family's reaction and adjustment to the results provided are important to address, particularly as research suggests that parents have increased stress in managing and parenting children with higher cognitive dysfunction relative to those with more minimal neurocognitive impact (Patel et al. 2013).

Postal and Armstrong (2013) note that through the feedback session, patients and families have the opportunity to more deeply understand their diagnoses, testing scores, and expected prognosis. They also suggest that through the process of providing feedback, neuropsychologists assist patients' understanding of particular neurocognitive syndromes in the broader real-world context. The neuropsychologist may be the first provider to integrate the patient's medical and personal history, academic or vocational difficulties, and assessment results and conceptualize these pieces to tell a more complete story. During these sessions, it is not uncommon for additional information to arise or for the neuropsychologist to receive further clarification on an existing issue. In some cases, the written report may be finalized after these details are integrated into the documentation.

In addition to verbal feedback, a written neuropsychological report is the primary vehicle for summarizing and communicating the results of the evaluation to patients and their families. It serves as a reference for families in the future as a document of their children's strengths and weaknesses, including impairments, and may be a tool for advocating for their child's needs. Please see Education in Chap. 11 for details about services that parents can advocate for. Therefore, it is especially important to understand that the language and professional "jargon" used in a report can be a barrier to a families' ability to interpret the results and should be used sparingly or avoided when possible. This can be the case even when parents have a university-level education (Cheung et al. 2014).

Feedback to the referring physician and the medical team involved in caring for the child is also necessary. It is important to help the team understand the child's functioning level for various reasons, ranging from feedback about the side effects experienced as a result of the treatment protocols used to preparing providers for the possibility of inconsistent treatment adherence due to forgetfulness or disorganization or even to help the provider tailor their communications to the "developmental age" and capacity of the child. Although this multidisciplinary feedback may take place in different formats across various work settings, it is often communicated in regular team meetings or more informal one-on-one conversations. Again, the written evaluation report becomes important as a communication tool with the medical team. There is not one "typical" style of a written report; length, amount of detail, and comprehensive nature of the report will vary. It is important, however, that reports include a summary and interpretation of results, address the referral question, and provide recommendations with relevant "next steps."

Finally, feedback provided to the school from the neuropsychological evaluation is essential. The recommendations and interventions formulated from the assessment can provide the scaffolding from which a more extensive and comprehensive educational plan can be devised. The unique insights provided from the evaluation often support a plan that is tailored to the specific needs of a student, often in the form of a 504 Accommodation Plan or Individualized Education Plan (IEP). Please see Chap. 11 on Education for more details. The plan is often best developed within the context of open communication between the family, school staff, and school administration. Without this open communication, procuring the appropriate services for children with cancer can be challenging because schools are often unaware of the specific disease-related neurocognitive and academic-related impairments experienced by this patient group. A case example of a childhood cancer survivor seen for clinical neuropsychological evaluation is presented below, as well as samples of questions typically asked in the neuropsychological interview.

Case Vignette

A right-handed, 22-year-old Hispanic and Caucasian male diagnosed at 16 years old with non-Hodgkin lymphoma of the bone and marrow is referred for a neuropsychological reevaluation by the survivorship clinic given concerns regarding his cognitive functioning and recommendations for college. The patient reported difficulties with executive functioning skills (i.e., sequencing tasks, working memory), maintaining attention, and processing speed. Memorization was also a new area of difficulty for him. These cognitive impairments were causing conflict with family members. The patient also reported significant anxious symptoms that presented physiologically (e.g., pain in his chest). He utilized spiritual coping (e.g., prayer) to manage his emotions. He reportedly drank socially but denied use of tobacco or other drugs.

He was born at 38 weeks' gestation with no reported pre- or perinatal complications. Developmental history was notable for a diagnosis of congenital hypotonia resulting in delayed motor skills. Speech and language developed normally. Medical history was also notable for a heart murmur and visual tracking difficulties. The patient was diagnosed with attention deficit hyperactivity disorder, inattentive type, as a child.

The patient underwent 8 months of treatment including cyclophosphamide, vincristine, prednisone, triple intrathecal therapy (methotrexate, hydrocortisone, cytarabine), and intrathecal systemic chemotherapy with cytarabine and etoposide. He was taking multivitamins, calcium, and an over-the-counter medication for attention problems, but no prescribed medications.

Box 10.3 Sample Questions Asked in the Clinical Interview

General clinical interview	*Question examples*
Purpose of the evaluation	Do you understand why your child's oncologist referred them for a neuropsychological evaluation?
Presenting cognitive complaints	Do you have specific concerns about your child's learning or thinking skills? Can you clarify the specific challenges your child is having? When did these concerns begin or when were they first brought to your attention? Have the difficulties worsened over time or stayed at about the same level? Have others noticed these challenges as well (e.g., teachers, other family members, caregivers)? Is there anything that seems to help your child in minimizing or managing these difficulties?
Neuropsychological domain	*Question examples*
Academic	Has there been a significant decline in your child's grades or performance at school? Is there difficulty in a particular subject area (e.g., reading, math)?
Attention	Is your child easily distracted or have difficulties focusing on the task at hand? Does your child require frequent repetition of instructions to complete a task correctly?
Executive functioning	Is your child routinely disorganized (e.g., lose or misplace personal items on a regular basis)? Does your child routinely turn in assignments late or wait to the last minute to complete them?
Processing Speed	Does it take your child longer than expected to respond to an instruction? Is your child routinely one of the last students to complete in-class assignments?
Visuospatial	Does your child find highly spatial activities (e.g., puzzles) difficult to complete independently? Are math concepts (e.g., geometry) particularly difficult for your child?
Language	Does your child exhibit challenges in expressing themselves verbally? Does your child seem to frequently have difficulty understanding what you ask them to do?
Memory	Does your child have difficulty remembering recent events? Does your child seem to forget details of recent conversations?

Family medical history was notable for chronic myelogenous leukemia, Parkinson's disease, diabetes type II, prostate cancer, multiple sclerosis, and coronary heart disease. Family mental health history was notable for severe depression, obsessive-compulsive disorder, and bipolar disorder.

Neuropsychological assessment included a clinical interview with the patient, collateral interview with the patient's mother completed with the patient's consent, one five-hour testing session, and feedback session. The patient required several breaks to maintain focus and he demonstrated occasional lapses in attention during the assessment. The results were considered to be a valid representation of his cognitive functioning approximately 5 years after completing treatment for non-Hodgkin lymphoma. He exhibited impairments in processing speed, sustained attention, and executive functioning (working memory, planning/organization, metacognition). He also evidenced a clinically elevated level of anxious symptoms and adaptive functioning impairments related to educational difficulties and parental conflict. The cognitive impairments significantly interfered with the patient's ability to acquire new information and greatly impacted his learning efficiency.

As a result of the evaluation, specific recommendations were crafted to meet the patient's educational needs in the college setting. He partnered with the office for students with disabilities at his institution for support with implementing the accommodations and interventions. Consultation for ADHD medication was also recommended for the patient at the time of the assessment given his long-standing history of attention difficulties potentially exacerbated by his previous cancer treatment.

Interventions to Prevent or Reduce Neurocognitive Late Effects

Interventions for neurocognitive late effects of pediatric cancer treatment include educational interventions, targeted cognitive remediation, pharmacologic therapy, and behavioral interventions. Educational interventions include school remediation/reentry programs, cognitive behavioral therapy, training in social skills or specific subjects, and use of computerized cognitive training. Provider and family advocacy is essential to access educational resources such as IEPs or classroom and testing accommodations (i.e., 504 plans) as part of school reintegration for survivors of childhood cancer. School reintegration programs vary widely across the USA and by clinical site. Hospital-based programs have largely been more comprehensive and have replaced workshops for peers and educators (Castellino et al. 2014). The proposed standard for school reintegration is staged programs organized by a counselor-liaison to advocate for and interpret neuropsychological evaluations and to coordinate resources in the community, home, and hospital (Nazem and Butler 2011). Please see Chap. 11 on Education for additional details.

Cognitive Remediation

Child-Directed, Clinic-Based Approach

Cognitive remediation therapy in children typically includes interventions that use metacognitive training in problem-solving and managing complex tasks through individualized self-monitoring of effectiveness followed by self-correction (Hardy et al. 2011). Evidence supports the beneficial effects of cognitive remediation in children after traumatic brain injury or stroke (Catroopa et al. 2009). Because of the similarities between cognitive deficits in traumatic brain injury and those observed in cancer-associated cognitive dysfunction, cognitive remediation therapy has been investigated in childhood survivors (Anderson and Catroppa 2005). A feasibility trial in survivors and caregivers showed statistically significant improvement in focused attention but not in arithmetic computation (Butler and Copeland 2002). A follow-up, multicenter randomized trial demonstrated a statistically significant improvement in academic achievement in the cognitive remediation therapy group following a 5-month intervention, compared with controls randomized to a wait list (Butler et al. 2008). Results are tempered by an equivalent improvement in neurocognitive functioning in the control arm, attributed to practice effect. Further, only 60 % of the children in the intervention group completed the prescribed treatment, and the beneficial effects were not sustained long term. A shorter, 15-session, clinic-based intervention with long-term survivors also showed benefits but reported low participation rates, attributed to the demands placed on parents to bring the child to the clinic while managing other responsibilities (Patel et al. 2009).

Following the earlier focus on remediating dysfunction in long-term survivors, a pilot study was conducted to explore if early intervention might prevent math declines in children with ALL. Children on therapy for ALL were randomized to intensive individualized training in math problem-solving or to standard care. While the standard care group had higher scores in applied mathematics at baseline, the intervention group improved such that it performed significantly better in applied mathematics and visual memory at the end of intervention and at 6-month follow-up. The standard care group did not improve in any area and declined in seven of 11 domains, illustrating the typical pattern of cognitive decline. Results from the pilot study demonstrated that early intervention is feasible and beneficial (Moore et al. 2012).

Computerized Training Approach

While clinic-based cognitive remediation has shown benefit in research studies, it is variably covered by insurance as a clinical service; hence, out-of-pocket cost limits access and in-person interventions may not be practical or desirable for families. Within this context, computerized cognitive training and remediation has been viewed as a highly desirable avenue to deliver intervention for cognitive deficits and has been studied in both brain-injured populations and, more recently, in childhood cancer survivors. Pilot trials of home-based, computerized brain training (e.g., Cogmed and Lumos Labs cognitive exercises) have demonstrated improvement in selected neurocognitive functions such as attention, memory, and visual processing skills, with some studies showing benefits from the parental perspective also, but without generalization to academic performance (Hardy et al. 2013; Kesler et al. 2011). More recently, a pilot computerized training program (Fast ForWord) to prevent reading delays was implemented while children with brain tumors were still undergoing therapy. The study demonstrated feasibility for prophylactic intervention but did not find significant differences in reading between the randomized groups (Palmer et al. 2014). A randomized trial of a home-based computerized training program targeting neurocognitive function is currently in evaluation as a feasibility study in childhood brain tumor patients following cranial radiation (NCT01503086).

Parent-Directed Approach

Given the limitations of clinic-based interventions directed at the child, a parent-directed intervention has been examined with the intent to indirectly benefit the child's learning and educational performance. Children of parents who received the eight-session skills training program showed significant improvement on selected academic measures and study skills compared to children of parents randomized to standard care. The study showed high adherence and perceived benefit among parents randomized to the intervention program (Patel et al. 2014b).

Pharmacologic Interventions

Deficits in attention are characterized as a modifiable domain in cognitive dysfunction according to current evidence (Reddick and Conklin 2010). Some aspects of cognitive dysfunction in survivors of pediatric cancer resemble that of attention deficit hyperactivity disorder, inattentive type (ADHD, inattentive type); however, many survivors do not fit the profile for inattention and/or hyperactivity. The most studied medication for treatment of ADHD, inattentive type, is a piperidine derivative, methylphenidate, a mixed dopaminergic-noradrenergic agonist, which enhances function of the fronto-striatal attentional network. Methylphenidate demonstrates a strong dose-response relationship on neurocognitive measures of vigilance, sustained attention, and reaction time in ADHD, inattentive type (Hanwella et al. 2011). Methylphenidate and other stimulant medications have been investigated in studies of childhood cancer survivors with cognitive dysfunction. Treatment with methylphenidate was found to result in improved sustained attention, social skills, and internalizing and externalizing behaviors; however, these benefits did not extend to improved academic performance (Conklin et al. 2009). Male gender, older age at treatment, and higher intellectual functioning at baseline predicted better response to methylphenidate in this later study.

An open-label trial for patients who demonstrated initial response to methylphenidate showed sustained responses after 12 months of continuation therapy, compared with those who did not receive methylphenidate. Parent, teacher, and patient reports were consistent in the treatment group, but not in the control group, where parents reported improvement and teachers and patients did not (Conklin et al. 2010). Based on these studies, the authors recommend that methylphenidate should be the standard of care for children with cognitive dysfunction who show measurable improvement after short-term use of methylphenidate.

Limitations of methylphenidate studies include cohorts that mix brain tumor and ALL survivors and short half-life of the drug. Importantly, a 5 % rate of dose-limiting side effects was noted with poorer tolerance in survivors of brain tumors compared to those with leukemia (Conklin et al. 2009; Thompson et al. 2001). A COG-randomized trial comparing

Adderall XR™ versus Concerta™ (ACCL0422A) was closed prematurely because of poor participant accrual, which is thought to be in part attributable to the appearance of black box warnings around the use of methylphenidate.

Modafinil, a dopaminergic CNS stimulant, is an alternative treatment to methylphenidate in ADHD, inattentive type. Although not approved by the Food and Drug Administration (FDA) for use in children under the age of 16, it is used off-label to treat narcolepsy, excessive daytime sleepiness, and ADHD, inattentive type (Castellino et al. 2014). Modafinil improved digit span, visual memory, and spatial planning capacity among adult volunteers with cancer, with enhanced benefit among those with lower cognitive capacity at baseline (Kaleita et al. 2006). COG is currently evaluating modafinil in a randomized trial among survivors of pediatric CNS tumors (NCT01381718).

Donepezil is an acetylcholinesterase inhibitor with beneficial effects on cognitive, behavioral, and functional symptoms in Alzheimer's and vascular dementias (Passmore et al. 2005). In a phase II, 24-week, open-label trial of 34 adults with primary brain tumors, donepezil (10 mg/day) resulted in improved attention, concentration, language function, verbal and figure memory, and mood (Rapp et al. 2004). These results formed the basis of an ongoing phase III trial in survivors of adult brain tumors (NCT00369785) and a feasibility trial in childhood brain tumor survivors (NCT00452868). Pilot data in the latter trial indicate good tolerance of the drug, with efficacy in improving executive function and memory over a 6-month, open-label trial (Castellino et al. 2012).

Gaps in Knowledge/Future Directions

As reviewed previously, neuropsychological evaluation is recommended as the standard of care for certain survivor populations who are at an increased risk of experiencing cognitive late effects of treatment. There are a number of cancer treatment centers that follow this guideline. However, to our knowledge, there is no set protocol that is implemented across institutions whereby different centers follow a uniform timeline for neuropsychological evaluations. This type of coordinated assessment approach could provide the opportunity for a large pool of data for future research endeavors. In addition, although neurocognitive screening measures have shown psychometric promise, larger initiatives to routinely integrate these tools into the clinic setting are just beginning and are lacking for broader diagnosis groups (e.g., leukemia). This is another area that is ripe for future growth, especially in the current dynamic health-care climate that calls for more time and resource-sensitive approaches.

Another area clearly in need of further research and consensus pertains to the area of intervention for neurocognitive dysfunction. As reviewed above, there are now several small studies using a variety of interventions and approaches suggestive of preliminary efficacy. Though this is encouraging, the next wave of research also will need to address how to translate the research-based programs into clinical care settings. As this process is initiated, it will also be important to concurrently evaluate the circumstances (disease, level of dysfunction, and patient/family characteristics) under which various intervention approaches or techniques are effective. We need further knowledge on the duration of any benefits and whether booster sessions are needed for benefits to endure over the long term. What is the dose of intervention required to obtain a minimally positive response in specific outcomes such as academic function? Is a single treatment approach (e.g., child-directed intervention) as effective as a combined treatment approach? It is also important to establish the optimal timing for various treatment approaches: during cancer therapy, soon after completion of therapy, or well into survivorship after deficits have emerged.

Clinical Pearls

- Survivors of acute lymphoblastic leukemia and brain tumors are especially susceptible to adverse cancer-related neurocognitive sequelae; however, children with other cancers may also experience similar difficulties and should be referred for neuropsychological evaluation if clinically indicated.
- Ongoing monitoring for children at risk to develop neuropsychological late effects following completion of cancer therapies is important to identify dysfunction and to facilitate intervention.
- Families need help in understanding their child's neurocognitive issues and establishing special education services at school.
- The degree of neurocognitive and behavioral impairments varies in magnitude based on disease, treatment, and individual factors; therefore, comprehensive neuropsychological evaluation needs to also consider information about the survivor's psychosocial history and functional status across multiple domains to develop a plan that includes a range of therapeutic and educational interventions.
- Yearly comprehensive neuropsychological evaluations may not be feasible or even necessary; consequently, a monitoring strategy that includes a detailed interview about the child's educational and developmental progress and/or abbreviated neurocognitive screenings may be useful in guiding referral for more comprehensive repeated evaluations.
- There is a growing body of intervention research showing preliminary efficacy in improving either cognitive or academic functioning to a modest degree, suggesting that referral to evidence-based, formal cognitive and educational intervention programs may be helpful.

References

Anderson V, Catroppa C (2005) Recovery of executive skills following paediatric traumatic brain injury (TBI): a 2 year follow-up. Brain Inj 19(6):459–470

Baron NM, Compton P, Patel SK, Jacob E et al (2013) Central nervous system injury and neurobiobehavioral function in children with brain tumors: a review of the literature. Cancer Nurs 36(2):E31–E47

Board of Directors, American Academy of Clinical Neuropsychology (2007) American academy of clinical neuropsychology practice guidelines for neuropsychological assessment and consultation. Clin Neuropsychol 21(2):209–231

Buizer AI, de Sonneville LMJ, Veerman AJP (2009) Effects of chemotherapy on neurocognitive function in children with acute lymphoblastic leukemia: a critical review of the literature. Pediatr Blood Cancer 52:447–454. doi:10.1002/pbc.21869

Butler RW, Copeland DR (2002) Attentional processes and their remediation in children treated for cancer: a literature review and the development of a therapeutic approach. J Int Neuropschol Soc 8(1):115–124

Butler RW, Copeland DR, Fairclough DL et al (2008) A multicenter, randomized clinical trial of a cognitive remediation program for childhood survivors of a pediatric malignancy. J Consult Clin Psychol 76(3):367–378

Castellino SM, Tooze JA, Flowers L et al (2012) Toxicity and efficacy of the pf the acetylcholinesterase (Ache) inhibitor donepezil in childhood brain tumor survivors: a pilot study. Pediatr Blood Cancer 59(3):540–547

Castellino SM et al (2014) Developing interventions for cancer-related cognitive dysfunction in childhood cancer survivors. J Natl Cancer Inst 106(8):1–16

Catroopa C, Anderson VA, Muscara F et al (2009) Educational skills: long term outcome and predictors following pediatric traumatic brain injury. Neuropsychol Rehabil 19(5):716–732

Cavell T (1990) Social adjustment, social performance, and social skills: a tri-component model of social competence. J Clin Child Psychol 19:111–122

Cheung L, Wakefield C, Ellis S et al (2014) Neuropsychology reports for childhood brain tumor survivors: implementation of recommendations at home and school. Pediatr Blood Cancer 61(6): 1080–1087

Children's Oncology Group: Long-term follow-up guidelines for survivors of childhood, adolescent and young adult cancers, Version 4.0. Children's Oncology Group, Monrovia, October 2013; Available on-line: www.survivorshipguidelines.org

Conklin HM, Lawford J, Jasper BW et al (2009) Side effects of methylphenidate in childhood cancer survivors: a randomized placebo-controlled trial. Pediatrics 124(1):226–233

Conklin HM et al (2010) Predicting methylphenidate response in long-term survivors of childhood cancer: a randomized, double-blind, placebo-controlled, crossover trial. J Pediatr Psychol 35(2):144–155

Conklin HM, Krull KR, Reddick WE et al (2012) Cognitive outcomes following contemporary treatment without cranial irradiation for childhood acute lymphoblastic leukemia. J Natl Cancer Inst 104: 1386–1395. doi:10.1093/jnci/djs344

Embry L, Annett R, Kunin-Batson A et al (2012) Implementation of multi-site neurocognitive assessments within a pediatric cooperative group: can it be done? Pediatr Blood Cancer 59(3):536–539

Gurney JG, Tersak JM, Ness KK, Landier W, Matthay KK, Schmidt ML (2007) Hearing loss, quality of life, and academic problems in long-term neuroblastoma survivors: a report from the Children's Oncology Group. Pediatrics 120(5):e1229–e1236

Gurney JG, Krull KR, Kadan-Lottick N et al (2009) Social outcomes in the childhood cancer survivor study cohort. J Clin Oncol 27:2390–2395

Hanwella R, Senanayake M, de Silva V (2011) Comparative efficacy and acceptability of methylphenidate and atomoxetine in treatment of attention deficit hyperactivity disorder in children and adolescents: a meta-analysis. BMC Psychiatry 11:176

Hardy KK, Hostetter SA, Bonner MJ (2011) Empirically supported intervention strategies for pediatric cancer patients with or at risk for neurocognitive deficits. In: Holcroft R (ed) Treatment strategies—oncology. The Cambridge Research Center, London, pp 84–88

Hardy KK, Willard VW, Allen TM, Bonner MJ (2013) Working memory training in survivors of pediatric cancer: a randomized pilot study. Psychooncology 22:1856–1865

Imbach P, Kuhne Th, Arceci R (eds) (2006) Pediatric oncology. Springer, Heidelberg

Kadan-Lottick NS, Zeltzer L, Liu Q, Yasui Y et al (2010) Neurocognitive functioning in adult survivors of childhood non-central nervous system cancers. J Natl Cancer Inst 102(12):881–893

Kahalley LS, Conklin HM, Tyc VL et al (2013) Slower processing speed after treatment for pediatric brain tumor and acute lymphoblastic leukemia. Psychooncology 22(69):1979–1986

Kaleita TA, Wellisch DK, Graham CA et al (2006) Pilot study of modafinil for treatment of neurobehavioral dysfunction and fatigue in adult patients with brain tumors. J Clin Oncol 24(18S):1503

Kesler SR, Lacayo NJ, Jo B (2011) A pilot study of an online cognitive rehabilitation program for executive function skills in children with cancer-related brain injury. Brain Inj 25(1):101–112. doi:10.3109/02699052.2010.536194

Krull K, Gioia G, Ness K et al (2008a) Reliability and validity of the childhood cancer survivor study neurocognitive questionnaire. Cancer 113(8):2188–2197

Krull K, Okcu M, Potter B et al (2008b) Screening for neurocognitive impairment in pediatric cancer long-term survivors. J Clin Oncol 26(25):4138–4143

Krull KR, Sabin ND, Reddick WE et al (2012) Neurocognitive function and CNS integrity in adult survivors of childhood Hodgkin lymphoma. J Clin Oncol 30(29):3618–3624

Krull KR, Bhojwani D, Conklin HM, Pei D et al (2013a) Genetic mediators of neurocognitive outcomes in survivors of childhood acute lymphoblastic leukemia. J Clin Oncol 31(17):2182–2188

Krull KR, Brinkman TM, Li C et al (2013b) Neurocognitive outcomes decades after treatment for childhood acute lymphoblastic leukemia: a report from the St Jude lifetime cohort study. J Clin Oncol 31:4407–4415. doi:10.1200/JCO.2012.48.2315

Kun LE (1997) General principles of radiation therapy. In: Pizzo PA, Poplack DM (eds) Principles and practice of pediatric oncology, 3rd edn. Lippincott-Raven, Philadelphia, pp 289–321

Moleski M (2000) Neuropsychological, neuroanatomical, and neurophysiological consequences of CNS chemotherapy for acute lymphoblastic leukemia. Arch Clin Neuropsychol 5:603–630

Moore IM, Hockenberry MJ, Anhalt C et al (2012) Mathematics intervention for prevention of neurocognitive deficits in childhood leukemia. Pediatr Blood Cancer 59(2):278–284

Moyer KH, Willard VW, Gross AM et al (2012) The impact of attention on social functioning in survivors of pediatric acute lymphoblastic leukemia and brain tumors. Pediatr Blood Cancer 59:1290–1295. doi:10.1002/pbc.24256

Nathan P, Patel S, Dilley K et al (2007) Guidelines for identification of, advocacy for, and intervention in neurocognitive problems in survivors of childhood cancer: a report from the children's oncology group. Arch Pediatr Adolesc Med 161(8):798–806

Nazem KJ, Butler RW (2011) Neuropsychological rehabilitation for survivors of childhood and adolescent brain tumors: a view of the past and a vision for a promising future. J Pediatr Rehabil Med 4(1):37–46

Nelson MB, Macey PM, Harper RM et al (2014) Structural brain alterations in children an average of 5 years after surgery and chemotherapy for brain tumors. J Neurooncol 119:317–326

Noll RB, Patel SK, Embry L et al (2013) Children's Oncology Group's 2013 blueprint for research: behavioral Science. Pediatr Blood Cancer 60(6):1048–1054. doi:10.1002/pbc.24421, Epub 2012 Dec 19

Packer RJ, Meadows AT, Rorke LB et al (1987) Long-term sequelae of cancer treatment on the central nervous system in childhood. Med Pediatr Oncol 15(5): 241–253

Palmer SL, Goloubeva O, Reddick WE et al (2001) Patterns of intellectual development among survivors of pediatric medulloblastoma: a longitudinal analysis. J Clin Oncol 19(8):2302–2308

Palmer SL, Armstrong C, Onar-Thomas A et al (2013) Processing speed, attention, and working memory after treatment for medulloblastoma: an international, prospective, and longitudinal study. J Clin Oncol 31:1–10

Palmer SL, Leigh LL, Ellison SC et al (2014) Feasibility and efficacy of a computer-based intervention aimed at preventing reading decoding deficits among children undergoing active treatment of medulloblastoma: results of a randomized trial. J Pediatr Psychol 39(4): 450–458

Passmore AP, Bayer AJ, Steinhagen-Thiessen E (2005) Cognitive, global, and functional benefits of donepezil in Alzheimer's disease and vascular dementia: results from large-scale clinical trials. J Neurol Sci 229–230: 141–146

Patel SK, Lai-Yates JJ, Anderson JW et al (2007) Attention dysfunction and parent reporting in children with brain tumors. Pediatr Blood Cancer 49:970–974. doi:10.1002/pbc.21151

Patel SK, Katz ER, Richardson R et al (2009) Cognitive and problem solving training in children with cancer: a pilot project. J Pediatr Hematol Oncol 31(9):670–677

Patel SK, Wong A, Cuevas M et al (2013) Parenting stress and neurocognitive late effects in childhood cancer survivors. Psychooncology 22(8):1774–1782. doi:10.1002/pon.3213, Epub 2012 Oct 25

Patel SK, Peters BB, Bell T et al (2014a) Parent involvement and neurocognitive functioning in childhood cancer survivors. J Behav Health 3(1):43–52. doi:10.5455/jbh.20131222084318

Patel SK, Ross P, Cuevas M et al (2014b) Parent-directed intervention for children with cancer-related neurobehavioral late effects: a randomized pilot study. J Pediatr Psychol 39(9):1013–1027, pii: jsu045

Peterson CC, Johnson CE, Ramirez LY et al (2008) A meta-analysis of the neuropsychological sequelae of chemotherapy-only treatment for pediatric acute lymphoblastic leukemia. Pediatr Blood Cancer 51: 99–104. doi:10.1002/pbc.21544

Phipps S, Rai SN, Leung W-H et al (2008) Cognitive and academic consequences of stem-cell transplantation in children. J Clin Oncol 26:2027–2033. doi:10.1200/JCO.2007.13.6135

Postal K, Armstrong K (2013) Feedback that sticks: the art of effectively communicating neuropsychological assessment results. Oxford University Press, Oxford

Pulsifer MB, Delgado I, Tarbell K et al (2010) Neurocognitive outcomes after proton radiation for pediatric brain tumors. J Clin Oncol 28(suppl):112s, abstr 680

Rapp SR, Rosdhal R, D'Agostino RB et al (2004) Improving cognitive functioning in brain irradiated patients: a phase II trial of an acetylcholinesterase inhibitor (donepezil). Neuro Oncol 6:357

Reddick WE, Conklin HM (2010) Impact of acute lymphoblastic leukemia therapy on attention and working memory in children. Expert Rev Hematol 3(6):655–659

Reddick WE, Glass JO, Helton KJ et al (2005) A quantitative MR imaging assessment of leukoencephalopathy in children treated for acute lymphoblastic leukemia without irradiation. AJNR Am J Neuroradiol 26:2371–2377

Robinson KE, Kuttesch JF, Champion JE et al (2010) A quantitative meta-analysis of neurocognitive sequelae in survivors of pediatric brain tumors. Pediatr Blood Cancer 55:525–531

Sanders JE, Hoffmeister PA, Storer BE et al (2010) The quality of life of adult survivors of childhood hematopoietic cell transplant. Bone Marrow Transplant 45:746–754. doi:10.1038/bmt.2009.224

Schulte F, Barrera M (2010) Social competence in childhood brain tumor survivors: a comprehensive review. Support Care Cancer 18:1499–1513. doi:10.1007/s00520-010-0963-1

Schwartz AL, Nail LM, Chen S et al (2000) Fatigue patterns observed in patients receiving chemotherapy and radiotherapy. Cancer Invest 18:11–19

Smedler AC, Ringden K, Bergman H, Bolme P (1990) Sensory-motor and cognitive functioning in children who have undergone bone marrow transplantation. Acta Paediatr Scand 79:613–621

Thompson SJ, Leigh L, Christensen R et al (2001) Immediate neurocognitive effects of methylphenidate on learning-impaired survivors of childhood cancer. J Clin Oncol 19(6):1802–1808

Trask C, Welch J, Manley P et al (2009) Parental needs for information related to neurocognitive late effects from pediatric cancer and its treatment. Pediatr Blood Cancer 52(2):273–279

von der Weid NX (2008) Adult life after surviving lymphoma in childhood. Support Care Cancer 16(4):339–345

Waber DP, Turek J, Catania L et al (2007) Neuropsychological outcomes from a randomized trial of triple intrathecal chemotherapy compared with 18 Gy cranial radiation as CNS treatment in acute lymphoblastic leukemia: findings from Dana-Farber Cancer Institute ALL Consortium Protocol 95–01. J Clin Oncol 25:4914–4921. doi:10.1200/JCO.2007.10.8464

Warris LT, van den Heuvel-Eibrink MM, den Hoed MAH et al (2014) Does dexamethasone induce more neuropsychological side effects than prednisone in pediatric acute lymphoblastic leukemia? A systematic review. Pediatr Blood Cancer 61:1313–1318. doi:10.1002/pbc.24988

Wong CS, Van Der Kogel AJ (2004) Mechanisms of radiation injury to the central nervous system: implications for neuroprotection. Mol Interv 4:273–284

Zebrack B, Gurney J, Oeffinger K et al (2004) Psychological outcomes in long-term survivors of childhood brain cancer: a report from the childhood cancer survivor study. J Clin Oncol 22:999–1006

Educational Issues: The Impact of Cancer in the Classroom

11

Christine L. Trask and Catherine C. Peterson

Educational Issues for Children with Cancer

In addition to family, school is one of the largest influences on children. It is a place for cognitive growth and learning, as well as a place for social relationships and development of self-concept and self-esteem. Treatment for cancer can create unique needs and challenges for school-aged children. There are educational needs for children who are currently in treatment for cancer, as well as needs for children who are childhood cancer survivors. While in treatment, the focus is often on ways to support a child's ongoing attendance or involvement at school. In contrast, following treatment, there is often increasing focus on specific learning needs that typically are direct sequelae of treatment. When examining these issues, however, it is important to recognize that cancer is a heterogenous disease with marked variability in outcome and associated features and that interventions and strategies will also need to take into account a child's developmental level. Loman and Vincent (2002) have suggested that children at highest academic risk include those with CNS-involved diseases, those with frequent or extended absences, those with a premorbid history of learning difficulties, and children who speak English as a second language. As a result, clinicians will need to consider the potential risk factors for each individual child, as well as the stage of treatment, to assess educational needs. Moreover, in addition to supporting the child with cancer, the clinician often also needs to consider the needs of the family and needs of school personnel.

C.L. Trask, PhD, ABPP (✉)
Department of Psychiatry and Human Behavior, Rhode Island Hospital/The Warren Alpert Medical School of Brown University, 593 Eddy Street, Physician's Office Building #430, Providence, RI 02903, USA

Department of Psychiatry and Human Behavior, School of Brown University, Providence, RI 02903, USA
e-mail: ctrask@lifespan.org

C.C. Peterson, PhD
Department of Psychology, Eastern Michigan University, 361F Science Complex, Ypsilanti, MI 48197, USA
e-mail: cpeter39@emich.edu

The Laws and Policies behind School-Based Services and Accommodations

In order to support a child with cancer within the educational system, it is important to understand the legal statutes that protect and support children at school. Children with cancer can be eligible for services and/or accommodations given their health condition. In particular, if there are deficits or issues identified from their health condition and they are impacting a child's performance at school, there are several federal laws within the United States that provide support and services.

A.N. Abrams et al. (eds.), *Pediatric Psychosocial Oncology: Textbook for Multidisciplinary Care*,
DOI 10.1007/978-3-319-21374-3_11

This includes the Individuals with Disabilities Education Act (IDEA) of 1997 and 2004, the Rehabilitation Act (section 504), the Americans with Disabilities Act (1990), and No Child Left Behind (2001).

The IDEA was initiated in 1975 as the Education for All Handicapped Children Act, which later became IDEA. The last amendment was issued in 2004, and the final regulations for school-aged children published in 2006. This most recent version was called the Individuals with Disabilities Education Improvement Act (IDEIA). This law provides free and appropriate public education ("FAPE") for children with disabilities from ages 3 to 21 in the least restrictive environment "LRE." As a result, this law applies to children from preschool through high school. Services can be provided up until age 22, as long as a student remains in high school. After a student graduates or leaves high school, they are no longer covered under IDEIA. For younger children, an amendment, public law 99–457, provides for early intervention services for children from birth to age 3.

In general, to receive special education services, children must meet criteria for classification under a disability. The law recognized 13 areas of disability, including intellectual disability/mental retardation, hearing impairment, deafness, speech/language disability, vision impairment, emotional disability, orthopedic impairment, autistic spectrum disorders, traumatic brain injuries, other health impairment, specific learning disability, co-occurring deafness/blindness, and multiple disabilities. For children who have been treated for childhood cancer, they may be eligible as a child with a health impairment and may also be identified as a child with a disability in another area, including a specific learning disability, hearing impairment, vision impairment, traumatic brain injury, or orthopedic impairment. Of note, the child's disability must be the reason for lack of adequate progress in school. IDEA provides for *services,* including specialized instruction, speech therapy, occupational therapy, physical therapy, adaptive physical education, counseling, and extended school year services. Once an individual education plan (IEP) is initiated, parents have specific rights, including regular and mandatory opportunities for review and modification of the IEP. The child's progress towards IEP goals must be monitored and reported to parents. In addition, IEPs must be reviewed at least annually, and the child must also be reevaluated at least once every 3 years. One of the significant changes in the revision of the Individuals with Disabilities Education Act (IDEA) in 2004 was related to the identification of children with a specific learning disorder. A learning disorder can be recognized in several areas, including: oral expression, listening comprehension, written expression, basic reading skills, reading fluency skills, reading comprehension, mathematics calculation, and mathematics problem solving. Previously, specific learning disabilities were recognized when a child exhibited a discrepancy between measured intellectual abilities and measured academic skills. The revision of IDEA in 2004 allowed states to abandon the discrepancy model for identification of a learning disorder and to base decisions on a child's response to scientific research-based intervention or use an alternative research-based procedure. In particular, response to intervention (RTI) is an approach that focuses on ecological validity, with direct repeated measurement of a child in the classroom, rather than reliance on neuropsychological test results. As noted in No Child Left Behind (2001), states were mandated to complete yearly assessments of all students in order to ensure that children were making adequate progress, resulting in testing routinely being done in the classroom. Moreover, to be classified as a child having a specific learning disability, academic delays must not be the result of inadequate instruction, limited English proficiency, economic or environmental disadvantage, cultural factors, intellectual disability, emotional disturbance, or a hearing, vision, or motor disability. As a result, for individuals evaluating or advocating for childhood cancer survivors, it is particularly important to understand the model an individual state is using to determine eligibility for services.

In contrast to services provided under IDEA, section 504 of the Rehabilitation Act of 1973, reauthorized in 2004, can provide *accommodations* to children who are not eligible for a formal IEP. Under this law, the definition of a disability is broader and is noted to be an "impairment which substantially limits one or more of such person's major life activities, such as learning…" Moreover, there are no age restrictions for accommodations under section 504, and therefore, these plans can continue in college settings. In addition, accommodations under a 504 plan do not have to be reviewed annually and are not monitored by the federal government for compliance, and formal assessment procedures are not required to obtain accommodations. Of note, this law applies to programs or activities that receive federal financial assistance, such as public schools.

Similar to section 504, the Americans with Disabilities Act (1990) notes that people with disability shall receive "reasonable accommodations" and cannot be discriminated against. The ADA extends the rights from section 504 to the private sector and applies to programs and facilities, regardless if they receive federal financial assistance, and extends into vocational settings. Similarly, provisions under the ADA of 1990 do not have any age restrictions. Although IDEA does not cover students in college, accommodations can be provided at college under section 504 and ADA. It is important to note, however, that these laws do not mandate that a student's performance be "optimized," but rather reach the standard of an "average person."

Educational Issues during Cancer Treatment

Education is often initially disrupted at the time of diagnosis and treatment. There can be unique physical, social-emotional, and cognitive issues that need to be addressed within the school system (see Table 11.1). In particular, children may be physically unable to attend school during this time, and school absences can be a primary concern. In addition, there may be side effects or immediate sequelae of treatment, such as fatigue, nausea, hair loss, and/or motor weakness, that can impact school functioning.

Table 11.1 Examples of needs of children with cancer at school

Physical
Attendance impacted by fatigue, nausea/vomiting
Potential mobility issues in the school
Susceptibility to infection
Social-emotional
Concerns related to body image, such as hair loss, limb loss, scars
Reduced opportunity to participate in school activities
Cognitive
Reduced attention/concentration related to physical illness

Absences

For children between the ages of five and 18, school is one of the largest components of their time. When children are diagnosed with cancer, however, treatment often significantly interferes with their participation at school. Depending on the type of treatment and side effects, children may experience significant disruption in both their social relationships at school and their academic education (Bruce et al. 2012; Gurney et al. 2009). Fatigue, nausea, vomiting, and immune compromise are specific issues that confront many children during treatment. Physical limitations to attendance are likely to be most pronounced shortly after diagnosis and in the initial stages of treatment. For example, one small study (Sullivan et al. 2001) found that patients missed between 27 and 170 days of school after diagnosis. Prevatt, Heffer, and Lowe (2000) reported that childhood cancer patients miss 40 days of school per year while in active treatment. Although treatments have evolved and more care is provided on an outpatient basis, there is limited information about current attendance rates of students in the United States while in active treatment. Disruptions to school attendance, however, also appear to persist after completion of treatment. In a study from Canada, French and colleagues (2013) studied absenteeism in survivors, 2 or more years after the end of treatment. Survivors missed significantly more days of school than the control group and averaged 11 absences per year, with 1.4 absences related to hospital visits, in comparison to an average of 5 absences per year for healthy controls in the school district. Moreover, absences were associated with difficulties with physical activity, pain, and energy level by patient report.

Moreover, it is important to be mindful of the impact of cumulative school absences. For children with frequent absences, a common response has been to consider grade retention. For example, Barrera et al. (2005) reported 21 % of a sample of childhood cancer survivors were retained versus 9 % in their control group. Research has suggested that grade retention may have some short-term benefit in academic performance, but this benefit disappears over time. Moreover, "social promotion" or the policy to advance a child to the next grade to maintain peer connections has also not been associated with long-term benefit (National Association of School Psychologists, Position Statement 2011). Rather, it is more important for education professionals to identify the child's specific learning needs and find ways to provide the needed educational experiences.

When medically unable to attend school, educational needs can be addressed through individual tutoring, as well as hospital-based classrooms, where available. When children have prolonged absences from school due to medical needs, they can be eligible for tutoring services. It is important to know that there may be a minimum number of consecutive days the child must be absent before they are eligible for tutoring services. Another issue often raised with tutoring is the limited number of hours that are typically provided (Bessell 2001; Sullivan et al. 2001). Clinicians may need to think creatively and form collaborative relationships to help supplement educational instruction during treatment. For example, as described by Ortlieb (2008), it may be fruitful for medical centers to explore partnerships with nearby universities training teachers. As part of a practicum or preservice experience, student teachers may be paired with patients to provide additional instructional support, and students can receive additional teaching opportunities. Online and computer-based learning programs may be another resource to provide patients with greater access to educational material.

In addition to educational needs, children also have social needs related to school absences. For children who are not medically able to attend school, it is important to explore avenues to continue their sense of community with their classroom. This can be done by creating weekly newsletters that outline activities in the classroom; letters from classmates; use of technology, such as sharing Care pages or Skype sessions; or posting a picture of the child in the classroom (see Table 11.2). For example, Monkey In My Chair is a charitable organization that provides a stuffed "monkey" to hold the child's place in the classroom, as well as an online portal that allows sharing of pictures and documents between the child and the classroom. In addition, Fox (2009) described the role of a laptop and webcam to help a homebound cancer patient "attend" class, with provision of a laptop and an agreement with the local telephone company for free home internet installation and a reduced service rate. There have also been several charities that have been created that can support these strategies by providing laptop computers to childhood cancer patients, such Hopecam (http://www.hopecam.org/) or Laptops of Love (http://laptopsoflove.com/). Moreover, there are also innovations exploring the use of technology to create a more

Table 11.2 Strategies for supporting social connections with school during active treatment

Develop a weekly newsletter outlining activities or lessons from the classroom
Encourage students to write letters or draw pictures to share with the patient
Videotape a class event to share with the student
If feasible, identify a few students to visit the patient and deliver items from the class
Explore the role of technology and social media to help keep the patient connected with the classroom (e.g., set up Skype session, have the classroom "Tweet" comments during the day, share the patient's Care page with the classroom)
Consider assigning reading selections or, for younger children, doing a read aloud, related to the patient's cancer experience

interactive experience for the child, such as a remote-controlled robot that would allow the child to "move" within the school environment (see http://www.vgocom.com/remote-student). These connections to school are critically important as adolescents with a childhood-onset chronic illness who have a strong connection to their school have been found to be more likely to graduate from college (Maslow et al. 2012).

School Reintegration Programs

When the child is ready to return to the classroom, it can be helpful to plan and organize this transition. Clinicians from medical treatment centers need to form a collaborative relationship with the school community to help bridge the gap to the school (see Table 11.3). During this time, a 504 plan may be instituted to accommodate for some of these issues, such as a reduced class day or provision of an extra set of books to reduce the demands to carry heavy loads (see Table 11.4 for additional examples). In particular, it is important to work with school nurses to discuss and identify any medical needs the child might have at school, such as restrictions in activities, need for access to water, or notification of infectious illnesses in the school. Similarly, when a child returns to school, it is essential for the teacher to know and understand the child's diagnosis, treatment, prognosis, and potential neurocognitive late effects (Gartin and Murdick 2009). Teachers often have to address and help students cope with absences, as well as maintain their academic progress and deal with potentially altered appearance (Best et al. 2005). See Fig. 11.1 for an example of an educational summary that can be used to help facilitate communication between medical providers and school personnel. Summaries of a child's diagnosis, treatment, and educational needs should be shared with the school when the child is first returning to school. This would typically be shared with the "point person," such as the school nurse or school psychologist, who is coordinating the child's return to school. Parents may also choose to share it with teachers or other school-based personnel working with their child.

In addition to identification of needed services and accommodations, a school re-integration plan typically includes supportive counseling for children and families, as well as an educational program for school personnel and/or peers and regular contact between the hospital and medical providers. Many hospitals utilize Child Life specialists, social work services, or psychology services to provide an educational session to the child's class or school. This program is often tailored to the child's developmental level and is created with input from the child and family. The

Table 11.3 Strategies to facilitate reentry to school

Identify a "point person" to act as a liaison between the medical and academic settings
Develop brief reports or communication methods that can provide child-specific information related to disease, medications, restrictions on activities, "action plans," and specific learning concerns
When the student returns to the classroom, encourage the teacher to identify a peer that can help familiarize the patient with classroom routines and provide social support
Help identify modifications that can be made to allow participation by the patient. For example, for a child with significant physical fatigue, encourage teachers to provide opportunities for peers to play cards or board games with the child during recess
Try to structure clinic visits to minimize absences from school, such as consolidating and coordinating multiple specialty visits during 1 day
If absences become excessive, assess for potential emotional, social, and family factors that may be contributing to school avoidance

Table 11.4 Common accommodations during treatment

Provision of home-based tutoring
Modified school day to address reduced endurance and fatigue
Reduced homework, modified assignments
Extended time for tests or classwork or projects
Quick communication about communicable diseases in the classroom
Permission to wear a hat or scarf to deal with hair loss
Unrestricted access to water and/or the bathroom
Early dismissal from class to provide extra time to navigate the hallways without peers present
Provision of an extra set of books in order to eliminate the need to carry books from school to home

EDUCATIONAL SUMMARY OF CANCER TREATMENT

Name:	Sex:	Date of Birth:
Grade:	School:	

CANCER DIAGNOSIS		
Diagnosis:	Date of Diagnosis:	Date Therapy Completed:

CHEMOTHERAPY: ☐**Yes** ☐**No** *If yes, complete chart below*	
Methotrexate	
Cytarabine	
Carboplatin	
Cisplatin	
Vincristine	

RADIATION ☐ Yes ☐ No *If yes, complete chart below*	
Site/Field (e.g., brain, chest, pelvis)*	Total Dose** (Gy)***

HEMATOPOIETIC CELL TRANSPLANT ☐Yes ☐No *If yes, answer question below*
Was this patient ever diagnosed with chronic graft-versus-host disease (cGVHD)? ☐**Yes** ☐**No**

Fig. 11.1 Educational summary of cancer treatment

SURGERY ☐Yes ☐No *If yes, complete chart below*	
Procedure	Site (if applicable, e.g., brain)

ONCOLOGY CARE PROVIDERS		
Role	**Name**	**Contact information**
Oncologist		
Nurse Practitioner		
Social Worker		
Educational Specialist		
Neuropsychologist		
Psychologist/Therapist		
Speech Therapist		
Occupational Therapist		
Physical Therapist		
Surgeon		
Other		

PHYSICAL NEEDS/CONCERNS ☐Yes ☐No If yes, complete chart below; Check all that apply							
Needs medical attention	Yes			Yes			Yes
Fever >101			Pain management			Mouth sores	
Bleeding, including nosebleeds			Fatigue			Hearing loss	

Fig. 11.1 (continued)

Vomiting			Hair loss			Vision impairment	
Dark urine			Seizures			Heart damage	
Presence of contagious diseases			Weight loss			Liver damage	
			Susceptibility to infection			Kidney damage	
Other issues:			Increased need for water			Other:	
Central Venous Catheter/Port			Bathroom access				
Other medical devices			Gastrointestinal issues				

COGNITIVE NEEDS/CONCERNS ☐Yes ☐No If yes, complete chart below; Check all that apply	
Cognitive/Neuropsychological Testing completed by:	Date Completed:
AREAS OF COGNITIVE CONCERN	

Weakness	Yes		Weakness	Yes		Weakness	Yes

Fig. 11.1 (continued)

General intellectual abilities			Language			Processing Speed	
Reading			Visual-Spatial			Organizational Skills	
Writing			Fine Motor			Attention	
Math			Penmanship			Memory	

SOCIO-EMOTIONAL NEEDS/CONCERNS ☐Yes ☐No *If yes, complete chart below; Check all that apply*							
	Yes			Yes			Yes
Anxiety			Social withdrawal			Reduced frustration tolerance	
Depression			Social immaturity			Hyperactivity/impulsivity	
Self-Esteem			Body image issues			Anger	

Summary prepared by:	Date prepared:

Fig. 11.1 (continued)

primary focus of this session is to help educate peers and teachers, as well as decrease the "stigma" or fear that can be associated with childhood cancer. The process for developing a reentry program is presented in Table 11.5. Further details about reentry programs are described in *Educating the Child with Cancer: A Guide for Parents and Teachers* (2003) by the Candlelighters Childhood Cancer Foundation.

Provision of an organized education program directed towards teachers and peers has been helpful in facilitating school reentry (Leigh and Miles 2002). Although formal research is limited, studies of comprehensive school reintegration programs reported improvements in self-concept, interpersonal relationships, and behavioral functioning (Katz et al. 1988, 1992). In particular, Helms and colleagues (2014) conducted a meta-analysis of the six identified studies of school reentry programs and found benefit in academic achievement and reduced levels of depression, but there was not a significant improvement in social competence. Prevatt and colleagues (2000) identified characteristics of effective reintegration programs, including identification of a "point person" to coordinate services for the child with cancer, provide consultation between medical specialists to school personnel, and assist with school reentry education program for peers in the classroom.

Table 11.5 Steps to develop a school reentry presentation

Obtain the child and family's consent and input
Determine the preferred audience (e.g., teachers, peers in classroom, peers from the grade)
Determine if the child wants to be present and/or participate during the presentation
Typical content areas will include: general information about cancer, specific information about the child's type of cancer and its treatment, presence of a central line or port, other medical devices, any possible changes in appearance, any possible changes in behavior, what students can do to help support the child
Review the content to be discussed and determine if there is anything the child does not want presented
Review the plan with school personnel and identify a location for the presentation

Research has continued to examine potential essential components of school reentry programs, including greater attention to some of the social needs. As noted by Butler and Haser (2006), fear of peer rejection has been identified as the main reason children struggle to return to school. Individual research studies have suggested that school reentry programs with a social component are associated with reduced behavioral problems and improved sense of social competency (Barrera and Schulte 2009; Varni et al. 1993). Moreover, the Rehabilitation including Social and Physical activity and Education with Children and Teenagers with Cancer (RESPECT) was recently initiated in Denmark (Thorsteinnsson et al. 2013) to study the benefit of ambassador-facilitated educational, physical, and social interventions. A unique aspect of this program was to identify and develop two peer "ambassadors" who would not only share experiences from school with the patient but also join the patient in some of the hospital-based experiences, such as the hospital school program and hospital meals, in order to better understand the patient's experience. The importance of developing peer supports is underscored in a qualitative study of five adolescents with a variety of cancers. Larouche and Chin-Peuckert (2006) noted teens reported a theme of using friends as "peer shields" to help them cope with body image issues related to treatment, with four of the five acknowledging that concerns about body image impacted their desire to return to school.

School Avoidance/School Refusal

For some children, a prolonged absence from school due to health-related needs can lead to school avoidance or school refusal. As conceptualized by Kearney (2008), school refusal can manifest as frequent absences, chronic tardiness, or generalized dread related to attending school. The presence of significant anxiety, particularly separation anxiety and generalized anxiety, as well as depression, can be a significant risk factor for school avoidance (Kearney and Albano 2004; Lyon and Cotler 2007). School refusal may serve to help children avoid situations that can elicit anxiety or depression, avoid social rejection, avoid evaluative situations, increase attention from others, and pursue other pleasurable activities, such as watching television or playing videogames (Kearney 2008). It is important to identify the specific factors for an individual child that are contributing to school avoidance behaviors in order to guide treatment; however, the primary treatment recommendation is to have the child return to school as soon as possible and avoid providing support for ongoing absences (Fremont 2003). Treatment can include child-directed cognitive-behavioral interventions, including relaxation training and exposure-based practice; parent-directed intervention, such as establishment of a contingency management system; and pharmacological treatments for underlying anxiety or depression (Kearney and Bensaheb 2006). In addition, it is important to provide increased social supports at school, address any potential underlying learning issues, and educate parents about the importance of regular school attendance.

Impact of Neurocognitive Late Effects

After completion of treatment, many family members and educators may feel that cancer is a thing of the past. Certain types of pediatric cancers and treatments, however, are associated with late effects, which emerge in the years following completion of treatment. These late effects include neurocognitive changes that are linked to educational issues, such as increased difficulty on school-related subjects (Spinelli 2003). As noted earlier, childhood cancer survivors are more likely to repeat a grade, receive special education services, and have lower overall educational attainment (Vance and Eiser 2002; Gerhardt et al. 2007; Moore et al. 2009). For example, as noted in a survey from the Childhood Cancer Survivor Study (CCSS), although the majority of survivors of a childhood CNS malignancy graduated from high school, they completed fewer years of education than their siblings (Ellenberg et al. 2009). In general, childhood cancer survivors are less likely to graduate from high school or attend college (Oeffinger et al. 2006; Mulrooney et al. 2008). In another study of a heterogeneous sample of childhood cancer survivors, 25 % qualified for special education services versus 8 % of a sibling control group (Mitby et al. 2003). Similarly, 23 % of childhood cancer survivors are reported to utilize special education services (Gorin and McAuliffe 2008). In addition, other research has suggested that 40–50 % of survivors of acute lymphoblastic leukemia (ALL) and up to 70–80 % of survivors of CNS malignancies will be eligible for special education services at some point (Nathan et al. 2007).

Risks and Related Features of Neurocognitive Late Effects

These educational outcomes are related to underlying cognitive changes that can emerge related to treatment effects. See Chap. 10 for a more in-depth discussion of neurocognitive late effects (NCLE). In general, research has reflected significant neurocognitive deficits, which are influenced by the type of cancer, treatment-related variables, and patient-related variables. For example, children with brain tumors are at greatest risk for NCLE, followed by children treated for leukemia and non-Hodgkin's lymphoma. Similarly, cranial radiation treatment is associated with greater risk for cognitive change, followed by use of intrathecal chemotherapies. Younger age of diagnosis and female gender have also been identified as potential risk factors. For those that experience NCLE, specific neurocognitive weaknesses, such as greater reported difficulties in task efficiency, emotional regulation, and memory functioning, were associated with lower educational attainment (Ellenberg et al. 2009).

There have been several recent meta-analyses of neuropsychological sequelae of childhood cancer, often with additional educational endpoints. For example, Campbell and colleagues (2007) reviewed 28 empirical studies of children treated for acute lymphocytic leukemia. In general, survivors of leukemia had poorer performance across measures of intellect and academic skills in comparison to healthy or illness controls. Similarly, Peterson and colleagues (2008) conducted a meta-analysis of 13 studies of children treated with only chemotherapy without radiation for leukemia and found similar patterns of weaknesses in intellectual indices, as well as reading and math skills in comparison to controls.

Deficits were similar or larger when examined with children with brain tumors. As noted in a meta-analysis by Robinson et al. (2010) utilizing information from 39 empirical studies of 1,318 children with brain tumors from 1992 to 2009, there was a medium-to-large effect size in general intellectual abilities, with an accompanying, but smaller, effect size in academic. Another meta-analysis by de Ruiter et al. (2013) of 710 children with brain tumors reported in 29 studies from 1999 to 2011 found similar large effects for general intellectual abilities and visual-analytic skills. Scores were lower in association with treatment with cranial radiation, use of chemotherapy, and longer time since diagnosis.

Academically, math has generally been found to be the area of greatest weakness for childhood cancer survivors (Harshman et al. 2012; Barrera et al. 2005). In particular, children treated for ALL have also shown specific deficits in arithmetic (Brown et al. 1992). For children with posterior fossa brain tumors (Mabbott et al. 2005), there may be a greater range of educational weaknesses, and research has reflected reduced academic performance in spelling, reading, and mathematics.

Needs in the Schools

These educational issues present a unique challenge to educators and school personnel. Given the significant advances in treatment, there are an increasing number of childhood cancer survivors in school settings. It has been estimated that in a large high school, at any given time, there are likely two or three students who are childhood cancer survivors (Kadan-Lottick et al. 2010). Despite this increasing population, there is little research available related to school psychologists' or teachers' knowledge or needs related to working with childhood cancer survivors. An initial presentation of results of an anonymous survey of members of the National Association of School Psychologists (Trask and Faust 2011) examined issues related to school psychologists' knowledge, training, and experience in dealing with NCLE. Based on 73 respondents from 27 states, school psychologists reported having very low levels of knowledge of NCLE and having very limited formal training about NCLE. Results suggested that treatment centers need to bridge the gap between hospital programs and the school community. For example, the Internet was rated as being the most frequently used source of information about NCLE for school psychologists, whereas physicians and nurses in medical centers were rated as being used less often. Information from the Internet was rated as being more easily accessed, generally more helpful, and equally as reliable as information gained from physicians and nurses. Similar to research with school psychologists, other research has reported that teachers do not rate themselves as knowledgeable about cancer and its treatment (Brown et al. 2011). This is an important endeavor, as other researchers (Nabors and Lehmkuhl 2004) have noted that improving teachers' knowledge can empower them in their role teaching children with cancer.

Impact of NCLE on the Family

One of the challenges for a clinician is to determine the timing and focus of discussions with parents about potential neurocognitive late effects from cancer treatment. As noted by Trask and colleagues (2009) in a survey of parents of childhood cancer survivors, they have a high need for information about potential cognitive changes and their educational impact, both during treatment and after completion of treatment. Parents with higher levels of distress reported wanting to receive this information sooner and closer to the time of diagnosis. Nevertheless, there was still 12 % of the sample who did not want any additional information. Moreover, Zebrack and Isaacson (2012) noted that adolescent and young adult cancer patients have specific concerns about issues related to returning to school/work but vary significantly in the amount and type of information they wish to receive. In general, there continues to be a need for clinicians to be sensitive to and flexible in the timing of discussions related to the potential education impact of treatment.

For those children who develop NCLE, many also struggle with associated emotional distress or behavioral dysregulation (see Chap. 15 for review of psychological outcomes and quality of life), and it is important to recognize that these patterns of school difficulties, learning deficits, and cognitively mediated dysregulation symptoms can be extremely stressful for parents to manage. Many families report that management of their child's cognitive and academic struggles leads to ongoing strain, as they find that they need to help their child with their work more, advocate for their child's academic needs, explain to school personnel the details of NCLE, and sometimes carefully reconsider their child's overall ability level and long-term potential. Research has supported the stress and burden that these parents typically report. For example, in childhood cancer survivors, the presence of executive weaknesses, particularly related to behavioral regulation, is related to increased parental stress (Patel et al. 2013). The ongoing behavior management and school advocacy demands on parents may result in increased and chronic strain for parents, and given the link between survivor academic difficulties and family conflict (Ach et al. 2013), it follows that NCLE likely have a broad effect on the entire family system of the survivor. Peterson and Drotar (2006) presented a family systems-based model illustrating how the childhood cancer survivor presents a pattern of NCLE and psychological difficulties, and these child characteristics interact in a dynamic and reciprocal manner with family factors, such as family functioning, caregiver burden, and caregiver psychological functioning (Peterson and Drotar 2006; see Fig. 11.2). These patterns of family functioning are also influenced by potential contributing factors, such as premorbid family functioning, responsiveness of the school, and the growth and development of the child over time. Therefore, it is important for clinicians

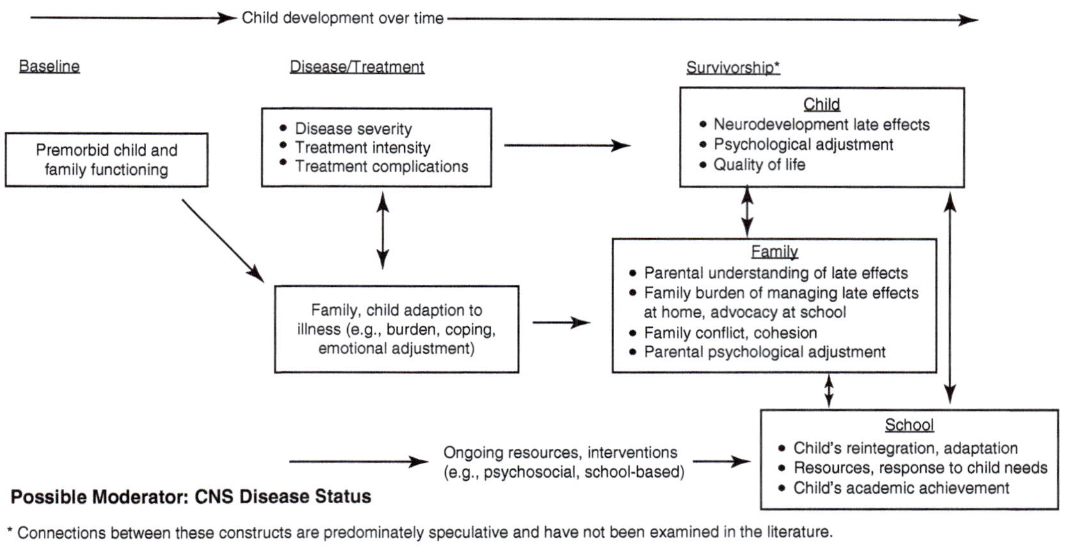

Fig. 11.2 Peterson and Drotar's theorized integrated model of NCLE and family functioning in survivors of pediatric cancer (Peterson and Drotar, *Clinical Child Psychology and Psychiatry*, 11(3):352, copyright 2006. Reprinted by permission of SAGE)

providing long-term follow-up care to families to recognize the ongoing nature of how the survivor's cognitive abilities and school difficulties may interact with parent stress and overall family strain, even long after the cancer itself is in remission.

Research from both the childhood cancer survivor population (Hocking et al. 2011; Patel et al. 2014a) and other pediatric populations (e.g., traumatic brain injury; Taylor et al. 1999) has indicated that family factors and parenting behaviors may actually influence the manifestation of the cognitive deficits in the child. For example, a family that is more cohesive and supportive of one another is more likely to be able to provide the supports and resources to help the child reintegrate into school successfully, advocate for appropriate services at school, and provide that child with the academic and emotional support to promote the best possible outcomes in the face of cognitive deficits. Considering the dynamic nature of the family system, however, it is also important to note that these patterns evolve over time, and the child's abilities may play a strong predictive role in how the family adapts to the educational issues. For example, it may be that children with relatively stronger compensatory mechanisms and coping skills of their own are perhaps more likely to succeed in school, thereby reducing the overall sense of strain and caregiver burden placed on the family system. In sum, the child, family, and school personnel are regularly interacting over the course of many years in an effort to understand and successfully manage late effects of treatment in survivors throughout their academic and early employment career. It is therefore important to recognize that the severity, compensatory mechanisms, functional impairment, and accommodations of the NCLE can play a significant role in understanding how a survivor's family continues to experience distress and burden long after active treatment has ended.

In addition to considering a family-focused approach to understanding the impact of NCLE, Peterson and Drotar's family systems model (2006) can also be applied to understanding the potential for family-based or parenting-based interventions to ameliorate adverse outcomes for survivors. For example, Patel and colleagues (2014b) focused their intervention specifically on parent training to promote academic strategies and pro-learning behaviors in childhood cancer survivors with late effects and found some significant benefits for parent pro-learning behaviors and moderate effects on improving children's academic outcomes. A clinical and research approach that considers the wide-ranging impact of NCLE on the families of survivors, as well as the survivors themselves, may lead to more targeted, effective interventions and ultimately may yield improved outcomes of interventions and other supportive services provided in long-term survivor care.

Identifying Children with Educational Needs

One of the challenges is to accurately and efficiently determine which survivors will need interventions or supports at school. The Children's Oncology Group (COG) recommends that high-risk survivors be screened for neurocognitive weakness when they transition into a survivorship program, regardless of patient- or parent-reported concerns. COG also recommends that any survivor who has experienced prolonged school absences or who is experiencing school-related difficulties be evaluated, regardless of diagnosis or risk category (Nathan et al. 2007). In addition to an initial or baseline assessment, it has also been recommended that children treated for CNS cancer receive biennial comprehensive neuropsychological assessments (Armstrong and Briery 2004). Assessments should include measures of academic functioning, as well as measures of processing speed, attention, executive functions, memory, language, and visual abilities (Katz and Madan-Swain 2006). Also see Chap. 10 for recommendations related to assessments for neurocognitive late effects. In addition to neurocognitive weaknesses, childhood cancer survivors may also experience other late effects or associated side effects from treatment that can interfere with their participation and success at school, including hearing loss, vision impairment, fatigue, and motor coordination deficits. Specialized assessments by audiology, speech/language therapists, ophthalmology, and physical therapy may also be essential to understand the needs of childhood cancer survivors. The Association of Higher Education and Disability (AHEAD 2005) has identified seven elements which should be present in documentation of a disability evaluation in order to obtain supports while in higher education (See Table 11.6). Barriers to attainment of adequate neurocognitive assessment for survivors include a lack of adequately trained professionals, insurance limitations, and concerns from survivors and/or parents about being identified or "labeled" as having a special education need. In order to obtain needed assessment for survivors, clinicians should examine resources in their areas (see Table 11.7). Comprehensive neuropsychological assessments may be available at medical settings, as well as in private practice. For survivors who do not have access to neuropsychologists, school psychologists may be helpful, particularly for assessing academic issues and helping identify appropriate cognitive supports. Given concerns about the limited resources for assessment, as well as the increased use of computerized assessments for concussion management, there has also been interest in the use of computerized batteries to assist with screening childhood cancer survivors (Ullrich and Embry 2012). In addition to barriers related to access to professionals, concerns about the interpretation of assessments may also be a significant barrier. For example, Cheung and colleagues (2014), examining the implementation of recommendations provided in assessments, found that only 60 % of the families in their study actually shared a copy of the report with the school. This information is essential for school personnel if they are going to intervene with a child.

Table 11.6 Essential components of documentation (AHEAD 2005)

The credentials of the evaluator
A diagnostic statement of disability
A description of the methodology or procedure for assessment
A description of functional limitations
A description of the expected progress
History of current and past accommodations and services
Recommendations for current accommodations

Interventions: Developmental Considerations

When working with a pediatric population, it is particularly important to be mindful of developmental considerations for a given child (see *Yardsticks: Children in the Classroom Ages 4–14*, third edition, (2007) by Chip Wood for a more detailed discussion of children's developmental needs within an educational environment). In particular, interventions should be tailored to a child's developmental stage. For example, children in Kindergarten may learn best through play and hands-on activities. Treatment effects that impact mobility, or exploration and manipulation of small objects, may be particularly problematic and may need to be the focus of intervention at

Table 11.7 Resources for neurocognitive assessments

	School psychologist	Neuropsychologist	Computerized assessments
Pros	Direct observation of child at school Increased familiarity with demands of school Costs covered by school	Comprehensive assessment of memory and executive functioning Understanding of brain behavior relationships Can be an advocate	Faster, easier to complete Less dependent on having trained personnel available Better designed for serial assessments
Cons	May have limited knowledge or experience with childhood cancer Not mandated to assess	Costs Limited providers in some areas, long waiting lists May or may not be covered by insurance	Requires trained professional to interpret Questions about validity Limited availability of programs

this age. In contrast, by the middle to end of third grade, there are greater expectations for sustained attention and organization in work. Executive deficits may be revealed at this time, and children may struggle to keep up with the pace of work and work efficiently. By age 14, there is increased demand for efficient note-taking skills, management of long-term projects, and inferential reasoning skills.

Interventions: Specific Educational Interventions – Math

There are different interventions or approaches that are most helpful for specific types of learning challenges, such as math. For children with specific learning disability in math, they have shown improvement when provided with interventions that provide explicit and systematic instruction (National Math Advisory Panel 2008), such as those with "clear teacher demonstrations, scaffolded instruction, guided practice, academic feedback, and cumulative review" (Doabler et al. 2012). In particular, in a meta-analysis, Gersten and colleagues (2009) reviewed 11 studies and found that explicit instruction and use of heuristics was associated with improved math achievement, whereas there was no evidence of efficacy for peer-assisted instruction. Similarly, in a meta-analysis conducted by Zheng, Flynn, and Swanson (2012), math problem solving was enhanced by explicit instruction, with components of instruction that included advance organizers, skill modeling, explicit practice, fading prompts/providing help as necessary, elaboration, task reduction, questioning, and providing and reminding students to use strategy cues.

In addition to research of children with learning disabilities in general, there is also a small body of research based on childhood cancer survivors. In examining instructional approaches specifically with childhood cancer survivors, Moore and colleagues (2012) reported on the efficacy of a math intervention for children with leukemia treated by chemotherapy, comparing baseline performance 12 months after completion of induction therapy to a post-intervention assessment done 1 year later and a follow-up assessment done an additional 12 months later. Individualized instructional support, with a specific problem-solving component and a multimodal approach, was provided 1–2 hours per week. Results reflected improvements in math skills for the intervention group in comparison to a standard of care group. There were also improvements seen in visual working memory.

Interventions: Specific Educational Interventions – Writing

Specific writing disorders can be related to handwriting and/or spelling and compositional skills. Interventions and supports for handwriting are often directed by occupational therapists and can include specific penmanship instruction (e.g., a specific curriculum such as Handwriting without Tears) and the use of assistive technology, such as keyboarding, voice dictation, and other software (Freeman et al. 2004). Use of explicit instruction in sound-symbol relationships and sound-letter patterns is associated with improvements in basic spelling skills (Berninger et al. 2006). There have also been strategies developed to improve student's structure in writing (Walker et al. 2005) or organization in writing (Graham and Harris 2003).

Interventions: Specific Educational Interventions – Reading

The majority of research on intervention for specific learning disabilities has focused on reading instruction, and there is more information available about the efficacy of interventions. In particular, reading instructional programs, such as Orton-Gillingham, Lindamood Phoneme Sequencing Program, Phono-Graphix, and FastForWord have been studied. The key components of effective instruction include phonological awareness, sound-symbol association, syllables, morphemes, syntax, and semantics via direct, systematic, sequenced instruction (Lyon et al. 2006). Moreover, Slavin and colleagues

(2011) found that one-to-one tutoring, focusing on phonics, with certified teachers was the most effective strategy.

Interventions: Other Neuropsychological Approaches

Cognitive remediation interventions typically utilize repeated practice or exercises to attempt to improve a specific cognitive domain while also providing instruction in strategies to compensate for these deficits. Many cognitive remediation programs target enhancing attention and memory skills, which are believed to underlie difficulties in academic skill development (Armstrong 2003). For example, the Cognitive Remediation Program by Butler and colleagues has shown some benefit for improvement in attention, as well as academic achievement and social skills, for childhood cancer survivors (e.g., Butler 1998; Butler and Copeland 2002; Butler et al. 2008). Similarly, Patel and colleagues (2009) noted improvements in academic skills with the use of one-on-one counseling in behavioral study skills, metacognitive strategies, information processing strategies, and academic mastery techniques. Some cognitive remediation programs have utilized computerized training (e.g., Cogmed). Hardy and colleagues (2013) noted improved visual working memory skills following weekly Cogmed sessions for 3 months, which was also associated with improvements in parent-reported learning difficulties. For deficits in attention, the role of stimulant medication (e.g., Conklin et al. 2010; Daly and Brown 2007), as well as neurofeedback (e.g., de Ruiter et al. 2013), has also been the attention of research studies. Although stimulant medication has been associated with improvements in attention of childhood cancer survivors, it has also been associated with some increased side effects, particularly for girls and those with lowered intellectual abilities, and it has not been consistently associated with improved academic performance (Conklin et al. 2009). See Chap. 10 for further discussion of interventions for neurocognitive deficits.

Interventions: Strategies to Improve Organization and Retention of Information

In addition to formal treatments or interventions, there are also multiple strategies that students can use in the classroom. This includes specific note-taking techniques (e.g., Cornell Note-Taking, Guided Notes). For example, Haydon and colleagues (2011) conducted a review of the use of guided notes, a technique in which a teacher provides a handout with an outline of the lecture with key elements omitted that the student must list for and fill in to the outline. In general, across studies, students appeared to retain more information and obtain higher scores on tests and quizzes. Similarly, another technique is to try to "prime attention" or "preteach" by reviewing key terms or concepts before the material is presented in class.

Interventions: The Role of Technology

There are multiple different types of software or applications that can be beneficial for childhood cancer survivors. For example, for a student with ongoing peripheral neuropathy impacting handwriting, access to a voice dictation word-processing system can be beneficial to improve efficiency and endurance for writing. The Family Center on Technology and Disability provides a guide and examples of assistive technology devices (see www.fctd.info). There are also ever-increasing applications to help provide memory prompts, assist with organization of work or assignments, create flashcards, help with time management, and support note-taking. Reviews of specific apps have been published by Palmer (2013) and Prupas (2011), as well as through the National Center for Learning Disabilities. Computer-based tutoring programs have been shown to be nearly as effective as "human tutoring" (VanLehn 2011). Computer programs have also been used to help remediate educational weaknesses, such as to increase oral reading fluency and task engagement (Clarfield and Stoner 2005).

Interventions: Advocacy and Parental Involvement

One of the strongest predictors of academic achievement in children remains parents' expectations and involvement. In particular, meta-analyses (Fan and Chen 2001; Hill and Tyson 2009) found that parental involvement was associated with school achievement, with higher parental expectations for academics being associated with greater long-term success (Mistry et al. 2009). When factors of parental involvement have been examined, however, a high or excessive degree of parental control and academic pressure is associated with negative academic outcomes (Karbach et al. 2012). Rather, parents with a high degree of involvement, but a low degree of behavioral control/greater autonomy granting, were associated with higher academic achievement, particularly in adolescence (Kramer 2012). The importance of autonomy has been noted in typically developing children, as well as children with disabilities (Doren et al. 2012).

Parents also have to struggle with managing their child's needs for involvement based on the child's developmental level. Initially, parents will be the primary educational advocate for a child. It is important for them to receive guidance and support for this role. For example, there are many documents and pieces of information (see Table 11.8) that are important for them to maintain. At the start of the school year, it can be helpful to provide classroom teachers with a brief summary of the educational needs (see Table 11.9) for the child. As the child ages, the responsibility for advocacy would be shifted gradually to the child. For example, the child might initially provide feedback to the parents on the summary, then the child would begin to write the summary with parent support. The goal would be that by the end of high school, the child would be able to create the summary independently and have experience with sharing and discussing it with their teachers.

As previously noted, there is an interaction between the family system and the child's functioning. It is important for the psychosocial clinician to also consider the parents' coping and support when addressing educational needs. For example, increased familial conflict and decreased familial support were associated with delays in academic achievement for survivors of childhood brain tumors (Ach et al. 2013). In particular, child and parental stress was significantly related to impairments in the child's school and work (Hile et al. 2014). Moreover, parenting stress, rather than parental overprotectiveness, was associated with poorer behavioral and social outcomes for children with cancer (Colletti et al. 2008).

Table 11.8 Documents for parents to keep for educational planning

Report cards
Results of standardized testing completed at school
Neuropsychological test results
Copies of notes from school meetings
Copies of 504 plans and IEPs
Results of college entrance scores
Copies of communications with school personnel
List of questions or concerns, with noted responses or answers
Phone numbers for key educational personnel and educational consultants

Table 11.9 Elements of an educational summary

A picture of the child
The child's diagnosis, types of treatments, and any identified treatment effects
A brief bullet list of the child's strengths as a learner, as well as areas of need
Identify if there is a formal IEP or 504 plan
Note the most essential accommodations or helpful strategies to promote success at school for the child

Case Vignette: 504 Plan

Following completion of treatment, a 15-year-old boy with a pineal gland tumor treated with cranial radiation and chemotherapy was noted to have some hearing loss related to his chemotherapy treatment. He had historically been a very strong student and had never previously received any special education services. His mother, who was a single parent, was struggling to determine if the changes in academic performance were related to the stressors of his cancer, which might be expected to

Table 11.10 Clinician's role related to educational needs

To support the child
During treatment, minimize school absences
Plan and implement a school reentry program
Be aware of risk factors for neurocognitive late effects and educational difficulties
Identify patients at risk for educational difficulties
Actively and systematically screen at risk groups for educational issues
Identify resources within the hospital or community, such as:
Neuropsychologists or psychologists who can conduct neurocognitive evaluations
Psychiatrists, psychologists, or social workers who can conduct psychological assessments and provide mental health treatments
Speech, audiology, occupational therapy (OT), physical therapy (PT) professionals to do assessments and provide services
Assistive technology programs
Tutoring services
Help advocate for needed special education services and accommodations
Monitor patients educational progress throughout survivorship
To support the parent
Consider parents' needs for information about potential educational impact of cancer treatment
Educate parents about children's rights in education
Identify local resources that can provide educational support and advocacy guidance for parents
Help establish appropriate expectations for parents for children's academic achievement
To support the school
Work collaboratively with school personnel to provide information about the child's illness, treatment, and expected course
Provide regular educational sessions for school personnel to increase knowledge and understanding of the educational impact of childhood cancer

remit, or if they were physiologically related to his tumor and its treatment. In particular, she was uncertain if attainment of a college degree continued to be an appropriate expectation for him. Results of a screening neuropsychological assessment reflected significant isolated weaknesses in memory functioning within the context of average to high average intellectual and academic skills. Although he had some hearing loss, weaknesses in memory were greater for visual material, suggesting that hearing was not a significant reason for his academic difficulties. He received classroom-based accommodations under a 504 plan, with a diagnosis of a cognitive disorder, not otherwise specified, which would correspond to the eligibility category of "other health impairment." Although his condition impacted his performance at school, he was not felt to require specialized instruction or specific services, such as speech therapy or occupational therapy. As a result, a 504 plan, instead of an IEP, was created to provide accommodations including exemption from rote memorization tasks and permission to have "open book" or use of notes for examinations; permission to use an electronic planner/calendar at school, with "alarms" for scheduled activities or as homework reminders; and preferential seating to reduce potentially interfering background noises. With these accommodations, he successfully completed high school and was accepted to college, where he has been succeeding with ongoing supports.

Case Vignette: IEP

A 13-year-old boy with a premorbid history of ADHD and a history of T-cell lymphoma, diagnosed at age 11, was treated with cranial radiation (1,800 cGy) and chemotherapy, including intrathecal methotrexate. He missed a substantial amount of 6th and 7th grade. Given some of his pre-existing social difficulties related to ADHD, as well as his lengthy absence, a school reentry presentation was particularly helpful to help foster peers' understanding and empathy. A neuropsychological evaluation reflected a significant relative weakness in visual processing speed in contrast to average verbal and visual reasoning abilities on intellectual testing. Academic skills testing reflected difficulty in integrated writing skills and speeded tasks of academic fluency. Other neuropsychological findings included weakness in visual-spatial organizational skills. An IEP was initiated to provide individualized instructional services related to writing, as well as classroom-based accommodations, such as extended time for exams and modifications of assignments to reduce written demands. School-based counseling services were also provided to help support social skills and facilitate peer-based relationships.

Conclusion

Children with cancer may have unique educational needs. In addition to support for the child directly, clinicians' roles also include psychosocial assessment of the survivor and family and providing support to the larger family and school community (see Table 11.10). During treatment, the clinician may need to help monitor and minimize school absences, as well as support ongoing participation in school-based activities. Accommodations under a 504 plan may be particularly helpful in supporting a child with cancer at school and school reentry programs. Specific educational presentations to the class and identification of a "point person" or liaison between the hospital and the school are often a primary focus during treatment. After completion of treatment, the clinician's focus turns to potential neurocognitive or educational late effects from treatment. It is essential for clinicians to understand the potential risks and develop effective screening practices, not just for the child, but also for the larger family and school systems. Families may need support and guidance about how to manage educational issues and advocate for their child. Helping families accurately understand their child's cognitive needs and abilities may serve to form more appropriate expectations for a child's academic performance, which may enhance outcomes. Similarly, school personnel need to be informed about potential risks for the educational impact of childhood cancer and its treatment, as well as potential strategies to support the child at school. By addressing a child's educational needs, in addition to their physical health, clinicians can make a profound impact on a child's future and success.

Clinical Pearls

Ongoing participation in school is an important part of childhood. Efforts to minimize children's absences, maintain their connection with peers, and facilitate their return to the classroom are essential.

If children experience significant neurocognitive changes related to treatment that interfere with their performance at school, they may be entitled to special education services, as described and managed through an IEP. For children who do not require specific services, such as specialized instruction, they may be eligible for accommodations under a 504 plan.

It is important for clinicians to collaborate with school personnel, to educate them about neurocognitive or educational needs of childhood cancer survivors, and to understand the specific models and requirements for special education services and accommodations.

Clinicians need to support and educate parents to advocate for their children's education needs and help identify appropriate resources for families in the community.

Educational Resources

Organizations – see Chap. 25 for general cancer resources

Wrightslaw Special Education Law and Advocacy at wrightslaw.org

US Department of Education at www.ed.gov

Resources for Parents

The American Cancer Society (2011) Children diagnosed with cancer: returning to school

Keene N (2003) Educating the child with cancer: a guide for parents and teachers. American Childhood Cancer Organization

Leukemia and Lymphoma Society (2005) Learning and living with cancer: advocating for your child's educational needs [brochure]. Leukemia and Lymphoma Society, White Plains

McDougal S (1997) Children with cancer: effects and educational implications. Accessed via the following website: www.ped-onc.org/cfissues/backtoschool/cwc.html

Resources for Teachers

Leeney SN, Katz ER (2005) Cancervive parent's and teacher's guide for kids with cancer. Cancervive, Los Angeles

Leukemia and Lymphoma Society. The Trish Green Back-to-School Program for Children

Peckman V (1993) Children with cancer in the classroom. Teaching Exceptional Children, volume 26, pages 26–32

The Royal Marsden NHS Foundation Trust and the Specialist Schools and Academies Trust (2008) Pupils with cancer: a guide for teachers. The Royal Marsden NHS Foundation Trust, London

Spinelli CG (2004) Dealing with cancer in the classroom: the teacher's role and responsibilities. Teaching Exceptional Children, volume 36, pages 14–21

Books to Share with Other Students in the Classroom

Cooper H (2012) Jacob has cancer: his friends want to help. American Cancer Society

Gaynor K (2008) The famous hat. Special stories

Gosselin K (2001) Taking cancer to school. JayJo Books

Klett A (2002) The amazing Hannah, look at everything I can do! Candlelighters Childhood Cancer Foundation

Meyers B, Mays LC (2011) The long and short of it: a tale about hair. American Cancer Society

Schultz C (1990) Why, Charlie Brown, why. Leukemia and Lymphoma Society

Acknowledgments The authors thank Megan Adriance for her collaboration in the development of a survey of school personnel related to neurocognitive late effects (NCLE). They also thank Michael Anderson for his input related to classroom dynamics.

References

Ach E et al (2013) Family factors associated with academic achievement deficits in pediatric brain tumor survivors. Psychooncology 22:1731–1737

Americans with Disabilities Act of 1990. Pub L. No. 101–336, 104 Stat 328

Armstrong FD (2003) Cognitive late effects of childhood cancer and treatment: issues for survivors. National Cancer Policy Board, Institute of Medicine and National Research Council, National Academies of Science commissioned background paper (www.ion.edu/ncpb) for National Cancer Policy Board (2003) In: Hewitt M, Weiner SL, Simone JV (eds) Childhood cancer survivorship: improving care and quality of life. The National Academies Press, Washington, DC

Armstrong FD, Briery BG (2004) Childhood cancer and the school. In: Brown RT (ed) Handbook of pediatric psychology in school settings. Laurence Erlbaum, Mahwah, NJ, pp 263–281

Association of Higher Education and Disability (AHEAD) (2005) Elements. http://ahead.org/resources/best-practices-resources/elements. Accessed 30 Sept 2014

Barrera M, Schulte F (2009) A group social skills intervention program for survivors of childhood brain tumors. J Pediatr Psychol 34(10):1108–1118. doi:10.1093/jpepsy/jsp018

Barrera M, Shaw AK, Speechley KN et al (2005) Educational and social late effects of childhood cancer and related clinical, personal, and familial characteristics. Cancer 104:1751–1760. doi:10.1002/cncr.21390

Berninger VW et al (2006) Modeling phonological core deficits within a working memory architecture in children and adults with developmental dyslexia. Sci Stud Read 10:165–198

Bessell AG (2001) Children surviving cancer: psychosocial adjustment, quality of life, and social experiences. Excep Child 67(3):345–359

Best SJ, Heller KW, Bigge JL (2005) Teaching individuals with physical or multiple disabilities. Pearson, Upper Saddle River

Brown RT et al (1992) Chemotherapy for acute lymphocytic leukemia: cognitive and academic sequelae. J Pediatr 121:885–889

Brown MB, Bolen LM, Brinkman TM et al (2011) A collaborative strategy with medical providers to improve training for teachers and children with cancer. J Educ Psychol Consult 21:149–165. doi:10.1080/10474412.2011.571478

Bruce BS, Newcombe J, Chapman A (2012) School liaison program for children with brain tumors. J Pediatr Oncol Nurs 29:45–54

Butler RW (1998) Attentional processes and their remediation in childhood cancer. Med Pediatr Oncol S1:75–78

Butler RW, Copeland DR (2002) Attentional processes and their remediation in children treated for cancer: a literature review and the development of a therapeutic approach. J Int Neuropsychol Soc 8:115–124

Butler RW, Haser JK (2006) Neurocognitive effects of treatment for childhood cancer. Ment Retard Dev Disabil Res Rev 12:184–191

Butler RW et al (2008) Interventions to improve neuropsychological functioning in childhood cancer survivors. Dev Disabil Res Rev 14:251–258. doi:10.1002/ddrr.33

Campbell LK et al (2007) A meta-analysis of the neurocognitive sequelae of treatment for childhood acute lymphocytic leukemia. Pediatr Blood Cancer 49:65–73. doi:10.1002/pbc.20860

Cheung LLT et al (2014) Neuropsychology reports for childhood brain tumor survivors: implementation of recommendations at home and school. Pediatr Blood Cancer 61:1080–1087

Clarfield J, Stoner G (2005) The effects of computerized reading instruction on academic performance of students identified with ADHD. School Psychol Rev 34(2):246–254

Colletti CJM et al (2008) The relationship of parent overprotection, perceived vulnerability, and parenting stress to behavioral, emotional, and social adjustment in children with cancer. Pediatr Blood Cancer 51:269–274

Conklin HM et al (2009) Side effects of methylphenidate in childhood cancer survivors: a randomized placebo-controlled trial. Pediatrics 124(1):226–233

Conklin HM et al (2010) Predicting methylphenidate response in long-term survivors of childhood cancer: a randomized, double-blind, placebo-controlled, crossover trial. J Pediatr Psychol 35:144–155

Daly BP, Brown RT (2007) Management of neurocognitive late effects with stimulant medication. J Pediatr Psychol 32:1111–1126

De Ruiter MA, van Mourik R, Schouten-van Meeteren AYN, Grootenhuis MA, Oosterlaan J (2013) Neurocognitive consequences of a paediatric brain tumour andits treatment: a meta-analysis. Dev Med Child Neurol 55(5):408–417. doi:10.1111/dmcn.12020

Doabler CT, Fien H, Nelson-Walker NJ, Baker SK (2012) Evaluating three elementary mathematics programs for presence of eight research-based instructional design principles. Learn Disabil Q 35(4):200–211. doi:10.1177/0731948712438557

Doren B, Gau JM, Lindstrom LE (2012) The relationship between parent expectations and postschool outcomes of adolescents with disabilities. Except Child 79(1):7–23

Education for All Handicapped Children Act of 1975. Pub L. No. 94–142. 89 Stat 773

Ellenberg L, Liu Q, Gioia G et al (2009) Neurocognitive status in long-term survivors of childhood CNS malignancies: a report from the childhood cancer survivor study. Neuropsychology 23(6):705–717. doi:10.1037/a0016674

Fan X, Chen M (2001) Parental involvement and students' academic achievement: a meta-analysis. Educ Psychol Rev 13:1–22. doi:10.1023/A:1009048817385

Fox C (2009) More than machines. T H E J 36(6):23–26

Freeman AR, MacKinnon JR, Miller LT (2004) Assistive technology and handwriting problems: what do occupational therapists recommend? Can J Occup Ther 71(3):150–160

Fremont WP (2003) School refusal in children and adolescents. Am Fam Physician 68:1555–1560

French AE, Tasngaris E, Barrera M et al (2013) School attendance in childhood cancer survivors and their siblings. J Pediatr 162:160–165

Gartin BC, Murdick NL (2009) Children with cancer: school related issues. Phys Disabil: Educ Relat Serv 27:19–36

Gerhardt CA, Dixon M, Miller KC et al (2007) Educational and occupational outcomes among survivors of childhood cancer during the transition to emerging adulthood. J Dev Behav Pediatr 28(6):448–455

Gersten R, Chard DJ, Jayanthi M et al (2009) Mathematics instruction for students with learning disabilities: a meta analysis of instructional components. Rev Educ Res 82:1202–1242

Gorin SS, McAuliffe P (2008) Implications of childhood cancer survivors in the classroom and the school. Health Educ 109(1):25–48. doi:10.1108/09654280910923363

Graham S, Harris KR (2003) Students with learning disabilities and the process of writing: a meta-analysis of SRSD studies. In: Swanson HL, Harris KR, Graham S (eds) Handbook of learning disabilities. Guilford Press, New York, pp 323–341

Gurney JG, Krull KR, Kadan-Lottick N et al (2009) Social outcomes in the Childhood Cancer Survivor Study cohort. J Clin Oncol 27:2390–2395

Hardy KK, Willard VW, Bonner MJ (2013) Computerized cognitive training in survivors of childhood cancer: a pilot study. J Pediatr Oncol Nurs 28:27–33

Harshman LA et al (2012) Population-based exploration of academic achievement outcomes in pediatric acute lymphoblastic leukemia survivors. J Pediatr Psychol 37(4):458–466. doi:10.1093/jpepsy/jsr119

Haydon T, Mancil GR, Kroeger SD et al (2011) A review of the effectiveness of guided notes for students who struggle learning academic content. Prev School Fail 55(4):226–231. doi:10.1080/1045988X.2010.548415

Helms AS, Schmeigelow K, Brok J et al (2014) Facilitation of school re-entry and peer acceptance of children

with cancer: a review and meta-analysis of intervention studies. Eur J Cancer Care. doi:10.1111/ecc.12230
Hile S, Erickson SJ, Agee B, Annett RD (2014) Parental stress predicts functional outcome in pediatric cancer survivors. Psychooncology 23:1157–1164
Hill NE, Tyson DF (2009) Parental involvement in middle school: a meta-analytic assessment of the strategies that promote achievement. Dev Psychol 45(3):740–763. doi:10.1037/a0015362
Hocking MC, Barnes M, Shaw C et al (2011) Executive function and attention regulation as predictors of coping success in youth with functional abdominal pain. J Pediatr Psychol 36:64–73
Individuals with Disabilities Education Act of 1997. Pub L No. 105–17. 20 USC 1401
Individuals with Disabilities Improvement Act of 2004. Pub L No. 108–446. 20 USC 1400
Kadan-Lottick NS, Zeltzer LK, Liu Q et al (2010) Neurocognitive functioning in adult survivors of childhood non-central nervous system cancers. J Natl Cancer Inst 102:881–893
Karbach J, Gottschlin J, Spengler M et al (2012) Parental involvement and general cognitive ability as predictors of domain-specific academic achievement in early adolescence. Learn Instruct 23:43–51
Katz ER, Madan-Swain A (2006) Maximizing school, academic, and social outcomes in children and adolescents with cancer. In: Brown RT (ed) Comprehensive handbook of childhood cancer and sickle cell disease: a biopsychosocial approach. Oxford University Press, New York, pp 313–338
Katz ER, Rubenstein C, Hubert N, Blew A (1988) School and social reintegration of children with cancer. J Psychosoc Oncol 6:123–140
Katz ER, Varni JW, Rubenstein CL et al (1992) Teacher, parent, and child evaluative ratings of a school reintegration intervention for children with newly diagnosed cancer. Child Health Care 21:69–75
Kearney CA (2008) School absenteeism and school refusal behavior in youth: a contemporary review. Clin Psychol Rev 28:451–471
Kearney CA, Albano AM (2004) The functional profiles of school refusal behavior: diagnostic aspects. Behav Modif 28:147–161
Kearney CA, Bensaheb A (2006) School absenteeism and school refusal behavior: a review and suggestions for school-based health professionals. J Sch Health 76:3–7
Keene N (2003) Educating the child with cancer: a guide for parents and teachers. Candlelighters Childhood Cancer Foundation, Kensington
Kramer KZ (2012) Parental behavioural control and academic achievement: striking the balance between control and involvement. Res Educ 88:85–98
Larouche SS, Chin-Peuckert L (2006) Changes in body image experienced by adolescents with cancer. J Pediatr Oncol Nurs 23:200–209
Leigh LD, Miles MA (2002) Educational issues for children with cancer. In: Pizzo PA, Poplack DG (eds) Principles and practice of pediatric oncology, 4th edn. Lippincott, Williams & Wilkins, Philadelphia, pp 1463–1476
Loman P, Vincent N (2002) School reintegration: current trends and future directions. Presentation at a meeting of the Children's Oncology Group, St. Louis
Lyon AR, Cotler S (2007) Toward reduced bias and increased utility in the assessment of school refusal behavior: the case for diverse samples and evaluations of context. Psychol Sch 44:551–565
Lyon GR, Fletcher JM, Fuchs K et al (2006) Learning disabilities. In: Mash E, Barkley R (eds) Treatment of childhood disorders, 3rd edn. Guilford, New York, pp 512–591
Mabbott DJ, Spiegler BJ, Greenberg ML et al (2005) Serial evaluation of academic and behavioral outcome after treatment with cranial radiation in childhood. J Clin Oncol 23(10):2256–2263
Maslow G, Haydon AA, McRee AL, Halpern CT (2012) Protective connections and educational attainment among young adults with childhood-onset chronic illness. J Sch Health 82:364–370
Mistry R, McCarthy WJ, Yancey AK et al (2009) Resilience and patterns of health risk behaviors in California adolescents. Prev Med 48:291–297
Mitby PA et al (2003) Utilization of special education services and educational attainment among long-term survivors of childhood cancer: a report from the Childhood Cancer Survivor Study. Cancer 97: 1116–1126
Moore JB, Kaffenberger C, Goldberg P et al (2009) School reentry for children with cancer: perceptions of nurses, school personnel, and parents. J Pediatr Oncol Nurs 26(2):86–99
Moore IM, Hockenberry MJ, Anhalt C et al (2012) Mathematics intervention for prevention of neurocognitive deficits in childhood leukemia. Pediatr Blood Cancer 59:278–284. doi:10.1002/pbc.23354
Mulrooney DA et al (2008) Twenty years of follow-up among survivors of childhood and young adult acute myeloid leukemia. Cancer 112:2071–2079
Nabors LA, Lehmkuhl HD (2004) Children with chronic medical conditions: recommendations for school mental health clinicians. J Dev Phys Disabil 16:1–15
Nathan PC, Patel SK, Dilley K et al (2007) Guidelines for identification of, advocacy for, and intervention in neurocognitive problems in survivors of childhood cancer. Arch Pediatr Adolesc Med 161(8):789–806
National Association of School Psychologists (2011) Grade retention and social promotion (position statement). National Association of School Psychologists, Bethesda
National Math Advisory Panel (2008) Foundations for success: the final report of the national mathematics advisory panel. U.S. Department of Education, Washington, DC
No Child Left Behind (NCLB) Act of 2001 (2002) Pub L. No. 107–110, 115, Stat. 1425
Oeffinger KC et al (2006) Chronic health conditions in adult survivors of childhood cancer. N Engl J Med 355:1572–1582

Ortlieb E (2008) Empowering preservice teachers through tutoring chronically ill cancer patients. Education 128(3):477–485

Palmer R (2013) The top 10 iPad apps for special education. In: T.H.E Journal. http://www.specialneedsdigest.com/2013/06/the-top-10-ipad-apps-for-special.html. Accessed 30 Sept 2014

Patel SK et al (2009) Cognitive and problem solving training in children with cancer: a pilot project. J Pediatr Hematol Oncol 31:670–677

Patel SK, Wong AL, Cuevas M et al (2013) Parenting stress and neurocognitive late effects in childhood cancer survivors. Psychooncology 22:1774–1782. doi:10.1002/pon.3213

Patel SK, Peters BB, Bell T et al (2014a) Parent involvement and neurocognitive functioning in childhood cancer survivors. J Behav Health 3:43–52

Patel SK, Ross P, Cuevas M et al (2014b) Parent-directed intervention for children with cancer-related neurobehavioral late effects: a randomized pilot study. J Pediatr Psychol 39(9):1013–1027. doi:10.1093/jpepsy/jsu045

Peterson CC, Drotar D (2006) Family impact of neurodevelopmental late effects in survivors of pediatric cancer: review of research, clinical evidence, and future directions. Clin Child Psychol Psychiatry 11:349–366. doi:10.1177/1359104506064980

Peterson CC et al (2008) A meta-analysis of the neuropsychological sequelae of chemotherapy-only treatment for pediatric acute lymphoblastic leukemia. Pediatr Blood Cancer 51:99–104. doi:10.1002/pbc.21544

Prevatt FF, Heffer RW, Lowe PA (2000) A review of school reintegration programs for children with cancer. J School Psychol 38:447–467

Prupas A (2011) There's a special app for that-part 9: apps for college/university students with learning disabilities. In: Inov8 educational consulting. http://www.inov8-ed.com/2011/07/theres-a-special-app-for-that-part-9-apps-for-col. Accessed 30 Sept 2014

Rehabilitation Act of 1973 as amended by Pub L No. 110–325, 29 USC 701 et seq

Robinson KE et al (2010) A quantitative meta-analysis of neurocognitive sequelae in survivors of pediatric brain tumors. Pediatr Blood Cancer 55:525–531. doi:10.1002/pbc.22568

Slavin RE, Lake C, Davis S et al (2011) Effective programs for struggling readers: a best-evidence synthesis. Educ Res Rev 6:1–26

Spinelli CG (2003) Educational and psychosocial implications affecting childhood cancer survivors: what educators need to know. Phys Disabil: Educ Relat Serv 21:49–65

Sullivan NA, Fulme DL, Zigmond N (2001) School: the normalizing factor for children with childhood leukemia: perspectives of young survivors and their parents. Prev School Fail 46:4–13. doi:10.1080/10459880109603338

Taylor HG, Yeates KO, Wade SL et al (1999) Influences on first-year recovery from traumatic brain injury in children. Neuropsychology 13:76–89

Thorsteinnsson T et al (2013) Study protocol: rehabilitation including social and physical activity and education in children and teenagers with cancer (RESPECT). BMC Cancer. doi:10.1186/1471-2407-13-544

Trask CL, Faust M (2011) Neurocognitive late effects: the need for greater outreach to the schools. Psychooncology 20(s1):75

Trask CL, Greene Welch JJ, Manley P et al (2009) Parental needs for information related to neurocognitive late effects from pediatric cancer and its treatment. Pediatr Blood Cancer 52:273–279. doi:10.1002/pbc.21802

Ullrich NJ, Embry L (2012) Neurocognitive dysfunction in survivors of childhood brain tumors. Semin Pediatr Neurol 19:35–42. doi:10.1016/j.spen.2012.02.014

Vance YH, Eiser C (2002) The school experience of the child with cancer. Child Care Health Dev 28:5–19

VanLehn K (2011) The relative effectiveness of human tutoring, intelligent tutoring systems, and other tutoring systems. Educ Psychol 46(4):197–221. doi:10.1080/00461520.2011.611369

Varni JW, Katz ER, Colegrove R et al (1993) The impact of social skills training on the adjustment of children with newly diagnosed cancer. J Pediatr Psychol 18:751–767

Walker B, Shippen ME, Alberto P et al (2005) Using the "expressive writing" program to improve the writing skills of high school students with learning disabilities. Learn Disabil Res Pract 20:175–183

Wood C (2007) Yardsticks: children in the classroom from 4–14, 3rd edn. Northeast Foundation for Children, Turner Falls

Zebrack B, Isaacson S (2012) Psychosocial care of adolescent and young adult patients with cancer and survivors. J Clin Oncol 30:1221–1226

Zheng X, Flynn LJ, Swanson HL (2012) Experimental intervention studies on word problem solving and math disabilities: a selective analysis of the literature. Learn DisabilQ36(2):97–111.doi:10.1177/0731948712444277

12 Adolescents and Young Adults with Cancer: A Biopsychosocial Approach

Brad Zebrack, Sheila Judge Santacroce, Pandora Patterson, and Alexandra Gubin

Rapid and significant human development characterizes adolescence and young adulthood. New social demands and ongoing cognitive and emotional maturation coincide with neuroendocrine changes and sexual development making this a stressful yet exciting phase of life. Adolescence and young adulthood are also times when developmental and health trajectories can be derailed by significant challenges to physical, psychological, and social well-being. These challenges are experienced quite differently by older adolescents and young adults (AYAs) in their 20s and 30s and have distinct behavioral implications, when compared to children and older adults.

Cancer is one example. It is the leading cause of death from disease for young people aged 15–29 years in the United States (Bleyer et al. 2006). Only accidents, homicide, and suicide claim more young lives than cancer. Cancer incidence peaks during the first 5 years of life with a second peak occurring during adolescence and early adulthood, most prominently in males. About five times as many people are diagnosed with cancer during the second 20 years of life as they are during the first two decades of life (National Cancer Institute 2015).

The types and prevalence of malignancies that occur in AYAs differ from those occurring in pediatric and older adult populations and vary as age increases from 15 to 39 years. The most prevalent cancers among the AYA population include leukemias, lymphomas, germ cell tumors (including testicular cancer), sarcomas, central nervous system tumors, melanoma, and colorectal, liver, cervical, breast, and thyroid cancer (http://www.cancer.gov/cancertopics/aya/types). Among 25- to 39-year-olds, the prevalence of breast cancer

B. Zebrack, PhD, MSW, MPH (✉)
University of Michigan School of Social Work, 1080 S. University, Room 2778, Ann Arbor, MI 48109-1106, USA
e-mail: zebrack@umich.edu

S.J. Santacroce, PhD, RN, CPNP, FAANP
School of Nursing, The University of North Carolina at Chapel Hill, Carrington Hall CB#7460, Chapel Hill, NC 27599-7460, USA

P. Patterson, PhD
CanTeen Australia and Cancer Nursing Research Unit, Sydney University, CanTeen Australia, GPO Box 3821, Sydney, NSW 2001, Australia
e-mail: Pandora.Patterson@canteen.org.au

A. Gubin, MSW, LCSW-C
Department of Pediatric Oncology, The Sidney Kimmel Comprehensive Cancer Center at Johns Hopkins, Baltimore, MD USA

Ulman Cancer Fund for Young Adults, Johns Hopkins Bloomberg Children's Center, 1800 Orleans Street, Room 11365, Baltimore, MD 21287, USA
e-mail: agubin1@jhmi.edu

A.N. Abrams et al. (eds.), *Pediatric Psychosocial Oncology: Textbook for Multidisciplinary Care*, DOI 10.1007/978-3-319-21374-3_12

and melanoma increases (Bleyer et al. 2006). These early breast cancers tend to be aggressive, with an excess rate of death for AYAs, and particularly African American women, compared to older women (Johnson et al. 2013). Less than 5 % of cancers in 15- to 29-year-olds have been attributed to a family cancer syndrome (Bhatia and Sklar 2002), and environmental factors appear to affect AYAs differentially.

In general, a biopsychosocial approach to care acknowledges that biological, psychological (i.e., emotions, cognitions), social (i.e., environment, economics, culture), and behavioral processes are interrelated in shaping human responses to disease (Engel 1977). For example, disparities in survival outcomes for AYAs with cancer may be a function of some or all of the following factors: differential biologic tumor response, delays in diagnosis and initiation of treatment, environmental exposures, genetic susceptibility, access to clinical trials, and health insurance (Bleyer 2011). Young peoples' brains and related neuroendocrine functions are still "under construction" and not fully developed until they are well into their twenties. The regulation of impulse control, which is controlled by the frontal lobes, develops last with the greatest changes occurring between puberty and adulthood. AYAs are physiologically underdeveloped in the areas that control impulses, foresee consequences, and temper emotional responses to environmental stressors. The amygdala, which develops before the frontal lobes, is responsible for impulsive and aggressive behavior, and its dominance makes AYAs less likely than mature adults to give due consideration to their behavior and its consequences. The brain is most vulnerable when young people are most likely to experiment with drugs or alcohol. Furthermore, when confronted with chronic health conditions, AYAs are often likely to resist adherence to medical recommendations (Patton et al. 2012). However, since the AYA brain is plastic and amenable to change, intervening with AYAs has great potential to shape cognition function and lifelong health behaviors.

AYAs engage in a myriad of developmental tasks associated with physiological, psychological, and social maturation, such as establishing autonomy from parents; developing a personal set of values and identity; establishing and reinforcing peer relationships, particularly intimate and sexual relationships; and obtaining adequate preparation to join the workforce. Prevalence of mental health disorders is highest during young adulthood, with 15 % of 18- to 29-year-olds having reported a history of major depressive disorder, 21 % reporting a mood disorder, and 30 % reporting any anxiety disorder (National Institute of Mental Health 2005; Kessler and Wang 2008). Coupled with risks for mood and other mental disorders, adolescents and young adults are primed to experience profound emotional distress, including anxiety and depression, when faced with a life-threatening event such as cancer. Anxiety and depression can have negative implications on the quality of life and even survival outcomes of AYAs with cancer including an increase in physical pain, potential for nonadherence with treatment, and higher disease morbidity (Lauer 2015). Post-traumatic stress symptoms and post-traumatic stress disorder have been associated with young adult survivors of childhood cancer (Rourke et al. 2007). In comparison to older adult cancer patients, adolescents and young adults lack the range of coping tools and life experiences, and this makes them particularly vulnerable to emotional distress (Lauer 2015; Trevino et al. 2012). Mental health professionals should provide routine screening of emotional distress and psychosocial adjustment to cancer for every newly diagnosed AYA patient, early in the cancer diagnosis. After accidents and homicide, suicide is the 3rd leading cause of death for young people aged 15–24 years (Lizardi et al. 2010).

Other complicating social and environmental factors may be history of substance use, child abuse, and poverty. Substance use is one of the largest contributors to morbidity and mortality among AYAs. Fifty-five percent of adolescents report having been drunk by 12th grade, and 28 % of 18- to 24-year-olds report binge drinking (5+ drinks in the last 2 weeks) (Centers for Disease Control and Prevention 2012). Prevalence rates are high for alcohol abuse (14 %), drug abuse (11 %), and any substance abuse disorder (17 %) among 18- to 29-year-olds (Kessler and Wang 2008).

Overall, 3–18 % of children in the United States have been sexually abused before the age of 12 (United States Department of Health and Human Services 2013). Around the world, 20 % of females and 8 % of males have suffered some form of sexual abuse before age 18 years (Pereda et al. 2009). The emotional and behavioral responses to sexual abuse and other traumatic experiences can exacerbate during adolescence or young adulthood and be expressed as unsafe sexual behavior, drug/alcohol abuse, psychiatric symptoms, and low levels of self-esteem (Lalor and McElvaney 2010). These risk factors can complicate disease management and adherence to therapy for AYAs diagnosed with cancer.

Twenty-one percent of children age 18 years and younger in the United States live in poverty (Felner and DeVries 2013). AYAs who grow up in poverty will likely continue to experience adverse events that can increase the likelihood of comorbid medical and psychosocial problems. Once these problems develop, AYAs who are impoverished can experience limited and disparate access to health care and other resources that address the constellation of biopsychosocial challenges. On the other hand, AYAs who have experience negotiating early life stressors can be resilient to adverse effects of later life stressors.

Case Vignette Substance Abuse

After meeting with a 16-year-old male with a premorbid history of opioid addiction and new diagnosis of acute lymphoblastic leukemia, the oncology team collaborated with the hospital's adolescent medicine service to develop a structured pain medication plan and behavioral regimen for the patient. A primary goal of the patient's pain plan was to provide clinically appropriate pain relief with the least amount of opiates. In order to maintain close monitoring of the patient's pain medication use, the oncology team became the sole prescribers of pain medication for this patient. Opioid medication was introduced only during potentially more painful points of treatment including surgical procedures such as a bone marrow biopsy and for debilitating side effects of treatment such as mucositis. The oncology team engaged the patient and his mother in the development and execution of a written behavioral contract signed by the patient and his mother. Some of the core stipulations of the contract included the following:

The patient would actively engage in his health care by continuing to participate in cancer treatment and outpatient substance treatment.

The oncology team would be the only health-care providers to prescribe pain medication to the patient.

The patient's mother would dispense his pain medication and monitor his use outside of the hospital setting.

His mental health-care needs were met by ensuring that he continued to work with the outpatient substance abuse counselors as well as the oncology social worker to address the risk of substance abuse relapse during the course of his illness and strategies for coping with stress. Effective psychosocial models utilized with this patient included cognitive behavioral therapy and motivational interviewing. Complementary modalities of managing pain such as meditation, deep breathing exercises, and yoga were also used. Throughout his treatment, the oncology team assessed the patient's pain with a focus on any potential drug-seeking behaviors.

Experiencing Cancer as an AYA

Understanding the biological, psychological, and social contexts of AYAs' lives and the interface between adolescent and young adult development and cancer is critical for the delivery of optimal care for this age-defined population. Cancer-related issues such as premature confrontation with mortality, changes in physical appearance, increased dependence on parents, disruptions of social life and school/employment because of treatment, and loss of reproductive capacity become particularly distressing (Zebrack and Isaacson 2012) and have the potential to exacerbate or complicate self-management of cancer-related symptoms, treatment side effects, and adherence to medical recommendations including medications, health-care appointments, and lifestyle modifications (Butow et al. 2010). While healthy peers are experiencing typical adolescence and young adulthood, AYAs are hospitalized or become homebound, often under the watchful eyes of hypervigilant parents and clinicians. They lack privacy and may become isolated from their peer group. Ultimately, most are unable to experience a "normal" adolescent life (Jones 2008). Confronting the adversities of cancer also has the potential to promote AYA maturation and psychosocial development. It exposes them to ideas, people, and opportunities for renewed esteem and confidence, identity transformation, and enriched knowledge about their body, empathy for others, and interest in health-related career paths (Lehmann et al. 2014; Phillips and Jones 2014).

Caring for AYAS with Cancer

Optimal assessment, care planning, and treatment across a continuum of care must occur with the understanding that maturation and development is co-occurring and that life disruptions can put AYAs at risk for lasting psychological, emotional, and social complications. To enhance care for AYAs, health-care professionals must cultivate their own clinical skills to help AYAs successfully cope with the challenges of cancer and the extent to which cancer influences their social worlds, particularly with regard to substance use/abuse, fertility, sex and sexuality, dying, and death. Quality cancer care for AYAs is dependent upon their needs being addressed by providers particularly trained to do so and should include mental health providers (e.g., social workers, psychologists, and psychiatrists, psychiatric mental health nurse practitioners), fertility specialists, nutritionists, music and art therapists, physical therapists, sexual health counselors, and palliative care teams.

Key Components of AYA Care

There exists an essential and unique set of medical and psychosocial aspects of care for AYAs for which age-appropriate clinical approaches and interventions are essential.

Family-Centered Care

Family-centered care provides an important model for how to best support adolescents and young adults with cancer, and particularly in the area of medical decision-making. A core component of family-centered care is an acknowledgment of various levels of engagement of families within the patient's medical care (Institute for Patient- and Family-Centered Care 2010). This is an especially relevant concept in the care of AYAs who, while flexing a sense of independence and autonomy, also seek input and support from others in the navigation of their medical care.

AYAs and Family of Origin

Many AYA patients remain or return to the family home during treatment and rely on their parents for tangible assistance and emotional support to an extent that can be inconsistent with previously held personal expectations and developmental norms. Thus, being mindful of the developmental challenges that AYA cancer can pose for parents and AYA siblings is critical. Family support and cohesiveness can be important contributors to positive adjustment. Family functioning has been identified as the single best predictor of distress, with poorer family functioning predictive of greater distress and suboptimal treatment adherence (Kondryn et al. 2011; Zebrack 2011).

Given the strong influence of family functioning, the provision of family-focused care is essential in the form of providing psychosocial support information and needs assessments where possible. In cases where poor family functioning is identified, additional support and assessment should be provided along with referrals to psychosocial care providers (e.g., oncology social workers) where appropriate. Health professionals should identify potential risk and protective factors in terms of family functioning as well as family-related concerns so that appropriate levels of support can be provided (see Table 12.1).

AYAs as Parents

Some AYA patients will already be parents when they are diagnosed with cancer. Pressing concerns include when, how, and how much to tell their children about the cancer diagnosis as well as changes in the parent's appearance and family routines. Parents, especially single parents with cancer, will also worry about who can help care for their children during treatment or

Table 12.1 Family risk factors and the promotion of protective factors

Family risk factors	Promoting protective factors
Closed communication, e.g., family members are not kept informed and there are limited opportunities for involvement and discussion in decision-making	Encourage *open communication* among family members; keeping each other informed provide opportunities for negotiation and open decision-making
Avoidance of sharing of feelings, e.g., there is an overemphasis on positive thinking or fear that sharing feelings may upset or worry others	Teach family members to *express feelings* and feel comfortable doing so
Unbalanced cohesion, e.g., families may be enmeshed and may be dependent and reactive to each other, relying heavily on each other for support	Work with the family to achieve *healthy boundaries*; remaining close to each other, but also maintaining their own independence
Low levels of adaptability, e.g., difficulty accepting or adapting to change	Increase *psychological flexibility* among family members allowing them to respond and reorganize themselves well in times of change/stress
Loss of familiarity, e.g., disruptions to family life over an extended period of time can bring instability and lack of familial support	Work with the family to *restore* previous family activities and priorities. Also allow for the possibility to develop *new ways of being* as a family
Lack of a social support network, e.g., families who are socially isolated are likely to rely heavily/exclusively on immediate family members for emotional and practical support	Promote the *development of, and access to, a social support network* to provide adequate emotional and practical support outside of the immediate family
Parental distress, e.g., parents experiencing elevated levels of psychological distress, finding it difficult to adjust and cope with the difficulties a cancer diagnosis brings	Foster *effective parental adjustment* by assisting parents to be aware of their levels of distress and to seek psychological assistance where needed; provide coping strategies and increase psychological flexibility to allow acceptance of their situation
Financial instability (existing or as a result of the cancer diagnosis), e.g., due to medical costs, time out of work, travel	Link family with *financial services* to assist in ameliorating the financial impact associated with the cancer diagnosis
Poor parenting skills, e.g., focus on negative behaviors with little acknowledgment of positive behaviors, inconsistent discipline techniques, and expectations placed on each young person	Encourage *parenting competence* by teaching effective and consistent disciplining and monitoring of AYAs, good conflict resolution skills, and reinforcement of positive behaviors
Preexisting stressors, e.g., mental health issues, domestic violence, drug and alcohol issues, or care duties of other family members	Address stressors to nurture a *stable family environment* where additional stressors are well managed. This may involve referring to other services as appropriate

Source: Supporting adolescent and young adult siblings of cancer patients: the family context. Retrieved from https://www.canteen.org.au/media/63525/RTPIssue1_Paper.pdf. Permission obtained to adapt material (CanTeen Australia 2011b)

if they do not survive their cancer. AYA patients who are parents can benefit from specific guidance about how to talk with their children about cancer and what to watch for in terms of signs of child distress (Maynard et al. 2013). More information about addressing AYA parent's concerns about their children can be found at www.mghpact.org.

Managing and Comprehending Information

Health-care providers should ask AYAs directly about how they would prefer to receive this information, be it verbal, written, and audiovisual instruction. Doing so becomes one way to restore a sense of control to AYAs, for whom lost control and autonomy are major challenges. The main topics AYA patients want information about are their cancer and its treatment, the decision-making process, the health-care system, and survivorship issues such as what can be done to manage persistent, worsening, or late adverse effects (Palmer et al. 2007; Zebrack 2008). Many AYAs also want information about healthy diet, exercise, infertility, complementary and alternative approaches, and insurance. Addressing AYAs' information needs requires health professionals to (1) use a caring manner and understandable language, (2) allow time for AYAs to process information, (3) not assume AYAs are confident to ask questions, and (4) expect AYA and parent concerns to differ (Palmer et al. 2007). Many AYAs independently access cancer-related information and support online. With online usage prevalent in this age group, the development of evidence-based, developmentally appropriate Web-based information for AYA patients is essential. For example, the website www.nowwhat.org.au supports young people affected by cancer, whether they are dealing with their own or an immediate family member's cancer. This website sets an international benchmark, combining access to professional counselors and youth-specific information and providing interactive, personalized online peer support community (Patterson et al. 2014).

Patient-Provider Relationships and Communication

The quality of the patient-provider relationship and therapeutic bond, specifically between the oncologist and AYA patient, has been shown to demonstrate a great impact on the psychosocial well-being of the patient, which, in turn, can have implications on treatment adherence and quality of life (Trevino et al. 2013). Special consideration of how information is communicated is essential to AYA patients who will engage most effectively with providers who present information in a direct yet genuine, non-authoritative manner (Trevino et al. 2013). Clinicians should demonstrate a sense of self-awareness and exhibit a clear sense of professional boundaries when working with AYAs, who might be inclined to question authority. Flexibility and patience on the part of the clinician are critical to the development of a trusting patient-provider relationship.

AYA health communications and collaborative decision-making can be sensitive issues. Some AYAs prefer to be shielded from discussions about their cancer, treatment options, and potential late effects and/or to assume a dependent position with regard to decision-making. Others want a prominent or fully independent role. Respecting AYAs' preferences for autonomy can be agonizing for their parents. AYAs over age 18 years are legal adults in the United States and are expected to provide informed consent for both their medical treatment and participation in biomedical research. Their parents are deemed to have no rights to their health information without specific patient agreement, which could be a blanket agreement or vary by the nature and complexity of the decision being made.

AYAs under age 18 years should be engaged in health communications and decision-making and asked to provide assent. Although most AYAs lack experience to guide communications and decisions about cancer treatment and rely heavily on parental advice about how to proceed, others prefer to function independently of their parents. Parents, however, can feel responsible to protect and advocate for their children and thus struggle with their child and their child's clinician over access to health information and control of decisions and other aspects of care.

Clinicians must determine, as early as feasible, the extent to which the AYA patient wishes to involve parents in health communications and treatment decision-making and then acknowledge that these wishes may change over time. Health-care providers must be mindful of the potential conflict and tension that might arise between AYAs and their families in decisions concerning medical care (Grinyer 2009). Should a patient wish for an individual(s), such as a parent or spouse/partner, to have access to her medical information, the treating health-care provider should implement procedures (Health Insurance Portability and Accountability Act (HIPAA) release form in the United States) and establish specific parameters for doing so. One approach is for the clinician to give information to the patient first and then, with patient permission and to the extent specified, to parents or other designated individuals with the patient together (Grinyer 2003). This approach also provides AYAs with opportunities to hear complex and significant information repeated and to learn from parent questions. However, it is also important to note that there may be a history of problems between a parent and child that will complicate the AYA's cancer experience. Assessment is required to determine the best approach for integrating parents and other individuals into AYA care. This approach can also promote development of an open, trusting health-care relationship between AYAs, their social network members, and their oncology care providers.

Case Vignette : Patient-Provider Communication and Shared Decision-Making

A 22-year-old woman received chemotherapy and radiation for a brain tumor. During the course of her treatment, she took a medical leave from college and moved home to live with her mother, who served as her primary caregiver. The patient's parents were divorced. The patient included her mother in the initial discussions with the patient's primary medical team in order to review her diagnosis and proposed treatment plan. From the outset, it was evident that the patient displayed a full range of capacity to make medical decisions. Following the consultation, the social worker met with the patient individually to perform a psychosocial assessment. The primary goal of the interview was to educate the patient about her legal rights to make medical decisions and the confidential and protected nature of her health information. Moreover, the social worker aimed to glean an understanding of the patient's communication style and preferences. The following questions were posed to the patient:

How do you learn best (i.e., verbal, written, and audiovisual formats)?
How much information would you like to know about your medical condition?
With whom have you engaged in the past when making important decisions, such as those concerning your health?
Are there others with whom you wish to have access to your medical information?

The patient stated that while she would be in charge of her health care, she wanted her mother to be engaged in all levels of her care from daily medical rounds to meetings with the medical team about changes in her medical condition and treatment planning. Moreover, the young woman was emphatic that she did not wish for her father, from whom she was estranged, to have access to her medical information or be involved in any aspect of her care. To formalize the patient's wishes about who could be granted access to her health information, the social worker facilitated the implementation of a HIPAA release form, which established that her mother could have access to her health information. A copy of this document was included in the patient's medical records so that health-care providers were properly informed of her wishes.

Clinical Trials

Pediatric and adult settings can each lack opportunities for AYA enrollment in clinical trials, particularly trials that consider the unique biology and behavior of some AYA cancers. Much of the improvement that has been made in survival rates for children with cancer has been attributed to their high rates of enrollment in national collaborative or institutional clinical trials. More than 60 % of pediatric cancer patients in the United States (most under the age of 15 years) are treated on research protocols (http://www.childrensoncologygroup.org/index.php/what-is-a-clinical-trial; accessed 13 Feb 2015). In contrast, 10–15 % of 15- to 19-year-olds and about 2 % of 20- to 29-year-olds with cancer are enrolled in such trials in the United States (Bleyer et al. 2006), with similar low figures observed in other Western countries (Fern and Whelan 2010; Ferrari et al. 2008). While disparities in clinical trial participation for 20- to 29-year-olds are similar across racial and ethnic groups, gender disparity with lower male participation stands out (Fern and Whelan 2010).

Some psychosocial barriers to AYA enrollment in clinical trials include intense emotional responses to the cancer diagnosis; lack of experience making important decisions, especially medical decisions; concerns about further loss of control and quality of life due to clinical trial requirements; lack of information about available clinical trials or complexity of the information; beliefs that community providers can offer the same level of care, monitoring, and services as what they would receive through clinical trial participation; misconceptions about clinical trials and fears of being "treated as a guinea pig"; and the costs that can be associated with being treated outside the local community (Buchanan et al. 2014). AYAs, however, report that they participate in clinical trials for both the therapeutic benefits that they hope to accrue for themselves and as a means to help other people like them (Miller et al. 2013). AYAs might need assistance identifying clinical trial options, comprehending trial requirements and implications and, for those who want to participate in a trial, ongoing emotional and practical support for accessing the trial and adhering to its requirements. Without improving AYA access and participation in clinical trials, improving medical outcomes for AYA cancer patients will continue to be limited.

Psychosocial Screening, Assessment, and Care Planning

A biopsychosocial approach requires the use of developmentally appropriate assessment tools to identify AYAs at risk for psychosocial distress or other conditions that may disrupt their care or compromise survival and quality of life. Given the dearth of instruments available (Wakefield et al. 2013), an *AYA Oncology Psychosocial Care Manual* (CanTeen Australia 2011a) was developed which includes an AYA-modified version of the National Comprehensive Cancer Network (NCCN) Distress Thermometer and Psychosocial Problem Checklist (areas related to practical, family, emotional, social, physical information) and a comprehensive assessment of cancer experience inclusive of physical systems review, family, education, employment, social activities, substance use (e.g., alcohol, drugs, tobacco), sexuality and sexual relationships, religious and spiritual beliefs, mental health, current stressors, strengths, and support. These instruments screen, assess, and assist in identifying patients at risk for psychosocial challenges managing their cancer (Evan and Zeltzer 2006; Hedstrom et al. 2006). Consideration should be given to acute stress symptoms along with risk factors including lower socioeconomic status, prior exposure to trauma, history of childhood adversity such as parental death, family psychiatric history, and protective factors such as social support and resilience that can affect AYAs' emotional responses to cancer and its treatment.

The screening tool, care plan, and assessment measure were developed to be administered at key time points along the AYA psychosocial care pathway, aiming to support the young person throughout their treatment by addressing current support needs and taking into consideration needs that may be most significant posttreatment for healthy survivorship. In addition to the screening and assessment tools, the *AYA Oncology Psychosocial Care Manual* includes a care plan *pro forma* to provide a means for clinicians to collate relevant screening and assessment information and develop a strategy to manage issues raised. It enables treating teams to identify patients at risk, monitor the progressive coping of the patient, identify areas of need requiring additional care and support, and guide counseling so that AYAs receive the support they need, even as their needs change (CanTeen Australia 2011a; Palmer et al. 2014). Table 12.2 outlines how the patient moves through the pathway as described in the *AYA Oncology Psychosocial Care Manual* (pp. 5–6) (CanTeen Australia 2011b).

The initial psychosocial assessment should also include attention to substance abuse risk factors including personal, family or peer group history of substance abuse (e.g., illicit drugs, prescription drugs, alcohol), and personal or family history of psychological problems especially depression. This is especially important since most AYA patients will be prescribed opioid therapy for cancer-related pain. Abuse risk factors are dynamic and must be carefully monitored over the cancer trajectory (Pergolizzi et al. 2012).

Table 12.2 The AYA psychosocial care pathway

Elements	Process
Initial Psychosocial Screen	Every young person should receive a psychosocial screen, ideally within 2 weeks of diagnosis and/or first treatment cycle. It identifies the level of distress currently experienced by the patient and the nature of such distress. Information should also be provided about clinical trials, support organizations, entertainment, home comforts, websites, alcohol and drug use, fertility preservation, communication tools, sexual health, educational support, and the lead clinician
Development of Care Plan	Within 2 weeks following the administration of the screening tool, a care plan based on the outcomes of the screening tool should be developed by the treating team in collaboration with the patient. It focuses on addressing the current needs of the patient through referral, information provision, further assessment, and/or standard patient management
Second Screen and Psychosocial Assessment	This is conducted once treatment is established. Approximately 8 weeks post diagnosis and/or treatment commencement is a significant period for the patient. Given it is often a time of changing and/or increasing need, a second screen is conducted. Resources permitting, it is beneficial for patients to also receive a full psychosocial assessment during this stage of their cancer journey to further inform care planning and the provision of psychosocial support
Development of Working Care Plan	While the template for the Working Care Plan is the same as that used for the initial care plan, the information documented differs due to the clinician's increased knowledge of the patient, their family, and environment. Developed within 2 weeks of the Second Screen and Psychosocial Assessment, the Working Care Plan should have further depth of detail than the initial care plan and incorporate patient-specific strategies to manage adherence, identify risks, and plan for survivorship
Progress Screen	A Progress Screen is conducted approximately 6 months post diagnosis and/or treatment commencement to address any changes in the patient's experience, illness trajectory, family, or environment throughout the cancer journey
Revision of Working Care Plan	Any changes in need identified by the Progress Screen should be incorporated into a revised care plan to allow continued patient support in a relevant and effective manner
Further Screening and Care Planning	Any further screening and care planning should take place at the clinician's discretion or the patient's request. At a minimum, this should occur at remission, recurrence, or progression. Additional time points to consider include changes in treatment, changes in treatment goals, treatment completion, and during significant times in the young person's life (e.g., moving into a new school year, relationship breakups, family breakdown)

CanTeen Australia (2011b)

Overall, AYAs are more likely to abuse opioids than adults (Pergolizzi et al. 2012), and opioid abuse can develop through experimentation or legitimate opioid use. AYAs who use more than one opioid concurrently seem to merit particularly close monitoring for abuse (Ehrentraut et al. 2013).

Treatment Adherence

Whether or not an AYA patient is eligible for or opts to enroll in a clinical trial, treatment adherence is a significant issue. Less than 90 % adherence to oral therapy has been associated with 3.9-fold higher risk of relapse among children and adolescents with acute lymphoblastic leukemia (Bhatia et al. 2012). Adolescents are among the groups at highest risk for suboptimal adherence to oral cancer therapy. One small study found that adolescents took less than 75 % of prescribed doses and had perfect adherence to their oral regimen post-stem cell transplant on fewer than 4 days per week (McGrady et al. 2014). Adolescent difficulties with adherence to oral therapy tend to become more pronounced over time (McGrady et al. 2014; Rohan et al. 2015). Adolescent adherence can be adversely affected by factors that include wanting to be like their peers, cognitive decline, and lower parental involvement (Buchanan et al. 2014; Malbasa et al. 2007). Factors associated with perfect adherence include having future-oriented goals, family support, and a second "overprotective" parent caregiver (Hullman et al. 2015).

Clinicians should expect that AYAs will have difficulties with adherence and that adherence will deteriorate over time (Bhatia et al. 2012). Means of assessing adherence include self-report, pharmacy records, pill counts, and laboratory tests such as leukocyte counts and drug metabolite assays. Self-report tends to overestimate adherence for reasons that include social desirability and recall bias. Clinicians can elicit more reliable self-reports by using nonjudgmental, understanding, and optimistic approaches that normalize less than perfect adherence and include questions about doses missed during specific time frames and the circumstances. Clinicians can also explore strategies to improve adherence and reinforce good adherence. Parents might help by obtaining and organizing medications and establishing reminder systems to maximize adherence (Malbasa et al. 2007). However, given their drive for independence, AYAs can be irritated by parental involvement. Also, parents with high demands on their time and low levels of social support might prematurely delegate sole responsibility for medication adherence to the AYA (Bhatia et al. 2012). Clinicians can coach AYAs in explicating what they need from their parents with regard to supporting positive health behaviors such as helping AYAs stay organized with medications and fostering engagement in decisions about medical care.

At diagnosis, health literacies and reading abilities in English and the AYA family's primary language also should be assessed. AYAs, and when applicable their parents and partners, should be encouraged to discuss their understandings of the disease and its prognosis, treatment goals, and beliefs about treatment efficacy and to define their roles and responsibilities in adherence considering AYA development and routines (Williams 2001). AYAs routinely should be provided with precise verbal and written information, in both English and their primary language, about the treatment that has been prescribed and copies of treatment calendars.

Information is not sufficient to promote optimal adherence. Regular reminders via mobile devices using Internet applications such as "Pillbox" and "MedCoach" could help promote AYA adherence by using the normative means that AYAs use to communicate and manage their lives (Santacroce and Crandell 2013). Reminders can be sent by short message service (SMS) or text messaging, or personal devices can be set to alarm or display an image at predetermined times when medication is due. Other possibilities include medication adherence-oriented applications that AYAs can download to their smartphones (e.g., MyMedSchedule) and provide means for recording doses and side effects (Dayer et al. 2013).

Technology and social media should not be overlooked as effective tools for addressing adherence in the adolescent and young adult population. For example, the videogame "Re-Mission," which conceptualizes chemotherapy as battling cancer, has been shown to improve adolescents' understanding of and engagement in cancer treatment (Kato et al. 2008). The facilitation of social media such as Facebook and Twitter, when utilized in a safe and HIPAA-compliant manner, also may serve as effective platforms of engagement with AYAs in medication adherence and other important aspects of cancer care.

Case Vignette : Medication Adherence
A 17-year-old female patient with acute lymphoblastic leukemia who was in the middle of her treatment regimen reported to her primary oncologist that she was no longer taking her oral chemotherapy medication as prescribed. The social worker met with her to explore the patient's attitudes and behaviors as they might relate to nonadherence. The patient talked about increased stress related to her returning to school and her mother working longer hours. With the transition back to school, the patient indicated a heightened sense of wanting to feel "normal" again and a desire to spend more time with friends. She endorsed the belief that continuing to take chemotherapy meant that she was still sick, an identity that she wanted desperately to break away from in an attempt to return to "normal." She also talked about "forgetting" to take her medication and about not being reminded to do so by her mom. After the meeting, the social worker met with the patient's mother to gain a better understanding of the family system. The patient's mother reported that her job had become more demanding and as a result, she was less focused on her daughter's medication adherence. Based on these separate encounters, the team decided to meet with the patient and her mother to address how to better support the patient's efforts toward improved medication adherence. Psychoeducation about the critical importance of medication adherence to overall survival was provided verbally and with educational pamphlets. In addition, medication organizational systems were suggested including a weekly pillbox and electronic medication calendars. Moreover, the social worker began to provide counseling to the patient on a regular basis to address her beliefs about her identity as a cancer patient and connected her with programs to meet other teens living with cancer, including the Ulman Cancer Fund for Young Adults and the Leukemia & Lymphoma Society.

Sex and Sexuality

The adolescent and early adult years represent a critical time in sexual development. A cancer diagnosis can seriously threaten onset of puberty, normative exploration of sexual practices and behaviors, and formation of gender identity and sexual orientation. Early menopause, infertility, fatigue, osteoporosis, and changes in cognition represent treatment-related side effects that can adversely impact AYAs' sexual function and practices as well as overall sense of self (Bolte and Zebrack 2008). Physical alterations to the body as a result of treatment such as scarring, weight loss/gain, and hair loss can adversely impact body image. In addition, self-esteem may be compromised by poor body image, lack of sufficient sexual knowledge, and increased difficulties relating to family, peers, and intimate partners (Evan et al. 2006). In turn, a positive identity and healthy social relationships can suffer and lead to a heightened sense of isolation and alienation (Bolte and Zebrack 2008). Moreover, impaired sexual development can increase emotional and psychological distress that, if left untreated, can have implications on overall quality of life (Canada et al. 2006).

The topic of sexual health should be included as part of the medical and psychosocial assessment early in the diagnosis. Of note, adolescents and young adults aged 15–24 comprise half of all new cases of sexually transmitted disease (STDs) (Centers for Disease Control and Prevention, 2014, 2012 Sexually Transmitted Diseases Surveillance, http://www.cdc.gov/std/stats12/adol.htm). Medical providers should be especially diligent about engaging AYA patients in a conversation about sexual history and safe sexual practices (Centers for Disease Control and Prevention 2011, 2014, www.cdc.gov/std/treatment/2010/clinical.htm).

Some AYAs interpret information about the risk for impaired fertility as meaning they will be unable to become pregnant or get someone pregnant. Furthermore, AYA patients and survivors may engage in risky sexual behavior to feel "normal," because they feel lonely, or to address worries about poor body image, sexual performance, and other aspects of sexuality as well as a sense of invincibility. These responses to AYA cancer can lead to unintended or high-risk pregnancy (Murphy et al. 2013). Therefore, AYAs also need information about how to protect their sexual health and prevent pregnancy until they are prepared to be a parent. Sexual health and safe sexual practices should also be presented within the context of infection control and potential for bleeding, as well as other potential health risks associated with engaging in sexual behaviors during certain points of cancer treatment (Lauer 2015). Males should be counseled to protect themselves from sexually transmitted diseases while neutropenic, to use condoms, and to not engage in oral sex. They should also use condoms for 2 weeks post chemotherapy to prevent exposing partners to chemotherapy. Female condoms and dental dams may also serve as protective barriers from protecting against chemotherapy exposure (Kelvin et al. 2014). Menstrual cycles during chemotherapy can pause or become irregular, and females should be made aware that this does not mean they are unable to get pregnant. Females should be counseled to use a reliable form of birth control throughout the treatment phase and to limit their risk of sexually transmitted infections that can further impair fertility by assuring that their male sexual partners wear condoms. AYA females should have a pregnancy test before therapy is initiated. Since pregnancy symptoms (e.g., nausea, vomiting, fatigue, cessation of menses) can also be caused by cancer therapy, pregnancy testing at the start of each treatment cycle can identify unrecognized pregnancy and limit the possibility of fetal exposures to chemotherapy.

In efforts to provide comprehensive oncology care to the AYA population, health-care professionals must acknowledge the normative and healthy sexual development of AYAs with cancer. The responsibility to address sexual health rests with the health-care providers, not the patient (Bolte and Zebrack 2008). However, research indicates that health-care providers do not routinely address the topic of sexual health with cancer patients as a result of a lack of knowledge about normative sexual development and behaviors and lack of comfort in communicating about this topic (Katz 2005).

The PLISSIT Model (Permission, Limited Information, Specific Suggestions, Intensive Therapy) is an effective tool that can be implemented to effectively assess, educate, and provide intervention in the sexual well-being of AYA cancer patients (Bolte and Zebrack 2008) as described below:

Permission Health-care providers should encourage patients to discuss their sexuality, a topic that many AYAs may lack proper knowledge about and feel reluctant or uncomfortable to bring up on their own. Health-care providers should be sensitive to patient confidentiality and privacy when engaging in a dialogue about sensitive information, such as sexual health. There should be the opportunity for the patient to meet alone with the provider unless the patient specifically indicates a desire for his loved ones to be present during a conversation about the patient's sexual health (Kelvin et al. 2014). When addressing sexual health, providers should use language that is empathic and accessible as a means to promote comprehension of medical concepts (Centers for Disease Control and Prevention 2011). Open-ended versus closed-ended questions can allow for patients to feel more comfortable to engage openly and honestly in a dialogue about sexual health. For example, in addressing current sexual activity, a provider might say, "How do you protect yourself when you have sex?" rather than, "You're using protection, right?"

Limited Information When addressing sexual matters with the AYA population, health-care providers should provide information and resources that educate patients about the implications of a cancer diagnosis on their sexual health. For the AYA cancer population in particular, safe sex practices should always be encouraged, for both protections against STIs and STDs as well as pregnancy. As mentioned in the Fertility section, some AYAs may recover from impaired fertility; thus, safe sexual practices should always be practiced during and following treatment.

Specific Suggestions

If indicated, health-care providers should offer specific suggestions on strategies to enhance sexual well-being and guide patients and their partners in a renewed set of expectations around sexuality and sexual behavior. For example, if an AYA female patient is struggling with body image issues related to hair loss, normalizing this experience for the patient by educating her that it is a common challenge for many other patients and also offering a specific suggestion as to how to address the issue, such as "Many patients find that wearing a wig, hat, or scarf can help make them feel more comfortable about their body and hanging out with friends," might serve as an effective approach.

Intensive Therapy For patients who have experienced physical side effects of treatment impacting sexual function, oncology providers should enlist the support of a gynecologist, urologist, physical therapist, endocrinologist, and other specialists who may be able to appropriately address sexual side effects of cancer treatment. In addition, as sexual changes can fuel emotional distress, it is important to consider the support of a mental health provider or sex therapist to guide the psychosocial adjustment and impact of a cancer diagnosis on sexuality. Psychoeducational interventions focused on sexual development and reproductive health issues have shown to be meaningful in the reduction of psychosocial distress in AYAs with cancer (Canada et al. 2006). Some helpful resources for patients and providers to consider include American Association of Sexuality Educators, Counselors, and Therapists (www.acog.org/patients), American Congress of Obstetricians and Gynecologists Information (www.acog.org/patients), Sexuality Information and Education Council of the United States (www.siecus.org), and American Cancer Society's *Sexuality for the Woman with Cancer* (http://bit.ly/1rTICty) and *Sexuality for the Man with Cancer* (http://bit.ly/1m5Houb).

Case Vignette : Sexuality and Fertility

A 24-year-old woman receiving treatment for Ewing sarcoma expressed a deep-seated desire to become pregnant during her cancer journey. She had preexisting mental health disorders, including borderline personality disorder and bipolar disorder, which made her more vulnerable to impulsive, risky behavior. Prior to the initiation of treatment, the patient was educated about the potential risk for infertility and was provided a listing of educational and supportive resources. The patient decided against cryopreservation due to conflict with religious beliefs. Throughout the course of treatment, the patient continued to manifest a strong desire to become pregnant and engaged in unsafe sexual practices. The medical team was proactive about regularly assessing the patient for unsafe sexual practices and provided her with education and information about the risks associated with such behavior including high-risk pregnancy, STIs/STDs, and increased risk of infection during periods when her neutrophil count was low from chemotherapy, as well as risk to the fetus related to chemotherapy. It became apparent that sexuality and fertility, specifically, were so highly connected to the patient's core fears about facing mortality. Getting diagnosed with a life-threatening illness during this particular stage of the patient's life, and facing mortality as a young adult, may have contributed to a desire to expedite life goals such as getting married and starting a family. The social worker addressed with the patient other life goals including returning to college and work and connected the patient to a psychologist and psychiatrist in the community to manage the ongoing mental health needs of the patient, which were magnified by the cancer. Shortly following completion of treatment, the patient's oncologist referred the patient to a gynecologist to address the patient's sexual health and reproductive capacity. About a year following completion of treatment, the patient became pregnant. Around this time, she also relapsed with cancer. The case highlights that safe sexual practices should be employed not only during the treatment phase but also during the period of time following treatment when the risk of relapse remains high.

Fertility

Having received information from clinicians about their cancer diagnosis and proposed treatment regimen, AYAs can experience great psychological urgency to start treatment (Keim-Malpass et al. 2013). For AYAs who will undergo therapies that can impair fertility, this urgency can be a barrier to consultation with a fertility specialist and fertility preservation. Other barriers to consultation and preservation include gatekeeping by clinicians and parents who underestimate the importance of fertility to AYAs or the risk of impaired fertility, not knowing what can be done to preserve fertility or feeling awkward addressing these sensitive issues.

When fertility is at risk, providers should discuss the risk and options for fertility preservation with the patient or parents as appropriate before treatment starts, answer questions about whether fertility preservation could adversely affect treatment outcomes, initiate referral to a reproductive specialist for those who are interested, document these discussions (Loren et al. 2013), and provide access to resources that can help address potential financial barriers to fertility preservation. An additional role for psychosocial experts is to help AYAs and their family members address distress related to risk for infertility (Loren et al. 2013).

Psychosocial providers play a critical role in fertility preservation. Effective psychosocial services for both sexes should include using a proactive approach to ensure that all AYA patients and, as applicable, their parents and partners receive information about the potential impact of cancer therapy on fertility through face-to-face discussion and educational materials (Crawshaw 2013). Clinicians' areas of expertise include, but are not limited to, the following: referrals to fertility specialists, counseling and guiding patients and families in the decision-making process in regard to fertility preservation, providing information and resources designed to help address potential financial barriers to fertility preservation, and fostering relationships within the community, specifically with fertility centers and long-term storage facilities of sperm, oocyte (egg), embryo, ovarian, and testicular tissue specimens.

Reliable sources of information about fertility preservation include LIVE*STRONG* (http://www.livestrong.org/we-can-help/fertility-services/), the Oncofertility Consortium, and National Comprehensive Cancer Network Guidelines for Patients: Caring for Adolescents and Young Adults. For health-care professionals, the following are recommended guidelines and resources: National Comprehensive Cancer Network Guidelines: Adolescent and Young Adult (AYA) Oncology, Fertility Preservation for Patients with Cancer: American Society of Clinical Oncology Guideline Update, and the Clinical Oncology Society of Australia (http://wiki.cancer.org.au/australia/COSA:AYA_cancer_fertility_preservation).

End of Life

AYAs living with a potentially life-limiting disease such as cancer have beliefs, values, and medical preferences about end-of-life care and wish to communicate this information with loved ones and health-care providers (Wiener et al. 2012). It is critical that health-care providers bring up the topic of end-of-life care preferences as early as is medically appropriate and continue this discussion through the course of treatment. Allowing AYAs the opportunity to engage in end-of-life care preferences can help to reestablish a sense of control and independence over their health care (Wiener et al. 2012). Moreover, guiding AYA patients as much as possible in a meaningful dialogue with their family members about advance care planning preferences can be beneficial to the overall psychosocial adjustment of a family coping with impending death (Lyon et al. 2013).

AYAs with advanced or terminal cancer have distinctive medical and psychosocial needs that are not adequately provided by either pediatric or adult palliative care services (Pritchard et al. 2011). A discussion group, as part of a larger workshop on AYAs with cancer, was held during 2010 in Toronto. Recommendations included the development of a specific AYA screening tool designed to detect increased anxiety or new symptoms and to initiate discussion about palliative or symptom care; set standards for palliative care in AYA patients and include in hospital accreditation; involve the palliative/symptom care team early in the disease trajectory to help manage clinically important symptoms that may not be associated with imminent death; establish specific AYA multidisciplinary palliative care teams that are flexible and can work in both pediatric and adult facilities, as well as a "virtual" environment to support AYAs being cared for at home; improve physical facilities in hospices and hospitals to meet the distinctive needs of AYAs who are terminally ill; and enhance support for palliative care at home by changing legislation to improve care benefits and developing "virtual, palliative care support teams" (Fernandez et al. 2011). Adequate provision of AYA palliative care and symptom management services will likely confer notable benefits to AYA and their families. The outcome of research exploring the written preferences for end of life is a tool, "Voicing My CHOiCES," which allows AYAs living with serious illnesses to plan their end-of-life care (Wiener et al. 2012). The tool, which is not a legally binding document, provides AYAs an opportunity to express and share their preferences for how they wish to be cared for as they approach the end of life and be remembered after their death. Guidance is provided on how to incorporate the tool into AYA care (Zadeh et al. 2015).

In addition to Voicing My CHOiCES, patients over the age of 18 years should also be encouraged to execute advance directives, which are legal documents that allow patients to elect a medical power of attorney and complete a living will. An advance directive aims to ensure that medical preferences and wishes be honored at end of life should a patient become unable to make decisions about their medical care. It is critical that end-of-life care preferences for clinical care, including pain management, spiritual support, and advanced directives, be documented in the electronic medical record.

Age-Appropriate Resources and Social Support

To minimize the disruption caused by the cancer experience and promote healthy development, young people with cancer need opportunities to participate in typical activities with peers as much as possible. To achieve this, the health-care environment must be flexible, for example, with scheduling treatments and clinical evaluations to minimize school and work disruptions, overnight visitation by romantic partners and friends during hospitalization, and use of technology to deliver cancer therapy, symptom management, and peer support in community settings.

Identifying and recognizing AYA strengths and support networks provides an important base to build upon and promote healthy growth and development. Taking this approach with young people can empower them to improve in areas in which they already feel confident and encourage them to tackle more difficult issues as their confidence builds. AYAs may need assistance in identifying their strengths, so explaining this concept and giving them examples can be helpful. Further, young people often have a support network of other people (including family members, friends, teachers, other services) in their lives. Encouraging AYAs to identify and seek assistance from supportive others is critical.

Quality of life in AYA patients has been shown to be largely a function of social support. Improving social support can be used as a strategy to mitigate the adverse influence of the cancer experience on body image, identity formation, emotions, coping skills, and occupational goals (Roberts et al. 1997). While parents are usually identified as a primary source of support, peers who have experienced cancer can also play important roles. Interventions that aim to enhance peer support can offer safety and encouragement not usually available to AYAs and promote their psychological adjustment.

Peer support provides AYA patients with opportunities to address mutual concerns and can also decrease feelings of social isolation, depression, and anxiety (Roberts et al. 1997). Participation in usual activities with friends and new cancer-related experiences can promote successful achievement of AYAs' developmental tasks. The positive effects of peer support and technology- and skill-based interventions, along with minimizing disruption to important social roles, cannot be underestimated, thereby helping AYAs overcome potential adverse effects of cancer on development by strengthening their internal and external coping resources (Zebrack and Isaacson 2012). Clinicians can enhance care to AYAs by being knowledgeable about, and referring AYA patients to, reputable organizations and online peer support programs. See Chap. 25 for specific resources.

Conclusion

Adolescent and young adult (AYA) patients often fall through a schism between pediatric oncology (mainly family focused and holistic) and adult oncology (mainly individual and disease focused) and, as a result of the disjuncture between these two worlds, bear the brunt of limited access to clinical trials and decreased quality of care (Ferrari et al. 2010). Neither the pediatric nor the adult models of care are ideally suited to the complex psychosocial needs of AYA patients. A comprehensive, multipronged effort is required to bridge the gap in the psychosocial care of AYA patients, to provide AYAs with the attention they require, and ultimately to eliminate the observed disparities in outcomes and supportive care services.

Clinical Pearls

- Adolescents and young adults with cancer face an intense, complex psychosocial experience that, if not properly addressed, can lead to diminished quality of life and potentially low survival outcomes. As such, psychosocial care is critical in the overall treatment plan in AYAs with cancer.
- The delivery of care and overall health-care environment for AYAs with cancer should honor the unique life stage of this patient population and promote opportunities for developmental milestones to be reached.
- Clinicians should aim to promote a sense of self-efficacy and control in AYAs and their families, which, in turn, may lead to a more positive engagement in cancer treatment.
- In order to effectively and appropriately engage AYA cancer patients in their health care, health-care providers need to be knowledgeable about adolescent and young adult development and normative behaviors. Moreover, providers should display comfort and an aptitude in communication about potentially uncomfortable topics such as sex and sexuality, fertility, substance use and abuse, and death and dying.

References

Bhatia S, Sklar C (2002) Second cancers in survivors of childhood cancer. Nat Rev Cancer 2(2):124–132

Bhatia S, Landier W, Shangguan M, Hageman L, Schaible A, Carter A et al (2012) Nonadherence to oral mercaptopurine and risk of relapse in Hispanic and non-Hispanic white children with acute lymphoblastic leukemia: a report from the Children's Oncology Group. J Clin Oncol 30:2094–2101

Bleyer A (2011) Latest estimates of survival rates of the 24 most common cancers in adolescent and young adult Americans. J Adolesc Young Adult Oncol 1(1):37–42. doi:10.1089/jayao.2010.0005

Bleyer A, O'Leary M, Barr R, Ries L (eds) (2006) Cancer epidemiology in older adolescents and young adults 15 to 29 years of age, including SEER incidence and survival: 1975–2000. National Cancer Institute, Bethesda, NIH Pub. no. 06–5767

Bolte S, Zebrack B (2008) Sexual issues in special populations: adolescents and young adults. Semin Oncol Nurs 24(2):115–119

Buchanan N, Block R, Smith A, Tai E (2014) Psychosocial barriers and facilitators to clinical trial enrollments and adherence for adolescents with cancer. Pediatrics 133:S123–S130

Butow P, Palmer S, Pai A, Goodenough B, Luckett T, King M (2010) Review of adherence-related issues in adolescents and young adults with cancer. J Clin Oncol 28(32):4800–4809. doi:10.1200/jco.2009.22.2802

Canada AL, Shover LR, Li Y (2006) A pilot intervention to enhance psychosexual development in adolescents and young adults with cancer. Pediatr Blood Cancer 49(6):824–828

CanTeen Australia (2011a) Adolescent and young adult oncology psychosocial care manual. CanTeen, Sydney

CanTeen Australia (2011b) Supporting adolescent and young adult siblings of cancer patients: the family context. Research to practice paper. CanTeen Australia, Sydney. https://www.canteen.org.au/health-professionals/research-and-evaluation/best-practice-projects/research-to-practice-paper-issue-1/. Accessed 28 July 2014

Centers for Disease Control and Prevention (2011) 2010 STD treatment guidelines, clinical prevention guidance, sexually transmitted diseases, treatment guidelines, 2010 retrieved 15 Jan 2015, from http://www.cdc.gov/std/treatment/2010/clinical.htm

Centers for Disease Control and Prevention (2012) Vital signs: binge drinking prevalence, frequency, and intensity among adults – United States, 2010. Morb Mortal Wkly Rep 61(1):14–19

Crawshaw M (2013) Psychosocial oncofertility issues faced by adolescents and young adults over their lifetime: a review of the research. Hum Fertil 16:59–63

Dayer L, Heldenbrand S, Anderson PJ, Gubbins P, Martin B (2013) Smartphone medication adherence apps: potential benefits to patients and providers. J Am Pharm Assoc 53:172–18

Ehrentraut J, Kern K, Long S, An A, Faughnan L, Anghelescu D (2013) Opioid misuse behaviors in adolescents and young adults in a hematology/oncology setting. J Pediatr Psychol 39:1149–1160

Engel G (1977) The need for a new medical model: a challenge for biomedicine. Science 196:129–136

Evan E, Zeltzer LK (2006) Psychosocial dimensions of cancer in adolescents and young adults. Cancer 107(7):1663–1671

Evan E, Kaufman M, Cook A, Zeltzer LK (2006) Sexual health and self-esteem in adolescents and young adults with cancer. Cancer 107(7 Suppl):1672–1679

Felner RD, DeVries ML (2013) Poverty in childhood and adolescence: a transactional-ecological approach to understanding and enhancing resilience in contexts of disadvantage and developmental risk. In: Goldstein S, Brooks RB (eds) Handbook of resilience in children. Springer, New York, pp 105–126

Fern LA, Whelan JS (2010) Recruitment of adolescents and young adults to cancer clinical trials – international comparisons, barriers, and implications. [Research Support, Non-U.S. Gov't]. Semin Oncol 37(2):e1–e8

Fernandez C, Fraser GAM, Freeman C, Grunfeld E, Gupta A, Mery LS, De Pauw S, Schacter B, Young Adults with Cancer, B (2011) Principles and recommendations for the provision of healthcare in Canada to adolescent and young adult–aged cancer patients and survivors. J Adolesc Young Adult Oncol 1(1):53–59

Ferrari A, Montello M, Budd T, Bleyer A (2008) The challenges of clinical trials for adolescents and young adults with cancer. [Review]. Pediatr Blood Cancer 50(5 Suppl):1101–1104

Ferrari A, Thomas D, Franklin ARK, Hayes-Lattin BM, Mascarin M, van der Graaf W, Albritton KH (2010) Starting an adolescent and young adult program: some success stories and some obstacles to overcome. J Clin Oncol 28(32):4850–4857. doi:10.1200/jco.2009.23.8097

Grinyer A (2003) Young adults with cancer: parent interactions with health care providers. Eur J Cancer 13:88–95

Grinyer A (2009) Contrasting parental perspectives with those of teenagers and young adults with cancer: comparing the findings from two qualitative studies. Eur J Oncol Nurs 13:200–206

Hedstrom M, Kreuger A, Ljungman G, Nygren P, von-Essen L (2006) Accuracy of assessment of distress, anxiety, and depression by physicians and nurses in adolescents recently diagnosed with cancer. Pediatr Blood Cancer 46:773–779

Hullman S, Brumley L, Schwartz L (2015) Medical and psychosocial associates of nonadherence in adolescents with cancer. J Pediatr Oncol Nurs 32:103–113

Institute for Patient- and Family-Centered Care (2010) Frequently asked questions: what is patient- and family-centered care? Retrieved 16 Dec 2014, from http://www.ipfcc.org/faq.html

Johnson RH, Chien FL, Bleyer A (2013) Incidence of breast cancer with distant involvement among women in the United States, 1976 to 2009. JAMA 309(8):800–805

Jones B (2008) Promoting healthy development among survivors of adolescent cancer. Fam Community Health Adv Adolesc Health 31(1):S61–S70

Kato PM, Cole SW, Bradlyn AS, Pollock BH (2008) A video game improves behavioral outcomes in adolescents and young adults with cancer: a randomized trial. [Multicenter Study. Randomized Controlled Trial. Research Support, N.I.H., Extramural. Research Support, Non-U.S. Gov't]. Pediatrics 122(2):e305–e317

Katz A (2005) The sounds of silence: sexuality information for cancer patients. J Clin Oncol 1:238–241

Keim-Malpass J, Baernholdt M, Erickson J, Ropka M, Schroen A, Steeves R (2013) Blogging through cancer: young women's persistent problems shared online. Cancer Nurs 36:163–172. doi:10.1097/NCC.0b013e31824eb879

Kelvin JF, Steed R, Jarrett J (2014) Discussing safe sexual practices during cancer treatment. Clin J Oncol Nurs 18(4):449–453

Kessler RC, Wang PS (2008) The descriptive epidemiology of commonly occurring mental disorders in the United States. Annu Rev Public Health 29:115–129

Kondryn HJ, Edmondson CL, Hill J, Eden TO (2011) Treatment non-adherence in teenage and young adult patients with cancer. Lancet Oncol 12:100–108

Lalor K, McElvaney R (2010) Child sexual abuse, links to later sexual exploitation/high-risk sexual behavior, and prevention/treatment programs. Trauma Violence Abuse 11(4):159–177

Lauer AL (2015) Treatment of anxiety and depression in adolescents and young adults with cancer. J Pediatr Oncol Nursing 1–6

Lehmann V, Grongvist H, Engvall G, Ander M, Tuinman M, Hagedoorn M, Sanderman R, Mattsson E, von Essen L (2014) Negative and positive consequences of adolescent cancer 10 years after diagnosis: an interview-based longitudinal study in Sweden. Psychooncology 23:1229–1235

Lizardi D, Thompson RG, Keyes K, Hasin D (2010) The role of depression in the differential effect of childhood parental divorce on male and female adult offspring suicide attempt risk. J Nerv Mental Dis 198(9):687–690

Loren A, Mangu P, Beck L, Brennan L, Magadalinski A, Partridge A, Quinn G, Wallace WH, Oktay K (2013) Fertility preservation for patients with cancer: American Society of Clinical Oncology clinical practice guideline update. J Clin Oncol 19:2500–2510

Lyon ME, Jacobs S, Briggs L et al (2013) Family-centered advance care planning for teens with cancer. JAMA Pediatr 167(5):460–467

Malbasa T, Kodish ED, Santacroce SJ (2007) Adolescent adherence to oral therapy for leukemia: a focus group study. J Pediatr Oncol Nurs 24:139–151

Maynard A, Patterson P, McDonald FEJ, Stevens G (2013) What is helpful to adolescents who have a parent diagnosed with cancer? J Psychosoc Oncol 31(6):675–697

McGrady ME, Williams SN, Davies SM, Pai AL (2014) Adherence to outpatient oral medication regimens in adolescent hematopoietic stem cell transplant recipients. Eur J Oncol Nurs 18(2):140–144

Miller V, Baker J, Leek A, Hizlan S, Rheingold S, Yamokoski A, Drotar D, Kodish ED (2013) Adolescent perspectives on phase I cancer research. Pediatr Blood Cancer 60:873–878

Murphy D, Klosky JL, Termuhlen A, Sawczyn KK, Quinn GP (2013) The need for reproductive and sexual health discussions with adolescent and young adult cancer patients. Contraception 88(2):215–220

National Cancer Institute (2015) A snapshot of adolescent and young adult cancers. Retrieved 17 Feb 2015, from http://www.cancer.gov/researchandfunding/snapshots/adolescent-young-adult

National Institute of Mental Health (2005) Mental illness exacts heavy toll, beginning in youth. Retrieved 15 Jan 2015, from http://www.nimh.nih.gov/news/science-news/2005/mental-illness-exacts-heavy-toll-beginning-in-youth.shtml

Palmer S, Mitchell A, Thompson K, Sexton M (2007) Unmet needs among adolescent cancer patients: a pilot study. Palliat Support Care 5(2):127–134

Palmer S, Patterson P, Thompson K (2014) A national approach to improving adolescent and young adult (AYA) oncology psychosocial care: the development of AYA-specific psychosocial assessment and care tools. Palliat Support Care 12(3):183–188

Patterson P, McDonald FEJ, Orchard P (2014) A new Australian online and phone mental health support service for young people living with cancer. [Article]. Australas Psychiatry 22(2):165–169. doi:10.1177/1039856213519144

Patton GC, Coffey C, Cappa C, Currie D, Riley L, Gore F, Degenhardt L, Richardson D, Astone N, Sangowawa AO, Mokdad A, Ferguson J (2012) Health of the world's adolescents: a synthesis of internationally comparable data. Lancet 379:1665–1675

Pereda N, Guilera G, Forns M, Gomez-Benito J (2009) The prevalence of child sexual abuse in community and student samples: a meta-analysis. Clin Psychol Rev 29:328–338

Pergolizzi J, Gharibo C, Passki S, Labhsetwar S, Taylor R, Pergolizzi J, Muller-Schwefe G (2012) Dynamic risk factors in the misuse of opioid analgesics. J Psychosom Res 72:443–451

Phillips F, Jones B (2014) Understanding the lived experience of Latino adolescent and young adult cancer survivors. J Cancer Surviv 8:39–48

Pritchard S, Cuvelier G, Harlos M, Barr R (2011) Palliative care in adolescents and young adults with cancer. Cancer 117(S10):2323–2328. doi:10.1002/cncr.26044

Roberts C, Piper L, Denny J, Cuddeback G (1997) A support group intervention to facilitate young adults' adjustment to cancer. Health Social Work 22(2):133–141

Rohan J, Drotar D, Alderfer M, Donewar C, Ewing L, Katz E, Muriel A (2015) Electronic monitoring of medication adherence in early maintenance phase treatment for pediatric leukemia and lymphoma: Identifying patters of non-adherence. J Pediatr Psychol 40:75–84

Rourke MT, Hobbie WL, Schwartz L, Kazak AE (2007) Posttraumatic stress disorder (PTSD) in young adult survivors of childhood cancer. Pediatr Blood Cancer 49(2):177–182

Santacroce SJ, Crandell J (2013) Feasibility and preliminary findings from a pilot study of allostatic load in adolescent-young adult (AYA) childhood cancer survivors and their siblings. J Pediatr Oncol Nurs 31:122–134

Trevino KM, Maciejewski PK, Fasciano K, Greer J, Partridge A, Kacel EL, Block S, Prigerson HG (2012) Coping and psychological distress in young adults with advanced cancer. J Support Oncol 10(3):124–130

Trevino KM, Fasciano K, Prigerson HG (2013) Patient-oncologist alliance, psychosocial well-being, and treatment adherence among young adults with advanced cancer. J Clin Oncol 31(13):1683–1689

United States Department of Health and Human Services (2013) Child maltreatment. National Institutes of Health: Bethesda, MD. 2012

Wakefield CE, Patterson P, McDonald FEJ, Wilson HL, Davis E, Sansom-Daly US (2013) Assessment of psychosocial outcomes in adolescents and young adults with cancer: a systematic review of available instruments. Clin Oncol Adolesc Young Adults 13:13–27

Wiener L, Zadeh S, Battles H, Baird K, Ballard E, Osherow J, Pao M (2012) Allowing adolescents and young adults to plan their end-of-life care. Pediatrics 130:1–9. doi:10.1542/peds.2012-0663

Williams AB (2001) Adherence to HIV regimens: 10 vital lessons. Am J Nursing 101:37–44

Zadeh S, Pao M, Wiener L (2015) Opening end-of-life discussions: how to introduce Voicing My CHOiCES, an advance care planning guide for adolescents and young adults. Palliat Support Care 13:591–599, Published online, 13 March, 2014

Zebrack BJ (2008) Information and service needs for young adult cancer patients. Support Care Cancer 16:1353–1360

Zebrack BJ (2011) Psychological, social, and behavioral issues for young adults with cancer. Cancer 117(S10):2289–2294. doi:10.1002/cncr.26056

Zebrack B, Isaacson S (2012) Psychosocial care of adolescent and young adult patients with cancer and survivors. J Clin Oncol 30(11):1221–1226. doi: 10.1200/jco.2011.39.5467

Pediatric Hematopoietic Stem Cell Transplantation: Psychosocial Assessment and Care

13

Kristin Bingen and Jennifer A. Hoag

Introduction to Hematopoietic Stem Cell Transplant

There are an ever growing number of successful hematopoietic stem cell transplants (HSCT) being conducted on an increasingly wide range of oncologic, hematologic, and immunologic conditions (Cairo and Heslop 2008). Despite the progress being made in curing life-threatening diseases, HSCT is still considered a high-risk procedure because of the treatment-related morbidity and mortality. There are two types of transplants, which is based on whether the patient receives her own hematopoietic stem or progenitor cells (autologous) or cells from a donor (allogeneic). Allogeneic cells are donated by another person (e.g., sibling, parent, or unrelated donor from the National Bone Marrow Registry) and attained from their bone marrow, peripheral blood, or umbilical cord.

Clinical indications for HSCT include malignancies, particularly in the case of cancer relapses or recurrences [e.g., relapsed acute lymphoblastic leukemia (ALL) or acute myeloid leukemia (AML)] as well as non-malignancies (e.g., immune deficiency disorders, bone marrow failure, severe aplastic anemia). Oncology patients who are referred for an HSCT likely have already experienced a lengthy illness and treatment course, which consisted of chemotherapy and other treatment-related side effects and hospitalizations, as is often the case with relapsed ALL and AML patients. This is in stark contrast to patients with non-malignancies referred to HSCT, such as aplastic anemia, who may not have had previous treatment experiences or hospitalizations or may present as asymptomatic prior to HSCT. Therefore, in these latter cases, the patient and family may be less well prepared or less likely to know what to expect.

Upon transplant hospitalization, the treatment includes several sequential phases beginning with the conditioning phase, followed by infusion and the engraftment process, which combined make up the acute phases of transplant hospitalization (approximately 4–6 weeks in total). The conditioning phase typically lasts 7–10 days and consists of myeloablative chemotherapy and, in some cases, is coupled with total body irradiation. The purpose of this phase is to destroy any remaining malignant cells, suppress the immune system to prevent rejection, and create marrow space. Nausea, vomiting, pain, and fatigue are common side effects that begin during this phase and continue throughout the admission. Patients also become blood and platelet transfusion dependent. Maintaining good

K. Bingen, PhD (✉) • J.A. Hoag, PhD
Division of Hematology/Oncology/Blood and Marrow Transplant, Department of Pediatrics, Medical College of Wisconsin, 8701 Watertown Plank Road, Milwaukee, WI 53226, USA
e-mail: kbingen@mcw.edu; jhoag@mcw.edu

A.N. Abrams et al. (eds.), *Pediatric Psychosocial Oncology: Textbook for Multidisciplinary Care*, DOI 10.1007/978-3-319-21374-3_13

nutrition is a common struggle and may require total parenteral nutrition. More recently, reduced intensity conditioning regimen transplants or "mini transplants" with lower doses of chemotherapy and radiation have been provided to more vulnerable patients who are not healthy enough to receive a myeloablative regimen prior to HSCT, in an effort to reduce toxicities that lead to morbidity and mortality.

The next phase is the bone marrow or stem cell infusion, which is infused through a central venous line over a period of 20–60 minutes, the process of which is similar to a blood transfusion. A primary potential side effect that can occur during the infusion is an anaphylactic reaction, thus requiring patients to be closely monitored during the infusion. A 2–4-week "waiting period" follows the infusion, during which the patient has no effective immune system and is very susceptible to infection. Additional symptoms during this phase include mucositis and fevers, with the primary treatment focus being symptom management. As the patient begins to demonstrate signs of engraftment (which is when the new immune system begins to grow and create new blood cells), mucositis begins to heal and infections resolve; however, for those that receive an allogeneic transplant, acute graft-versus-host disease (GVHD) can occur. GVHD occurs when the donor cells see the host cells as foreign and attack them. Skin, gut, liver, and lungs can be impacted and graded from mild to severe, with severe GVHD causing life-threatening symptoms. Chronic GVHD is defined as symptoms that last for or begin at least 100 days after transplant. GVHD is typically treated with steroids, which have a number of physical and emotional side effects. GVHD symptoms have a negative impact on the patient's health-related quality of life (HRQL), particularly in the physical and social domains (Clarke et al. 2008; Tanzi 2011). Patients with moderate to severe GVHD often require hospitalization for treatment to control their symptoms and manage their pain. Patients with GVHD often are socially isolated due to pain, debilitating diarrhea, risk for infection, and physical appearance changes related to steroid side effects (e.g., significant weight gain and swelling in the face, stomach, and limbs) and skin GVHD (severe itchiness, skin flaking, and severe body rashes).

Following discharge from transplant hospitalization, patients experience a lengthy recovery with an intensive outpatient regimen that can last from months to years. During this time, patients often receive intravenous (IV) hydration; take many medications which need to be frequently monitored and adjusted, including immunosuppressive medications; have dietary and activity restrictions and recommendations; and are socially isolated due to continued infection risk with a young immune system. Motivating good nutrition and adequate fluid intake as well as treatment adherence become primary focuses of intervention during recovery. Social isolation may last for 6 or more months post-HSCT depending upon the patient's transplant-related complications and immunosuppressed state. This isolation can be a primary stressor as patients struggle to cope with not being able to attend school or socialize with their friends in public areas despite feeling well.

Pre-HSCT Psychological Evaluation

Once a patient is recommended to receive a transplant by the HSCT team, HSCT candidates receive a comprehensive medical evaluation or "workup." Potential HSCT candidates receive a physical examination, blood tests, a bone marrow biopsy, as well as a number of tests to assess organ functioning to determine the patient's overall health status and appropriateness to undergo an HSCT. In addition to the medical workup, most pediatric HSCT centers require a psychosocial assessment prior to a patient receiving an HSCT, and, in fact, many health insurance companies will not approve coverage for an HSCT without one. A psychosocial provider (Sherman et al. 2004), with expertise in the psychosocial issues associated with pediatric HSCT, typically conducts pre-HSCT psychological evaluations. The purpose of these evaluations is not meant to make a determination as to whether a patient should have an HSCT or not but instead should serve to assess the patient and family's psychosocial functioning, stress and coping, HSCT knowledge and preparedness, and supportive care needs in order to best prepare and support the patient and family prior to, during, and after an HSCT. Taking a sensitive, supportive approach when conducting a pre-HSCT psychological evaluation can also serve to establish a therapeutic relationship with the patient and family, thereby making it more likely for the psychosocial provider to be successful in addressing any problems or crises that may arise during the transplant and recovery. Recommendations based upon results of the evaluation should be shared in written and/or verbal format with the HSCT team prior to the HSCT admission in order for the multidisciplinary team to (1) provide more education when there is a lack of or misunderstanding of the HSCT, (2) address any potential psychosocial or economic concerns or barriers raised prior to the HSCT that may negatively impact the success of the HSCT, and/or (3) ensure that appropriate supportive care services are in place for the patient and family prior to or at HSCT admission.

Optimal timing of the pre-HSCT psychological evaluation occurs after the patient and family meet with the HSCT oncologist for education but prior to the patient or parents formally consenting and assenting, when appropriate, to HSCT. The purpose of the psychological evaluation should be discussed with the parents and patient. Whenever possible, it is important for the psychosocial provider to meet with the patient and parents separately, particularly when the HSCT candidate is an adolescent, so each has the opportunity to freely share personal thoughts, feelings, and concerns.

There are a number of salient domains to assess during the pre-HSCT psychological evaluation, which are discussed below and summarized in Table 13.1, along with examples of quantitative measures that may be used to supplement semi-structured interview questions. In a survey of pediatric HSCT centers registered in the Pediatric Blood and Marrow Transplantation Consortium, psychosocial screening was typically assessed via interview with infrequent use of quantitative measures (Sherman et al. 2004). Sherman et al. (2004) recommend taking a qualitative and quantitative assessment approach. Development of validated measures specific to pediatric HSCT is needed.

Knowledge of HSCT and Ability to Consent or Assent

A primary focus of the assessment should be to ascertain the level of understanding patients and parents have about the HSCT and recovery process. Any questions, concerns, or gaps in knowledge, including misperceptions, should be addressed with further education provided by the HSCT team so that the patient and parents can provide informed consent and, when appropriate, assent to the HSCT (see Table 13.2 for educational tools and resources). In addition, having a developmentally appropriate understanding of the HSCT process better prepares children, adolescents, and young adults for the HSCT, which may help them cope or reduce anticipatory anxiety leading up to the transplant. For the patient, the extent of HSCT knowledge is dependent upon age or developmental level, and therefore, questions assessing the level of comprehension should be tailored accordingly. For example, younger to school-aged children want to be informed about how a treatment will make them feel in the present or immediate future, how the doctors and nurses will help them to feel better when ill, and who will take care of or be with them in the hospital. Therefore, for younger children, it is expected that they may understand the very basics of HSCT, such that they will be in the hospital for a long time, may feel sick at times, but will get medicine to help them feel better. In contrast, adolescents are typically able to cognitively understand the complexity and intensity of the HSCT process at a level similar to their parents and thus should be able to provide a more detailed description of the HSCT process.

When inquiring about the HSCT procedure, the psychosocial provider should gain a sense of whether the patient and parents understand the different phases of the transplant, including a

Table 13.1 Summary of patient and family assessment domains and measurement examples for pre-HSCT psychological evaluation

Assessment domain	Salient assessment factors	Examples of interview questions	Examples of measures tailored to individual patient needs
HSCT knowledge (informed consent/assent)	HSCT procedure Benefits vs risks Decision making/voluntariness Alternative treatment options Patient and parental HSCT responsibilities Length of hospitalization Recovery process	What is your understanding of what happens during transplant? What happens when you are first hospitalized (conditioning regimen); what happens next (HSCT infusion, engraftment)? How did you come to the decision of having a transplant? Who decided? What are some of the risks or potential side effects of transplant? Did the doctor tell you about any other treatment options besides transplant? What do you anticipate the experience will be for you during your hospitalization for your transplant? Tell me what you know about the recovery process after you are discharged from the hospital after transplant.	Open-ended interview questions
Psychosocial functioning	Current psychosocial distress (depression, anxiety, behavioral problems) HRQL Helpful vs unhelpful coping strategies Previous mental health history	Tell me about how you have been feeling emotionally. How have you been coping with your illness and treatment? Do you have any specific fears associated with medical procedures? What are you most concerned or worried about with HSCT? Have you ever seen a counselor or therapist for any reason? Have you ever been prescribed medications for your mental health?	*Internalizing and externalizing problems*: Achenbach System of Empirically Based Assessment (ASEBA; Achenbach and Rescorla 2001) Behavior Assessment System for Children – Second Edition (BASC-2; Reynolds and Kamphaus 2004) *HRQL*: Behavioral Affective and Somatic Experiences Scale (BASES; Phipps et al. 1994, 1999) Child Health Ratings Inventories (CHRIs Generic & HSCT module; Parsons et al. 2005) PedsQL™ (Varni et al. 2001) Functional Assessment of Cancer Therapy Quality of Life Measurement System (FACT-BMT; Cella et al. 1993) *Coping strategies*: Kidcope (children and adolescents; Spirito et al. 1988) Coping Strategies Inventory (Tobin et al. 1984) Ways of Coping (young adults; Folkman and Lazarus 1988)

Assessment domain	Salient assessment factors	Examples of interview questions	Examples of measures tailored to individual patient needs
Medical adherence	Past and current problems following the medical regimen Missed or errors in medication Pill-swallowing problems History of missed appointments	How difficult has it been to follow what the doctors and nurses tell you to do? Tell me how you do with swallowing pills. Do you ever have difficulty remembering when to take your medicine or which medicines to take?	BASES Compliance Scale (Phipps et al. 1994, 1999)
Social support and stressors	Quantity and quality of support Identification of primary support persons Types of support received Other stressors or barriers to HSCT (economic stressors)	Who supports you the most through treatment? Tell me how you would rate the level or quality of the support you receive. Tell me about other stressful situations in your life.	Multidimensional Scale of Perceived Social Support (Zimet et al. 1988) Life Event Scale (Adapted from the Social Readjustment Rating Scale; Holmes and Rabe 1967)
Family functioning and parental adjustment	Family structure Family expression of feelings with each other Family communication Family conflict/cohesion Past and current parental stress, coping, and psychological functioning Family mental health history Family role changes Parental employment issues	Who lives at home with you? How do you get along with your parent(s) and sibling(s)? How has your family life changed since being diagnosed? Who do you talk to in your family when you are stressed? For parent: Tell me how you are coping with your child's health and treatment. For young adult patient or parent: Is your employer or work environment supportive?	Family Environment Scale – 3rd Edition (Moos and Moos 1994) Impact on Family Scale (Stein and Riessman 1980) PAT2.0 (Pai et al. 2008) CHRIs – parent version (parent report of own health and child's health; Parsons et al. 2005) Coping Health Inventory for Parents (McCubbin et al. 1983) Sibling Relationship Questionnaire (Furman and Buhrmester 1985) Pediatric Parenting Stress Inventory (Devine et al. 2014)
Cognitive, academic, and vocational functioning	Past or current learning or cognitive problems School or vocational performance Educational or vocational services	Do you/your child or have you/your child ever received extra help in school? Do you/your child have an Individualized Education Plan or 504 Plan? What classes are you/your child really good at? What classes do you/your child have difficulty in?	Objective, standardized cognitive, and academic tests (see narrative section) Wechsler Scales of Intelligence (Wechsler 2004) or WASI-II (Wechsler 2011) Wide Range Achievement Test 4, Reading and Arithmetic Composites (academic screen; WRAT4; Wilkinson and Robertson 2006) COG ALTE07C1 abbreviated cognitive testing battery (Embry et al. 2012)

Table 13.2 Informational and supportive resources for pediatric HSCT

Support and resource programs	*Program description*	*Website address*
American Cancer Society	Provides information about pediatric and adult HSCT.	cancer.org
Blood & Marrow Transplant Clinical Trials Network	A multi-institutional clinical trials network for HSCT that offers clinical trial participation to HSCT patients in the United States.	https://web.emmes.com/study/bmt2/
Blood & Marrow Transplant Information Network	A support and informational resource for HSCT patients, survivors, and caregivers.	bmtinfonet.org
Imerman Angels	International program that provides patient to survivor and caregiver to caregiver connections for support.	imermanangels.org
Insights e-Community	Online social networking or discussion group to connect with other adolescents and young adults who are facing or have undergone an HSCT.	bethematch.org
National Bone Marrow Transplant Link	An information and resource program for patients who receive an HSCT and their families.	nbmtlink.org
National Cancer Institute	Provides information regarding pediatric HSCT using physician data queries (PDQ) or fact sheets about HSCT.	cancer.gov/cancertopics/pdq or cancer.gov/cancertopics/facts
National Marrow Donor Program; Be the Match	This program recruits potential bone marrow donors, maintains a registry of potential bone marrow donors, and facilitates the donor search and matching for a potential HSCT recipient. Be the Match is operated by the National Marrow Donor Program, which conducts research to improve HSCT outcomes and provides support and informational resources for patients and families.	bethematch.org
Pediatric Blood and Marrow Transplant Consortium	An international clinical trial group specifically focused on improving outcomes in pediatric HSCT through research and education	pbmtc.org
Educational resources	*Format*	*Available at*
Bone Marrow & Blood Stem Cell Transplants: A Guide for Patients (2012) by Susan K. Stewart	Book; Also available in Spanish.	bmtinfonet.org
Autologous Stem Cell Transplants: A Handbook for Patients (2012) by Susan K. Stewart	Book	bmtinfonet.org
Super Sam versus the Marrow Monsters	Animated DVD for children and their families. Also available in Spanish.	bethematch.org
Insights: Experiencing Transplant as a Young Adult	DVD for adolescents and young adults to learn about HSCT based upon other HSCT survivors' personal experiences.	bethematch.org
Me and My Marrow: A Kid's Guide to Bone Marrow Transplants (1999) by Karen Crowe	Children's book	www.us.astellas.com

general overview of the conditioning or preparative regimen (i.e., chemotherapy and total body irradiation versus chemotherapy only; number of days for conditioning), what occurs during the stem cell or bone marrow infusion (i.e., similar to an intravenous blood transfusion), and what happens after the infusion (i.e., waiting for engraftment, monitoring and treatment of infections or toxicities). Patients and parents typically describe the benefit of transplant to be a cure for their disease, whereas potential risks and side effects of HSCT are commonly discussed as death, symptoms such as nausea, pain, and/or fatigue, GVHD, infection, rejection or loss of graft, and/or long-term sequelae of treatment. Encouraging the patient and parents to discuss the process of arriving at the decision to choose an HSCT provides insight into the informed consent or assent process for the patient and family, such as whether the patient participated in the decision-making process, whether it was a mutual decision between the patient and parents, and what information or factors led them to the decision to proceed with HSCT. Patients and parents should understand any potential alternative options (e.g., palliative care) and therapies (e.g., chemotherapy only protocol) with associated benefits and risks of each option compared to HSCT. Patients and their parents should have awareness that they will be hospitalized for about 1 month and potentially longer based upon the patient's medical needs. To promote adherence, it is important for the patient and parents to understand what the oncologist expects of them during the HSCT hospitalization and recovery, such as taking multiple medications several times per day, bathing, mouth rinses, physical activity or therapy, and compliance with vitals. Finally, patients and parents should have an understanding of the length of the recovery process, number of outpatient clinic appointments per week and what those appointments will entail, and isolation expectations and duration. Semi-structured, open-ended patient interview questions (with parallel parent questions) aimed at assessing comprehension of each of these domains may best capture the depth of understanding (see Table 13.1 for sample interview questions).

Psychosocial Functioning of the HSCT Candidate

HSCT is an intensive treatment that is both physically and emotionally demanding. Not only do HSCT patients have to cope with painful procedures, treatment-related side effects such as nausea and vomiting, diarrhea and/or constipation, pain, fatigue, infertility, and worries about their health and survival, they also are isolated from school and friends and separated from family members during a lengthy hospitalization and recovery during which they are immunocompromised, all of which negatively impact their quality of life across physical, emotional, and social domains. Pediatric HSCT patients often experience increased distress and anxiety and lower health-related quality of life (HRQL) prior to their HSCT admission which extends through the acute phase of transplant and then begins to steadily improve 4–12 months post-HSCT before returning to baseline functioning by 1–3 years post-HSCT (Clarke et al. 2008; Packman et al. 2010; Tanzi 2011). Declines in social competence and self-esteem are also noted from pre- to 6 months post-HSCT (Phipps 2006). Risk factors for lower HRQL and negative psychosocial outcomes in HSCT recipients include older age at transplant, lower socioeconomic status, allogeneic (unrelated donor) transplant, presence of acute or chronic GVHD, pre-HSCT parental distress or maternal depressive symptoms, and pre-HSCT child distress or poor psychological functioning (Clarke et al. 2008; Packman et al. 2010; Tanzi 2011).

Given the multitude of HSCT stressors the pediatric recipient faces, it is important to assess the patient's current and past psychological functioning, stress, and coping prior to HSCT, but also intermittently about once per week (depending upon needs) during the acute and recovery phases of transplant. HSCT recipients should be screened for internalizing (i.e., depression, anxiety) and externalizing (i.e., oppositionality, inattention, hyperactivity) symptoms, which may impact coping with HSCT. Information also should be obtained regarding the patient's history of procedural distress, pain, and/or mood and behavioral side effects secondary to steroid treatment. An assessment of the patient's current HRQL also will help the psychosocial provider ascertain the severity of the impact that the patient's disease and previous treatment history has had in physical/functional, emotional, social, and practical domains. Screening may include both open-ended interview questions and quantitative questionnaires or checklists completed by the patient (when age appropriate) and parent, particularly for younger children (see Table 13.1 for examples of measures). There are a few validated measures that have been developed for pediatric patients who undergo an HSCT, primarily to evaluate HRQL in the HSCT setting [i.e., Behavioral, Affective, and Somatic Experiences Scale (BASES), Child Health Rating Inventories – HSCT module (CHRIs-HSCT), Functional Assessment of Cancer Therapy – BMT (FACT-BMT)]. A review of the patient's preexisting mental health conditions, past or current participation in counseling services, past or current psychiatric medications or hospitalizations, and family psychiatric history should be conducted. For adolescent and young adults, it is additionally important to screen for past and current cigarette smoking, tobacco use, alcohol/illicit drug use, sexual activity, and suicidality or self-injurious behaviors (see Chapter 4 on Assessment).

Coping Strategies

There is a dearth of information related to the use of effective coping strategies in pediatric HSCT. HSCT recipients report using multiple strategies to cope with HSCT-related stressors. It is important to inquire what strategies patients have used to help them cope with illness-related stress, including prior hospitalizations, which can be promoted during transplant. Coping strategies may be cognitive, behavioral, social, or spiritual. Common coping strategies reported in clinical practice include distraction, engaging in hospital-based activities, reading, watching TV or movies, staying connected to or being with friends and family, online social networking, talking to others, and relying on faith and prayer (see Chapters 5 and 6 on Coping and Psychotherapeutic Modalities, respectively). Patients should be encouraged to discuss what activities they will be engaging in their hospital rooms on a daily basis and what items they will be bringing with them during the HSCT hospitalization to keep them busy. Similarly, it is important to inquire about any previous experiences with hospitalizations. This will help the psychosocial provider ascertain whether the patient and family have firsthand knowledge of what to expect with lengthy hospitalizations and chemotherapy side effects.

Medical Adherence

HSCT patients and their parent(s) face a challenging, complicated outpatient medication regimen once they are discharged from the HSCT hospitalization. Evaluation of medical adherence is one of the most essential domains to assess prior to an HSCT because it has the potential to directly impact treatment-related complications and HSCT outcomes. Because of the complicated daily medication regimen and lengthy recovery process, problems with medical adherence are not uncommon. A recent study found that adolescents who have undergone HSCT have difficulty adhering to the outpatient medication regimen (McGrady et al. 2014). Psychosocial providers should inquire about any past or current problems with pill swallowing, following the medical care regimen, listening to or complying with the instructions by the HSCT team, or missed clinic appointments. Communication with the referring medical provider may also be a helpful source of information to identify any adherence concerns. Any factors that may have contributed to adherence problems should be identified and intervened upon as soon as possible.

Case Vignette

Kyle, a 16 year old with relapsed acute lymphoblastic leukemia (ALL), presented for a pre-HSCT psychological evaluation. During the evaluation, he disclosed having a complicated social and mental health history, including behavioral problems and placement in a foster care group home. Kyle was denied an HSCT at another hospital due to concerns about his mental health history. Adherence had not been reported as a problem. Utilizing a multidisciplinary team care approach, the patient was able to successfully receive an HSCT by proactively addressing his psychosocial and caregiving needs. Successful intervention approaches utilized with this patient included (1) establishing a team of consistent caregivers with whom he could develop positive, trusting relationships; (2) creating a daily schedule with age-appropriate activities; (3) providing clear, firm behavioral guidelines and expectations with rewards and consequences (i.e., privileges); and (4) participating in individual supportive psychotherapy, with goals of establishing a therapeutic relationship, utilizing cognitive-behavioral strategies to promote goal setting and positive behavioral choices as well as teaching anger and stress management techniques. Once discharged from the hospital after his HSCT, Kyle recovered for a period of time at an inpatient rehabilitation hospital.

Social Support and Stressors

Positive social support is a key factor in patients' coping with the stresses of HSCT (Bingen et al. 2012). Psychosocial providers should assess the level and quality of the support perceived by the patient and family and who is providing the most practical and emotional support to them. Support may be provided by a combination of family members, friends, school personnel, employer or coworkers, church or spiritual community, and/or neighborhood or surrounding community. Patients and families with limited support would benefit the most from consistent multidisciplinary supportive care services. Any stressors or barriers related to HSCT as well as non-HSCT stressors should be identified in order to potentially address or reduce these concerns prior to transplant whenever possible. For example, patients and their families often report financial strain related to previous medical treatment, potential loss of employment to care for the ill child, or health insurance problems, particularly for young adult patients who may be underinsured.

Family Functioning

Evaluation of family functioning should include obtaining information about the family constellation/structure, cohesiveness, conflict, and expressiveness as well as parental adjustment, parent-child relationships, and sibling relationships. In addition, the psychosocial provider should ascertain whether there have been any family role changes and disruptions in the family's daily life due to the patient's illness and treatment. For families who live a distance from the transplant center, it will be important to assess where they will be residing (e.g., Ronald McDonald House) and who will be taking care of the patient's siblings, when applicable. A qualitative assessment of pre-HSCT parental stress and coping and premorbid parental mental health history is crucial based upon previous research indicating that premorbid parental psychological functioning during the acute phase of transplant is a strong predictive factor in long-term parental adjustment after HSCT (Vrijmoet-Wiersma et al. 2009). Only parental and family history that is relevant to the child's HSCT should be sensitively documented in the child's medical records. Equally as important, both family and parental functioning prior to HSCT are predictive of child adjustment and HRQL after HSCT (Clarke et al. 2008; Packman et al. 2010; Tanzi 2011).

Cognitive, Academic, or Vocational Functioning

A comprehensive educational and cognitive assessment prior to HSCT can serve many purposes including determining the child's understanding of the HSCT, school needs during and after the HSCT, and reintegration after the

HSCT. As part of the pre-HSCT psychological evaluation and when insurance coverage permits, pediatric psychologists or neuropsychologists may also conduct cognitive and/or academic testing to directly evaluate HSCT candidates' functioning prior to HSCT, which can later serve as a comparison for future testing after HSCT to determine if there have been any cognitive changes over time. Due to HSCT workup time constraints as well as the patient's health at presentation, a comprehensive psychological or cognitive testing battery which would assess all domains that may be impacted by treatment may not be feasible. Because of this, an abbreviated testing battery is recommended to serve as a neurocognitive screen of the patient's current abilities (see Chapter 10 on Neurocognitive Issues).

Previous research has established that neurotoxic chemotherapy and radiation (particularly cranial radiation) can negatively impact cognitive functioning years after treatment, known as "cognitive late effects" (for review, see Mulhern and Butler 2006). However, due to methodological challenges such as small sample sizes from single transplant centers, it remains unclear as to whether the treatment regimen (myeloablative chemotherapy, total body irradiation, corticosteroid treatment for GVHD) for HSCT is a sole risk factor for development of cognitive late effects or an additive risk factor for patients who received chemotherapy (and is some cases radiation therapy) prior to HSCT,such as in the case of patients with ALL. In a review of longitudinal studies, Phipps (2006) concluded that there is low risk for development of cognitive or academic problems for children who receive an HSCT at or above the age of 6 years, but this risk may be increased for children who receive an HSCT when they are younger than 5 years old and, in particular, 3 years old or younger.

Research indicates that parental and child distress, HRQL, and adjustment fluctuate over the course of transplant and recovery (Clarke et al. 2008; Packman et al. 2010; Tanzi 2011; Vrijmoet-Wiersma et al. 2009) and therefore should be evaluated pre-, during, and post-HSCT. As a result, weekly assessments are recommended, even if only for a brief "check-in," during the acute and recovery phases of transplant, which can gradually become less frequent over time based upon supportive care needs and frequency of clinic appointments.

Clinical Interventions for Commonly Reported Psychosocial Issues in Pediatric HSCT

Procedural Anxiety and Pain

Children undergoing an HSCT frequently experience invasive and/or painful procedures, such as nasogastric (NG) tube placement, peripherally inserted central catheter (PICC) or central venous line dressing changes, and apheresis collection of stem cells. Managing pain and reducing procedural distress become important priorities for clinicians that provide supportive care. The following is a brief review of clinical interventions for pain and procedural anxiety; see Chapters 6 and 7 for a more comprehensive review.

Cognitive-behavioral interventions, including deep breathing and relaxation, distraction, psychoeducation, behavioral rehearsal, modeling, and imagery, have all been demonstrated to be efficacious in managing pain and anxiety during procedures (Kuppenheimer and Brown 2002; Packman et al. 2010). For more painful procedures, a combination of pharmacologic and psychological interventions may be needed to effectively reduce distress (Kazak et al. 1998).

Behavioral Concerns

Care plans are used during HSCT admissions to manage nonadherence (e.g., refusing to take medications), motivate cooperation (e.g., participating in physical therapy), and set the tone for expectations coming into a lengthy hospitalization. Ideally, care plans are created with the cooperation and input of all pertinent parties, including medical and nursing staff, psychosocial providers, parents, and patients. The care plan should be individualized for each patient's particular needs with developmental age and cultural considerations in mind. The care plan is meant to be a more comprehensive document than a reward program or behavioral management plan alone (although these may be included in a care plan). It also may include an overview of tasks that must be completed daily by the patient, formalize the role of daily structure or schedule from wake to bedtime, and set expectations for parental involvement. Care plans should be shared with families and documented in the medical record and a copy placed in the patient's room.

Case Vignette
Suzy, a 6-year-old girl with relapsed ALL, had numerous admissions for chemotherapy prior to proceeding with HSCT. During these admissions, Suzy often refused to take her medications. When urged to comply, Suzy would hit and kick staff. Although Suzy's parents were supportive of staff efforts to garner compliance, they would also get angry with staff when Suzy was upset. In anticipation of her HSCT, Suzy's transplant psychologist in conjunction with her parents created a sample care plan to help set appropriate expectations for her transplant (see Box 13.1).

Behavioral management plans to address specific behaviors may be part of the larger care plan. These plans follow the principles of behavioral modification and include specific expectations, along with rewards for successful completion of tasks. In the case of Suzy, a "behavior bucks" program was implemented whereby she earned a "behavior buck" each time she completed an assigned medical task (e.g., taking medication within 15 min). She was able to "go shopping" with her earned behavior bucks for small prizes (similar to prizes found in the treasure box at a doctor or dentist office) and privileges that were selected and priced for the plan. Behavior bucks were withheld and privileges withdrawn for nonadherent behavior.

The success of behavioral care plans during transplant hinges on the consistency with which they are followed among care providers over time. Before beginning any plan, there should be discussion about who will implement the plan (i.e., parents and/or hospital staff). If hospital staff will carry out the plan, communicating the plan and training the many staff that may be impacted is of the utmost importance.

Coping with Lengthy Hospitalization and Isolation

The stringency of isolation restrictions during HSCT admission varies by institution. Nevertheless, at a minimum, children undergo a lengthy, physically and emotionally demanding treatment during which time they are unable to attend school or participate in typical social activities. Cognitive-behavioral and supportive therapies may be utilized in reducing sadness and anxiety during the acute phase of hospitalization. Systematic research is needed before these therapies should be applied as standard of care.

Anecdotally, consistent care provided by a small team of primary nurses increases patient and family comfort and willingness to seek support and/or ask questions. Nurses that are more familiar with the psychosocial issues of a specific patient are better able to tailor their support efforts and provide increased consistency in implementing care plans. Daily schedules can be used effectively to increase predictability and establish routines during hospitalization.

Depending on transplant unit policies, visitation from family and friends can provide much needed support to the patient during long-term hospitalization. Some patients may benefit from connecting with transplant survivors, which can be facilitated by the psychosocial provider with both parties permission or through a national program, such as Imerman Angels (see Table 13.2).

The role of technology during HSCT is an understudied area. Texting, social media websites, video-sharing websites, and video chatting all offer ways for patients to receive encouragement and psychological support, socialize, seek information, and entertain themselves in ways that did not exist for patients a decade ago (see Chapter 19). Future research related to the uses and gratifications of technology is warranted.

Pill Swallowing

Throughout the HSCT admission, children are required to take medications orally. As the date of discharge nears, medications that were previously given intravenously are transferred to oral form. Most medications can be given in liquid form, but children complain of bad taste and large volume. Therefore, emphasis is placed on being able to swallow pills. This can be quite anxiety provoking for some children and lead to crying spells or avoidance in anticipation of having to take medication. If possible, pill swallowing should be taught well before the date of discharge as the pressure to learn a new skill under time constraints can increase distress and frustration.

The standard approach to teach pill swallowing is to use systematic desensitization utilizing placebo pills of various sizes. Candies, such as Tic Tacs and Mini M&Ms, are frequently used to mimic the different shapes and sizes of oral medications. Candies that are very light are not recommended as they have a tendency to float around the mouth rather than be swallowed. The clinician should begin by providing a brief explanation of the basic anatomy of the esophagus, including the ability to stretch around large amounts of food. Then, children should be taught to place the placebo pill on the back of their tongue. A sip of preferred liquid (i.e., water or milk; soda is discouraged as the carbonation can cause stomach upset that children can attribute to the pill) precedes swallowing the placebo. After several successes, children are gradually moved up to larger sized placebos until they are able to swallow candies that will resemble the size and shape of home medications.

There are times when the standard approach to pill swallowing proves ineffective. Pill swallowing aids, such as Pill Glide (a lubricated flavored spray) and pill cups that allow children to swallow water and a pill simultaneously, have been used with mixed results (Diamond and Lavallee 2010). Kaplan et al. (2010) demonstrated success utilizing a novel approach focused on head placement (see a training video at www.ucalgary.ca/research4kids/pillswallowing). Regardless of approach utilized, it is imperative to educate parents about the importance of keeping the environment calm during practice sessions and to handle failures with as much neutrality as possible.

Preparing for Discharge

Discharge discussions begin once children have demonstrated engraftment, are able to take oral medications, and are infection-free. Discharge is a time of ambivalence for parents and patients alike. On the one hand, families are excited to leave the hospital following a lengthy admission; on the other hand, they can be overwhelmed by the complex medical needs that they now must manage with more limited hospital support. Most institutions require parents to participate in a variety of teaching topics and demonstrate proficiency before they are able to be discharged. Having parents complete all medical care over a 24-hour period during the final days of hospitalization can increase competency and confidence. Nevertheless, parents continue to report high levels of stress as they prepare to take over their child's care. Normalization of their feelings and reassurance that they can reach someone by telephone day or night can be helpful in quelling some of the anxiety. In the early days following discharge, parents are also appreciative of the intensive follow-up that is required post-HSCT. Although difficult in certain settings, continuity of care between the inpatient and outpatient setting can also ease distress.

As families prepare to leave the hospital, it is also important to establish realistic expectations about the possibility of future hospitalizations given the immunocompromised state of the patient. This preparation can decrease feelings of guilt, frustration, and disappointment upon readmission.

Adherence at Home

The medical requirements following HSCT discharge are demanding and time consuming. There are medications to take throughout the day, dietary and activity restrictions, and caloric intake and fluid goals. Nonadherence can lower the chances of survival, increase risk of complications, and lead to poorer quality of life. Unfortunately there are no known adherence interventions created specifically for the HSCT population; however, because the demands of daily care are similar in complexity to some of the other pediatric chronic health conditions, one can extrapolate from interventions targeted at other chronic illness populations. Adolescents and young adults are particularly vulnerable to high rates of nonadherence because they are still developing independence and self-management skills, have different immediate priorities, have interrupted social support, and sometimes lack detailed knowledge of their treatment. Drotar (2013) recently proposed a comprehensive collaborative adherence promotion model that can be adapted for the adolescent and young adult population as described by Butow and colleagues (2010; see Table 13.3).

Table 13.3 HSCT adherence model

Develop a collaborative relationship and increase ownership in health by involving the patient in all HSCT-related discussions.
Discuss adherence throughout the course of treatment. Critical time points: discharge from the HSCT hospitalization, any time there is a change in treatment regimen (e.g., discontinuing intravenous fluids and increasing the need for oral intake), and when the patient takes over self-management.
Education is key! Discuss what each medication treats/prevents, how it works, and why it is important to take consistently. Highlight the importance of participating in HSCT follow-up care and continuing to follow isolation restrictions even after feeling better.
Ask how medication is managed at home and what strategies (e.g., pill box) are being utilized to facilitate adherence.
Acknowledge and normalize barriers to adherence (e.g., returning to school/work, changes in dosing, and adverse side effects). Flexibly and creatively strategize solutions (e.g., altering the timing of follow-up appointments that interfere with classes).
Establish a plan to monitor adherence (e.g., using laboratory values to test for therapeutic levels of cyclosporine and tacrolimus, frequency of medication refill requests).

Adapted from Drotar (2013) and Butow et al. (2010)

School Reintegration

Returning to school following an HSCT can be a difficult transition given the academic and social difficulties inherent in extended time away from the classroom due to medical isolation precautions. Additionally, treatment-related medical (e.g., fatigue) and neurocognitive late effects can have long-ranging impact on the successful return to school. While there are no school reintegration studies aimed at the HSCT population, interventions specific to pediatric cancer have primarily focused on improving communication between HSCT providers and school personnel, addressing academic needs through homebound education, and preserving social relationships during post-HSCT home isolation (Tadmor et al. 2012). Many patients benefit from a gradual return to school (e.g., half days) as well as supportive educational services (i.e., 504 Plan, Individualized Education Plan). Chapter 11 covers this topic in great detail.

Sibling Donors

When considering HSCT, physicians must consider the degree of human leukocyte antigen (HLA) "match" between donor and recipient; those with a strong degree of match are considered immunologically compatible. Siblings have a 25 % chance of being an HLA match with one another and, as such, are often the first to be considered for donation once the decision has been made to pursue an allogeneic HSCT as the treatment course. Matched sibling transplants also offer lower risk of GVHD, nonrelapse-related mortality, and equivalent, if not superior, rates of disease-free survival as compared to unrelated bone marrow and cord blood transplants (Zhang et al. 2012).

Donor Assessment

The decision to have one child undergo a non-therapeutic medical procedure for the benefit of another child has been discussed extensively in the literature and has been brought before the court system (Pentz et al. 2008; also see Chapter 17). Historically, parents have made the decision for a minor child to donate to his sibling because it was implied that children were unable to make such a decision for themselves. In a study examining hospital management of minor donors, Chan and colleagues (1996) found that 84 % of pediatric transplant centers allow parental consent as the only documentation necessary to permit a child to donate bone marrow. However, the method of sole parental consent has been questioned in the literature, suggesting that parents of minor children are conflicted decision makers for sibling donation (Pentz 2006; Ross and Glannon 2006).

Despite evidence to suggest that children as young as 9 years of age are able to make medical decisions on their own behalf (Weisz 1992; Weithorn and Campbell 1982), only two states – Alabama and Wisconsin – have written statutes that specifically address the issue of minor sibling donation. In Alabama, minors may consent to donation of their bone marrow once they have reached the age of 14 years or have been emancipated (ALA. CODE § 22-8-9, 2012). The Wisconsin law (WIS. STAT. ANN. §146.34, 2012) allows potential donors to assent as long as the transplant physician has informed the parent/donor about the benefits and risks to donor and recipient and alternative treatments to transplant. The minor also must be deemed the most acceptable donor, medically cleared to donate, and undergo a psychological and intellectual evaluation.

Studies have found that sibling donors do not feel as if they have a choice in the decision to donate (Packman et al. 1997; Pentz et al. 2014) and feel compelled to do it (MacLeod et al. 2003; Wiener et al. 2007). Even years after their donation, siblings may understand why they needed to donate but wish that they could have had more influence in coming to that conclusion for themselves.

Once the decision to donate has been made, many donors continue to be ambivalent toward the process; while they may feel proud to be the donor, many also report feeling very nervous about the idea of injections, pain, and possible harm during the procedure (Wiener et al. 2008). The literature focusing on the sibling donor's experience after donation is limited, but points to a number of consistent findings. In the months and years following donation, siblings retrospectively report experiencing feelings of anger, jealousy, guilt about being healthy, anxiety, sadness, and loneliness (Freund and Siegel 1986; Packman et al. 1997; Wiener et al. 2008; Wilkins et al. 2007).

The emotional impact of donation can be complicated by the health of the recipient sibling. Wiener and colleagues (2007) found that donor siblings of successful transplants without complications reported overall positive experiences, such as an increased closeness of the family and increased understanding of the recipient sibling's illness, while donor siblings of successful transplants with complications, such as GVHD, had negative experiences and felt responsible for the outcome of the transplant. Donor siblings of unsuccessful transplants resulting in the death of the recipient experienced feelings of blame, guilt, and anger.

As a result of the vague and/or nonexistent state laws governing minor donation, along with the known psychosocial risks of donation, the American Academy of Pediatrics (AAP 2010) created guidelines to direct the participation of minors as hematopoietic stem cell donors (see Table 13.4). The AAP further suggested that potential donors be assigned an advocate early in the process whom will help them understand the process of donation and protect their rights (see Table 13.5). The meeting with the donor consists of three primary goals: (1) determine ability and willingness to assent to donation, (2) minimize the emotional risks of donating, and (3) investigate the quality of the sibling relationship and potential likelihood of emotional benefits from donation. See Table 13.6 for a recommended assessment model.

Table 13.4 AAP guidelines for minor participation in hematopoietic stem cell donation

No medically equivalent histocompatible adult relative willing and able to donate
Strong personal and positive relationship between the sibling donor and recipient
Some likelihood that the recipient will benefit from transplant
Clinical, emotional, and psychosocial risks to the donor are minimized
Parental permission and donor assent are obtained

Table 13.5 Donor advocate

Role and training
Not involved in the care of the recipient
Trained in child development
Has knowledge of HSCT and donation
Process
Initial contact should be as soon as the donor begins the process of medical clearance to donate
Meetings with donor can be conducted jointly with caregiver, although separate interviews may yield more meaningful information

It is common for donors to voice misinformation or fears during the assessment. Most of these issues can be addressed by the donor advocate, although occasionally the donor may be referred back to the medical team for additional education. Very rarely, a sibling will report information that may make them an unsuitable candidate for donation, such as unwillingness to donate/coercion or a significant mental health history that places them at very high risk of emotional distress. In these cases, the transplant team, in conjunction with the donor advocate, must make a decision about whether to proceed. If available, an ethics consult can also be helpful in these cases.

Case Vignette

Megan, the 14-year-old sister of a boy with refractory ALL, was evaluated by a psychologist as a potential donor for her brother. During the evaluation, she reported feeling forced to donate her marrow because her parents said if she didn't she would be to blame if her brother died. The family history was complicated by parental divorce and reports of abuse and neglect in both households. Megan described her parents as physically abusive and emotionally unavailable. Megan had a history of depression and suicidal ideation and was being followed by a psychotherapist in the community. Based on the results of the pre-donation psychological evaluation, the HSCT team determined that she was at significant emotional risk and opted to proceed with a different course of treatment for her brother.

Intervention

A recently published multisite prospective study by Pentz and colleagues (2014) advocates for basic education for all potential sibling donors before HLA typing, more robust education for identified donors, and ongoing supportive follow-up in the post-transplant period. The donor assessment described above can serve as an initial therapeutic intervention because it normalizes the experiences and feelings of the donor, prepares them for the emotional experience of donation and recovery, and establishes guidelines for parents about when to seek additional psychotherapeutic support. Beyond the initial assessment, the donor advocate remains a resource for the family and ideally would provide supportive follow-up care; however, there are practical and emotional barriers to providing ongoing care to donors. Following donation, siblings return to their usual routine at home and school and become less available for intervention. Parents already busy at the bedside with the recipient may be unaware of any distress occurring at home or too emotionally taxed to manage less pressing issues. Donors, aware of parental stress, may be unwilling to burden them with additional concerns and try to manage their feelings on their own.

Table 13.6 Summary of minor sibling pre-donation psychological evaluation

Assessment goals	Salient assessment factors	Examples of interview questions	Examples of measures (time/resources permitting)
Determine ability and willingness to assent to donation	Donation procedure Decision making/voluntariness Alternative treatment options Ability to read assent/consent form	What is your understanding of the procedure to collect your stem cells/bone marrow? What do you expect for your recovery? How did you make the decision to donate? What were the most and least important factors in making this decision? When were you told that you could donate bone marrow to your sibling? What were your thoughts when you were told that you were a match for your sibling? If you decided not to be a donor for your sibling, what other options are available for your sibling?	WRAT4, Reading Composite (Wilkinson and Robertson 2006)
Minimize emotional risks of donating	Current psychosocial distress (depression, anxiety, needle phobia) Expectations for recipient's health Control and responsibility	Tell me about your previous experience with blood draws/IVs. What have you been told to expect for your sibling? What is the name of your sibling's illness? How responsible do you think you are for your sibling's health? How much control do you have over your sibling's health? Do you know what GVHD is? Explain your understanding of GVHD.	*Behavioral checklists* ASEBA Self-Report (Achenbach and Rescorla 2001) BASC-2 (Reynolds and Kamphaus 2004)
Investigate the quality of the sibling relationship and potential likelihood of emotional benefits from donation	Family functioning Sibling relationship (strength of foundation for personal connection)	What was your family like before your sibling got sick? What is it like now? What do you and your sibling like to do together? Name some of your sibling's friends.	Observation of sibling interaction
Educate caregivers	Donor psychosocial history Provide education and resources	What role has your child played in the decision to donate? How can you help your child feel more prepared for the procedure? What do you view as the psychosocial risks and benefits of donation? How can you support your child after donation knowing that your other child will be in the hospital and undergoing intensive medical treatment?	*Behavioral checklists* ASEBA Parent Proxy (Achenbach and Rescorla 2001) BASC-2 (Reynolds and Kamphaus 2004)

When a recipient dies or experiences significant complications (e.g., chronic GVHD), the likelihood of donor distress increases. In these cases, the donor advocate is encouraged to reach out to the donor to assess their need for additional support. This may include psychotherapeutic interventions by the donor advocate or referral to a local mental health provider.

Parent, Sibling, and Family Functioning

HSCT is not only stressful for the recipient, but it has a significant impact on the family as well. As a result, HSCT assessment and interventions should be family-centered throughout the HSCT care continuum. The following sections provide an overview of the impact of HSCT on parents, non-donor siblings, and the family as well as supportive care needs.

Parental Stress, Coping, and Adjustment

Parents are faced with a host of practical and emotional challenges when their child receives an HSCT. They are naturally worried about their child's health and well-being given the child's high-risk disease and the intensity of the HSCT regimen with potential severe or life-threatening treatment-related side effects or complications. They are concerned about whether the transplant "will work" to cure their child's disease. For patients who have an HLA-matched sibling, parents have the additional worry of the well-being of their child who donated. Employed parents may have to reduce their work hours or take a medical leave of absence to care for their child during and after HSCT, thereby creating a significant financial strain on the family. This is extremely burdensome in single-parent households in which there is only one income supporting the family, and a loss of employment may lead to a loss of health insurance for the HSCT recipient and family. In a two-parent household, one parent may be the "resident caregiver" during the HSCT hospitalization and outpatient recovery while the other parent may be working full-time to financially support the family. The primary breadwinner may feel guilty about not being able to care for their child as much as they would like, whereas the resident caregiving parent may feel overwhelmed with the full-time care responsibilities. While parents are trying to deal with all of these emotional and practical challenges, they may also be caring for other children and/or their own elderly parents. Parents struggle with trying to find alternative caregivers for their children when they are in the hospital with the HSCT recipient and are challenged to maintain some normalcy for their children such as attending school and participating in extracurricular activities and social events. Parents feel guilty about not being present or being less available for their other children while in the hospital caring for the HSCT recipient. This is a particular struggle for single-parent households or for families who live a long distance from the transplant center.

Given the number of HSCT-related stressors, it is important to assess parental stress and coping across the HSCT care continuum. Similar to the trajectory of child distress, a review of research of parents of children receiving HSCT found that the majority of parents reported significantly higher levels of distress (anxiety, depression, posttraumatic stress symptoms, somatic complaints) prior to and during the acute hospitalization phase of HSCT compared to normative group data, with distress levels decreasing over time especially between 3 and 6 months following transplant and returning to baseline or positive adjustment by 18 months post-HSCT (Vrijmoet-Wiersma et al. 2009). Despite this, a subset of parents is at risk for difficulty coping years after their child's HSCT. Risk factors for long-term parental distress were grouped into three categories: (1) factors related to the child's disease and treatment (transfers to the intensive care unit, higher number of hospitalizations 6 months after HSCT, and higher HSCT risk); (2) demographic factors (younger maternal age, lower socioeconomic status); and (3) parental stress and coping during the acute phase of HSCT or premorbid parental or child psychosocial functioning. Protective factors of parental distress included mothers with a more optimistic personality or who used coping strategies of acceptance, humor, and "putting reason before emotion" or parents who had a supportive family environment (Vrijmoet-Wiersma et al. 2009). Unfortunately, results of the reviewed studies are mainly generalizable to mothers as very few studies included fathers or had a small number of fathers as respondents.

Sibling Stress, Coping, and Adjustment

Far less is known about sibling adjustment and supportive care needs when a child receives an HSCT. Siblings who are not donors of HSCT recipients still have to cope with one or both parents being less physically or emotionally available because they are caring for their brother or sister in the hospital or at frequent clinic appointments during recovery. Siblings may need to stay with relatives or family friends and, as a result, may feel disconnected or displaced from their family. In addition, siblings may be less able to socialize with their friends or participate in extracurricular activities as they used to before their brother or sister became ill. In a review of the scant literature, Packman et al. (2010), who have conducted the majority of studies on siblings of HSCT recipients, concluded that siblings of HSCT patients experience a range of natural feelings but some report posttraumatic stress symptoms, anxiety, and low self-esteem. Siblings of HSCT recipients also expressed interruption in their "normal" family life, a lack of parental attention, limited understanding of transplant, feelings of loneliness, and a reliance on a faith in God to help them cope, which were thematic responses in qualitative studies that were reviewed (Packman et al. 2010).

Family Functioning

When a child undergoes an HSCT, many aspects of a family's life are disrupted. Families of children who receive an HSCT experience a reliance on supportive others for assistance, disrupted daily schedules and routines, changes in familial roles, economic strain, and separation or difficulty finding time to spend together as a family. Both positive (i.e., family cohesion) and negative (i.e., family conflict) family functioning have been shown to be predictive factors for parent and child outcomes in HSCT (Clarke et al. 2008; Phipps et al. 2005; Vrijmoet-Wiersma et al. 2009). There has been limited research on the impact of a child's HSCT on the family unit, with family functioning as the primary outcome. Jobe-Shields et al. (2009) found that higher parental depressive symptoms were associated with lower levels of family cohesion and expressiveness, and lower family conflict and greater family expressiveness was related to less severe illness-related distress reported by the child prior to HSCT. Pre-HSCT family cohesion and expressiveness served as protective factors against child illness-related distress when parents reported low depressive symptoms, but this was not the case when parents reported high depressive symptoms (Jobe-Shields et al. 2009), which highlights the importance of addressing the supportive care needs of parents and families when a patient receives an HSCT.

The impact of the child's HSCT on the parents' marital relationship is not known. Anecdotally, parents face reduced or limited time together as a couple (physical separation for some due to distance) because of their child's HSCT care demands, which can make communication and support difficult. Parents often have to cope with role changes in the family, which also may strain the relationship. Extrapolating from the few studies that have investigated the impact of childhood cancer on parents' relationship suggests that there is no elevation in divorce rates (Syse et al. 2010), but negative or positive changes may occur depending on factors such as time since diagnosis (minimal or positive changes in relationship the further out from diagnosis), communication between parents (quality and quantity), gender differences in stress and coping, and parental role changes (Da Silva et al. 2010).

Family-Based Interventions

Multidisciplinary supportive care of families, based upon family systems and stress and coping models, is necessary to provide comprehensive care that helps to reduce HSCT-related stress and enhance existing positive support systems and healthy coping strategies. For example, hospital-based social workers have the expertise necessary to assist parents or young adult patients as they apply for financial assistance, including Supplemental Security Income disability benefits, address health insurance and prescription medication issues, identify or arrange medical transportation, assist in filing for family medical leave, and complete advanced directives or power of health care agent documents.

Psychosocial providers should inform and connect families to local and national support programs and resources (see Table 13.2) and can advocate for support and assistance from the family's support system such as school personnel for the siblings (i.e., teacher, school psychologist, or guidance counselor) and employers for the parents, with the family's permission. Many parents and siblings express benefiting from being connected to other parents and siblings of children who have undergone HSCT. Referrals to support groups and family-based or sibling support camps should be provided, when available. Psychosocial providers also may initiate communication with another willing HSCT family whose child has received an HSCT at the transplant center in person, by telephone and email, or via online social networking (Facebook), or this connection may be facilitated through a national program such as Imerman Angels (see Table 13.2; see Chapters 25 and 11 on Resources and Education, respectively).

Importantly, psychosocial providers should provide family-centered care by providing supportive counseling to parents, siblings, and the family unit when an immediate family member is having difficulty coping with the child's HSCT, which may decrease short- and long-term negative family outcomes. Goals of supportive counseling may consist of strengthening and teaching healthy coping, problem-solving, and stress management strategies, teaching effective family communication skills, and encouraging self-care activities, such as eating healthy, taking regular breaks from the bedside for respite whenever possible, physical activity or exercise (even if it is a walk in or around the hospital), and good sleep hygiene. Referrals to community-based mental health providers may be necessary to address and treat premorbid mental health disorders. Hospital-based chaplains should also be accessible to meet their religious or spiritual needs or to help coordinate visits from their community-based church or spiritual leaders.

The majority of supportive care provided to families of children who undergo an HSCT is based upon anecdotal evidence in clinical practice. Despite family functioning being a strong contributing factor to parental and child distress or adjustment in HSCT, to date there have been only two published intervention studies that targeted parents of children undergoing HSCT (Lindwall et al. 2014; Streisand et al. 2000). Streisand et al. (2000) evaluated a one-session stress inoculation intervention for mothers ($N=22$) of children receiving an HSCT, who found no difference in parental stress between mothers who were randomly assigned the intervention compared to those who received the standard care. A more recent multisite randomized controlled study compared the parental benefit of a child targeted complementary therapy intervention (massage and humor therapy), a combined parent (massage and relaxation) and child intervention (massage and humor therapy), and standard of care (Lindwall et al. 2014). Results suggested no significant differences between groups in the areas of acute parental distress, positive affect, depression, or posttraumatic stress. Parents in all three groups demonstrated significant improvement over time across all domains, indicating that parental functioning decreases around the time of HSCT admission but returns to baseline functioning over time (Lindwall et al. 2014). Parsons and colleagues (2013) also recently completed a 6-month randomized controlled multisite study of a web-based support and education intervention for parents of pediatric HSCT recipients ($N=102$

intervention arm; $N=99$ control arm) known as HSCT-CHESS™ (Comprehensive Health Enhancement Support System) funded by the National Cancer Institute. Preliminary results indicated no intervention effect on parental emotional functioning at 6 months post-HSCT. However, parents who used the website though the 6-month intervention period had a significantly higher emotional functioning score (6.3 points higher; effect size = 0.32) compared to parents who were randomized to the intervention but did not actually use the website (Parsons et al. 2013).

Future Directions and Conclusion

Despite the significant inherent challenges of a lengthy HSCT hospitalization and recovery with a major disruption of normalcy and social isolation, most children, adolescents, and young adults and their families demonstrate resiliency and seem to recover over time from the distress they experience prior to and during the acute phase of transplant. However, a subset of patients and parents continue to struggle years after transplant. Therefore, it is important to understand the contributing risk and protective factors for HSCT outcomes in patients and families. Pre-HSCT functioning of the patient and family is a strong predictor of post-HSCT functioning based upon existing research, which highlights the importance of conducting a comprehensive psychological assessment prior to HSCT but also throughout the different phases of HSCT given our understanding of the trajectory of distress and HRQL. Despite the limited assessment tools developed for use in pediatric HSCT, consideration should be made for the inclusion of quantitative measures of psychosocial functioning and HRQL that have been validated with children, adolescents, and young adults in cancer and other chronic illness populations. Similarly, most clinical interventions that have been implemented in the pediatric HSCT setting are based upon "what works" or "what doesn't work" in clinical practice to support the patient and family. More research is needed to develop and evaluate interventions specific to the pediatric HSCT population, their parents, siblings, and families and/or determine the efficacy of existing interventions in cancer and other chronic illness for use in pediatric HSCT. Regardless, given the intensity and complexities of HSCT care, supportive care should be multidisciplinary, with care coordination and communication among providers, and family-centered and consistently delivered from inpatient to outpatient settings across the HSCT care continuum. Special attention also should be made for siblings, both donors and non-donors, and family functioning as a primary focus of research. Longitudinal, multisite studies with larger sample sizes are essential to gain a better understanding of siblings' natural reactions to changes in the family related to HSCT versus siblings at risk for psychosocial difficulties.

Clinical Pearls

- Psychosocial providers should have expertise in the unique stressors and supportive care needs of pediatric HSCT recipients and their families.
- Assessment and intervention should be family-centered given the impact of HSCT on patients, parents, and siblings.
- Sibling donors require an assessment and supportive care approach that takes into consideration their unique experience.
- Evidence-based psychosocial assessment and treatment specific to pediatric HSCT is needed.

Box 13.1: Sample HSCT Care Plan

The following plan has been created in collaboration with the HSCT team, nursing, supportive services, and Suzy's parents in order to help Suzy have a successful and safe transplant experience.

A. Suzy will have many new demands placed on her during her transplant. It is recommended that the following expectations be incorporated into a reward system so that she is motivated to participate in her care. The reward system will be created by parents and psychosocial providers.
   (a) Oral medications must be taken within 15 minutes regardless of parent presence. A timer can be set if this would be a helpful visual reminder for Suzy.
   (b) Suzy must sleep in her own bed every night, all night.
   (c) Mineral oil baths three times daily.
   (d) Clothing changed two times daily.
   (e) Mouth care to include brushing teeth two times a day and mouthwash four times a day.
   (f) Vitals every 4 hours. May be more often if medically necessary.
   (g) Participation in bedside education.
   (h) Participation in physical therapy.

B. If Suzy refuses to cooperate or becomes disrespectful toward nursing, parents are encouraged to leave the room and allow nursing to work individually with Suzy to complete her care.

C. A sleep/wake routine will help Suzy to maintain structure in her day. It will also guarantee better cooperation with early morning demands and help facilitate her transition back home after transplant. Sleep/wake routines have been shown to improve patient and parent quality of sleep.
   (a) At 9:30 PM, parents and/or nursing will remind Suzy that she needs to be in her bed with lights out and television off by 10:00 PM. This warning will help prepare her and allow her time to complete any bedtime cares (e.g., brushing teeth).
   (b) At 10:00 PM, lights and television must be turned off. If nursing enters the room after 10:00 PM and this has not happened, they will provide a verbal reminder and then turn off lights and television.
   (c) Parents and/or nursing will wake Suzy at 7:30 AM in preparation for 8:00 AM vitals and weight.
   (d) Napping during the day is permitted. However, daytime naps will be limited, particularly late afternoon naps when Suzy feels well, in order to facilitate better sleep routines at night.

D. Suzy is encouraged to play outside of her room as long as she is not on isolation precautions.

E. Good hygiene is of the utmost importance during transplant. Parents and Suzy are encouraged to handwash or sanitize every time they reenter the room. Food and drink should be fresh. All partially consumed food and drink should be thrown away. Suzy should not eat or drink after anyone else.

F. Parents are strongly encouraged to participate in morning rounds to help ensure that they understand the plan as presented by the team.

References

Achenbach TM, Rescorla LA (2001) Manual for the ASEBA school-age forms and profiles. University of Vermont Research Center for Children, Youth and Families, Burlington

Ala. Code 22-8-9 (2012) Consent of minor to donation of bone marrow; Consent by parent or legal guardian

American Academy of Pediatrics (2010) Policy statement – children as hematopoietic stem cell donors. Pediatrics 125(2):392–404

Bingen K, Kent MW, Rodday AM, Ratichek SJ, Kupst MJ, Parsons SK (2012) Children's coping with hematopoietic stem cell transplant: results from the journeys to recovery study. Child Health Care 41(2):145–161

Butow P, Palmer S, Pai A, Goodenough B, Luckett T, King M (2010) Review of adherence-related issues in adolescents and young adults with cancer. J Clin Oncol 28(32):4800–4809

Cairo MS, Heslop H (2008) Pediatric blood and marrow transplantation: state of the science. Bone Marrow Transplant 41:97

Cella DF, Tulsky DS, Gray G, Sarafian B, Linn E, Bonomi A, Silberman M, Yellen SB, Winicour P, Brannon J, Eckberg K, Lloyd S, Purl S, Blendowski C, Goodman M, Barnicle M, Stewart I, McHale M, Bonomi P, Kaplan E, Taylor S IV, Thomas CR Jr, Harris J (1993) The functional assessment of cancer therapy (FACT) scale: development and validation of the general measure. J Clin Oncol 11(3):570–579

Chan KW, Gajewski JL, Supkis D, Pentz R, Champlin R, Bleyer WA (1996) Use of minors as bone marrow donors: current attitude and management as survey of 56 pediatric transplantation centers. J Pediatr 128(5):644–648

Clarke SA, Eiser C, Skinner R (2008) Health-related quality of life in survivors of BMT for paediatric malignancy: a systematic review of the literature. Bone Marrow Transplant 42:73–82

Da Silva FM, Jacob E, Nascimento LC (2010) Impact of childhood cancer on parents' relationship: an integrative review. J Nurs Scholarsh 42(3):250–261

Devine KA, Heckler CE, Katz ER, Fairclough DL, Phipps S, Sherman-Bien S, Dolgin MJ, Noll RB, Askins MA, Butler RW, Sahler OJ (2014) Evaluation of the psychometric properties of the pediatric parenting stress inventory (PPSI). Health Psychol 33:130–138

Diamond S, Lavallee DC (2010) Experience with a pill-swallowing enhancement aid. Clin Pediatr 49(4):391–393

Drotar D (2013) Strategies of adherence promotion in the management of pediatric chronic conditions. J Dev Behav Pediatr 34(9):716–729

Embry L, Annett RD, Kunin-Baston A, Patel SK, Sands S, Reaman G, Noll RB (2012) Implementation of multi-site neurocognitive assessments within a pediatric cooperative group: can it be done? Pediatr Blood Cancer 59:536–539

Folkman S, Lazarus R (1988) Ways of coping questionnaire. Mind Garden, Palo Alto

Freund BL, Siegel K (1986) Problems in transition following bone marrow transplantation: psychosocial aspects. Am J Orthopsychiatry 56(2):244–252

Furman W, Buhrmester D (1985) Sibling relationship questionnaire. Child Dev 56:448–461

Holmes TH, Rabe RH (1967) The social readjustment rating scale. J Psychosom Res 11:213–218

Jobe-Shields L, Alderfer MA, Barrera M, Vannatta K, Currier JM, Phipps S (2009) Parental depression and family environment predict distress in children prior to stem-cell transplantation. J Dev Behav Pediatr 30(2):140–146

Kaplan BJ, Steiger RA, Pope J, Marsh A, Sharp M, Crawford SG (2010) Successful treatment of pill-swallowing difficulties with head posture practice. Paediatr Child Health 15(5):e1–e5

Kazak AE, Penati B, Brophy P, Himelstein B (1998) Pharmacologic and psychologic interventions for procedural pain. Pediatrics 102:59–66

Kuppenheimer WG, Brown RT (2002) Painful procedures in pediatric cancer: a comparison of interventions. Clin Psychol Rev 22:753–786

Lindwall JJ, Russell K, Huang Q, Zhang H, Vannatta K, Barrera M, Alderfer M, Phipps S (2014) Adjustment in parents of children undergoing stem cell transplantation. Biol Blood Marrow Transplant 20:543–548

MacLeod KD, Whitsitt SF, Mash EJ, Pelletier W (2003) Pediatric sibling donors of successful and unsuccessful hematopoietic stem cell transplants (HSCT): a qualitative study of their psychosocial experience. J Pediatr Psychol 28(4):223–231

McCubbin HI, McCubbin MA, Patterson JM, Cauble AE, Wilson LR, Warwick W (1983) CHIP-coping health inventory for parents: an assessment of parental coping patterns in the care of the chronically ill child. J Marriage Fam 45:359–370

McGrady ME, Williams SN, Davies SM, Pai AL (2014) Adherence to outpatient oral medication regimens in adolescent hematopoietic stem cell transplant recipients. Eur J Oncol Nurs 18(2):140–144

Moos R, Moos B (1994) Family environment scale manual: development, applications, research, 3rd edn. Mind Garden, Palo Alto

Mulhern RK, Butler RW (2006) Neuropsychological late effects. In: Brown RT (ed) Comprehensive handbook of childhood cancer and sickle cell disease: a biopsychosocial approach. Oxford University Press, New York, pp 262–278

Packman WL, Crittenden MR, Rieger JB, Schaeffer E, Bongar B, Cowan MJ (1997) Siblings perceptions of the bone marrow transplantation process. J Psychosoc Oncol 15:81–105

Packman W, Weber S, Wallace J, Bugescu N (2010) Psychological effects of hematopoietic SCT on pediatric patients, siblings and parents: a review. Bone Marrow Transplant 45(7):1134–1146

Pai ALH, Patino-Fernandez AM, McSherry M, Beele D, Alderfer MA, Reilly AT, Hwang WT, Kazak AE (2008) The psychosocial assessment tool (PAT2.0): psychometric properties of a screener for psychosocial distress in families of children newly diagnosed with cancer. J Pediatr Psychol 33(2):50–62

Parsons SK, Shih MC, Mayer DK, Barlow SE, Supran SE, Levy SL, Greenfield S, Kaplan SH (2005) Preliminary psychometric evaluation of the Child Health Ratings Inventories (CHRIs) and Disease-Specific Impairment Inventory-HSCT (DSII-HSCT) in parents and children. Qual Life Res 14:1613–1625

Parsons SK, Mayer DK, Ratichek SJ, Rodday AM, Syrjala KL, Davies S, Patel SK, Schwartz L, Kupst MJ, Bingen K, Guinan EC, McTavish F, Stewart S, Terrin N, Gustafson DH (2013) An eHealth program for parents of pediatric hematopoietic stem cell transplant (HSCT) recipients enhances parents' emotional functioning with continued use: results of the HSCT Comprehensive Health Enhancement Support System (CHESSTM) Study. Psycho-Oncology 22:100–101

Pentz R (2006) Duty and altruism: alternative analyses of the ethics of siblings bone marrow donations. J Clin Ethics 17(3):227–230

Pentz RD, Haight AE, Noll RB, Barfield R, Pelletier W, Davies S, Alderfer MA, Hinds PS (2008) The ethical justification for minor sibling bone marrow donation: a case study. Oncologist 13:148–151

Pentz RD, Alderfer MA, Pelletier W, Stegenga K, Haight AE, Hendershot KA, Dixon M, Fairclough D, Hinds P (2014) Unmet needs of siblings of pediatric stem cell transplant recipients. Pediatrics 133(5):e1156–e1162

Phipps S (2006) Psychosocial and behavioral issues in stem cell transplantation. In: Brown RT (ed) Comprehensive handbook of childhood cancer and sickle cell disease: a biopsychosocial approach. Oxford University Press, New York, pp 75–99

Phipps S, Hinds PS, Channell S, Bell GL (1994) Measurement of behavioral, affective, and somatic responses to pediatric bone marrow transplantation: development of the BASES scale. J Pediatr Oncol Nurse 11:109–117

Phipps S, Dunavant M, Jayawardene D, Srivastiva DK (1999) Assessment of health- related quality of life in acute in-patient settings: use of the bases instrument in children undergoing bone marrow transplantation. Int J Cancer 12:18–24

Phipps S, Dunavant M, Lensing S, Rai SN (2005) Psychosocial predictors of distress in parents of children undergoing stem cell or bone marrow transplantation. J Pediatr Psychol 30(2):139–153

Reynolds CR, Kamphaus RW (2004) BASC-2, behavior assessment system for children, 2nd edn. AGS Publishing, Circle Pines

Ross LF, Glannon W (2006) A compounding of errors: the case of bone marrow donation between non-intimate siblings. J Clin Ethics 17:220–226

Sherman AC, Simonton S, Latif U, Nieder ML, Adams RH, Mehta P (2004) Psychosocial supportive care for children receiving stem cell transplantation: practice patterns across centers. Bone Marrow Transplant 34:169–174

Spirito A, Stark L, Williams C (1988) Development of a brief coping checklist for use with pediatric populations. J Pediatr Psychol 13(4):555–574

Stein REK, Riessman CK (1980) The development of the impact on family scale: preliminary findings. Med Care 18:465–472

Streisand R, Rodrigue JR, Houck C, Graham-Pole J, Berlant N (2000) Brief report: Parents of children undergoing bone marrow transplantation: documenting stress and piloting a psychological intervention program. J Pediatr Psychol 25(5):331–337

Syse A, Loge JH, Lyngstad TH (2010) Does childhood cancer affect parental divorce rates? A population-based study. J Clin Oncol 28(5):872–877

Tadmor CS, Rosenkranz R, Ben-Arush MW (2012) Education in pediatric oncology: learning and reintegration into school. In: Kreitler S, Ben-Arush MW, Martin A (eds) Pediatric psycho-oncology: psychosocial aspects and clinic interventions, 2nd edn. Wiley-Blackwell, Chichester

Tanzi EM (2011) Health-related quality of life of hematopoietic stem cell transplant childhood survivors: state of the science. J Pediatr Oncol Nurs 28(4):191–202

Tobin DL, Holroyd KA, Reynolds RVC (1984) User's manual for the coping strategies inventory. Ohio University, Department of Psychology, Athens

Varni JW, Seid M, Kurtin PS (2001) PedsQL 4.0: reliability and validity of the pediatric quality of life inventory version 4.0 generica core scales in health and patient populations. Med Care 39:800–812

Vrijmoet-Wiersma CMJ, Kolk AM, Grootenhuis MA, Spek EM, van Klink JMM, Egeler RM, Bredius RGM, Koopman HM (2009) Child and parental adaptation to pediatric stem cell transplantation. Support Care Cancer 17:707–714

Wechsler D (2004) The Wechsler intelligence scale for children, 4th edn. Pearson Assessment, London

Wechsler D (2011) Wechsler abbreviated scale of intelligence, 2nd edn. Pearson Assessment, London

Weisz V (1992) Psycholegal issues in sibling bone marrow donation. Ethics Behav 2:185–201

Weithorn LA, Campbell SB (1982) The competency of children and adolescents to make informed treatment decisions. Child Dev 53:1589–1598

Wiener LS, Steffen-Smith E, Wayne AS (2007) Hematopoietic stem cell donation in children: a review of the sibling donor experience. J Psychosoc Oncol 25:45–66

Wiener LS, Steffen-Smith E, Battles HB, Wayne A, Love CP, Fry T (2008) Sibling stem cell donor experiences at a single institution. Psychooncology 17:304–307

Wilkins KL, Hons BS, Woodgate RL (2007) An interruption in family life: siblings' lived experience as they transition through the pediatric bone marrow transplantation trajectory. Oncol Nurs Forum 34(2):28–35

Wilkinson GS, Robertson GJ (2006) Wide range achievement test four professional manual. Psychological Assessment Resources, Lutz

Wis. Stat. 146.34 (2012) Donation of bone marrow by a minor.

Zhang M, Davies SM, Camitta BM, Logan B, Tiedemann K, Eapen M (2012) Comparison of outcomes after HLA-matched sibling and unrelated donor transplantation for children with high-risk acute lymphoblastic leukemia. Biol Blood Marrow Transplant 18:1204–1210

Zimet GD, Dahlem NW, Zimet SG, Farley GK (1988) The multidimensional scale of perceived social support. J Pers Assess 52:30–41

Palliative Care for Children with Cancer and Their Families

14

Abby R. Rosenberg, Joanne Wolfe, and Barbara L. Jones

What (and When) Is "Palliative Care?"

Case Vignettes

Logan (now 5 years old) was 2 when he was diagnosed with high-risk neuroblastoma. His mother recalls the first few weeks of his treatment. "We could barely understand the words being said, let alone make sense of his having cancer. Not knowing what to expect or how to protect him terrified me."

Melissa is a 17-year-old young woman with recurrent osteosarcoma. "When my cancer came back, I was trying to make some really hard decisions. My team asked me how I define quality of life, and I said 'being able to dance.' We kept talking about how to fit my values in with my medical decisions. It helped me figure out which treatments to try and how to balance my hopes and expectations."

Amy was 8 years old when she died of refractory leukemia. "No one will ever be 'prepared' for the death of their child," says her mother. "But our team helped us to be as ready as possible. First, they helped us decide how to spend our time. Then, they helped us understand what to expect. After that, they helped us to say 'goodbye.' Throughout, they were there, beside us, supporting us. Amy didn't suffer. She lived and was happy against all odds. For that I am grateful."

A.R. Rosenberg, MD, MS (✉)
Seattle Children's Hospital Cancer and Blood Disorders Center, Seattle, WA, USA

Clinical Research Division, Fred Hutchinson Cancer Research Center, Seattle, WA, USA

Treuman Katz Center for Pediatric Bioethics, Seattle Children's Research Institute, Seattle, WA, USA
e-mail: abby.rosenberg@seattlechildrens.org

J. Wolfe, MD, MPH
Department of Psychosocial Oncology and Palliative Care, Center for Outcomes and Policy Research, Dana-Farber Cancer Institute,
450 Brookline Avenue, Boston, MA 02215, USA

Department of Psychosocial Oncology and Palliative Care, Dana-Farber Cancer Institute,
Boston, MA, USA

Boston Children's Hospital, Boston, MA, USA
e-mail: joanne_wolfe@dfci.harvard.edu

B.L. Jones, PhD, MSW
School of Social Work, University of Texas at Austin, Austin, TX, USA

The Institute for Grief, Loss, and Family Survival, UT Austin School of Social Work,
1925 San Jacinto Blvd, Mail Stop D3500, Austin, TX 78712, USA
e-mail: barbarajones@mail.utexas.edu

A.N. Abrams et al. (eds.), *Pediatric Psychosocial Oncology: Textbook for Multidisciplinary Care*,
DOI 10.1007/978-3-319-21374-3_14

Children, adolescents, and young adults with cancer and their families face extraordinary challenges during their diagnostic and treatment periods, including uncertainty about prognosis, fears of death, disability, risks in treatment choices, disruptions of school and social activities, changes in peer relationships, family upheaval, and economic hardship. Regardless of their ultimate survival outcomes, most patients experience substantial physical and emotional suffering during and after their cancer experience, which, in turn, may have long-term effects on patients, families, and larger communities (Wolfe et al. 2000a; Kreicbergs et al. 2004a; Rosenberg et al. 2015).

Box 14.1: "What Is Palliative Care?"

The active total care of a patient's mind, body, and spirit, including:

- Managing distressing symptoms
- Establishing goals of care
- Facilitating decision-making and advance care planning
- Providing additional psychosocial and/or spiritual support
- Facilitating home-based care including hospice
- Providing bereavement support for families

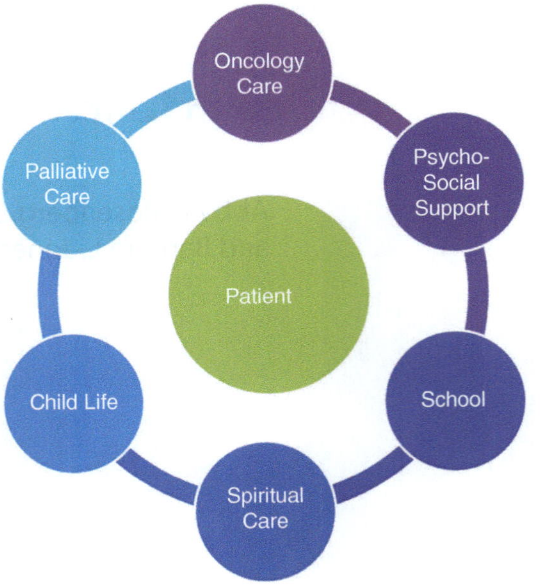

Fig. 14.1 Model of pediatric palliative care *approach* and *specialty*. Palliative care *approach* refers to interdisciplinary patient care that recognizes and meets the needs of the whole patient. Palliative care *subspecialty teams* fit within this approach and provide additional expertise (e.g., pain and symptom management, decision-making support, and/or advance care planning)

"Palliative care" refers to the active total care of a patient's body, mind, and spirit and therefore strongly complements the whole patient psychosocial care (WHO 2014). Although the term "palliative care" historically referred to care specific to patients at the end of life, its current definition is more holistic; it begins when illness is diagnosed and continues regardless of whether or not a child receives disease-directed treatment (WHO 2014). Pediatric palliative care (PPC) has emerged as both *an approach* and a *medical subspecialty* that improves the quality of life of patients and families facing the problems associated with life-threatening illness through prevention and relief of suffering (Fig. 14.1) (Wolfe and Sourkes 2011). Effectively integrating palliative care into the care of children with cancer requires a broad interdisciplinary perspective that includes the family and also makes use of available local and community resources. It may be provided in tertiary care facilities, community health centers, and children's homes.

Pediatric oncology care necessarily involves an interdisciplinary team, typically consisting of physicians, nurses, and psychosocial clinicians, as well as child life specialists, educators, chaplains, physical therapists, and subspecialty medical teams, depending on patient and family needs. While each member of the team has discipline-specific roles, all members are responsible for providing a steady presence, anticipatory guidance, assessment and relief of child and family distress, and response to questions and concerns. Palliative care teams also consist of multiple disciplines and provide additional perspective and skill, especially when prognosis is uncertain. PPC providers are trained to help children and families make choices consistent with their values and overall goals of care. They also have expertise in complex pain and symptom management, decision-making, and enabling patient quality of life despite the inherent restrictions of their illness.

The role and involvement of palliative care change over time. Early integration of oncology and PPC may facilitate patient and family adjustment, support, and comprehension of complicated and/or high-risk treatment plans. Later roles may include decision-making support for patients with poor prognoses, exploring overall goals of care, coordinating outpatient hospice care, and providing ongoing bereavement support.

For example, children with advanced cancer have high degrees of symptom burden and suffering from both physical and emotional causes (Wolfe et al. 2000a). Prognostic uncertainty is prevalent and patients' parents may be highly distressed (Rosenberg et al. 2013). For the more than 2000 children in the United States who die from their cancer each year (Onelov et al. 2007; Ries Lag et al. 1999), the anticipated time until death and how one should spend this time are often unclear. Clinical experience suggests that patients with some forms of incurable cancer may live for months to years; whereas others may be expected to die within weeks. All of these factors may inhibit mindful family decision-making and patient and family quality of life.

The empirical benefits of integrated palliative care include optimal pain and symptom management; better understanding of patient and family goals, values, and beliefs; stronger psychosocial and spiritual care; and improved patient and family quality of life. Many of these have been confirmed in the adult oncology literature. Among adults with terminal lung cancer, for example, palliative care has been associated with fewer physical symptoms, improved mood, and more accurate perceptions of prognosis. Patients who received standard oncology care integrated with palliative care survived longer than those who received oncology care alone, refuting presumptions that inclusion of palliative care would necessarily shorten patient's life expectancies (Temel et al. 2010). Multiple studies have suggested that palliative care involvement is associated with improved management of distressing symptoms, better communication, earlier recognition of prognosis, and fewer hospitalizations among other adult oncology populations (Greer et al. 2012; Bakitas et al. 2009; Epstein and Morrison 2012).

However, few studies have been conducted in pediatric oncology populations, and formal evidence of these benefits is sparse. In a study of over 24,000 children who died more than 5 days following an admission to a children's hospital, only 4 % received formal palliative care consultations. Those that did receive PPC consultations had fewer days in the hospital before death, received fewer medications, and were less likely to have invasive interventions or die in an intensive care unit (Keele et al. 2013). In pediatric oncology settings, increased focus on palliative care has resulted in improved advance care planning, including better preparation for end-of-life experiences and decreased pain among patients with advanced cancer (Wolfe et al. 2008).

Integrating palliative care into routine care for patients with advanced cancer is becoming more common in medical oncology settings but is unfortunately inconsistent in pediatric centers. Only 58 % of Children's Oncology Group institutions report having a formal PPC team (Dalberg et al. 2013; Johnston et al. 2008). Therefore, psychosocial clinicians may be responsible and have the opportunity to integrate the concepts of PPC into their care for children with cancer and their families. This PPC-inclusive approach provides a support system to help patients live as actively and as wholly as possible until death and to help families cope throughout the illness experience, bereavement, and beyond.

Caring for Children with Prognostic Uncertainty

Case Vignette

Jonah was 17 years old when his acute lymphoblastic leukemia came back for the first time. His doctors recommended a hematopoietic stem cell transplant (HSCT) as a potential curative option and explained that Jonah's disease was high risk and that chances for cure were less than 30 %.

Jonah and his family decided to proceed with the transplant. "Of course we would try it," said Jonah later. "I wanted to live, and 30 % was still good enough odds." During his months of treatment and recovery, he and his family remained optimistic he would survive, although each privately struggled with the angst of "what if it comes back?"

Unfortunately, Jonah's leukemia did come back. This time his doctors said his chances for cure were less than 5 %. "I didn't know what to do the second time around," he explained. "All of a sudden, the odds were really low. Part of me felt like the numbers couldn't be right and I should keep fighting, but another part said 'that's not how I want to live.'"

During the ensuing discussions, providers asked Jonah to articulate how he did want to live. As he came to understand that being home with his friends and family was most important to him, the decisions became more clear. "We decided to go with some oral chemotherapy that would slow the leukemia down, but not keep me in the hospital," he explained. "It took time for us to accept it, and there were times when I still couldn't. But we kept talking about my options, my goals, what my family hoped for, what mattered to us. That helped."

Prognostic Understanding and Communication

Several studies over the past decade have shown that there are discrepancies between physician and parent understanding of their child's cancer prognosis, both at diagnosis and when the illness is more advanced. For example, Wolfe et al. showed that providers tend to recognize the child as having no realistic chance for cure approximately 100 days before families do and approximately 200 days prior to the patient's death (Wolfe et al. 2000b). While this may be unsurprising (health-care personnel have prior training and experience recognizing incurable cancer), the discrepancy in recognition remains a critical issue in providing appropriate psychosocial care for patients and families. It is important that providers communicate to families when cure is unlikely as it influences when discussions regarding advance care goals and "do not resuscitate" (DNR) plans occur, with earlier communication leading to earlier discussions. Likewise, patients and families are more likely to endorse goals of "lessening suffering." Parents are then more prepared for their child's ultimate death, and physicians perceive the child's death as more peaceful (Wolfe et al. 2000b; Maurer et al. 2010).

In contrast, when parents are unaware of their child's impending death, children are more likely to die in the ICU and to receive cure-directed therapy that may impair their overall quality of life (and quality of death) (Valdimarsdottir et al. 2007). Parents with less time to prepare for their child's death are more likely to have long-term psychological morbidities (Valdimarsdottir et al. 2007; Lannen et al. 2008), poor physical health, and poor quality of life (Jalmsell et al. 2011). These findings suggest that effective parent-provider communication and promotion of concordance regarding prognosis and goals of care will improve patient and family experiences. Unfortunately, doing so is challenging.

Barriers to End-of-Life Communication

Parent Factors Parents of children with cancer tend to be more optimistic than their providers regarding the likelihood of cure both at the time of diagnosis (Mack et al. 2007a) and when cancer progresses or recurs (Mack et al. 2008; Rosenberg et al. 2014b). Parents with less education tend to have disproportionately poorer concordance with their medical team regarding cure likelihood

(Rosenberg et al. 2014b; Mack et al. 2007a). However, no studies (to date) have included sufficient numbers of participants to fully explore other demographic or cultural determinants of parent perspectives. Furthermore, evidence suggests that parents may not be willing to formally endorse their child's impending death (Rosenberg et al. 2014a). When parents of children with advanced cancer were asked what actions supported them in good parenting, they reported that knowing "all that can be done is being done" was the most important way that health-care professionals could support them (Hinds et al. 2009). Yet, in retrospect, parents may experience some decisional regret, especially when children experience high degrees of physical or emotional suffering at the end of life (Mack et al. 2008).

Relational Factors In retrospect, bereaved parents endorse relational aspects of care as indicators of high quality care. Specifically, higher parent ratings of physician care were associated with physicians giving clear information about what to expect in the end-of-life period, delivering information sensitively, speaking directly with the child, and preparing the parent for the child's death (Mack et al. 2005). In contrast, parents who become aware of their child's impending death during his last 24 hours report poorer communication and less satisfaction with their medical teams (Valdimarsdottir et al. 2007). Likewise, siblings of children with cancer are at greater risk for poor adjustment and long-term morbidities when they are not included in end-of-life discussions or preparation (Rosenberg et al. 2015). It follows that good communication is a key component of parent satisfaction and quality of care. See Chapter 2 for more information about communication.

Medical Factors Parent-provider concordance also may be associated with specific cancer types or medical interventions. For example, parents of children with leukemia have reported shorter awareness times prior to their child's death than parents of children with other types of cancer (Valdimarsdottir et al. 2007). Similarly, the first documentation of a child's unlikely cure is approximately 4 days prior to death for children on hematopoietic stem cell transplant (HSCT) services, compared to 84 days prior to death for children receiving standard hematology/oncology care (Ullrich et al. 2010a). These observations provide opportunities for intervention and suggest that families of children undergoing HSCT may need additional communication and decision-making support.

Medical Provider Factors Among oncology providers, personal distress may create a barrier to end-of-life communication. A majority of pediatric oncologists find breaking bad news highly stressful. Nearly a quarter of pediatric oncologists say it is "the worst part of the job," and more than half feel a personal sense of failure when cure is no longer possible (Hilden et al. 2001). Another barrier may be that providers wish not to "take away hope" or contribute to additional patient and parent distress. There is no evidence that open and realistic discussions of prognosis do either (Mack and Smith 2012). Rather, parents who know their child's anticipated trajectory are better able to cope and make decisions they feel are appropriate for their child, family, and values (Mack et al. 2007b).

High-quality prognostic communication may improve with clinician experience. Physicians who are older or more experienced tend to have higher rates of concordance with their patients' families regarding cure likelihood and goals of care (Mack et al. 2007a; Rosenberg et al. 2014b). While most providers report learning their communication skills through trial and error (Hilden et al. 2001), recent studies suggest that effective advance care communication skills can be taught (Back et al. 2007; Bylund et al. 2010).

Overcoming Barriers A critical component of effective communication is recognizing these barriers and understanding why they exist. The death of a child seems inherently unnatural. It is normal for parents to hold out hope for a cure, extended life, or a miracle. "Leaving no stone unturned" is an appropriate parent response (Bluebond-Langner et al. 2007). Recent evidence suggests that mild (e.g., outpatient, oral) cancer-directed therapy may be psychologically beneficial to children as well (Wolfe et al. 2015).

Providers are responsible for relaying information honestly and compassionately such that families may establish appropriate goals of care, make informed decisions, and fully support their child's whole well-being. Interdisciplinary staff may be helpful, if not necessary, for successful communication. Wolfe et al. have previously found that involvement of a psychosocial or PPC clinician in end-of-life care is associated with alignment of physician and parent prognostic understanding and likely patient and family experiences as a whole (Wolfe et al. 2000b).

Guidelines for Effective Communication regarding Prognosis and Goals of Care

Several strategies for effective communication have been described (Von Gunten et al. 2000; Baile et al. 2000; Beale et al. 2005; Makoul 2001), all of which include similar guiding principles and efforts to make a human connection with the child and family (Table 14.1). A simple but successful outcome of effective communication regarding prognosis or goals of care is when families are able to "expect the worst" (e.g., fully understand and anticipate potentially difficult experiences, including the child's death) while also "hoping for the best" (e.g., maintaining realistic hopes and goals while also identifying with their own good parent roles). This dual reality may, in turn, promote better patient and family coping, adjustment, and quality of life (Hill et al. 2013).

Decision-Making and Advance Care Planning

At more advanced stages of cancer, delineation of goals of care becomes a particularly important element of decision-making. When goals are clear, decisions regarding therapy may fall into place. For example, a parent whose goal is to "extend time with my child, without hope of cure" may decline intensive inpatient chemotherapy in favor of oral medications that can be administered at home. This alignment is especially true when clinicians apply models of shared decision-making, where exploring goals of care with patients and families may lead to discussions of how those goals may be best met (Waldman and Wolfe 2013).

Box 14.2: Phrases and Questions That May Elicit Goals of Care

Words that work: common phrases and questions used to elicit goals of care
Tell me about you (your child) as a person.
What is your understanding of your (your child's) illness?
In light of your understanding, what is most important to you?
What are you hoping for? What are your worries?
In times of difficulty, where do you find your strength? How well is that working for you?
What do you think has caused you (your child) to suffer the most?
What makes you (your child) most joyful?

Advance care planning (ACP) refers to the process of thinking about, talking about, and planning for future health care and end-of-life care. Engaging in ACP may be challenging for the same reasons it is difficult for patients, parents, and providers to discuss poor prognosis. In essence, preparing for a child's death may feel inherently unnatural and be plagued by emotional distress, avoidance, and uncertainty. Determining if, when, and to what extent pediatric and adolescent patients are included in ACP discussions may be an additional challenge. Parents and providers may want to protect their children and therefore deliberately shield them from difficult conversations (de Vries et al. 2010). However, children ages 14 years and older often have adult-level comprehension of their situation and the consequences of their decisions. Patients between 10 and 20 years old report that "thinking about their relationships with others" is the single most

Table 14.1 Guidelines for effective communication regarding prognosis and goals of care

Step	Practice	Examples
1.	Prepare for the discussion	Setting up the interview, planning the setting, establishing a protocol for communication, and determining who should be present (this should involve efforts to understand and respect a family's own needs and styles for communication, including when/how to involve the child him- or herself)
2.	Establish what the patient and family already know, as well as their objectives for the conversation	(For first-time interactions): "I have read your medical chart and learned about you, but it would help me to hear, in your own words, what is your understanding of what is happening with your child?" (For already established relationships):"I have some things I'd like to talk about today, but before I start, I'd like to know what you hope to discuss?"
3.	Deliver information	Explaining medical information according to the child's developmental status and the family's needs and choosing appropriate strategies, including assessments of family's understanding (these may also include obtaining an invitation from the patient/family)
4.	Respond to emotions	Listening attentively, maintaining openness, providing safe silence, and affirming the love and struggle that went into particular decisions
5.	Establish goals for care and treatment priorities	"As you think about what is ahead for your child, what is most important to you?" "What does good quality of life look like for your child?"
6.	Establish a plan	Evaluating understanding, summarizing, and delineating next steps. This step underscores the ongoing nature of the relationship, decisions being made, and supportive care

important factor in their choices regarding continued cancer treatment and goals of care (Hinds et al. 2005). Nearly all adolescents and young adults living with life-threatening illness report wanting to be able to choose and record the kind of treatment they do (and do not) want, how they want to be cared for, what they want to share with others, and how they want to be remembered (Wiener et al. 2012).

Evidence suggests patients as young as 3 years old are aware of their prognosis without being told (Bluebond-Langner 1978). Patients of all ages who are unaware or shielded may paradoxically feel greater distress or anxiety by "not knowing;" providing age-appropriate honest information may alleviate some patients' fears. When patients are present for initial discussions about diagnosis and prognosis, parent distress is significantly decreased (Mack et al. 2006). Likewise, among over 400 bereaved parents, none of those who talked to their child about death regretted having done so, but 27 % of those who avoided the topic regretted the lost opportunity (Kreicbergs et al. 2004b). The corollary is also true; nearly three quarters of parents did not experience regret. Most important, therefore, is to uncover and respect the family communication style.

One approach to gauge readiness for advance care planning is to ask patients and families: (1) whether talking about what would happen if treatment was no longer effective would be helpful, (2) whether talking about medical care plans ahead of time would be upsetting, and (3) whether they would be comfortable writing down/discussing what would happen if treatments were no longer effective (Wiener et al. 2008). Other more specific and age-appropriate instruments have also been developed and can help guide conversations and address critical elements of patient and family values, beliefs, goals, hopes, and worries (Table 14.2) (Zadeh et al. 2014; agingwithdignity.org).

Other types of anticipatory guidance should include discussions about the child's resuscitation status, preferred location of death, organ and/or tissue donation and autopsy, and funeral planning. Of note, many children who die from advanced cancer will not be candidates for organ donation due to concerns for disseminated cancer in body tissues. Other children only have isolated eligible tissues (e.g., their corneas). It is important to communicate to families who wish to donate that their preference is heard and honored, even if it cannot be met. Autopsy should be

Table 14.2 Examples of advance care planning tools

Age group	Tool name	Included concepts	Examples of activities
Pediatric	"My wishes"	How I want people to treat me How comfortable I want to be What I want my loved ones to know What I want my doctors and nurses to know	Drawing, storytelling, journaling
Adolescent and young adult	"Voicing my CHOiCES"	How I want to be comforted How I would like to be supported (so I don't feel so alone) Who I want to make my medical care decisions if I cannot make them on my own Types of life support I want or do not want What I would like my family and friends to know me My spiritual thoughts and wishes How I wish to be remembered	Detailed checklists of advance directives including delegated decision-makers and requests for "do not resuscitate" discussions, as well as open-ended storytelling, journaling, and directed writings
Adults (>18 years old)	"5 Wishes"	The person I want to make health-care decisions when I can't The kind of medical treatment I want (or don't want) How comfortable I want to be How I want people to treat me What I want my loved ones to know	Detailed checklists of advanced directives, legally binding in 42 states in the United States. Also includes open space for free writing and individual requests

Available at http://agingwithdignity.org/catalog

NB: These are three examples of commercially available guides for clinicians and health-care providers. Experience suggests these tools are most effective when completed with a provider who is familiar with them. The corresponding booklets need not be completed in one sitting; rather, various topics should be introduced when clinically indicated.

offered to every family. In a study of 30 bereaved parents, only 37 % recalled a conversation about autopsy, and 90 % of those who did not recall such conversations suggested they would have considered the procedure. The majority of parents indicated that discussions about autopsy would be appropriate when it is clear that cure is no longer possible, rather than at the time of their child's death. Furthermore, educating parents about the potential research, emotional, and clinical benefits of autopsy would enable their informed decision-making (Wiener et al. 2014). Parents who choose autopsy for their children often do so to advance medical knowledge and/or respect their child's wishes. Among 33 bereaved parents of children with brain tumors, none who requested autopsy regretted it, and 91 % stated they would make the same choice again (Baker et al. 2013). We have found that some parents may also find peace in knowing the definitive cause of their child's death, while others may decline because they feel that they "know" the cause. Either choice is appropriate.

PPC care team involvement can help facilitate ACP. If PPC providers were involved early in the cancer experience, they may have joined the primary psychosocial oncology team in helping the family with initial adjustments to cancer and to challenges that develop over time. Later PPC involvement may then feel more seamless in advanced stages of the illness (Waldman and Wolfe 2013). Studies have shown that changes in terminology (e.g., "advanced care team" or "supportive care team") may also lead to increased referrals, particularly later in the cancer experience (Dalal et al. 2011). Better description of palliative care as 'an added layer of support' may also enable its involvement. PPC expertise can help guide communication, enabling medical personnel to effectively and compassionately relay difficult concepts, thereby facilitating family understanding and, in turn, realistic expectations. Furthermore, PPC can assist with very difficult decision-making for parents, providers, and patients alike. Combined, PPC involvement may alleviate patient, parent, and provider suffering.

Continued Cancer-Directed Therapy and Phase I Clinical Trials

In advanced pediatric cancer, it is often unclear to what extent cancer-directed treatment will be effective. And as described above, it is natural for parents (and providers) to hold out hope for a cure and leave no stone unturned. This continued search for treatment options often includes consideration of enrollment in phase I clinical trials. Few studies, however, have described how parents or providers make decisions about experimental therapies. The goal of phase I research is to identify appropriate dosage and safety data for new drugs, not to demonstrate efficacy or to impact curability. It is unclear how many patients or parents are aware of this fact (Agrawal and Emanuel 2003). For example, the most common reason parents enroll in clinical research studies is to receive some direct medical benefit for their child; only 20 % report wanting to help future patients (Truong et al. 2011). Most adolescent patients hope enrolling in phase I studies will extend their lives (Miller et al. 2013), but many also endorse wanting to help other patients (Wendler et al. 2012). It is the responsibility of the interdisciplinary team to explore patients' and families' understanding of phase I research, their reasons for enrolling, and their hopes and other goals of care. Often, these conversations can be easily integrated into other decision-making and ACP discussions.

Patients with advanced cancer may also request continued, nonexperimental cancer-directed therapy, even when its efficacy is limited. This request may align with goals of care and parenting roles, as well as alleviate patient suffering and prolong time with family. Sometimes, however, cancer-directed therapy can directly impede quality of life, due to side effects, the need to be proximal to the hospital, restrictions in activities, and other clinical (or investigational study) requirements. Understanding patients' and/or families' specific values and goals of cancer-directed therapy therefore becomes more important over time. Eventually, quality of life may become a major factor in patient, parent, and provider decision-making, and providers must enable families to support the child's quality of life, perhaps by giving them permission to reframe their goals and responsibilities.

Concurrent Care Models

The integration of palliative care has never necessitated forgoing other forms of treatment; however, because families and providers may link palliative care and hospice with the cessation of cancer-directed therapy, referrals to palliative care may occur late. In the United States, this bias may extend from legislation passed in the 1980s, defining hospice as a Medicare benefit that required patients to have a prognosis of 6 months or less and because of limited reimbursement mechanisms also required patients to forgo continued cancer-directed therapy. Outside of the United States, hospice is a term used to describe a philosophy of care that focuses on alleviating the suffering of patients with advanced illness. It may also be used in association with a specific location for end-of-life services.

Hospice care for pediatric cancer patients remains largely underutilized in the United States, perhaps because it is associated with similar barriers to palliative care services (Fowler et al. 2006). One approach to promoting early and ongoing PPC involvement is the relatively new provision of palliative and hospice care concurrently with cancer-related therapies. In 2010, the United States implemented the Affordable Care Act (ACA) in an effort to expand population access to multiple medical services. Included in this program was a provision, Section 2303, termed the "Concurrent Care for Children" Requirement (CCCR), allowing publicly insured children with life-limiting illness to receive "curative" treatments like chemotherapy or dialysis concurrently with hospice care. The program has several notable limitations, including a stipulation that children receiving this benefit have a life expectancy of fewer than 6 months. While the program has the potential to allow children with high needs to receive complete end-of-life care at home, few states have successfully implemented models of concurrent care for pediatric cancer patients to date. The long-term effect of this critical change has yet to be measured (Bona et al. 2014).

Location of Death

As research and clinical efforts have focused on improving quality of palliative and end-of-life care for children with cancer, the location of their deaths has also received attention. In the United States, most children and families may choose between death at home (with or without hospice) and death in the hospital. Very few states offer free-standing hospice facilities. In contrast, the latter are more standard in the United Kingdom and Canada. In Canada, parents of children with cancer and their health-care providers tend to prefer home as their first choice for end-of-life care and for the location of their child's death (Kassam et al. 2014). Most importantly, however, is that families have the opportunity to plan the location of their child's death, because in doing so, they experience less decisional regret (Dussel et al. 2009).

One challenge in enabling children to die at home is concurrently meeting their pain and symptom management needs. Children may often return to the hospital for intractable symptom control or because parents become overwhelmed or exhausted while caring for them. Children who receive PPC services, however, are more likely to die in their or their parents' preferred location, providing another testament to the value of palliative care team integration in pediatric cancer care (Postier et al. 2014; Friedrichsdorf et al. 2015). Comprehensive end-of-life care should therefore address these preferences early, in order to plan and accommodate patient and/or family wishes.

Pain and Symptom Management

Pain and symptom management is often the initial or primary reason for a palliative care referral. Parents of children with cancer report that pain, emotional distress, fatigue, and nutrition "cause the most problems" during cancer treatment, and these problems are associated with parent and survivor distress (Heden et al. 2013; Poder et al. 2010; Rosenberg et al. 2013). The most commonly reported symptoms are fatigue, reduced mobility, pain, anorexia, nausea, vomiting, and disordered mood, and these are often intertwined (Jalmsell et al. 2006). Many physical symptoms have psychosocial components and vice versa (Wolfe et al. 2015). For example, 96 % of children experience fatigue in the last month of life, and suffering from fatigue is associated with additional suffering from pain, dyspnea, anxiety, sadness, fear, diarrhea, nausea, vomiting, and anorexia (Ullrich et al. 2010b).

Certain cancer types, treatment regimens, and patient-ages may be related to symptom complaints and their management. For example, patients with central nervous system (CNS) tumors have higher prevalence of neurocognitive deficits, impaired speech, or other motor dysfunctions (Jalmsell et al. 2006). Some studies suggest patients with leukemia or lymphoma report worse physical and psychosocial quality of life compared to those with solid non-CNS and CNS tumors, and recent HSCT is associated with worse psychosocial health (Tomlinson et al. 2011). Other studies suggest that patients with bone sarcoma have greater disability and inferior quality of life (Nagarajan et al. 2004; Barrera et al. 2012). Finally, patients diagnosed as adolescents and young adults may be at higher risk of depression, anxiety, and fatigue (Poder et al. 2010).

At the end of life, the prevalence of troubling symptoms is particularly high; 89 % of bereaved parents believe their children suffered "a lot" or "a great deal" in the last month of life (Wolfe et al. 2000b). Unfortunately, treatment of specific symptoms is frequently inadequate. For example, bereaved parents report their child received treatment for pain (80 %), dyspnea (70 %), or fatigue (20 %), but these treatments were successful in only 27, 16, and 5 % of cases, respectively (Wolfe et al. 2000a). Additionally, the symptoms that become the most distressing to parents are those which are persistently unrelieved (Pritchard et al. 2010), and parents are more likely to consider hastening their child's death if they believe their child is suffering (Dussel et al. 2010).

Alleviating suffering at the end of life is challenging in part because symptoms may become more refractory to standard interventions (Pritchard et al. 2008). However, studies suggest recent and progressive improvements. Comparing pediatric cancer patients who died in the early 1990s and those who died in the later 1990s and early 2000s, the latter cohort more commonly discussed hospice and/or DNR wishes, less commonly died in the ICU, and less commonly reported suffering from pain or dyspnea, and their parents more commonly felt prepared for the child's death (Wolfe et al. 2008). These strides may reflect more global awareness of child symptom burden, whole family psychosocial needs, and standard PPC involvement at the end of a child's life.

Financial Implications

Case Vignette
Carlos is 8 years old when his rhabdomyosarcoma recurs. He and his parents relocate to a new city with a large academic medical center to receive an experimental therapy. They understand his prognosis is poor but feel a need to exhaust all options regarding possible curative options. Moving has required that Carlos' mother quit her job to remain at the bedside. His father continues to work in their home community and care for Carlos' two older siblings. This has caused a great deal of social and financial hardship for the family, and they struggle to navigate what is best for their family.

The economic impact of pediatric cancer on patients' families can be profound and long lasting; however, formal investigation of this impact is relatively recent. Costs may relate to concrete medical expenses as well as unmeasured costs related to lost income, financial debt, work disruption, and other material hardships. For example, family spending may be redirected toward the pediatric patient's medical needs, thereby impacting patient and sibling recreational activities, education choices, diet, and lifestyle choices. These more intangible costs of cancer are independently associated with parent psychological distress, in turn affecting patient and family well-being (Rosenberg et al. 2013; Tsimicalis et al. 2011). Financial hardship is an additional and critical stressor that may contribute to poor outcomes including survivorship or morbidity (Lightfoot et al. 2012; Bona et al. 2015).

Among families of children with advanced cancer, 94 % report work disruptions and 42 % report that at least one parent had to quit work in order to care for their child. Twenty-seven percent reported "great economic hardship" due to their child's cancer. Families at or below 200 % of the federal poverty level (FPL) were disproportionately affected; half of the poorest families lost more than 40 % of their annual income compared with 5 % of the wealthiest families (Bona et al. 2014).

Similar findings have been described among bereaved families. Among families who were between 3 and 5 years bereaved, over 80 % reported work disruptions resulting from their child's cancer. Sixty percent of families lost at least 10 % of their total income, and 19 % of families lost more than 40 %. Again, poor families experienced the greatest proportional loss, and after accounting for income lost, 15 % of American families fell below the FPL (Dussel et al. 2011). Interdisciplinary teams must be mindful of these financial stressors and strive to provide appropriate support to patients and families. Meeting families' needs must include directed psychosocial support, as well as additional interventions to reduce the risk of economic hardship.

Spiritual Implications

The implications of spirituality and meaning-making in comprehensive cancer care for children are addressed in detail in Chapter 18.

However, supporting patient and family spirituality in advanced illness is critical in advanced cancer for several reasons: (1) It addresses existential questions that may predominate when patients approach death, such as "why did this happen?"; (2) it may be a driving force in helping families to cope with cancer; (3) it may be a source of hope and comfort, contributing to better acceptance of the child's impending death; and (4) it may guide family decision-making and goals of care (Hexem et al. 2011).

Comprehensive spiritual care is beyond the scope of most clinicians. Among adult cancer patients, 88 % say spirituality is important and 72 % say their spiritual needs are unmet by their medical team (Balboni et al. 2007). Approximately one-third of pediatricians understand spirituality is important, but fewer than 10 % ask their patients about it (Grossoehme et al. 2007). Common reasons for not discussing spirituality include providers feeling it "is not their role," worrying about offending the family, feeling personally uncomfortable with the topic, or having limited time and resources to do so (Curlin et al. 2007). Compared to the general public, pediatric oncologists are less likely to believe in God, attend religious services, or consider themselves moderately or more spiritual; in contrast, however, they more commonly believe in basic "religious truths" such as "do unto others as you would have done to yourself" than population norms (Ecklund et al. 2007).

The power of the medical team in supporting religious and spiritual beliefs is significant. In a multisite, prospective cohort study of adults with advanced cancer, high community religious support was associated with more intensive end-of-life care including death in the ICU. In contrast, high spiritual support from the medical team (meaning the medical team inquired and supported patients' spiritual wishes) was associated with greater receipt of hospice services and less intensive medical interventions such as cardiopulmonary resuscitation and ICU death (Balboni et al. 2013).

Relatively few studies have described the role of spirituality in end-of-life care for pediatric cancer patients, and findings regarding its import are conflicting. For example, some parents describe spiritual care as necessary, whereas others may feel angry at God or reject their prior beliefs and communities (Hexem et al. 2011). For these reasons, determining the role of spiritual support for the child and their family is especially challenging and warrants the involvement of chaplains in the interdisciplinary care team. Various models for integrating chaplaincy in pediatric palliative care have been proposed; which works best may depend on the setting and available resources (Fitchett et al. 2011).

Cultural Implications

Providing appropriate whole patient care for individuals with different life experiences, beliefs, values, languages, and notions of health care requires cultural awareness and humility. This is particularly important in advanced illness. There is paucity of literature describing the cultural considerations for pediatrics in general, let alone for pediatric patients with advanced cancer.

Dealing with the potential or real loss of a child is extremely challenging in any culture; however, specific cultural influences may further complicate PPC involvement (De Trill and Kovalcik 1997). Nearly 40 % of health-care providers have identified cultural differences as a frequent barrier to adequate palliative care (Davies et al. 2008). For example, Latino families may hesitate to integrate palliative care strategies because their cultural beliefs tend to imply that parents must exhaust all possible options, regardless of the potential for success (Thibodeaux and Deatrick 2007). The underutilization of palliative care services among ethnic minorities has been described and often attributed to the lack of familiarity with the terminology, language barriers, religious differences, distrust of medical systems, physician factors, and other factors (Wiener et al. 2013).

A systematic review of the available literature identified seven distinct themes regarding the influence of culture on pediatric palliative care (Wiener et al. 2013). First, cultural norms and customs affect family decision-making styles and should therefore be integrated into all discussions from the time of diagnosis. These may include traditions of consulting with community or family elders, deference to family boundaries (including the role of the child-patient in decision-making), and gender. Second, religious faith may mandate certain practices or customs at the end of life, including the presence of clergy, death rituals, decisions about autopsy, and discussions about the afterlife and/or reincarnation. Providers should inquire about these customs early and endeavor to support and respect them.

Third, language differences may create significant barriers to quality medical care, including end-of-life care. These barriers are more complicated than simple medical interpretation, although trained medical interpreters are imperative. Rather, cultural nuances can have profound impact on family experience and the degree of therapeutic alliance between families and providers. For example, reluctance to discuss end-of-life care may stem from belief that acknowledging the child's impending death will, in fact, hasten it (Liu et al. 1999). In such cases, unsuspecting providers may, in fact, cause parental anxiety by attempting to bring up the topic. Likewise, nonverbal communication styles have their own implications. Some cultures see touching a patient's head as compassionate, whereas others see it as intrusive or disrespectful (Washington 2011). Providers should endeavor to understand their patients' and families' cultural beliefs in order to avoid offense and to foster cooperative, successful communication.

Fourth, various cultures may have opposing views of the inclusion of children in care planning. While Western philosophy recommends that parents openly and truthfully communicate with their children, particularly their adolescents and young adults, nondisclosure of a child's life-threatening diagnosis is acceptable, if not preferred, in multiple other cultures (Elwyn et al. 1998). Fifth, cultural and language barriers may create challenges in the assessment of pain and symptom complaints (Anderson et al. 2000). The perception, experience, and preferred treatment of pain all vary by culture (Davidhizar and Giger 2004). Sixth, there are cultural differences in the meaning behind pain, illness, suffering, and death. For example, suffering may be a mechanism for atoning for sins in this or a former life and may therefore be necessary to gain entry into heaven or to avoid pain in future lives (Davidhizar and Giger 2004; Mazanec and Tyler 2003). Seventh, cultural differences may dictate where children die. Among Chinese individuals, some believe death at home is bad luck, whereas others believe that if a child dies in the hospital, his soul would be lost (Mazanec and Tyler 2003). Likewise, the public versus private display of grief may be guided by cultural perspectives. In all of these cases, cultural competency is critical to providing optimal clinical and psychosocial care.

Geographic barriers also exist and these are particularly important because over 90 % of global childhood cancer deaths occur in low- or middle-income countries (Wolfe 2011). While awareness of PPC (and how to deliver it) has improved in developed nations, the rest of the world has not seen such strides. The children who die in underdeveloped nations will therefore do so without basic cancer care or pain relief (Delgado et al. 2010). Barriers to care include delays in diagnosis, limited access to curative therapies and pain management and opioids in particular, insufficient or undertrained staff, and other financial, social, or geographic barriers (Clemens et al. 2007).

To overcome these barriers, the World Health Organization (WHO) has defined palliative care as a human right (WHO 2014). The organization has continued to lobby to make this issue a priority and is working to facilitate partnerships within and across nations to provide appropriate training, resources, and services to children who die from serious illness (Delgado et al. 2010).

When Death Is Imminent

Case Vignette

Emily, an 8-year-old girl, was diagnosed with a diffuse intrinsic pontine glioma several months ago. She initially received palliative radiation therapy in order to slow the progression of her tumor. Now, her symptoms have again worsened and her death seems imminent. She suffers from persistent headache pain, which is being treated by her home hospice team. Her parents and siblings are suffering, too. They worry she will suddenly stop breathing and that they will not be present to say goodbye. They ask about what to expect, how they can continue to support her, and how they should include her friends and siblings in her final days.

Death is dynamic and influenced by physiologic processes such as the underlying disease process, concurrent physical health, nutrition, and mental status, as well as less understood spiritual and emotional factors. PPC aspires to enable a "better" death experience for the child and their family. This aspiration implies pain and symptom control as well as preparation for the death itself. It is therefore important that providers recognize when death is imminent and communicate to families what to expect.

Family members may hesitate to leave the bedside, for fear that their child will die in their absence. As such, it can be helpful to guide families in recognizing signs of impending death. To introduce the topic, we recommend simply asking whether it would be helpful to know more about what to expect as the child is dying. The following discussion should be clear and concise; however, it is also important to warn parents that it may not be possible to know the exact moment when death will occur. We have observed that some children choose the moment of their death; some choose to die when their parent is not present as a last effort to protect the parent from further suffering, while others seem to wait until needed family members are present to say "goodbye." Sharing these observations may provide additional comfort to families.

Common signs of impending death are progressive and include weakness, fatigue, loss of appetite, inattention or disorientation to time, urinary incontinence or retention, low blood pressure, mottling or cooling of the skin, agitation, delirium, and coma. One of the most distressing signs to parents may be changes in respiratory patterns including noisy breathing (often mislabeled as "death rattle") and Cheyne-Stokes respirations. The latter are characterized by oscillation between shortness of breath and non-breathing, with fluctuations in the depth of respirations. When describing these anticipated patterns to parents, it is important to remind them also that children do not suffer during these respiratory patterns, nor are they painful to the patient.

Most children die peacefully, especially when experienced clinicians provide their care. Rare circumstances, however, can result in the child experiencing sudden, high distress. These include tension pneumothorax, airway obstruction, bowel obstruction, hemorrhage, and seizure and may require more invasive treatment strategies to alleviate suffering. Although it may be challenging to describe these circumstances to patients and families, it is important to be transparent about the possible circumstances and discuss how they might be managed.

There are times at the end of a child's life when discontinuing medical interventions becomes appropriate. For example, the drive to eat and drink wanes as death approaches. Experience with adults suggests they do not feel hunger or thirst (Dalal et al. 2009); however, parents may feel great anxiety in minimizing their child's nutrition. Furthermore, if they do elect to limit their child's fluids and nutrition, they should be counseled on the expected changes in their child's appearance in order to minimize their reactive distress.

Another example of limiting medical intervention is when ventilatory support is discontinued. This is one of the most common ways children die in the ICU and often follows a consensus that ventilator dependence is irreversible and continued ventilatory support will not result in a meaningful quality of life. Following withdrawal from the ventilator, most children die within hours to days. Before withdrawing, however, families should be informed of all potential outcomes, including the possibility that their child *will* take a breath and even survive. In any of these difficult cases, it is helpful to provide reassurance to parents and families that they have made the best decision possible for their child (Feudtner et al. 2015).

Finally, there are numerous activities that families may engage in during the final periods of their child's life (as well as immediately afterward). These include legacy-building projects that contribute to family memories and provide comfort. Examples include prints or molds of the child's hands and feet, obtaining a lock of hair, making a memory box or book, and taking photographs or videos. It is important to offer a variety of possibilities in order to find those that appeal to individual family members while also respecting a family's decision to decline.

In summary, caring for a dying child is an intimate and emotional experience that involves great privilege. Meeting the needs of patients and families is critical during the time leading up to and following the child's death and requires an interdisciplinary approach (Fig. 14.2).

Bereavement

The death of a child has a profound and lasting impact on parents, siblings, family, and the community. When a child dies, the entire family is thrust into an often overwhelming period of bereavement and suffering. In fact, death of a child is known to be a predictor for complicated mourning and grief (Enright and Marwit 2002; Kacel et al. 2011; Meert et al. 2011). Bereaved parents experience increased risk of depression, posttraumatic stress, prolonged grief, suicidal ideation, isolation, physical health decline, and behavioral health concerns (Rosenberg et al. 2012; Vega et al. 2014). While some of these outcomes are normal and cannot necessarily be prevented, bereaved parents are also at increased risk for prolonged grief disorder (PGD), which may include symptoms of extended physical and psychological distress, sleep disturbances, and poorer health outcomes (Prigerson et al. 2009). Grief reactions of parents have been shown to persist longer and have more intensity than grief experienced due to loss of spouse or parent (Kacel et al. 2011). In one study, bereaved parents were shown to have higher overall rates of mortality from both natural and unnatural causes (Li et al. 2003). There is also evidence that parental grief reactions of mothers and fathers may differ based on both sociocultural norms and the intensity of the caregiving experience (Alam et al. 2012). While there is a depth of research about the clinical presentation of bereavement following the death of a child, there is less evidence of empirically based interventions to support parents in the hospital after the death of a child.

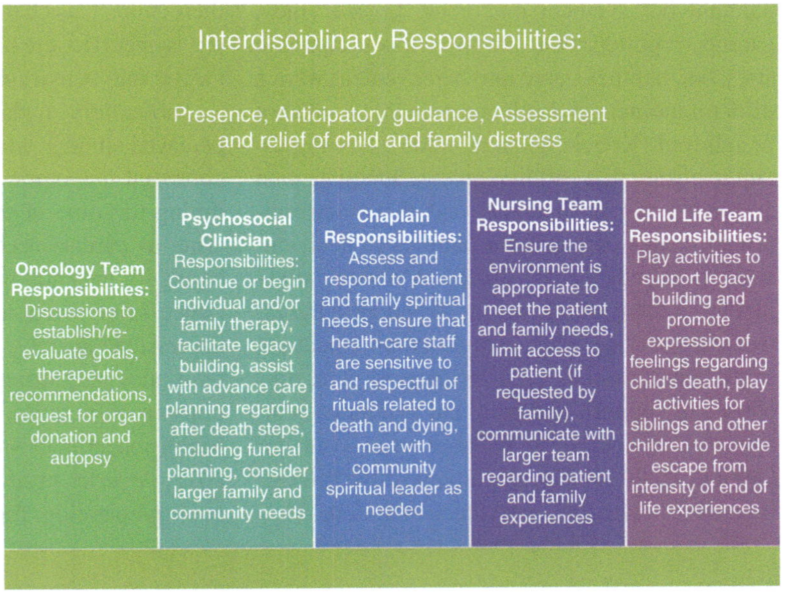

Fig. 14.2 Suggested interdisciplinary roles when caring for imminently dying children

A recent review by Donovan et al. of hospital-based bereavement services identified the importance of transitional bereavement support for families after the death of a child (Donovan et al. 2015). The most common interventions being offered included phone support at significant time points, educational materials, group programs, sibling camps, remembrance programs, and post bereavement visits (Donovan et al. 2015). In the aggregate, these hospital-based bereavement services provided the following benefits for bereaved families: feeling cared for and supported, building a new community, and improved coping and personal growth. Additionally, staff found meaning and satisfaction from providing bereavement support to families after the death of a child. While bereavement services in hospitals are often underfunded and difficult to sustain, the positive impact on parental grief and staff satisfaction suggest that hospitals should consider mechanisms to provide such services (Donovan et al. 2015).

Parents report that decision-making at the end of life is one of the most stressful aspects of treatment, and studies have shown that communication with health-care professionals can mitigate aspects of parental bereavement (Maurer et al. 2010). Therefore, how health-care teams provide care during life may greatly impact parental bereavement outcomes. In one study, parents reported that the two most common stressors that they carry into bereavement were a difficult moment at death and pain that could not be relieved (Kreicbergs et al. 2005). It is important to ensure that children receive adequate pain and symptom management and that interdisciplinary teams partner with families in decision-making (Hinds et al. 2012). A recent study identified the positive impact of pediatric palliative care services that include communication, shared decision-making, continuity of care, psychosocial support, and pain and symptom management on long-term parental grief (van der Geest et al. 2014). Specifically, positive interaction with health-care providers including communication, continuity of care and parental involvement, and symptom management showed a significant impact. Most parents report that care is better when physicians and health-care providers provide honest information with sensitivity, give clear expectations at the end of life, communicate directly with the child, and prepare the family for the death of the child (Mack et al. 2005).

Assessing for bereaved parents' needs following the death of the child may help professionals design programs to address their distress (Meert et al. 2010). Despite the intensity, length, and difficulty of parental grief, parents do survive and begin to regain a sense of their life without their child (Kreicbergs et al. 2004a; Vega et al. 2014). This process may be enhanced by providing psychosocial support and counseling to parents during their child's last month of life (Kreicbergs et al. 2007). Grief is a long and agonizing process, but parents report that being able to assign a sense of meaning to the experience and to the child's life can assist them in their recovery (Vega et al. 2014). In fact, recent grief theory and interventions support the importance of helping parents maintain continuing bonds with their deceased child, recognizing that grief is a lifelong process (Davies 2004; Klass 2006). In addition, most parents appreciate continued contact and communication with those who cared for their child. This challenges our health-care delivery system to create models of care that can extend into bereavement.

Particularly underserved are the needs of bereaved siblings who may suffer long-term psychosocial outcomes. Siblings often feel isolated during the time of treatment of their brother or sister as parents need to focus their energies on caring for the child who is ill. Siblings may experience grief reactions that include guilt, anger, depression, anxiety, and confusion. In the long term, they may struggle with substance use, relationship difficulties, and other behavioral and health concerns (Foster et al. 2012; Gerhardt et al. 2012; Alderfer et al. 2010). Siblings report that poor preparation for the death, dissatisfaction with communication, no chance to say goodbye, and negative impact of the cancer on their familial relationships contribute to higher distress (Rosenberg et al. 2015). Providing integrated psychosocial and/or PPC services to siblings during treatment and into bereavement may assist with these outcomes.

Despite the demonstrated need for parental and sibling grief interventions following the death of a child to cancer, the evidence of how to intervene is still unclear and inconclusive. Treatments for grief can include support from hospital staff during and beyond the illness, interpersonal therapy, cognitive behavioral therapy, group support, family-focused grief therapy, Internet and online support, and combined psychopharmacological treatments (Kacel et al. 2011). In supporting families following the death of a child, health-care systems should ensure that the team is fully staffed with behavioral healthcare providers such as psychologists, social workers, and child life specialists who can continue to work with the family after the death and can provide grief-specific interventions and community referrals to sustain the family in their grief process.

Summary

In summary, palliative care for children with cancer and their families involves an integrated interdisciplinary approach throughout the illness course. Pediatric palliative care uses psychosocial approaches to facilitate communication and advance care planning, holistic approaches to ease symptom distress and enhance well-being and quality of life in children and their families, and support anticipatory grief and bereavement. Such care is provided by the primary psychosocial oncology team from the time of diagnosis of cancer. As cancer advances or circumstances become more complex, children, families, and primary oncology clinicians may also benefit from the added support of a pediatric palliative care service.

Clinical Pearls

- "Palliative care" refers to the active total care of a patient's body, mind, and spirit.
- The prognostic uncertainties of pediatric cancer demand attention to ongoing communication, decision-making support, and, potentially, advance care planning.
- Children with advanced cancer and their families are at risk for additional physical, emotional, and spiritual suffering.
- Interdisciplinary providers have important and specific roles to play in providing support for both patients and families when death is imminent.

Pediatric palliative care can seamlessly complement the services available to patients and families in overwhelming situations, helping to alleviate their distress and promote their quality of life.

References

Agingwithdignity.Org. Aging with dignity. http://www.agingwithdignity.org/catalog

Agrawal ME, Emanuel EJ (2003) Ethics of phase 1 oncology studies: reexamining the arguments and data. JAMA 290:1075–1082

Alam R, Barrera M, D'agostino N et al (2012) Bereavement experiences of mothers and fathers over time after the death of a child due to cancer. Death Stud 36:1–22

Alderfer MA, Long KA, Lown EA et al (2010) Psychosocial adjustment of siblings of children with cancer: a systematic review. Psychooncology 19:789–805

Anderson KO, Mendoza TR, Valero V et al (2000) Minority cancer patients and their providers: pain management attitudes and practice. Cancer 88:1929–1938

Back AL, Arnold RM, Baile WF et al (2007) Efficacy of communication skills training for giving bad news and discussing transitions to palliative care. Arch Intern Med 167:453–460

Baile WF, Buckman R, Lenzi R et al (2000) SPIKES-A six-step protocol for delivering bad news: application to the patient with cancer. Oncologist 5:302–311

Baker JN, Windham JA, Hinds PS et al (2013) Bereaved parents' intentions and suggestions about research autopsies in children with lethal brain tumors. J Pediatr 163:581–586

Bakitas M, Lyons KD, Hegel MT et al (2009) Effects of a palliative care intervention on clinical outcomes in patients with advanced cancer: the Project ENABLE II randomized controlled trial. JAMA 302:741–749

Balboni TA, Vanderwerker LC, Block SD et al (2007) Religiousness and spiritual support among advanced cancer patients and associations with end-of-life treatment preferences and quality of life. J Clin Oncol 25:555–560

Balboni TA, Balboni M, Enzinger AC et al (2013) Provision of spiritual support to patients with advanced cancer by religious communities and associations with medical care at the end of life. JAMA Intern Med 173:1109–1117

Barrera M, Teall T, Barr R et al (2012) Health related quality of life in adolescent and young adult survivors of lower extremity bone tumors. Pediatr Blood Cancer 58:265–273

Beale EA, Baile WF, Aaron J (2005) Silence is not golden: communicating with children dying from cancer. J Clin Oncol 23:3629–3631

Bluebond-Langner M (1978) The private worlds of dying children. Princeton University Press, Princeton

Bluebond-Langner M, Belasco JB, Goldman A et al (2007) Understanding parents' approaches to care and treatment of children with cancer when standard therapy has failed. J Clin Oncol 25:2414–2419

Bona K, Dussel V, Orellana L et al (2014) Economic impact of advanced pediatric cancer on families. J Pain Symptom Manage 47(3):594–603

Bona K, London WB, Dongjing G, Abel G, Lehmann L, Wolfe J (2015) Prevalence and impact of financial hardship among New England pediatric stem cell transplantation families. Biol Blood Marrow Transplant 21(2):312–318

Bylund CL, Brown R, Gueguen JA et al (2010) The implementation and assessment of a comprehensive communication skills training curriculum for oncologists. Psychooncology 19:583–593

Clemens KE, Kumar S, Bruera E et al (2007) Palliative care in developing countries: what are the important issues? Palliat Med 21:173–175

Curlin FA, Lawrence RE, Odell S et al (2007) Religion, spirituality, and medicine: psychiatrists' and other physicians' differing observations, interpretations, and clinical approaches. Am J Psychiatry 164:1825–1831

Dalal S, Del Fabbro E, Bruera E (2009) Is there a role for hydration at the end of life? Curr Opin Support Palliat Care 3:72–78

Dalal S, Palla S, Hui D et al (2011) Association between a name change from palliative to supportive care and the timing of patient referrals at a comprehensive cancer center. Oncologist 16:105–111

Dalberg T, Jacob-Files E, Carney PA et al (2013) Pediatric oncology providers' perceptions of barriers and facilitators to early integration of pediatric palliative care. Pediatr Blood Cancer 60:1875–1881

Davidhizar R, Giger JN (2004) A review of the literature on care of clients in pain who are culturally diverse. Int Nurs Rev 51:47–55

Davies R (2004) New understandings of parental grief: literature review. J Adv Nurs 46:506–513

Davies B, Sehring SA, Partridge JC et al (2008) Barriers to palliative care for children: perceptions of pediatric health care providers. Pediatrics 121:282–288

De Trill M, Kovalcik R (1997) The child with cancer. Influence of culture on truth-telling and patient care. Ann N Y Acad Sci 809:197–210

De Vries MC, Wit JM, Engberts DP et al (2010) Pediatric oncologists' attitudes towards involving adolescents in decision-making concerning research participation. Pediatr Blood Cancer 55:123–128

Delgado E, Barfield RC, Baker JN et al (2010) Availability of palliative care services for children with cancer in economically diverse regions of the world. Eur J Cancer 46:2260–2266

Donovan LA, Wakefield CE, Russell V et al (2015) Hospital-based bereavement services following the death of a child: a mixed study review. Palliat Med 29:193–210

Dussel V, Kreicbergs U, Hilden JM et al (2009) Looking beyond where children die: determinants and effects of planning a child's location of death. J Pain Symptom Manage 37:33–43

Dussel V, Joffe S, Hilden JM et al (2010) Considerations about hastening death among parents of children who die of cancer. Arch Pediatr Adolesc Med 164:231–237

Dussel V, Bona K, Heath JA et al (2011) Unmeasured costs of a child's death: perceived financial burden, work disruptions, and economic coping strategies used by American and Australian families who lost children to cancer. J Clin Oncol 29:1007–1013

Ecklund EH, Cadge W, Gage EA et al (2007) The religious and spiritual beliefs and practices of academic pediatric oncologists in the United States. J Pediatr Hematol Oncol 29:736–742

Elwyn TS, Fetters MD, Gorenflo W et al (1998) Cancer disclosure in Japan: historical comparisons, current practices. Soc Sci Med 46:1151–1163

Enright BP, Marwit SJ (2002) Diagnosing complicated grief: a closer look. J Clin Psychol 58:747–757

Epstein AS, Morrison RS (2012) Palliative oncology: identity, progress, and the path ahead. Ann Oncol 23(Suppl 3):43–48

Feudtner C, Walter JK, Faerber JA et al (2015) Good-parent beliefs of parents of seriously ill children. JAMA Pediatr 169(1):39–47

Fitchett G, Lyndes KA, Cadge W et al (2011) The role of professional chaplains on pediatric palliative care teams: perspectives from physicians and chaplains. J Palliat Med 14:704–707

Foster TL, Gilmer MJ, Vannatta K et al (2012) Changes in siblings after the death of a child from cancer. Cancer Nurs 35:347–354

Fowler K, Poehling K, Billheimer D et al (2006) Hospice referral practices for children with cancer: a survey of pediatric oncologists. J Clin Oncol 24:1099–1104

Friedrichsdorf SJ, Postier A, Dreyfus J et al (2015) Improved quality of life at end of life related to home-based palliative care in children with cancer. J Palliat Med 18(2):143–150

Gerhardt CA, Fairclough DL, Grossenbacher JC et al (2012) Peer relationships of bereaved siblings and comparison classmates after a child's death from cancer. J Pediatr Psychol 37:209–219

Greer JA, Pirl WF, Jackson VA et al (2012) Effect of early palliative care on chemotherapy use and end-of-life care in patients with metastatic non-small-cell lung cancer. J Clin Oncol 30:394–400

Grossoehme DH, Ragsdale JR, Mchenry CL et al (2007) Pediatrician characteristics associated with attention to spirituality and religion in clinical practice. Pediatrics 119:e117–e123

Heden L, Poder U, Von Essen L et al (2013) Parents' perceptions of their child's symptom burden during and after cancer treatment. J Pain Symptom Manage 46:366–375

Hexem KR, Mollen CJ, Carroll K et al (2011) How parents of children receiving pediatric palliative care use religion, spirituality, or life philosophy in tough times. J Palliat Med 14:39–44

Hilden JM, Emanuel EJ, Fairclough DL et al (2001) Attitudes and practices among pediatric oncologists regarding end-of-life care: results of the 1998 American Society of Clinical Oncology survey. J Clin Oncol 19:205–212

Hill DL, Miller VA, Hexem KR et al (2013) Problems and hopes perceived by mothers, fathers and physicians of children receiving palliative care. Health Expect. doi:10.1111/hex.12078, epub 20 May 2013

Hinds PS, Drew D, Oakes LL et al (2005) End-of-life care preferences of pediatric patients with cancer. J Clin Oncol 23:9146–9154

Hinds PS, Oakes LL, Hicks J et al (2009) "Trying to be a good parent" as defined by interviews with parents who made phase I, terminal care, and resuscitation decisions for their children. J Clin Oncol 27:5979–5985

Hinds PS, Oakes LL, Hicks J et al (2012) Parent-clinician communication intervention during end-of-life decision making for children with incurable cancer. J Palliat Med 15:916–922

Jalmsell L, Kreicbergs U, Onelov E et al (2006) Symptoms affecting children with malignancies during the last month of life: a nationwide follow-up. Pediatrics 117:1314–1320

Jalmsell L, Onelov E, Steineck G et al (2011) Hematopoietic stem cell transplantation in children with cancer and the risk of long-term psychological morbidity in the bereaved parents. Bone Marrow Transplant 46:1063–1070

Johnston DL, Nagel K, Friedman DL et al (2008) Availability and use of palliative care and end-of-life services for pediatric oncology patients. J Clin Oncol 26:4646–4650

Kacel E, Gao X, Prigerson HG (2011) Understanding bereavement: what every oncology practitioner should know. J Support Oncol 9:172–180

Kassam A, Skiadaresis J, Alexander S et al (2014) Parent and clinician preferences for location of end-of-life care: home, hospital or freestanding hospice? Pediatr Blood Cancer 61:859–864

Keele L, Keenan HT, Sheetz J et al (2013) Differences in characteristics of dying children who receive and do not receive palliative care. Pediatrics 132:72–78

Klass D (2006) Continuing conversation about continuing bonds. Death Stud 30:843–858

Kreicbergs U, Valdimarsdottir U, Onelov E et al (2004a) Anxiety and depression in parents 4–9 years after the loss of a child owing to a malignancy: a population-based follow-up. Psychol Med 34:1431–1441

Kreicbergs U, Valdimarsdottir U, Onelov E et al (2004b) Talking about death with children who have severe malignant disease. N Engl J Med 351:1175–1186

Kreicbergs U, Valdimarsdottir U, Onelov E et al (2005) Care-related distress: a nationwide study of parents who lost their child to cancer. J Clin Oncol 23:9162–9171

Kreicbergs UC, Lannen P, Onelov E et al (2007) Parental grief after losing a child to cancer: impact of professional and social support on long-term outcomes. J Clin Oncol 25:3307–3312

Lannen PK, Wolfe J, Prigerson HG et al (2008) Unresolved grief in a national sample of bereaved parents: impaired mental and physical health 4 to 9 years later. J Clin Oncol 26:5870–5876

Li J, Precht DH, Mortensen PB et al (2003) Mortality in parents after death of a child in Denmark: a nationwide follow-up study. Lancet 361:363–367

Lightfoot TJ, Johnston WT, Simpson J et al (2012) Survival from childhood acute lymphoblastic leukaemia: the impact of social inequality in the United Kingdom. Eur J Cancer 48:263–269

Liu JM, Lin WC, Chen YM et al (1999) The status of the do-not-resuscitate order in Chinese clinical trial patients in a cancer centre. J Med Ethics 25:309–314

Mack JW, Smith TJ (2012) Reasons why physicians do not have discussions about poor prognosis, why it matters, and what can be improved. J Clin Oncol 30:2715–2717

Mack JW, Hilden JM, Watterson J et al (2005) Parent and physician perspectives on quality of care at the end of life in children with cancer. J Clin Oncol 23:9155–9161

Mack JW, Wolfe J, Grier HE et al (2006) Communication about prognosis between parents and physicians of children with cancer: parent preferences and the impact of prognostic information. J Clin Oncol 24:5265–5270

Mack JW, Cook EF, Wolfe J et al (2007a) Understanding of prognosis among parents of children with cancer: parental optimism and the parent-physician interaction. J Clin Oncol 25:1357–1362
Mack JW, Wolfe J, Cook EF et al (2007b) Hope and prognostic disclosure. J Clin Oncol 25:5636–5642
Mack JW, Joffe S, Hilden JM et al (2008) Parents' views of cancer-directed therapy for children with no realistic chance for cure. J Clin Oncol 26:4759–4764
Makoul G (2001) The SEGUE Framework for teaching and assessing communication skills. Patient Educ Couns 45:23–34
Maurer SH, Hinds PS, Spunt SL et al (2010) Decision making by parents of children with incurable cancer who opt for enrollment on a phase I trial compared with choosing a do not resuscitate/terminal care option. J Clin Oncol 28:3292–3298
Mazanec P, Tyler MK (2003) Cultural considerations in end-of-life care: how ethnicity, age, and spirituality affect decisions when death is imminent. Am J Nurs 103:50–58; quiz 59
Meert KL, Donaldson AE, Newth CJ et al (2010) Complicated grief and associated risk factors among parents following a child's death in the pediatric intensive care unit. Arch Pediatr Adolesc Med 164:1045–1051
Meert KL, Shear K, Newth CJ et al (2011) Follow-up study of complicated grief among parents eighteen months after a child's death in the pediatric intensive care unit. J Palliat Med 14:207–214
Miller VA, Baker JN, Leek AC et al (2013) Adolescent perspectives on phase I cancer research. Pediatr Blood Cancer 60:873–878
Nagarajan R, Clohisy DR, Neglia JP et al (2004) Function and quality-of-life of survivors of pelvic and lower extremity osteosarcoma and Ewing's sarcoma: the Childhood Cancer Survivor Study. Br J Cancer 91:1858–1865
Onelov E, Steineck G, Nyberg U et al (2007) Measuring anxiety and depression in the oncology setting using visual-digital scales. Acta Oncol 46:810–816
Poder U, Ljungman G, Von Essen L (2010) Parents' perceptions of their children's cancer-related symptoms during treatment: a prospective, longitudinal study. J Pain Symptom Manage 40:661–670
Postier A, Chrastek J, Nugent S et al (2014) Exposure to home-based pediatric palliative and hospice care and its impact on hospital and emergency care charges at a single institution. J Palliat Med 17:183–188
Prigerson HG, Horowitz MJ, Jacobs SC et al (2009) Prolonged grief disorder: psychometric validation of criteria proposed for DSM-V and ICD-11. PLoS Med 6:e1000121
Pritchard M, Burghen E, Srivastava DK et al (2008) Cancer-related symptoms most concerning to parents during the last week and last day of their child's life. Pediatrics 121:e1301–e1309
Pritchard M, Burghen EA, Gattuso JS et al (2010) Factors that distinguish symptoms of most concern to parents from other symptoms of dying children. J Pain Symptom Manage 39:627–636
Ries Lag SM, Gurney JG, Linet M, Tamra T, Young JL, Bunin GR (eds) (1999) Cancer incidence and survival among children and adolescents: United States SEER Program 1975–1995. National Cancer Institute, Bethesda
Rosenberg AR, Baker KS, Syrjala K et al (2012) Systematic review of psychosocial morbidities among bereaved parents of children with cancer. Pediatr Blood Cancer 58:503–512
Rosenberg AR, Dussel V, Kang T et al (2013) Psychological distress in parents of children with advanced cancer. JAMA Pediatr 167(6):537–543
Rosenberg AR, Dussel V, Orellana L et al (2014a) What's missing in missing data? Omissions in survey responses among parents of children with advanced cancer. J Palliat Med 8:953–956
Rosenberg AR, Orellana L, Kang TI et al (2014b) Differences in parent-provider concordance regarding prognosis and goals of care among children with advanced cancer. J Clin Oncol 32(27):3005–3011
Rosenberg AR, Postier A, Osenga K et al (2015) Long-term psychosocial outcomes among bereaved siblings of children with cancer. J Pain Symptom Manage 49(1):55–65
Temel JS, Greer JA, Muzikansky A et al (2010) Early palliative care for patients with metastatic non-small-cell lung cancer. N Engl J Med 363:733–742
Thibodeaux AG, Deatrick JA (2007) Cultural influence on family management of children with cancer. J Pediatr Oncol Nurs 24:227–233
Tomlinson D, Hinds PS, Bartels U et al (2011) Parent reports of quality of life for pediatric patients with cancer with no realistic chance of cure. J Clin Oncol 29:639–645
Truong TH, Weeks JC, Cook EF et al (2011) Altruism among participants in cancer clinical trials. Clin Trials 8:616–623
Tsimicalis A, Stevens B, Ungar WJ et al (2011) The cost of childhood cancer from the family's perspective: a critical review. Pediatr Blood Cancer 56:707–717
Ullrich CK, Dussel V, Hilden JM et al (2010a) End-of-life experience of children undergoing stem cell transplantation for malignancy: parent and provider perspectives and patterns of care. Blood 115:3879–3885
Ullrich CK, Dussel V, Hilden JM et al (2010b) Fatigue in children with cancer at the end of life. J Pain Symptom Manage 40:483–494
Valdimarsdottir U, Kreicbergs U, Hauksdottir A et al (2007) Parents' intellectual and emotional awareness of their child's impending death to cancer: a population-based long-term follow-up study. Lancet Oncol 8:706–714
Van Der Geest IM, Darlington AS, Streng IC et al (2014) Parents' experiences of pediatric palliative care and the impact on long-term parental grief. J Pain Symptom Manage 47:1043–1053
Vega P, Rivera MS, Gonzalez R (2014) When grief turns into love: understanding the experience of parents who have revived after losing a child due to cancer. J Pediatr Oncol Nurs 31:166–176

Von Gunten CF, Ferris FD, Emanuel LL (2000) The patient-physician relationship. Ensuring competency in end-of-life care: communication and relational skills. JAMA 284:3051–3057

Waldman E, Wolfe J (2013) Palliative care for children with cancer. Nat Rev Clin Oncol 10:100–107

Washington UO (2011) End of life culture clues. http://depts.washington.edu/pfes/CultureClues.htm

Wendler D, Abdoler E, Wiener L et al (2012) Views of adolescents and parents on pediatric research without the potential for clinical benefit. Pediatrics 130:692–699

WHO (2014) World Health Organization (WHO) definition of palliative care. www.who.int/cancer/palliative/definition/en/

Wiener L, Ballard E, Brennan T et al (2008) How I wish to be remembered: the use of an advance care planning document in adolescent and young adult populations. J Palliat Med 11:1309–1313

Wiener L, Zadeh S, Battles H et al (2012) Allowing adolescents and young adults to plan their end-of-life care. Pediatrics 130:897–905

Wiener L, Mcconnell DG, Latella L et al (2013) Cultural and religious considerations in pediatric palliative care. Palliat Support Care 11:47–67

Wiener L, Sweeney C, Baird K et al (2014) What do parents want to know when considering autopsy for their child with cancer? J Pediatr Hematol Oncol 36:464–470

Wolfe J (2011) Recognizing a global need for high quality pediatric palliative care. Pediatr Blood Cancer 57:187–188

Wolfe JHP, Sourkes B (2011) Textbook of interdisciplinary pediatric palliative care. Elsevier Saunders, Philadelphia

Wolfe J, Grier HE, Klar N et al (2000a) Symptoms and suffering at the end of life in children with cancer. N Engl J Med 342:326–333

Wolfe J, Klar N, Grier HE et al (2000b) Understanding of prognosis among parents of children who died of cancer: impact on treatment goals and integration of palliative care. JAMA 284:2469–2475

Wolfe J, Hammel JF, Edwards KE et al (2008) Easing of suffering in children with cancer at the end of life: is care changing? J Clin Oncol 26:1717–1723

Wolfe JOL, Cook EF, Ullrich C, Kang T, Rosenebrg AR, Geyer JR, Feudtner C, Dussel V (2015) Symptoms and distress in children with advanced cancer: prospective patient-reported outcomes from the PediQUEST study. J Clin Oncol 33(17):1928–1935

Zadeh S, Pao M, Wiener L (2014) Opening end-of-life discussions: how to introduce Voicing My CHOiCES, an advance care planning guide for adolescents and young adults. Palliat Support Care 13(3):591–599

15 Psychosocial Care for Pediatric Cancer Survivors

Cori C. Liptak, Candice Chow, Eric S. Zhou, and Christopher J. Recklitis

Introduction

Due to tremendous medical advances, most children diagnosed with cancer today will be successfully treated. Approximately 80 % of the 13,500 children diagnosed with cancer annually in the United States will become long-term survivors (Mariotto et al. 2009; Howlader et al. 2013; Smith et al. 2010), resulting in an estimated half a million survivors of childhood cancer by 2020 (Robison and Hudson 2014). In response to this growing population of long-term survivors, research has helped to shed light on the challenges experienced by survivors and has allowed survivorship providers to develop supportive and empirically informed care interventions.

The goal of this chapter is to provide a useful guide for clinicians working within the field of pediatric cancer survivorship. We will provide an overview of the research on psychosocial outcomes in childhood cancer survivorship, being mindful of the typical developmental challenges experienced within the general population. Given the variability in childhood cancers and individual differences in children, our presentation of topics is not intended to be exhaustive, but rather to provide an introduction to the most common issues that arise for long-term survivors of childhood cancers. We also present case examples that integrate challenges that may be encountered during early survivorship and their impact on development and outcomes over time within this population and describe clinical recommendations and interventions to be considered.

Cancer Survivorship as a Stressor

The diagnosis and treatment of cancer is an extraordinary time of challenge and represents, for most families, one of the most stressful and frightening experiences they will ever encounter. Treatments are often physically and emotionally arduous, and the illness typically disrupts the child's normal school and social and developmental context. While many patients show signs of psychological distress or acute stress reactions at some point during their treatment (Sawyer et al. 2000; Patenaude and Kupst 2005), many will successfully adapt to these challenges and be

C.C. Liptak, PhD (✉) • C. Chow, PhD
Department of Psychosocial Oncology and Palliative Care, Dana-Farber/ Boston Children's Cancer and Blood Disorders Center, 450 Brookline Ave, Boston, MA 02215, USA
e-mail: Cori_Liptak@dfci.harvard.edu; Candice_Chow@dfci.harvard.edu

E.S. Zhou, PhD • C.J. Recklitis, PhD, MPH
Perini Family Survivors' Center,
Dana-Farber Cancer Institute, 450 Brookline Ave, Boston, MA 02215, USA
e-mail: eric_zhou@dfci.harvard.edu; Christopher_Recklitis@dfci.harvard.edu

A.N. Abrams et al. (eds.), *Pediatric Psychosocial Oncology: Textbook for Multidisciplinary Care*,
DOI 10.1007/978-3-319-21374-3_15

able to establish positive psychological outcomes both during and after treatment (Zeltzer et al. 2009; Hudson et al. 2003b; Michel et al. 2010). For many patients and families, the completion of treatment is associated with mixed emotions including celebration and uncertainty (Haase and Rostad 1994). As patients and families establish a 'new normal' following the stress of cancer treatment, it can be a challenge to reestablish roles and adjust to a new family dynamics (Duffey-Lind et al. 2006). Individual identities need to be redefined, which can be difficult when the family structure has been so heavily attuned to the "sick child" (Labay et al. 2004; Bjork et al. 2011). In addition, the stressors that were present during treatment (e.g., finances and anxiety about recurrence) remain, yet the structure and support offered from providers at the treating institution change. Managing the loss of providers, adapting to new expectations (e.g., work and school), and coping with uncertainty can present a challenge to even the most well-adjusted individual. Therefore, providing education and support prior to and during the transition to off-treatment can be helpful in addressing these challenges. Providing individually tailored information for patients and families based on the diagnosis, treatment, and psychological risk factors has the potential to mitigate maladaptation during this critical transitional period (Duffey-Lind et al. 2006). Despite these challenges, most survivors adapt relatively well upon completion of treatment, yet there are a number of risk factors for psychological maladjustment and notable late effects that are critical for a clinician to monitor during the psychosocial care provided for childhood cancer survivors and their families.

Psychological Distress

Given that fewer than 5 % of all cancer survivors are survivors of *childhood* cancer, collaborative research efforts have been required to yield studies of large cohorts of survivors treated at multiple centers (Michel et al. 2010; Hawkins et al. 2008; Robison et al. 2002). Making use of standardized assessments of outcomes in these large samples, these studies have attempted to overcome the limitations common in smaller investigations at individual treatment sites (e.g., poor generalizability, lack of power, selection bias). Inclusion of psychological outcome data from a control group of nontreated siblings has addressed the questionable adequacy of normative comparison data that limited many previous studies, making data from the Childhood Cancer Survivor Study (CCSS) (Robison et al. 2002), the Swiss Childhood Cancer Survivor Study (SCSS) (Kuehni et al. 2012), and the St. Jude Lifetime Cohort Study (SJLIFE) (Hudson et al. 2011) extremely valuable.

Overall, results from the CCSS and other large survivor cohort studies have demonstrated that while most survivors do not experience significant impairments in mental health functioning, 17 % do, and survivors are more than twice as likely to have elevated levels of psychological symptoms as compared to their siblings (Hudson et al. 2003b; Zeltzer et al. 2009). Increased risk for anxiety and depression symptoms based on adult self-report and parent-report for younger survivors (Hudson et al. 2003b; Michel et al. 2010) has been indicated in both the CCSS and SCCS cohorts. Parents of child and adolescent survivors in the CCSS, for example, report that as many as 18 % of survivors have significant symptoms of anxiety and depression and that 20 % or more have problems with attention, antisocial behavior, and impaired social competence (Schultz et al. 2007). Similarly, 17 % of adult male survivors and 23 % of adult female survivors in the CCSS report general impairments in mental health-related quality of life (Zeltzer et al. 2009). Survivors in the CCSS have also been found to have elevated rates of suicidal ideation (Recklitis et al. 2010) and posttraumatic stress symptoms (Stuber et al. 2010). Studies using the SJLIFE cohort have begun to identify particular risk factors for elevated emotional distress including cancer-related pain, socioeconomic status, and learning or memory difficulties (Oancea et al.

2014) (cognitive late effects of treatment are covered in more detail in Chapter 10). Survivors of central nervous system (CNS) tumors are a cohort of patients that have been identified as having increased risk for psychological distress. In a study of adolescent and young adult survivors of CNS tumors, Liptak et al. (2012) found that on a self-report measure, 17 % of adolescents had elevations in distress and 34 % of young adult survivors endorsed items consistent with elevated depressive symptomatology period.

Research continues to provide strong evidence that psychological distress and adaptive problems are not uncommon in adult survivors of childhood cancers. However, it is important to note that this research focuses almost solely on the prevalence of psychological *symptoms* rather than diagnosable psychiatric *disorders*. This is indicative of both the relative difficulty of measuring psychiatric disorders in survey research and with the desire to report on psychological distress rather than exclusively on psychiatric diagnosis. Appreciating this distinction has important implications both for understanding the research on survivors' psychological late effects and for planning appropriate assessment and intervention programs. Some survivors with elevated symptoms of distress may not have symptoms of sufficient severity or with associated impairments to qualify for a particular diagnosis, and others may have severe symptoms that do not coincide with the patterns derived from the study of mental illness. Clinicians desiring to address psychological distress in this population should adopt a symptom-based focus rather than only seeking to identify and treat diagnosable mental disorders. In order to ensure a broad assessment of functioning, the National Comprehensive Cancer Network (NCCN) and others have strongly encouraged clinicians to assess, target, and intervene on psychological and behavioral symptoms that cause subjective distress, whether or not a psychiatric diagnosis is present (Network 2003; Holland et al. 2010; Kornblith 1998).

Case Vignette : Don, a 34-Year-Old Survivor of Rhabdomyosarcoma

Medical History: Don was diagnosed with rhabdomyosarcoma at age 10 and treated with intensive chemotherapy, which included drugs known to confer risk of long-term heart problems in some patients. He is referred for a psychological assessment in the context of a worsening cardiac condition.

Psychosocial Adaptation: Don is an outgoing and charismatic person who has been a successful businessman since he started his first business in college. He is single, has a large group of friends, and has been active in community organizations. Changes in his cardiac test results were noted by his physicians for several years, though Don has been able to continue his regular activities until the past year. Now he is often fatigued and cannot maintain his usual schedule of work and social activities. He is very worried about the likely diagnosis of heart failure and feels depressed at the thought he will become "an invalid." He can't believe it and notes that "after everything I went through, this is what I get!" He is particularly frustrated and angry with his cardiac care, feeling that he is getting worse and "no one seems to care." He makes frequent visits to the pediatric cancer follow-up clinic even though he knows the adult cardiology specialists are best suited to help him. Don feels helpless as a medical patient and notes, "I can talk to anyone, negotiate and wheel and deal my way around a boardroom or a bar room—why can't I talk to these doctors?" Over the course of a few therapy sessions, Don comes to realize he is treating his cardiac specialists with the same deference and awe he had toward his oncologist at age 10 and is expecting to have his cardiac care plan completely mapped out and managed. Unlike his cancer care, which was aimed at cure and followed a highly specific treatment protocol, his cardiac condition is chronic and there is no definitive treatment plan. This realization helps him become more active in his medical care, and he comes to feel more like "himself," as a competent assertive adult. He selects a new cardiologist with whom he feels he can have a good relationship. He is initially reluctant to join a support group for cardiac patients; however, when he does eventually join, he engages very actively and becomes something of a "leader" in the group, eventually using it to help him face his fears of losing the work and other activities that give his life meaning.

Comment: The onset of serious treatment-related conditions can arouse intense feelings for survivors. While Don exhibited symptoms of helplessness, hopelessness, sadness, and irritability, his symptom profile did not meet the criteria for a major depressive episode. However, if providers had not paid attention to his distressing symptoms and referred him for appropriate intervention, his mood difficulties would likely have worsened. In addition to the emotional issues anyone is facing with a serious medical condition, survivors may find themselves recalling and even re-experiencing some aspect of their childhood illness which can complicate efforts to cope with the new illness. Don's case is remarkable both because he regressed so profoundly into a child's role which increased his feelings of being overwhelmed and because with guidance he was able to recognize his situation and overcome it so quickly.

Social Outcomes and Interpersonal Relationships

Although many childhood cancer survivors are able to adapt and experience success within the domains of school, work, and interpersonal functioning, some experience impairments in their ability to attain developmental milestones in these areas (Maurice-Stam et al. 2007). There are circumstances in which even relatively minor changes in neurocognitive functioning can have a significant impact on a survivor's adaptation and can increase their risk of psychosocial issues. Learning difficulties, combined with symptoms of depression or anxiety, can create even greater barriers to success around social roles and have a negative impact on academic performance, employment, and interpersonal relationships. In addition to learning issues, the ongoing medical follow-up needed and the real possibility of additional medical problems are other stressors survivors must manage in the context of trying to maintain "real-world" expectations.

The literature has highlighted the neurocognitive issues associated with CNS treatment, with patients who have received radiation therapy or intrathecal chemotherapy being at greatest risk for learning difficulties. The CCSS data has indicated that the utilization of special education services is significantly higher for survivors (23 %) when compared to sibling controls (8 %). Patients with brain tumors, Hodgkin's disease, and leukemia and patients diagnosed before the age of 5 are identified as being at highest risk for needing special education services (Gurney et al. 2009). These findings are similar to the results of a Canadian cohort study in which survivors were reported as more likely to be retained, to need special education programs, and to have educational problems when compared to controls. Patients who had been treated for CNS tumors, leukemia, and neuroblastoma were identified as groups with significant risk factors around educational achievement (Barrera et al. 2005). Anticipatory guidance and support to parents of children who meet particular risk factors can be incredibly helpful at the time patients and families are transitioning off-treatment. Psychoeducation around special education and advocacy has the potential to empower parents, allow them to play a role in helping school personnel understand the impact of treatment on learning, and get children access to appropriate educational supports as early as possible (Northman et al. 2014). Educational needs of childhood cancer survivors are discussed in more detail in Chapter 11.

Case Vignette : Anna, a 26-Year-Old Leukemia Survivor

Medical History: Anna was treated at age 3 for acute lymphoblastic leukemia with chemotherapy and cranial radiation. At age 26, Anna is referred for a psychological assessment because of reported depression symptoms, frustration with her work and school ambitions, and conflict with her parents.

Psychosocial Adaptation: Anna denies most symptoms of depression but writes at the end of a depression screening measure, "It's not that I am suicidal, it's just that sometimes I think it would be better if I had not survived the leukemia." On interview, she describes a history of school problems starting in the 7th grade that took many years to be addressed. Anna feels her parents were slow to advocate for an evaluation, because they did not want to admit that she is "damaged goods." Anna began college hoping to study accounting but found this to be too challenging, even with supportive education services. She left college after 3 years with only 2 years of credits. Currently, she lives with her parents and works part-time at a local bookstore. Her sisters have graduate degrees and work in financial services as do both of her parents. She is disappointed with herself and angry that her parents are disappointed in her.

Over many months of therapy, Anna works on mourning the losses associated with her treatment including the loss of learning potential and changes in her relationship with her family. She also acknowledges that it is not her family's judgments that are most problematic but rather her own and makes use of cognitive-behavioral strategies to alter her own harsh self-criticisms. Whereas previously she either went to school taking a full load of challenging courses or dropped out and declared herself a failure, Anna is now able to devise a plan to take single college courses supplemented by tutoring and learning supports. She comes to see this plan not as admitting to being "damaged goods," but as a useful strategy for achieving her goal of graduating from college. Anna also has to confront the fact that as angry as she is with her parents, she chooses to remain dependent on them and to serve as a distraction from their longstanding marital conflict. Eventually, Anna chooses to leave the family home. She remarks with humor, "If I had known how great it would feel, I would have divorced my parents years ago."

Comment: Many survivors' learning problems may not come to light until many years after treatment, and even families who are knowledgeable of treatment late effects may be resistant to acknowledging them because of stigma. This case is unusual for the high level of family conflict that became associated with Anna's learning difficulties, but it is a good example of the role of preexisting family problems and the extent to which cancer treatment and medical late effects can become entwined with individual and family dynamics

From Recklitis and Liptak (2015)

The multifaceted issues faced by survivors of childhood cancer can also have a notable impact on the individual's social and psychosexual development (Roberts et al. 1998). The toxicity of cancer-directed treatments can often put these young patients at elevated risk for the development of sexual dysfunction and infertility in later life (Tromp et al. 2011; Green et al. 2009, 2010; Jacobs and Pucci 2013; Kenney et al. 2012). In addition, some physical effects of cancer treatment such as short stature, neurocognitive deficits, and poor physical functioning also may contribute to problems in social outcomes and development of intimate relationships (Janson et al. 2009; Kunin-Batson et al. 2011; Ness et al. 2005). Survivors of childhood cancer report more limited sexual behavior in the form of less frequent masturbation, communication with friends about sex, longer delays before dating, lower marriage rates (Pastore et al. 2001; Frobisher et al. 2010), and reduced interest in and satisfaction with sexual activities (Bober et al. 2013; Gurney et al. 2009; van Dijk et al. 2008; Sundberg et al. 2011; Hall et al. 2012).

While developing intimate and sexual relationships presents challenges for many young adults, survivors of childhood cancer may in addition need to confront ways in which their body image, sexual function, or fertility have been affected by cancer. Although the impact of oncology treatments on sexuality and fertility may be discussed in the consent and assent process at all ages, these issues become more relevant as survivors reach adolescence and young adulthood. Even under the best of circumstances, when these issues are talked about openly as part of treatment and follow-up care, survivors who are entering into a new romantic relationship have to take new risks such as talking with their partner about their concerns or possibly seeking medical consultation about sexual function or fertility. Despite these challenges, they are likely to be interested in engaging in sexual activities and may benefit from receiving age-appropriate information and counseling regarding their sexual development concerns (Hall et al. 2012; Morgan et al. 2010; Kelly 2013; Zebrack 2009). It is not uncommon for young adult survivors to have questions regarding their sexual functioning and fertility and to need assistance around how to communicate concerns to their partner. In limited research, it appears that a psychosocial intervention can help to improve sexual knowledge and body image and decrease anxiety related to sexual issues in this population (Canada et al. 2007).

Case Vignette : Tina, a 17-Year-Old Lymphoma Survivor

Medical History: Tina was diagnosed at 8 with lymphoma and had a long course of treatment, which included radiation and chemotherapy. She relapsed at age 14 and underwent a stem-cell transplant.

Psychosocial Adaptation: At 16, Tina returned to high school after missing a significant amount of school post-transplant. Despite being extremely bright and an excellent student in middle school, she experienced difficulty upon reentry to high school post-transplant—something she attributes to her cancer experience and its aftermath. "I was not really depressed or anything during my treatment. I was a pretty happy camper considering, but I look back and think of that time as my 'lost years.' When I returned to school after my first treatment, it was an easy transition and my parents were able to advocate for what I needed academically. I came back as the 'hero' and felt very well received by peers. But I relapsed and the second time has been so much more challenging. When I left school, everyone was starting to play spin the bottle, and when I got better and came back, it was like everyone was dating and having sex. I couldn't figure out what I missed and what I was supposed to do about talking to other kids, much less dating." Tina spoke about her understanding that she should be developing more independence from her parents but had such ambivalence about that process, particularly given all the medical visits following her transplant. "It seemed like none of my friends needed their parents anymore, but I still had to rely on mine for a lot of things like doctor's visits and keeping on top of my medications. I was glad they were there for me, but I also didn't want them to always be hovering over me and wondering if I was OK." Tina was overwhelmed with the college application process. She developed significant anxiety, particularly around the reality that she would need to be more independent from her parents. She began to smoke marijuana as a way to fit in socially and relax. She stated, "Drinking and drugging turned out to be a great way to break the ice and try to fit in. It also helped me manage the sense of panic that I felt every time I thought about the future. I know I am not the first person to screw up. Believe me, I knew all the other screw-ups, but I see now that cancer really messed with my adolescence in ways I never understood. I realized that I was not yet prepared to go to college and needed time to work on myself." Eventually Tina started psychotherapy and was treated for depression and anxiety, with a family intervention that helped her and her parents address the issues related to Tina's cancer, her substance use, and her desire to be both supported by and distinctly separate from her parents.

Comment: Tina's case demonstrates the extent to which a prolonged illness can effectively remove a child from the normal social and developmental context. Even as Tina coped well with the challenges of her treatment initially, her social and psychological development was significantly disrupted, particularly as a result of her relapse. When she returned to "normal" life and was comparing herself to peers, she was confronted with the significant differences between herself and others. Perhaps because of her long treatment and the extended period of isolation after her transplant, the family dynamics created by the circumstances made Tina's posttreatment adjustment more challenging than for most survivors

Adapted from Recklitis and Liptak (2015)

Employment

Given the issues cancer survivors may experience as a result of neurocognitive deficits or ongoing medical concerns, it is not surprising that finding and maintaining employment can be a challenge (Strauser et al. 2010). Employment is an important determinant of a survivor's quality of life and has significant implications for independence, self-esteem, family and social relationships, and health insurance coverage. Results from the CCSS indicate that survivors with poor physical health are eight times more likely to be unemployed than healthy survivors, with health-related concerns reported as the primary barrier to employment (Kirchhoff et al. 2010, 2011). The risk for unemployment increases in relation to the chronic medical conditions experienced by survivors post-therapy; this is particularly important given that 73 % of the CCSS survivors reported at least one chronic medical condition 30 years after cancer diagnosis (Oeffinger et al. 2006). Moving beyond the sole impact of physical health, research from the SJLIFE cohort demonstrated that treatment intensity, age at diagnosis, and physical health indirectly affect career readiness via impact on emotional functioning and vocational identity (Strauser et al. 2014). While survivors of childhood cancer are twice as likely to be unemployed when compared to healthy controls, survivors of pediatric brain tumors had a fivefold risk of being unemployed compared with other childhood cancer survivors (Strauser et al. 2013). Emotional issues, visual problems, and hearing problems were all identified as health conditions that affected or impeded a survivor's ability to work. Physical functioning limitations, such as an inability to operate a motor vehicle, further highlight the significant impact that disability can have on employability.

Case Vignette : John, a 27-Year-Old Brain Tumor Survivor

Medical History: John was diagnosed at the age of 8 and underwent a partial resection of a midbrain tumor followed by radiation therapy. At the age of 11, he developed a seizure disorder requiring ongoing medication. His neurocognitive profile demonstrates an average IQ, with variability in performance. Significant problems with impulsivity, organization, processing speed, and memory were noted.

Psychosocial Adaptation: John attended a high school program which emphasized vocational instruction as well as independent living skills. John graduated from the program at 22 and secured a job working in the culinary field. He was extremely proud of his employment status but clearly challenged by the demands of working in a fast-paced environment. John was able to live independently but required supervision from his parents around finances. He had some close friends and dated but had significant insecurity about his neurocognitive status. With his family and medical providers, he would frequently apologize for asking questions and ask if what he said was "dumb." John viewed his brain tumor history as a significant barrier, stating, "Why would anyone want to spend time with me?" or "Once someone finds out the truth about me, they will leave." His dissatisfaction with his social functioning often led to suicidal ideation with no plan or intent. John consistently presented to his brain tumor follow-up appointments with symptoms of depression and was treated with antidepressant medication and psychotherapy in the community. At age 26, John began to experience sudden and progressive hearing loss secondary to his radiation therapy. This was extremely upsetting for him and he began to experience significant anxiety associated with his overall well-being, asking, "Am I going to go blind too?" At the same time, he experienced two additional losses, first when he was laid off from his job and then when the woman he had been dating ended the relationship. In response to these multiple stressors, John attempted suicide by overdosing on a number of his medications. Subsequently, he participated in an intensive day treatment program and was followed closely for individual therapy and psychopharmacology. He moved into his parents' home in order to be adequately supervised and has been challenged by finding satisfying employment opportunities.

Comment: This case demonstrates how the dynamic relationship between medical, neurocognitive, and psychosocial issues can severely impact quality of life. Loss of employment for John was a significant stressor that compounded ongoing medical and emotional difficulties. The change in his level of independence as a result of the job loss and suicide attempt was a significant setback for John developmentally and severely impaired his ability to return to his previous level of functioning. An inability to find satisfying employment, despite advocacy and assistance from family, demonstrates how the complexity of late effects experienced within this population can interfere with the attainment of appropriate social roles.

Risk Factors

Researchers have attempted to identify key risk factors for psychological distress in survivors of childhood cancer. Since the relevance of specific risk factors can vary across types of cancer, age groups, and even social and cultural contexts, an exhaustive review of risk factors is beyond the scope of this chapter. Instead, we present an overview of the risk factors most important for understanding and assessing childhood cancer survivors along with our interpretation of the ways in which these factors may influence development and adaptation in individual survivors. Risk factors can be an important guide to assessing and monitoring survivors; however, it is critical to appreciate that the course of cancer survivorship is dynamic and individuals who may initially present with no risk factors require ongoing monitoring and evaluation as their risk status and emotional outcomes can change significantly over time.

In terms of demographic factors associated with psychological adjustment, female survivors have been found to be more likely to report psychological problems (Hudson et al. 2003b; Zeltzer et al. 2008), which is consistent with what has been noted in general populations (McLean and

Anderson 2009; Piccinelli and Wilkinson 2000). This suggests the possibility that females may be more vulnerable to distress or, alternatively, more willing to report psychological problems when they occur. Other demographic variables such as lower income, lower education, disability status, and unmarried status have been associated with poor psychological and quality of life outcomes (Hudson et al. 2003b; Zeltzer et al. 2008), but it is important to note that these factors may be both the result of and contributors to poor psychological adaptation. For example, depression would be expected to impair functioning in a way that makes it difficult for survivors to thrive in work and school environments, while problems with work and the stress of low income would also be expected to contribute to depression (Johnson et al. 1999). Although the precise directionality of the relationships between these sociodemographic variables and psychological adaptation in cancer survivors may not be known, the correlational relationships nevertheless aid in identifying groups of survivors who should be considered at higher risk. Psychiatric history and premorbid functioning are also important to consider, as these are known to be associated with poor outcomes after cancer (Parker et al. 2003; Schag et al. 1994). Similarly, extreme emotional or behavioral reactions that occurred during treatment suggest increased vulnerability to future psychological distress and should be considered risk factors for future adjustment problems.

Specific aspects of a child's cancer and cancer treatments are also thought to increase risk for long-term psychological adjustment problems. The literature supports the concept that more intensive treatments result in later adjustment problems if they increase distress or developmental disruption at the time of treatment, impede the child's ability to learn or acquire certain skills, or increase risk for medical late effects such as cognitive limitations, physical limitations, physical disfigurement, second cancers, or chronic conditions. Radiation therapy, which can disrupt normal development of treated areas in later life, has been associated with psychological problems, poor functional outcomes, and reduced quality of life, though the effects are different across types of radiation and types of cancers (Zeltzer et al. 2009). Cranial radiation, for example, can cause neurocognitive late effects, while pelvic radiation can cause problems with growth, mobility, and fertility, and both of these radiation fields have been found to increase the risk of adaptation problems later in life (Zeltzer et al. 2009; Speechley et al. 2006). Similarly, chemotherapy generally and more intensive chemotherapy regimens have also been associated with a greater likelihood of impaired quality of life and psychological functioning (Hudson et al. 2003a; Zebrack et al. 2002; Schultz et al. 2007). Within cancer-related factors, a brain tumor diagnosis has consistently been found to be associated with psychological symptoms, poor functional outcomes, and poor quality of life (Zeltzer et al. 2009; Recklitis et al. 2010). This association is likely due to the negative impact that CNS tumors and associated treatments can have on learning and educational and social skills later in life. Survivors of bone tumors have also been found to be at higher risk for psychosocial problems in some studies, which may reflect the impact of physical mobility problems and pain on both physical and emotional qualities of life (Ness et al. 2008). Several studies have not found a relationship between age of diagnosis and later adjustment (Zeltzer et al. 2008; Recklitis et al. 2010), indicating that no particular age group at the time of diagnosis should be considered at increased risk. Nonetheless, clinicians working with individual survivors should consider how age at the time of treatment may have affected survivors differently by disrupting their developmental course and making them more sensitive to the effects of specific treatments. For example, those diagnosed at younger ages may be less likely to recall their treatment and less likely to identify as "survivors" than those diagnosed in their teenage years (Casey et al. 2010).

Survivors with multiple medical problems have been found to report more psychological distress (Zebrack et al. 2004; Zeltzer et al. 2008), and a study of suicidal ideation among survivors (Recklitis et al. 2010) showed that poor health outcomes, including pain, are associated with greater likelihood of reporting suicidal ideation even after adjusting for depression. Survivors with poor physical health are also noted to be less likely to be employed and married or have medical insurance and more likely to have low educational attainment and at least one major medical condition (Zeltzer et al. 2008). This too is consistent with previous research indicating that medical problems, especially chronic conditions that are likely to interfere with routine functioning, are associated with significant psychological morbidity. Because survivors are likely to be diagnosed with chronic conditions at a much younger age than their peers (Oeffinger et al. 2006), they may have fewer coping resources, and their educational, career, and relationship plans may be more vulnerable. Having developed a chronic condition at a young age, many survivors of childhood cancer feel unfairly burdened, a sentiment sometimes expressed by, "I am too young for this!" Some survivors find the diagnosis of a treatment-related condition extremely anxiety provoking, raising fears that they may never feel at ease with their health again, especially if the new condition is chronic and unlikely to be cured. "It's not over when it's over," is a phrase commonly heard from survivors expressing a feeling of resignation that they are still not free from the negative impact of cancer despite having been cured of their disease (Table 15.1).

Periods of Vulnerability

While physical and psychological adjustment often improves after completion of cancer therapy, subsequent life periods and transitions can be associated with greater vulnerability to psychological distress and adaptive problems. From a developmental perspective, Erikson's theory of adolescent development (Erikson 1968) provides a useful framework for understanding how each new developmental period offers opportunities for reworking unresolved issues related to cancer. As cognitive capacities increase and social relationships change, the survivor may be prompted to think about their cancer experience in new ways. For most survivors, this reworking of the cancer experience may be subtle and lead to a sense of growth, but for others, there is the possibility that aspects of the cancer experience may reemerge later in life and, at times, lead to poor adaptation and to the development of psychological symptoms. Most survivors will pass through these vulnerable periods without significant distress; however, even those who had a sustained period of healthy recovery and good psychosocial adjustment are at a greater risk for new problems with psychological adaptation at particular life junctures.

For some survivors, the completion of therapy itself is an unexpectedly stressful time. Survivors who are greatly relieved to complete their medical regimen may also feel some anxiety around the sudden decrease in medical oversight, as well as some apprehension about leaving the "patient role" to return to the expectations of school and society. In some cases, survivors and their families speak of treatment as being such a central focus of their lives that it is only after its completion that they really process some of the emotional components of the cancer; this may lead to an increased sense of loss or depression. If the

Table 15.1 Factors associated with adjustment problems after childhood cancer

Personal factors	Disease factors	Physical factors
Female gender	Brain tumor or CNS-directed therapy	Poor health status
Preexisting conditions—mental illness, functional limits	Prolonged or intense treatments (e.g., bone marrow transplant)	Chronic medical conditions
Limited education or income	Cranial or pelvic radiation	Pain or disfigurement
Lack of social support	Residual disease/recurrence	Functional limitations (e.g., ambulation, communication)
Life stressors (e.g., divorce, unemployment)	Problems adjusting or adhering to treatment (e.g., medication nonadherence, substance abuse, extreme emotional distress)	Difficulties in self-care (e.g., dressing, eating, bathing)
Disabled status		

From Recklitis and Liptak (2015)

survivor has had a long treatment period during which they interacted predominantly with adults, they may upon the completion of treatment feel ill at ease with peers and unfamiliar with the latest trends within their peer group. For many young cancer survivors, the experience of returning to their regular school or peer group can feel bewildering, as they move from a context where they are the focus of intense attention and concern to being just one of the crowd. For young children, this loss of special status may present in the form of behavioral challenges (e.g., defiance, tantrums, withdrawal) as they react to the reintroduction of expectations and consequences that may have been suspended during the illness and attempt to adjust to a "new normal" (Labay et al. 2004; Bjork et al. 2011). For teenagers, difficulties during this transition period can include feeling isolated and misunderstood. In particular, patients who were treated for CNS tumors are less likely to be nominated as a best friend and are perceived as more sick, fatigued, and absent from school in relation to comparison peers (Vannatta et al. 1998).

Many survivors welcome an opportunity to move to a new school or living situation where their cancer history is not widely known as they feel it helps them move past being "the kid with cancer." For some, however, moving into a new environment means having to give up a special status they may not have recognized they had, as well as the onslaught of new concerns about how and when to disclose their cancer history. As one 22-year-old survivor, John recalls, "When I got to college, I was just one of a sea of new students. I thought that would be great, but the work was really hard, and I started to realize I wasn't prepared. My teachers and tutors in high school had cut me a lot of slack because of my cancer, and suddenly that help and support was all gone. Then when I tried to get to know people, it seemed like cancer always came up. What sports did I play, what was that scar from— inevitably I had to keep "coming out" as a cancer survivor and that was weird. At home, everyone knew me and I had never once had to tell anyone I had cancer, but in college, I was on my own and some people had really weird reactions. It became a big problem for me adjusting to college, and I ended up seeing a counselor first at the cancer center and then at school" (Recklitis and Liptak 2015).

Other major life changes, even very positive ones, can also prompt some new reflection about their health and questions of whether their cancer history can be a liability. For example, taking on a major new job role, starting a new relationship, and becoming a parent can be times that survivors find themselves worrying or reflecting on their health. As one survivor put it, "I never really thought much about my cancer, but when I got pregnant, it all came up. For 20 years, the fear that I might get sick again was way in the back of my head, and I did not even know it. Once I found out I was going to be a mom, it all came up and I kind of freaked out. I had to educate myself, see my doctors, and make sure I was really healthy and taking care of myself" (Recklitis and Liptak 2015) (Table 15.2).

Table 15.2 Common periods of vulnerability

Life transitions		
	Transition off-treatment	
		Decreased contact with medical professionals
		Greater integration with home and school routines
		Increased expectations and loss of special status
	Moving to a new environment	
		Loss of special status
		Question of disclosing cancer history
		Need to reestablish academic accommodations in new school system
	Career changes	
		Questions about insurance and employability
	Developing intimate relationships	
		Questions about disclosing cancer history
		Concerns about body image, sexuality, and fertility
Health related		
	Medical care and information	
		Regular medical follow-up and surveillance
		Cancer or other serious illnesses diagnosed in a friend or family member
		Notable cancer-related media event
	Physical health changes	
		Change in health status or functional status
		New diagnosis of medical condition
		Recurrence of cancer or secondary cancer

From Recklitis and Liptak (2015)

Case Vignette : Maria, a 22-Year-Old Survivor of a Low-Grade Brain Tumor

Medical History: Maria was diagnosed with a low-grade glioma at the age of 7 and was treated with chemotherapy and radiation.

Psychosocial Adaptation: As a result of her tumor and medical treatments, Maria suffers from multiple late effects including cognitive deficits, growth hormone deficiency, and left-sided weakness. Partially as a result of these very apparent challenges, Maria has had difficulty initiating and maintaining age-appropriate social relationships. She relies heavily on her parents for both emotional support and financial support. Maria strongly identifies herself as a cancer survivor; the majority of her nonacademic activities revolve around volunteering for her treating hospital, attending camps for cancer patients and survivors, and engaging in organized social activities for cancer survivors. She talks about being seen as "different" and "less than" her more successful and physically attractive siblings and cousins. Maria will be graduating from community college this year and presents with significant anxiety and ruminative worry around this transition. As a result, she initiated mental health services at her treating hospital, citing that the providers at the cancer center are "the only people who understand my medical history and what I am going through." During a brief course of treatment, Maria encountered difficulties utilizing cognitive-behavioral strategies to address her anxiety. Despite reassurance from her family that their support would continue well beyond college, Maria continued to perseverate on how she would cope with independence and adulthood after graduating. Maria arrived to most sessions reporting chronic low mood and was frequently tearful throughout sessions. After approximately eight sessions, psychopharmacological intervention as well as more intensive, community-based treatment was recommended. Maria's mood and anxiety have now stabilized with the help of medication. In addition, she is receiving services from a community-based therapist who can provide a more appropriate level of mental health care than what can be offered through the cancer center.

Comment: Maria's case demonstrates how the cognitive, developmental, and physical late effects of cancer can lead to feelings of isolation and hopelessness, particularly during crucial times of transition. For most young adults, the completion of college is a time of both excitement and anxiety, but for survivors who so clearly benefit from the structure of school, the uncertainty about the future can highlight limited coping resources and exacerbate preexisting psychological difficulties. Maria's connection to the cancer center allowed her to accept the initial psychological support offered and incorporate the recommendations made by her team that more intensive community-based interventions would be of benefit.

Psychosocial Care in the Context of Survivorship

After completion of cancer therapy, pediatric cancer patients typically continue to have regular oncology follow-up visits, though the frequency of visits decreases over time depending on the patients' diagnoses and individual needs. For our discussion of psychosocial care for survivors, we focus on the needs of long-term survivors who are no longer being regularly seen by an oncology provider and are generally 2 or more years from completion of cancer therapy. In some treatment settings, these survivors will continue to be followed by their treating clinical team, but in others, they may be provided with additional survivorship services or transferred to a specialized survivorship clinic inside or outside of their treatment center. Regardless of the type of setting where these long-term survivors are being seen, they are typically seen only once a year, and psychosocial care makes up one small but important part of the agenda for the annual survivorship visit. In providing psychosocial care to childhood cancer survivors, part of the conceptual and practical challenge is to consider what psychosocial services will be provided and how they will be integrated into survivorship care more broadly.

Conceptually, psychosocial care in the survivorship setting can be viewed as a bridge between the oncologic care and the specialized mental health care that can be provided in the community, similar to models of mental health services adapted for primary medical care settings (Collins 2010; Knapp and Foy 2012; Mental health: Integrated approach 2012). As discussed, most survivors adapt well after completion of cancer treatment and will not require psychosocial interventions, but identifying those survivors or families who do require mental health services is a priority. Cancer centers understandably assign most of their limited psychosocial resources to care for on-treatment families, and many families live at a considerable distance from their cancer center, two practical factors that strongly influence the scope of psychosocial care that can be successfully delivered in the survivorship context. While delivering a full range of specialty mental health services in the survivorship setting is not practical or necessary, utilizing behavioral health expertise is important to help identify and support those survivors with psychosocial needs and to arrange for community-based services (e.g., outpatient mental health, school-based services, community-based support groups, or government agencies). For the majority of survivors who are generally adapting well, the goal is to provide supportive services, education, and anticipatory guidance to address any subclinical adjustment problems and prevent the need for specialized behavioral services in the future. For the minority of survivors with active psychosocial needs, the goal is to identify these needs and refer them to appropriate services. The specific types of services offered to survivors may vary considerably, but this combination of bringing selected psychosocial services to the survivorship medical care setting and referring out to community-based care is common to most programs.

Through adapting models of behavioral health care for primary care settings (Collins 2010; Mental health: Integrated approach 2012; Knapp and Foy 2012), we have identified three central aims for optimal psychosocial care in the cancer survivorship setting:

1. Supporting the oncology provider in identifying survivors with significant psychosocial needs
2. Collaborating with oncology providers to assess and manage survivors' psychosocial needs
3. Referring survivors for psychosocial care in the community

Supporting oncology providers in identifying survivors with psychosocial needs may be the most important of these three aims since survivors have infrequent clinic visits and needs not identified are likely to remain unaddressed and may intensify over time. Oncologists and nurse practitioners are usually the first providers who assess survivors' psychosocial needs, both because psychosocial function is an important element of holistic care and because most survivorship programs will not be able to provide an individual assessment with a mental health professional for each survivor. Even when psychosocial providers do not personally assess each survivor who comes into the clinic, they can improve case identification in a clinic by helping determine the needs most important to assess (e.g., cognitive, emotional, social) and, in conjunction with the medical team, develop a system for identifying those needs. This may include developing administrative procedures to ensure that all survivors coming in for a clinic visit are offered a standardized psychosocial

Table 15.3 What do you say? Conversation starters for medical providers

Outside of your physical health, how are you doing?
What about your mood? Everyone has bad days, but is your mood very down or depressed for more than a day or two at a time?
How about feeling really tense or anxious—is that a problem for you?
When you filled out the emotional health questions, did any of those questions seem to apply to you?
Are there certain goals you are working on in your school/work/personal life?
Survivors sometimes tell me they think their treatment changed the way they look or how they feel about their body—is that something you ever think about?
Do you find yourself thinking about cancer frequently? Do these thoughts ever bother you or get in the way of your sense of pleasure/sleep/daily functioning?
Sometimes when people are feeling really burdened, they tell me they feel hopeless or like they are not sure life feels worth living—do you ever feel that way?
Is there anything else about how you are feeling or getting along at home, school, or work we should discuss?

Adapted from Recklitis and Liptak (2015)

assessment, for example, by including questions about psychosocial function (e.g., anxiety, depression, school, and social functioning) and health behaviors (e.g., exercise, smoking, alcohol, and substance use) on the health history or intake forms used in the clinic. In addition, psychosocial providers can talk with medical providers about how they can routinely inquire about psychosocial function during survivorship visits and even provide sample questions or coaching about how to sensitively raise these topics (see Table 15.3). Integrating psychosocial assessment into existing clinic procedures increases efficiency and may also destigmatize potentially sensitive topics by making them a routine part of survivorship care.

Use of Standardized Rating Scales

In some settings, psychosocial clinicians may also help implement self-report symptom rating scales that ask survivors or their parents to report on emotional health, behavior problems, and school difficulties. While screening measures should not be relied on as the sole source of psychosocial information, they can be efficient tools for collecting information and starting the conversation about psychosocial health. To be practical for clinical settings and minimize survivor burden, brief measures (<20 items) have generally been favored, though there is likely to be a trade-off between brevity on the one hand and accuracy and scope on the other. Short measures can have limited scope, however, so that only one or two symptom domains (e.g., fatigue, pain, depression) may be covered. In addition, very brief scales (<5 items) can have limited psychometric properties, and longer scales may be more successful at differentiating between significant and nonsignificant levels of distress. The one-item distress thermometer has been widely used in cancer patients, but reports of its sensitivity to clinical distress have varied across populations and studies with cancer survivors indicating it may not be well suited for this population (Recklitis et al. 2007; Merport et al. 2012). In selecting a self-report screening measure, providers should consider instruments that focus on problems likely to be most relevant to their particular population. In many survivor groups, depression and anxiety will be common concerns and because studies show cancer survivors are at higher risk for suicidal thoughts and behaviors, some consideration should be given to including feelings of hopelessness and suicidal thoughts. In some survivor groups, other symptom areas such as cognitive problems and substance abuse may be more relevant to assess, and each of the selection of screening measures should be tailored to the survivor population being followed. In our center, we have found that both survivors and parents are open to using these checklist measures, and they can be readily integrated into a survivorship visit (Recklitis et al. 2003; Liptak et al. 2012). Parent report measures are most useful for younger survivors (<10) who may be burdened by a paper-and-pencil form. Parent report may also be useful for assessing behavioral and school problems in survivors across ages. In adolescent and young adult patients, self-report measures are especially useful for assessing internalizing symptoms like anxiety, depression, social isolation, and hopelessness, as these may not be fully appreciated by parents (Recklitis et al. 2003; Liptak et al. 2012).

Whenever self-report rating scales are applied to cancer survivors, caution should be exercised in interpreting these measures as they are applied to cancer survivors. Reliability and validity of tests will vary in different populations, and several studies have indicated that previously validated tests may operate differently or require different cut-off scores to be used in cancer patients or survivors (Johnson et al. 1996; Zabora et al. 2001; Recklitis and Rodriguez 2007). Until research on cancer survivors has provided specific validation of the instrument and clinical cut-off scores in cancer survivors, clinicians should carefully consider how to interpret both negative and positive screening results and should work closely with a mental health consultant familiar with clinical screening tools to select and implement this kind of screening in a clinical environment. These measures alone may not be sufficient for evaluating psychosocial needs of individual survivors, but they can help inform the psychosocial assessment process in a number of ways. For example, using these forms routinely with all survivors reminds health-care providers to discuss psychosocial concerns they might otherwise neglect, and it allows at least some survivors an outlet for reporting on problems they may not bring up unless directly asked (Recklitis et al. 2003; Liptak et al. 2012). Being available to consult with medical providers and to provide assessment of individual survivors is itself a critical component of psychosocial care in the survivorship setting and also supports the first goal of problem identification. Oncology providers are often invested in talking with patients about their psychosocial needs but may be reticent to do so without an efficient means for providing follow-up for problems that may be identified. Ideally, mental health clinicians should be available to provide both individual care and group care in the survivorship setting. This may include support groups or psychoeducational programs, consultation to providers or survivors about community resources, and follow-up assessments for identified problems. In some cases, the psychosocial clinician may see survivors in a scheduled appointment similar to what would be provided in an outpatient mental health setting, but the model of survivorship care encourages clinicians to be very flexible in how, when, and where they deliver care. Depending on the need and practical considerations of a particular clinic visit, clinicians may see survivors for brief visits (15–30 min) at the time of a medical visit, with or without family members or medical providers present, and may use telephone and e-mail contact as a way of providing information, ongoing monitoring, or following up on a referral plan. To illustrate our approach to assessment, supportive care, and referral, below we provide a description of a typical psychosocial visit that might occur when a survivor is referred for psychosocial assessment. While many survivorship visits will follow this approach, it is also important to appreciate that psychosocial care can be delivered in a variety of ways, some of which are quite brief and have targeted goals. For example, survivors who are not reporting any significant distress but are interested in finding a community-based resource, such as a smoking cessation group, a book on effective parenting, or a survivor support group, may have information provided to them in a brief, informal interaction or in a follow-up phone call or e-mail.

During the Survivorship Visit

The clinician meeting the cancer survivor should enter the appointment with the primary aim of conducting a brief assessment and triaging any identified psychosocial needs. It is important that the clinician not be burdened with the expectation that they must complete a comprehensive psychological evaluation during the visit. As survivors often wait for professionals to initiate the discussion of psychosocial challenges, the experience of meeting with a clinician for the purposes of discussing their psychosocial needs can often be one of the first times that they have had the opportunity to raise such concerns (LAF 2004; Detmar et al. 2000; Greenberg 2004). Therefore, the clinician should utilize the survivorship visit as an opportunity to ascertain where the patient's psychosocial needs may be best met and how to encourage the patient to initiate recommended services.

Immediately prior to the visit with the patient, it is standard practice to acquire as much information as possible from as many different sources available about the patient's status including the reason for the referral. The opportunity to have a brief conversation with the referring provider offers a rich understanding of the specific patient's needs. Consulting with the oncology provider prior to seeing the patient, either in person or over the telephone, should be prioritized. Second, in some clinical settings, there may be psychosocial questions that are already integrated into patient medical history forms. The use of self-report measures can contribute to good clinical care as they provide a less intimidating venue for the patient to endorse clinical concerns and can act as helpful cues to initiate conversations. However, clinicians must remain wary of both the potential for false positives and the minimization of symptoms on self-report. While in many cases, the psychosocial clinician can obtain a sense of the clinical needs prior to meeting the patient, there is not always a clear sense of why the patient may have requested your services. The survivorship visit presents a unique opportunity during which the patient may be returning to a trusted medical facility, and this can facilitate their seeking psychosocial support.

During the visit, there are a number of key thinking points for the clinician to consider. This list is not intended as a comprehensive assessment of survivors' emotional health, but rather areas that the clinician can think about as they discuss the survivor's evolving adjustment:

- What are the primary presenting symptoms?
- When was the onset of the presenting symptoms? Were there any identifiable precipitants?
- What is the patient's history of mental health disturbances and/or treatment?
- What is the level of current impairment? Is there a need for immediate triage?
- Are there comorbid physical health issues that are relevant to consider?
- Does the patient have relevant cancer treatment-related late effects? For example, are they experiencing cardiac, hormonal, or neurological disturbances that may be impacting their psychosocial function?
- Is the patient taking any medications that may be affecting their mood state?
- Did the patient experience any developmental challenges as a result of their cancer diagnosis and treatment? For example, did they miss extended periods of school that may have impacted their social development?
- How are the patient's current sleeping habits and appetite?
- Is the patient actively engaged in work/school activities?
- Does the patient have concerns related to her social and family relationships?
- Does the patient have a support network that they can rely upon?

Initiating a conversation about psychosocial challenges in a medical setting may be uncomfortable. Psychosocial providers can frame their role as providing an integrative survivorship evaluation in collaboration with the oncology staff. In this role, the psychosocial clinician supports the oncology team in ensuring that mood-related issues do not impact the patient's quality of life and vice versa. As patients may not be accustomed to psychosocial services in an oncology setting, they may believe that they are limited to reporting physical health issues; it is the psychosocial provider's role to help separate physical from psychosocial needs. Whenever written assessment is used, reviewing responses and discussing them directly with the survivor is essential. By way of introduction, a provider may simply ask, "When you completed the questions about mood and emotional functioning, did any of those questions seem to apply to you?" The provider can then quickly scan the responses to the self-report items and inquire about any that were endorsed.

One challenge during psychosocial visits is the extent to which parents and caregivers play a role in the ongoing care of an adolescent or young adult survivor. Unless there is a clear clinical reason to do otherwise, we suggest starting with the entire family but letting family members know that they may be asked to step out for some part of the meeting so that the individual survivors can be met with alone. This will provide an opportunity to observe interactions and potentially obtain valuable information about family dynamics that may play a role in the patient's psychosocial functioning. It is important that the focus remains on patient-related issues as there is the possibility that parents may use this meeting as an outlet for their individual concerns. Though these challenges can certainly play a role in parents' ability to facilitate support for the survivor, it is important that the survivor has the opportunity to focus on his current needs. Particularly for adolescents and young adults, and those who are adequately developed both cognitively and emotionally, it is important to meet with them privately after disclosing confidentiality limitations. An individual assessment with the adolescent or young adult survivor can provide critical information about their well-being as well as any challenges they may feel uncomfortable disclosing in the presence of family members.

Though the assessment is often limited to the survivorship visit, it is not uncommon that a clinician will require additional follow-up to fully explore the survivor's needs and how best to guide them in aftercare. While conducting the assessment, one should consider whether to seek consultation from the survivor's oncology team or with other medical staff in order to clarify presenting concerns. In addition, it is also within reason to request that the patient return for a follow-up visit if possible. It will be important that one outlines the importance of returning for further evaluation and provides aims for a follow-up meeting.

Case Vignette : Sarah, a 23-Year-Old Survivor of Osteosarcoma

Medical History: Sarah was diagnosed with osteosarcoma at the age of 14 and treated with surgery and chemotherapy. Fortunately for Sarah, she has experienced relatively limited physical late effects of treatment.

Psychosocial Adaptation: Sarah, now a bright, articulate, 23-year-old survivor, comes to a routine survivorship clinic visit and reports to her oncology nurse practitioner feelings of depressed mood, lack of energy, and problems sleeping. She was treated 5 years ago in a college counseling center for depression. A social worker in the survivorship clinic sees Sarah for 30 min in the survivorship clinic for an interview and makes the following assessment and recommendation: Sarah's depression is not currently severe as she is working and maintaining most social activities and her symptom reports on a rating scale and in person suggest moderate depression. She has active supports from her roommates and has no current or past suicidal ideation or impulses and no hopelessness, so the need for treatment is not urgent or emergent. Sarah is worried about her depression but ambivalent about returning to treatment and unsure of how to access mental health care now that she is living on her own. In their discussion, it becomes clear that Sarah is ambivalent about returning to talk therapy but more open to restarting her antidepressant medication. The social worker suggests that as a first step Sarah contact her PCP to discuss medication for her symptoms and that she and Sarah follow up in 4 weeks by phone to see if Sarah has seen her PCP and to reassess her symptoms. Sarah seems relieved that she can do something about her depression without getting back into talk therapy and agrees. The social worker ends the session by giving Sarah her card with contact information, a teaching sheet about how to access outpatient mental health services, and also an informational flyer about support groups for people with depression including suicide prevention hotlines. The next day, the social worker copies the nurse practitioner on an e-mail she sends Sarah reiterating the plan and encouraging Sarah to contact her prior to the 4-week follow-up point if needed. After 4 weeks, the social worker calls and e-mails Sarah as agreed to, and Sarah reports she has restarted her antidepressant medication and is hopeful she will be feeling better soon. The social worker leaves a phone message and an e-mail offering to follow up with Sarah again in person or by phone but does not hear back from Sarah. At Sarah's next annual oncology follow-up visit, the social worker briefly joins the nurse practitioner, and together, they ask about her depression. Sarah reports she is continuing to take her antidepressant medication as prescribed by her PCP and that her symptoms have improved. She acknowledges that she has "issues" on her mind and that she will return to counseling to deal with them "someday." The social worker praises Sarah's ability to get herself the care she needs and offers to be available in the future if Sarah is looking for additional support or counseling.

Comment: Sarah's case is typical in that mild to moderate depressive symptoms are common in the general population and in young adult cancer survivors. Psychosocial intervention for Sarah is briefer than it would be in a mental health clinic and may take place with a medical provider in the room. The goal here is not to provide her with specialty mental health care, but to decide if she needs it. Because Sarah is verbal and relatively high functioning, a focal assessment of her depression can be completed in a short period of time using an interview and a symptom rating scale. Similarly, with some support and instruction from the social worker, Sarah is able to advocate for her needs and arrange a visit with her PCP. Some survivors would require a more in-depth assessment and would be less successful at implementing recommended follow-up, but many survivors like Sarah can make use of brief interventions to make important changes. Like many young adults, Sarah is not sure she wants to follow through on all recommended care (i.e., talk therapy in addition to medication), and the team responds to this by recognizing her autonomy and offering future opportunities to revisit her choices.

Following the Survivorship Visit

Depending on the severity of symptoms reported, the evaluating clinician may choose to implement particular interventions, including psychoeducation and consultation, brief in-clinic treatment, or referral to community-based services as appropriate. For mild and/or transient symptoms, psychoeducation and regular monitoring of symptoms may be sufficient. For example, survivors may present to clinic visits with increased worry around the time of their appointment due to a fear of disease recurrence. Health-related concerns will likely differ by disease group and length of time since diagnosis, with concerns about recurrence appearing more prominently in those with a history of CNS disease in comparison with other types of pediatric cancer. The psychosocial provider can intervene during the survivor's clinic visit by normalizing these fears, ensuring that all of the survivor's medical questions are answered, reviewing strategies for stress reduction, and providing information regarding when to seek additional assistance from a mental health provider. For survivors seeking interventions for mild symptoms (e.g., transient worry, mild adjustment challenges), referrals to support groups, primary care, or school-based supports may also be appropriate.

For the smaller proportion of survivors who present with persistent or more severe symptoms of psychological distress, additional steps may need to be taken. In addition to psychoeducation and regular monitoring of symptoms, these patients may require further psychological assessment, beyond what is feasible in the context of a brief clinic visit. Additional consultation and assessment can therefore be provided in a separate follow-up session or sessions. Patients with more severe symptoms may benefit from community-based mental health referrals or from referrals to primary care, the latter of which can then triage to additional in-network psychology/psychiatry providers. Patients should be provided with recommendations regarding the type and modality of therapy likely to be most efficacious for their presenting difficulties.

When considering community-based mental health referrals, the type of provider (e.g., psychologist, psychiatrist, social worker, counselor) and the intervention recommended (e.g., individual therapy, group therapy, psychotropic medication, cognitive-behavioral therapy) will depend on the presenting issues. While it can be difficult to identify community-based mental health providers who are familiar with childhood medical illness and the unique needs of cancer survivors, providers with some familiarity in this area are preferred. Survivors of pediatric cancer can present with a myriad of psychological challenges; behavioral and cognitive concerns often overlap with one another and can create a complex presentation (Kahalley et al. 2013). If a provider with some knowledge of the needs of cancer survivors cannot be identified, communication between the survivor's medical team and the mental health provider may be very beneficial, particularly if the survivor's difficulties stem from medical or neurocognitive late effects of their cancer treatment. For many survivors, information about the possible costs of mental health treatment and insurance coverage is essential to the decision-making process and increases adherence to recommendations for treatment.

It should be noted that adolescent and young adult survivors often have unique psychological needs that are distinctly different from those of pediatric and older adult survivors (e.g., concerns about financial independence, health-care transitions, limited interest in psychological intervention, parental involvement, etc.) (D'Agostino and Edelstein 2013). Referrals for psychological treatment should therefore be made with special consideration of the survivor's age and developmental level. While accessibility of quality services can be a challenge, there is work being done to increase the availability of survivorship care in settings that are convenient for this population (e.g., college health centers) (Forehand et al. 2014). Providing adolescents and young adults with information regarding some of the common challenges that their age group faces can be a helpful way to normalize distress and to create an avenue for problem solving. Because this group in particular may not be amenable to psychological intervention, the clinician should be open to respecting the patient's autonomy and to creatively exploring areas for intervention. Please refer to Table 15.4 for additional resources that may provide guidance around follow-up and community-based resources.

Future Directions in Psychosocial Care for Survivors

The recognition of psychological vulnerabilities of childhood cancer survivors has led to efforts to extend psychosocial care beyond the active treatment phase. The extension of psychosocial care to a new population of long-term survivors inevitably brings about changes in the focus, setting, and methods of delivering care, many of which have been summarized in this chapter. Survivorship care is still a relatively new and rapidly developing area of psychosocial cancer care, and novel approaches to delivering survivor care are currently being developed and investigated. In particular, there are many efforts to develop novel interventions that are well suited to the needs and interests of young adult survivors. Low-intensity interventions (Bennett-Levy et al. 2010; Health 2011) designed to require limited time commitment may be particularly appealing to the broad group of survivors who are looking for additional education or support but do not have serious psychiatric symptoms and may not live near their cancer center. Similarly survivors may be more open to interventions that are labeled as educational and health promoting, as these may fit better with our contemporary culture that emphasizes "wellness," and may avoid potential stigma of seeking mental health care. For example, day-long conferences, expressive writing interventions, online support groups, and video sharing have all been piloted as potential methods for addressing young survivors' needs for emotional support. Research on these interventions is quite limited, but studies of their outcomes are sorely needed if these interventions are going to be incorporated into standard care and made available to survivors who may benefit from them. Even more commonly used interven-

Table 15.4 Available follow-up resources for survivors with psychological concerns

Challenge	Referral resources
Financial limitations	Hospital/clinic finance department (e.g., insurance, bill paying) Social security or public welfare programs Advocacy groups (e.g., Livestrong.org Foundation, Healthcare For All) Local agencies and resources (e.g., food bank, shelters)
Problems with employment or school	Information on Family and Medical Leave Act and Americans with Disabilities Act Advocacy groups (e.g., Livestrong.org, Cancer Legal Resource Center) Public or private rehabilitation programs Appropriate evaluation or rehabilitation services (e.g., physical therapy, occupational therapy, neurocognitive testing)
Problems managing medical care	Refer to primary care for evaluation Disease-specific education and information (e.g., diabetes teaching sheets) Disease/condition-specific support group (e.g., American Chronic Pain Association, Fertile Hope) Cancer survivors' resources (e.g., Lance Armstrong Foundation, National Coalition for Cancer Survivorship)
Change in health behaviors	Education on health protection/promotion (e.g., smoking cessation teaching sheet) Primary/specialty care for evaluation (e.g., nutritionist) Local services (e.g., smoking cessation, weight loss program, Alcoholics Anonymous)
Coping with isolation or emotional concerns	Local support groups Advocacy groups (e.g., Livestrong.org, National Coalition for Cancer Survivorship) Organizations offering support groups (e.g., the Wellness Community, CancerCare, Cancer Hope Network) Disease-specific programs (e.g., Living Beyond Breast Cancer, Support for People with Oral, Head and Neck Cancer) Local mental health professionals for evaluation and treatment accessed through national organizations (e.g., American Psychosocial Oncology Society, American Psychological Association, National Association of Social Workers)

tions such as traditional support groups and methods for screening and referring survivors for mental health care often have limited empirical support, underscoring the need for more outcomes research for all interventions that are aimed at psychosocial care of childhood cancer survivors.

One of the significant challenges facing both medical care and psychosocial care of survivors is the limited capacity for pediatric specialty centers to provide this care (Freyer 2010). As patients get older, they may age out of pediatric oncology clinics, move away from their initial cancer center, or develop physical or mental health problems more appropriately managed outside of pediatric specialty care. As a result, childhood cancer survivors who are not connected to specialized survivorship programs may experience significant barriers to receiving appropriate interventions even when demonstrating clinically significant symptoms of distress (Dieluweit et al. 2010; Kahalley et al. 2013). Similar challenges exist for addressing survivors' medical needs (Freyer 2010), and making high-quality aftercare accessible to all survivors will likely require rethinking models of delivering care survivorship. For psychosocial providers, this may mean developing procedures for offering referral support to survivors or primary care providers, even for survivors not currently seen at the cancer center, and developing educational and support services survivors can access remotely using the telephone and Internet. Some national resources such as CancerCare and the American Psychosocial Oncology Society currently use the telephone to provide counseling or to make referrals for community-based in-person counseling to cancer survivors. At our center, we are piloting the use of video-conferencing technology to deliver stress reduction interventions and cognitive-behavioral interventions for insomnia to cancer survivors (Zhou et al. 2014). There has been increasing interest across hospitals to improve intervention accessibility for cancer patients by using technological means (Kuijpers et al. 2013; Bantum et al. 2014; Emmons et al. 2013). The need to extend psychosocial care for survivors beyond specialty oncology programs is a clear challenge, and web and mobile technologies offer the possibility of efficiently delivering programs to survivors at a distance. We anticipate that educational, supportive, and even diagnostic and psychotherapeutic interventions for cancer survivors using mobile technology will become more popular in the next decade and that with creative approaches to intervention development and rigorous outcomes research, these programs may prove useful for disseminating supportive care consistently to all childhood cancer survivors.

Clinical Pearls

- Psychosocial screening in survivors of childhood cancer needs to assess the prevalence of psychological *symptoms* as well as potential rather than diagnosable psychiatric *disorders*. It is the psychosocial clinician's role to assess, target, and intervene on psychological and behavioral symptoms that cause subjective distress, whether or not a psychiatric diagnosis is present.
- Risk factors can be an important guide to assessing and monitoring survivors; however, it is critical to appreciate that the course of cancer survivorship is dynamic and individuals who may initially present with no risk factors require ongoing monitoring and evaluation as their risk status and emotional outcomes can change significantly over time.
- Psychosocial clinicians must be flexible in how, when, and where they provide assessment and intervention to survivors, depending on the setting and model of care.

References

Bantum EO, Albright CL, White KK, Berenberg JL, Layi G, Ritter PL, Laurent D, Plant K, Lorig K (2014) Surviving and thriving with cancer using a Web-based health behavior change intervention: randomized controlled trial. J Med Internet Res 16(2):e54. doi:10.2196/jmir.3020

Barrera M, Shaw AK, Speechley KN, Maunsell E, Pogany L (2005) Educational and social late effects of childhood cancer and related clinical, personal, and familial characteristics. Cancer 15;104(8):1751–160

Bennett-Levy J, Richards D, Farrand P, Christensen H, Griffiths K, Kavanagh D, Klein B (2010) Oxford guide to low intensity CBT interventions. Oxford University Press, Oxford

Bjork M, Nordstrom B, Wiebe T, Hallstrom I (2011) Returning to a changed ordinary life–families' lived experience after completing a child's cancer treatment. Eur J Cancer Care 20(2):163–169. doi:10.1111/j.1365-2354.2009.01159.x

Bober SL, Zhou ES, Chen B, Manley PE, Kenney LB, Recklitis CJ (2013) Sexual function in childhood cancer survivors: a report from Project REACH. J Sex Med 10(8):2084–2093. doi:10.1111/jsm.12193

Canada AL, Schover LR, Li Y (2007) A pilot intervention to enhance psychosexual development in adolescents and young adults with cancer. Pediatr Blood Cancer 49(6):824–828. doi:10.1002/pbc.21130

Casey R, Zwemer E, Recklitis CJ (2010) Is survivor identity associated with physical and behavioral health?: results from Project REACH. In: Poster presented at the National Cancer Institute Conference on Cancer Survivorship Research, Washington, DC

Collins C (2010) Evolving models of behavioral health integration in primary care. Milbank Memorial Fund, New York

D'Agostino NM, Edelstein K (2013) Psychosocial challenges and resource needs of young adult cancer survivors: implications for program development. J Psychosoc Oncol 31(6):585–600. doi:10.1080/07347332.2013.835018

Detmar SB, Aaronson NK, Wever LD, Muller M, Schornagel JH (2000) How are you feeling? Who wants to know? Patients' and oncologists' preferences for discussing health-related quality-of-life issues. J Clin Oncol 18(18):3295–3301

Dieluweit U, Debatin KM, Grabow D, Kaatsch P, Peter R, Seitz DC, Goldbeck L (2010) Social outcomes of long-term survivors of adolescent cancer. Psychooncology 19(12):1277–1284

Duffey-Lind EC, O'Holleran E, Healey M, Vettese M, Diller L, Park ER (2006) Transitioning to survivorship: a pilot study. J Pediatr Oncol Nurs 23(6):335–343. doi:10.1177/1043454206293267

Emmons KM, Puleo E, Sprunck-Harrild K, Ford J, Ostroff JS, Hodgson D, Greenberg M, Diller L, de Moor J, Tyc V (2013) Partnership for health-2, a web-based versus print smoking cessation intervention for childhood and young adult cancer survivors: randomized comparative effectiveness study. J Med Internet Res 15(11):e218. doi:10.2196/jmir.2533

Erikson EH (1968) Identity: youth and crisis. Norton & Co., Oxford

Forehand RL, Williamson RS, Russo GS, Pyle SJ, Meacham LR (2014) College health as a partner in the care of pediatric cancer survivors. J Am Coll Health 62(7):506–510

Freyer DR (2010) Transition of care for young adult survivors of childhood and adolescent cancer: rationale and approaches. J Clin Oncol 28(32):4810–4818. doi:10.1200/JCO.2009.23.4278

Frobisher C, Lancashire ER, Winter DL, Taylor AJ, Reulen RC, Hawkins MM (2010) Long-term population-based divorce rates among adult survivors of childhood cancer in Britain. Pediatr Blood Cancer 54(1):116–122. doi:10.1002/pbc.22290

Green DM, Kawashima T, Stovall M, Leisenring W, Sklar CA, Mertens AC, Donaldson SS, Byrne J, Robison LL (2009) Fertility of female survivors of childhood cancer: a report from the childhood cancer survivor study. J Clin Oncol 27(16):2677–2685. doi:10.1200/JCO.2008.20.1541

Green DM, Kawashima T, Stovall M, Leisenring W, Sklar CA, Mertens AC, Donaldson SS, Byrne J, Robison LL (2010) Fertility of male survivors of childhood cancer: a report from the Childhood Cancer Survivor Study. J Clin Oncol 28(2):332–339. doi:10.1200/JCO.2009.24.9037

Greenberg DB (2004) Barriers to the treatment of depression in cancer patients. J Natl Cancer Inst Monogr 32:127–135. doi:10.1093/jncimonographs/lgh019

Gurney JG, Krull KR, Kadan-Lottick N, Nicholson HS, Nathan PC, Zebrack B, Tersak JM, Ness KK (2009) Social outcomes in the Childhood Cancer Survivor Study cohort. J Clin Oncol 27(14):2390–2395. doi:10.1200/JCO.2008.21.1458

Haase JE, Rostad M (1994) Experiences of completing cancer therapy: children's perspectives. Oncol Nurs Forum 21(9):1483–1492; discussion 1493–1484

Hall AE, Boyes AW, Bowman J, Walsh RA, James EL, Girgis A (2012) Young adult cancer survivors' psychosocial well-being: a cross-sectional study assessing quality of life, unmet needs, and health behaviors. Support Care Cancer 20(6):1333–1341

Hawkins MM, Lancashire ER, Winter DL, Frobisher C, Reulen RC, Taylor AJ, Stevens MC, Jenney M (2008) The British Childhood Cancer Survivor Study: Objectives, methods, population structure, response rates and initial descriptive information. Pediatr Blood Cancer 50(5):1018–1025. doi:10.1002/pbc.21335

Health NCCfM (2011) Generalised anxiety disorder in adults: management in primary, secondary and community care. British Psychological Society, London

Holland J, Andersen B, Breitbart W, Compas B, Dudley M, Fleishman S, Fulcher C, Greenberg D, Greiner C, Handzo G, Hoofring L, Jacobsen P, Knight S, Learson K, Levy M, Loscalzo M, Manne S, McAllister-Black R, Riba M, Roper K, Valentine A, Wagner L, Zevon M, Panel NDM (2010) Distress management. J Natl Compr Canc Netw 8(4):448–485

Howlader N, Noone AM, Krapcho M, Garshell J, Neyman N, Altekruse SF, Kosary CL, Yu M, Ruhl J, Tatalovich Z, Cho H, Mariotto A, Lewis DR, Chen HS, Feuer EJ, Cronin KA (2013) SEER Cancer Statistics Review, 1975–2010, vol 2013 (based on November 2012 SEER data submission). National Cancer Institute, Bethesda

Hudson MM, Mertens AC, Yasui Y, Hobbie W, Chen H, Gurney JG, Yeazel M, Recklitis CJ, Marina N, Robison LR, Oeffinger KC (2003a) Health status of adult long-term survivors of childhood cancer: a report from the Childhood Cancer Survivor Study. J Am Med Assoc 290(12):1583–1592

Hudson MM, Mertens AC, Yasui Y, Hobbie W, Chen H, Gurney JG, Yeazel M, Recklitis CJ, Marina N, Robison LR, Oeffinger KC, Childhood Cancer Survivor Study Investigators (2003b) Health status of adult long-term survivors of childhood cancer: a report from the Childhood Cancer Survivor Study. JAMA 290(12):1583–1592. doi:10.1001/jama.290.12.1583

Hudson MM, Ness KK, Nolan VG, Armstrong GT, Green DM, Morris EB, Spunt SL, Metzger ML, Krull KR, Klosky JL, Srivastava DK, Robison LL (2011) Prospective medical assessment of adults surviving childhood cancer: study design, cohort characteristics, and feasibility of the St. Jude Lifetime Cohort study. Pediatr Blood Cancer 56(5):825–836. doi:10.1002/pbc.22875

Jacobs LA, Pucci DA (2013) Adult survivors of childhood cancer: the medical and psychosocial late effects of cancer treatment and the impact on sexual and reproductive health. J Sex Med 10(Suppl 1):120–126. doi:10.1111/jsm.12050

Janson C, Leisenring W, Cox C, Termuhlen AM, Mertens AC, Whitton JA, Goodman P, Zeltzer L, Robison LL, Krull KR, Kadan-Lottick NS (2009) Predictors of marriage and divorce in adult survivors of childhood cancers: a report from the Childhood Cancer Survivor Study. Cancer Epidemiol Biomarkers Prev 18(10):2626–2635

Johnson LC, Murphy SA, Dimond M (1996) Reliability, construct validity, and subscale norms of the Brief Symptom Inventory when administered to bereaved parents. J Nurs Meas 4(2):117–127

Johnson JG, Cohen P, Dohrenwend BP, Link BG, Brook JS (1999) A longitudinal investigation of social causation and social selection processes involved in the association between socioeconomic status and psychiatric disorders. J Abnorm Psychol 108(3):490–499

Kahalley LS, Wilson SJ, Tyc VL, Conklin HM, Hudson MM, Wu S, Xiong X, Stancel HH, Hinds PS (2013) Are the psychological needs of adolescent survivors of pediatric cancer adequately identified and treated? Psychooncology 22(2):447–458. doi:10.1002/pon.3021

Kelly D (2013) Developing age appropriate psychosexual support for adolescent cancer survivors: a discussion paper. J Sex Med 10(Suppl 1):133–138. doi:10.1111/jsm.12048

Kenney LB, Cohen LE, Shnorhavorian M, Metzger ML, Lockart B, Hijiya N, Duffey-Lind E, Constine L, Green D, Meacham L (2012) Male reproductive health after childhood, adolescent, and young adult cancers: a report from the Children's Oncology Group. J Clin

Oncol 30(27):3408–3416. doi:10.1200/JCO.2011.38.6938
Kirchhoff AC, Leisenring W, Krull KR, Ness KK, Friedman DL, Armstrong GT, Stovall M, Park ER, Oeffinger KC, Hudson MM, Robison LL, Wickizer T (2010) Unemployment among adult survivors of childhood cancer: a report from the childhood cancer survivor study. Med Care 48(11):1015–1025. doi:10.1097/MLR.0b013e3181eaf880
Kirchhoff AC, Krull KR, Ness KK, Armstrong GT, Park ER, Stovall M, Robison LL, Leisenring W (2011) Physical, mental, and neurocognitive status and employment outcomes in the childhood cancer survivor study cohort. Cancer Epidemiol Biomarkers Prev 20(9):1838–1849. doi:10.1158/1055-9965.EPI-11-0239, 1055–9965.EPI-11-0239 [pii]
Knapp PK, Foy JM (2012) Integrating mental health care into pediatric primary care settings. J Am Acad Child Adolesc Psychiatry 51(10):982–984. doi:10.1016/j.jaac.2012.07.009
Kornblith A (1998) Psychosocial adaptation of cancer survivors. In: Holland JC (ed) Psycho-oncology. Oxford University Press, New York, pp 223–254
Kuehni CE, Rueegg CS, Michel G, Rebholz CE, Strippoli MP, Niggli FK, Egger M, von der Weid NX, Swiss Paediatric Oncology G (2012) Cohort profile: the Swiss childhood cancer survivor study. Int J Epidemiol 41(6):1553–1564. doi:10.1093/ije/dyr142
Kuijpers W, Groen WG, Aaronson NK, van Harten WH (2013) A systematic review of web-based interventions for patient empowerment and physical activity in chronic diseases: relevance for cancer survivors. J Med Internet Res 15(2):e37. doi:10.2196/jmir.2281
Kunin-Batson A, Kadan-Lottick N, Zhu L, Cox C, Bordes-Edgar V, Srivastava DK, Zeltzer L, Robison LL, Krull KR (2011) Predictors of independent living status in adult survivors of childhood cancer: a report from the Childhood Cancer Survivor Study. Pediatr Blood Cancer 57(7):1197–1203. doi:10.1002/pbc.22982
Labay LE, Mayans S, Harris MB (2004) Integrating the child into home and community following the completion of cancer treatment. J Pediatr Oncol Nurs 21(3):165–169
LAF (2004) LIVESTRONG poll finds nearly half of people living with cancer feel their non-medical needs are unmet by their healthcare system. Lance-Armstrong Foundation. http://www.livestrong.org. Accessed 14 July 2005
Langeveld NE, Ubbink MC, Last BF, Grootenhuis MA, Voute PA, De Haan RJ (2003) Educational achievement, employment and living situation in long-term young adult survivors of childhood cancer in the Netherlands. Psychooncology 12(3):213–225
Liptak C, Manley P, Recklitis CJ (2012) The feasibility of psychosocial screening for adolescent and young adult brain tumor survivors: the value of self-report. J Cancer Surviv 6(4):379–387. doi:10.1007/s11764-012-0237-7
Mariotto AB, Rowland JH, Yabroff KR, Scoppa S, Hachey M, Ries L, Feuer EJ (2009) Long-term survivors of childhood cancers in the United States. Cancer Epidemiol Biomarkers Prev 18(4):1033–1040. doi:10.1158/1055-9965.EPI-08-0988
Maurice-Stam H, Grootenhuis MA, Caron HN, Last BF (2007) Course of life of survivors of childhood cancer is related to quality of life in young adulthood. J Psychosoc Oncol 25(3):43–58. doi:10.1300/J077v25n03_03
McLean CP, Anderson ER (2009) Brave men and timid women? A review of the gender differences in fear and anxiety. Clin Psychol Rev 29(6):496–505. doi:10.1016/j.cpr.2009.05.003, S0272-7358(09)00067-1 [pii]
Mental health: integrated approach (2012) Health Serv J 122(6323):S8–11. http://www.ncbi.nlm.nih.gov/pubmed/23390718
Merport A, Bober SL, Grose A, Recklitis CJ (2012) Can the distress thermometer (DT) identify significant psychological distress in long-term cancer survivors? A comparison with the Brief Symptom Inventory-18 (BSI-18). Support Care Cancer 20(1):195–198. doi:10.1007/s00520-011-1269-7
Michel G, Rebholz CE, von der Weid NX, Bergstraesser E, Kuehni CE (2010) Psychological distress in adult survivors of childhood cancer: the Swiss Childhood Cancer Survivor study. J Clin Oncol 28(10):1740–1748. doi:10.1200/JCO.2009.23.4534
Morgan S, Davies S, Palmer S, Plaster M (2010) Sex, drugs, and rock 'n' roll: caring for adolescents and young adults with cancer. J Clin Oncol 28(32):4825–4830. doi:10.1200/JCO.2009.22.5474
Ness KK, Mertens AC, Hudson MM, Wall MM, Leisenring WM, Oeffinger KC, Sklar CA, Robison LL, Gurney JG (2005) Limitations on physical performance and daily activities among long-term survivors of childhood cancer. Ann Intern Med 143(9):639–647, doi:143/9/639 [pii]
Ness KK, Gurney JG, Zeltzer LK, Leisenring W, Mulrooney DA, Nathan PC, Robison LL, Mertens AC (2008) The impact of limitations in physical, executive, and emotional function on health-related quality of life among adult survivors of childhood cancer: a report from the Childhood Cancer Survivor Study. Arch Phys Med Rehabil 89(1):128–136
Network NCC (2003) Distress management clinical practice guidelines. J Natl Compr Canc Netw 1:344–374
Northman L, Ross S, Morris M, Tarquini S (2014) Supporting pediatric cancer survivors with neurocognitive late effects: a model of care. J Pediatr Oncol Nurs. doi:10.1177/1043454214554012
Oancea SC, Brinkman TM, Ness KK, Krull KR, Smith WA, Srivastava DK, Robison LL, Hudson MM, Gurney JG (2014) Emotional distress among adult survivors of childhood cancer. J Cancer Surviv 8(2):293–303
Oeffinger KC, Mertens AC, Sklar CA, Kawashima T, Hudson MM, Meadows AT, Friedman DL, Marina N, Hobbie W, Kadan-Lottick NS, Schwartz CL, Leisenring W, Robison LL (2006) Chronic health con-

ditions in adult survivors of childhood cancer. N Engl J Med 355(15):1572–1582. doi:10.1056/NEJMsa060185

Parker PA, Baile WF, de Moor C, Cohen L (2003) Psychosocial and demographic predictors of quality of life in a large sample of cancer patients. Psychooncology 12(2):183–193. doi:10.1002/pon.635

Pastore G, Mosso ML, Magnani C, Luzzatto L, Bianchi M, Terracini B (2001) Physical impairment and social life goals among adult long-term survivors of childhood cancer: a population-based study from the childhood cancer registry of Piedmont, Italy. Tumori 87(6):372–378

Patenaude AF, Kupst MJ (2005) Psychosocial functioning in pediatric cancer. J Pediatr Psychol 30(1):9–27

Piccinelli M, Wilkinson G (2000) Gender differences in depression. Critical review. Br J Psychiatry 177:486–492

Recklitis C, Liptak C (2015) Psychological challenges and adaptation in long-term survivors of childhood cancer. In: Mucci GA, Torno LR (eds) Handbook of long term care of the childhood cancer survivor. Springer, New York. 978-1-4899-7583-6

Recklitis CJ, Rodriguez P (2007) Screening childhood cancer survivors with the brief symptom inventory-18: classification agreement with the symptom checklist-90-revised. Psychooncology 16(5):429–436. doi:10.1002/pon.1069

Recklitis C, O'Leary T, Diller L (2003) Utility of routine psychological screening in the childhood cancer survivor clinic. J Clin Oncol 21(5):787–792

Recklitis CJ, Licht I, Ford J, Oeffinger K, Diller L (2007) Screening adult survivors of childhood cancer with the distress thermometer: a comparison with the SCL-90-R. Psychooncology 16(11):1046–1049. doi:10.1002/pon.1212

Recklitis CJ, Diller LR, Li X, Najita J, Robison LL, Zeltzer L (2010) Suicide ideation in adult survivors of childhood cancer: a report from the Childhood Cancer Survivor Study. J Clin Oncol 28(4):655–661. doi:10.1200/JCO.2009.22.8635

Roberts CS, Turney ME, Knowles AM (1998) Psychosocial issues of adolescents with cancer. Soc Work Health Care 27(4):3–18. doi:10.1300/J010v27n04_02

Robison LL, Hudson MM (2014) Survivors of childhood and adolescent cancer: life-long risks and responsibilities. Nat Rev Cancer 14(1):61–70. doi:10.1038/nrc3634

Robison LL, Mertens AC, Boice JD, Breslow NE, Donaldson SS, Green DM, Li FP, Meadows AT, Mulvihill JJ, Neglia JP, Nesbit ME, Packer RJ, Potter JD, Sklar CA, Smith MA, Stovall M, Strong LC, Yasui Y, Zeltzer LK (2002) Study design and cohort characteristics of the Childhood Cancer Survivor Study: a multi-institutional collaborative project. Med Pediatr Oncol 38(4):229–239

Sawyer M, Antoniou G, Toogood I, Rice M, Baghurst P (2000) Childhood cancer: a 4-year prospective study of the psychological adjustment of children and parents. J Pediatr Hematol Oncol 22(3):214–220

Schag CA, Ganz PA, Wing DS, Sim MS, Lee JJ (1994) Quality of life in adult survivors of lung, colon and prostate cancer. Qual Life Res 3(2):127–141

Schultz KA, Ness KK, Whitton J, Recklitis C, Zebrack B, Robison LL, Zeltzer L, Mertens AC (2007) Behavioral and social outcomes in adolescent survivors of childhood cancer: a report from the childhood cancer survivor study. J Clin Oncol 25(24):3649–3656. doi:10.1200/JCO.2006.09.2486

Smith MA, Seibel NL, Altekruse SF, Ries LA, Melbert DL, O'Leary M, Smith FO, Reaman GH (2010) Outcomes for children and adolescents with cancer: challenges for the twenty-first century. J Clin Oncol 28(15):2625–2634. doi:10.1200/JCO.2009.27.0421

Speechley KN, Barrera M, Shaw AK, Morrison HI, Maunsell E (2006) Health-related quality of life among child and adolescent survivors of childhood cancer. J Clin Oncol 24(16):2536–2543. doi:10.1200/JCO.2005.03.9628

Strauser D, Feuerstein M, Chan F, Arango J, da Silva Cardoso E, Chiu CY (2010) Vocational services associated with competitive employment in 18–25 year old cancer survivors. J Cancer Surviv 4(2):179–186. doi:10.1007/s11764-010-0119-9

Strauser D, Wagner S, Wong AW, O'Sullivan D (2013) Career readiness, developmental work personality and age of onset in young adult central nervous system survivors. Disabil Rehabil 35(7):543–550. doi:10.3109/09638288.2012.703754

Strauser D, Klosky JL, Brinkman TM, Wong AW, Chan F, Lanctot J, Ojha RP, Robison LL, Hudson MM, Ness KK (2014) Career readiness in adult survivors of childhood cancer: a report from the St. Jude Lifetime Cohort Study. J Cancer Surviv. doi:10.1007/s11764-014-0380-4

Stuber ML, Meeske KA, Krull KR, Leisenring W, Stratton K, Kazak AE, Huber M, Zebrack B, Uijtdehaage SH, Mertens AC, Robison LL, Zeltzer LK (2010) Prevalence and predictors of posttraumatic stress disorder in adult survivors of childhood cancer. Pediatrics 125(5):e1124–1134. doi:10.1542/peds.2009-2308, 125/5/e1124 [pii]

Sundberg KK, Lampic C, Arvidson J, Helstrom L, Wettergren L (2011) Sexual function and experience among long-term survivors of childhood cancer. Eur J Cancer 47(3):397–403. doi:10.1016/j.ejca.2010.09.040

Tromp K, Claessens JJ, Knijnenburg SL, van der Pal HJ, van Leeuwen FE, Caron HN, Beerendonk CC, Kremer LC (2011) Reproductive status in adult male long-term survivors of childhood cancer. Hum Reprod 26(7):1775–1783. doi:10.1093/humrep/der113

van Dijk EM, van Dulmen-den Broeder E, Kaspers GJ, van Dam EW, Braam KI, Huisman J (2008) Psychosexual functioning of childhood cancer survivors. Psychooncology 17(5):506–511. doi:10.1002/pon.1274

Vannatta K, Gartstein MA, Short A, Noll RB (1998) A controlled study of peer relationships of children surviving brain tumors: teacher, peer, and self ratings. J Pediatr Psychol 23(5):279–287

Zabora J, BrintzenhofeSzoc K, Jacobsen P, Curbow B, Piantadosi S, Hooker C, Owens A, Derogatis L (2001) A new psychosocial screening instrument for use with cancer patients. Psychosomatics 42(3):241–246

Zebrack B (2009) Information and service needs for young adult cancer survivors. Support Care Cancer 17(4):349–357. doi:10.1007/s00520-008-0469-2

Zebrack BJ, Zeltzer LK, Whitton J, Mertens AC, Odom L, Berkow R, Robison LL (2002) Psychological outcomes in long-term survivors of childhood leukemia, Hodgkin's disease, and non-Hodgkin's lymphoma: a report from the Childhood Cancer Survivor Study. Pediatrics 110(1 Pt 1):42–52

Zebrack BJ, Gurney JG, Oeffinger K, Whitton J, Packer RJ, Mertens A, Turk N, Castleberry R, Dreyer Z, Robison LL, Zeltzer LK (2004) Psychological outcomes in long-term survivors of childhood brain cancer: a report from the childhood cancer survivor study. J Clin Oncol 22(6):999–1006. doi:10.1200/JCO.2004.06.148

Zeltzer LK, Lu Q, Leisenring W, Tsao JC, Recklitis C, Armstrong G, Mertens AC, Robison LL, Ness KK (2008) Psychosocial outcomes and health-related quality of life in adult childhood cancer survivors: a report from the childhood cancer survivor study. Cancer Epidemiol Biomarkers Prev 17(2):435–446. doi:10.1158/1055-9965.EPI-07-2541

Zeltzer LK, Recklitis C, Buchbinder D, Zebrack B, Casillas J, Tsao JC, Lu Q, Krull K (2009) Psychological status in childhood cancer survivors: a report from the Childhood Cancer Survivor Study. J Clin Oncol 27(14):2396–2404. doi:10.1200/JCO.2008.21.1433

Zhou ES, Vrooman LM, Manley PE, Recklitis CJ (2014) Adapting cognitive-behavioral treatment for insomnia to a cancer survivorship program. Paper presented at the American Cancer Society Biennial Cancer Survivorship Research Conference, Atlanta

Integrative Care in Pediatric Oncology

16

Olle Jane Z. Sahler, Hilary McClafferty, and Marilyn A. Rosen

Pediatric integrative oncology is the intentional combining and coordinating of *conventional* and *evidence-based complementary therapies* into the overall treatment plan developed by the pediatric oncology team with the family. In contrast, according to the National Center for Complementary and Alternative Medicine (NCCAM http://nccam.nih.gov), alternative medicine refers to therapies used outside the mainstream biomedical model. Alternative therapies are not covered in this chapter.

The core principles of integrative medicine are as follows: (1) focus on the individual's innate healing response, (2) emphasis on the therapeutic relationship between patient and provider, (3) consideration on the whole person (body, mind, spirit) and all elements of lifestyle, (4) emphasis on health promotion, and (5) the use of all appropriate evidence-based therapies, both conventional and complementary.

As cancer and its treatment take a profound toll on children and caregivers, many families independently turn to complementary therapies to help support their children. Reasons include a desire to improve overall health and to mitigate treatment side effects and related conditions (e.g., fatigue, anxiety, depression, pain, nausea). Other reasons include a desire to explore all possible treatment options, maximize nutrition, reduce stress, and to offer all possible comfort and support throughout treatment including end-of-life. Prevalence reports of pediatric oncology patients using complementary therapies vary from 17 to 84 % primarily because of lack of standardized definitions (Ndao et al. 2013; Myers et al. 2005). To reduce confusion, the classifications developed by the NIH/NCCAM Advisory Board will be used in this chapter.

Many therapies have been found to support the natural healing process and are less invasive and sometimes less costly than comparable conventional medicine approaches. Consumer interest has significantly outpaced conventional medical education and training about complementary modalities. For example, in a survey of 90 pediatric oncologists, 99 % felt it was important to know what type of therapies their patients were using;

O.J.Z. Sahler, MD (✉)
Division of Hematology/Oncology, Golisano Children's Hospital @ Strong, University of Rochester School of Medicine and Dentistry, 601 Elmwood Avenue, PO Box 777, Rochester, NY 14642-8777, USA
e-mail: oj_sahler@urmc.rochester.edu

H. McClafferty, MD, FAAP
Departments of Pediatrics and Medicine, University of Arizona, PO Box 245153, Tucson, AZ 85724, USA
e-mail: hmcclafferty@email.arizona.edu

M.A. Rosen, MLS
Research Librarian (ret) Edward G. Miner Library, University of Rochester Medical Center, 601 Elmwood Avenue, Rochester, NY 14642, USA
e-mail: marilyn.rosen@gmail.com

A.N. Abrams et al. (eds.), *Pediatric Psychosocial Oncology: Textbook for Multidisciplinary Care*, DOI 10.1007/978-3-319-21374-3_16

however, fewer than 50 % asked their patients about use because of perceived lack of knowledge and time. Yet, over half of respondents expressed concern about possible harm especially from special diets, supplements/vitamins, and chiropractic treatment (Roth et al. 2009). Recently, the field of integrative medicine has been supported by better-defined research priorities (Briggs and Killen 2013), increased research funding, and organizations like the Consortium of Academic Health Centers for Integrative Medicine (http://www.imconsortium.org/).

The complementary therapies that might be considered in an integrative approach are presented in Table 16.1. No study has explored the usage of every possible modality. However, several practices are frequently reported including prayer, relaxation/imagery, supplements, massage, exercise, herbal medicines/teas, megavitamins/minerals, and special diets (McLean and Kemper 2006).

Why is an integrative approach developed with the oncology team preferable to independent use of complementary therapies?

Clear and open communication is critical to full disclosure of all therapies being used. This reduces the risk of unintended interactions (e.g., between drugs and supplements), a major concern of conventional providers. Good communication can also lead to consideration of an expanded range of therapies to accompany conventional treatment. Participating in such discussions enhances patients' self-efficacy, which may positively affect healing; addresses facts as well as uncertainty about treatment options; and more accurately informs the patient about the risks/benefits of the proposed therapies (Roth et al. 2009).

NCCAM suggests ways to begin the conversation at http://nccam.nih.gov/timetotalk. These "Time to Talk" pages include tip sheets for various topics, such as "5 tips on safety of mind and body practices for children and teens." These tip sheets include known evidence for the use of the modalities they cover. "Time to Talk" materials can be downloaded or ordered.

Table 16.1 NCCAM classifications of complementary therapies with selected examples

Practice	Examples
Whole medical systems	Naturopathy, Ayurveda, traditional Chinese medicine
Mind–body medicine	Meditation, prayer, mental healing, creative arts therapy (art, music, dance, writing)
Biologically based practices	Dietary supplements, botanical medicine
Manipulative and body-based practices	Chiropractic, osteopathy, massage
Energy therapies	Biofield therapies (Qigong, Reiki, therapeutic touch), bioelectromagnetics

Common Ethical Issues regarding Integrative Approaches

As in any medical encounter, ethical and legal considerations arise in integrative pediatric oncology treatment, especially if parents choose to forego conventional treatment in favor of an alternative therapy they perceive to be less toxic or dangerous. Kemper and colleagues have developed a table of efficacy and safety that can be used to evaluate any conventional or complementary therapy (Table 16.2).

Clinical decision making is complicated by the lack of research data currently available about complementary therapies, which introduce considerable uncertainty into specific clinical situations. The following guiding principles are especially applicable (Gilmour et al. 2011b).

- *Beneficence*: promote the well-being of the patient, regardless of the domain of medicine being considered.
- *Non-malfeasance*: "do no harm."
- *Patient autonomy*: does the patient have enough information to make an informed decision?

Training

A major challenge in developing an integrative oncology management plan is the variability of training, credentialing, and licensing in the

Table 16.2 Below is a 2×2 table illustrating an approach to evaluating a therapy based on efficacy and safety

		Efficacy	
		Yes	No
Safety	Yes	Use/recommend	Tolerate
	No	Monitor closely	Advise against

various modalities. Families and physicians must be well informed about the following issues (Gilmour et al. 2011a):

- Does sufficient evidence exist to suggest there is therapeutic benefit to using a particular modality?
- What are the practitioner's qualifications and pediatric experience?
- Is the practitioner's scope of practice clear?
- Is the proposed integrative treatment plan clear?
- Is consent for treatment informed?
- What is the duration of the trial of treatment?
- Will good quality treatment records be made available to the entire team of providers?

Integrative medicine is an evolving area. Board certification in IM for US physicians became available through a national certifying body in 2014. Fellowship training will be required for Board eligibility. Previously, the American Board of Integrative Holistic Medicine offered certification. Additional opportunities are available by modality. For example, the American Hypnosis Association offers in-person and online certification courses and seminars. Many training programs in nursing, psychology, dentistry, social work, and medicine offer courses in mindfulness training. The National Certification Commission for Acupuncture and Oriental Medicine (NCCAOM) offers accelerated courses in acupuncture for physicians and nurses leading to the designation of NCCAOM Diplomate of Acupuncture.

While the body of evidence supporting IM is growing, an ongoing challenge in pediatric integrative oncology is lack of focused clinical outcomes research in children. The following sections provide an overview of selected integrative pediatric oncology treatment approaches; these sections are not designed to offer an exhaustive review.

Framing an IM Approach to the Pediatric Oncology Patient

Elements of an integrative approach are tailored to the patient's needs and may include one or more of the following categories.

Nutrition	Spirituality	Whole medical systems approaches
Dietary supplements	Sleep	Environmental exposures
Mind–body medicine	Physical activity	Relationships/social support

An IM approach to pediatric oncology patients has the potential to align with the Children's Oncology Group 2013 blueprint for research in several key areas including quality of life (QOL), nutrition, and approaches to reduce nausea and vomiting (Sung et al. 2013).

Selected topics will be discussed below using case vignettes.

Nutrition

Case Vignette

A 13- year-old boy is undergoing treatment for Ewing sarcoma. His parents are concerned about his weight loss and the quality of food he is getting in the hospital. They ask if they can bring him whole foods from home.

Nutrition is a critical component of cancer treatment and a foundation of IM treatment. Poor nutrition decreases survival rates, response to treatment, and quality of life and increases time in the hospital (Bauer et al. 2011; Brinksma et al. 2012). The primary goals of an integrative nutrition plan are maintenance of existing body stores of healthy tissue, minimization of wasting due to illness and treatment side effects, support of age-appropriate growth, reduction of inflammation, and maintenance of good QOL (Bauer et al. 2011). Challenging confounding factors include presence of a hypermetabolic and pro-inflammatory state due to tumor metabolism, anorexia and cachexia, hormonal or other metabolic disruptions, stage of illness, infection, treatment regimen, and individual susceptibility to malnutrition. Unfortunately, the hypermetabolic state is often not reversible, even with adequate caloric supplementation. In addition, different malignancies have been associated with specific nutritional states. For example, children with solid tumors are at higher risk of undernourishment compared to children receiving high-dose steroids or cranial radiation, who are at high risk for fat accumulation, insulin resistance, and possible metabolic syndrome. Multimodal treatment regimens add to the complexity of nutrition management as each treatment may result in different or overlapping toxicities (Bauer et al. 2011).

The Mediterranean diet is a mainstay of IM and consists of a primarily plant-based diet with ample vegetables and fruits, whole grains, lean proteins with an emphasis on fish, low-fat dairy, and beverages and spices with potent anti-inflammatory and antioxidant properties. One study in 117 adult survivors of childhood leukemia showed that adherence to a Mediterranean diet pattern was associated with lower adiposity, waist circumference, body mass index, and odds of developing metabolic syndrome (Tonorezos et al. 2013). Few studies exist on the benefit of this diet pattern in patients undergoing treatment.

A concern about the use of the Mediterranean diet during cancer treatment is the potential of naturally antioxidant-rich foods to interfere with certain types of treatment especially anthracyclines, platinum-containing agents, alkylating agents, and radiation therapy, which act against cancer cells by generating free radicals. While no data exist to support outright interference with therapy, some sources, such as the American Cancer Society, recommend not exceeding 100 % of the RDA for antioxidant-type vitamins such as vitamins C and E during treatment (Doyle et al. 2006).

Case Vignette
The vegetarian parents of a 7-year-old boy with neuroblastoma being treated with chemotherapy and radiation ask about including raw and unprocessed foods (honey, sprouts) to promote cellular recovery.

NCI guidelines regarding food safety are consistent in recommending no raw foods that have not been packaged and then thoroughly washed; no foods from salad bars, buffets, sidewalk vendors, potlucks, delis, or bulk food bins; no fish, oysters, shellfish, or eggs that have not been thoroughly cooked (no sushi or cookie dough); no sprouts; no whole pieces of poultry not cooked to 180° or ground poultry cooked to 165°; and no beef, pork, lamb, or venison not cooked to 160°. All milk, yogurt, cheese, other dairy products, fruit juices, and honey should be pasteurized (National Cancer Institute 2014c).

For these vegetarian parents who are eager to help boost their child's immune system, the best approach is to provide a varied diet that contains adequate protein from cooked tofu, beans, and nuts; mono- and polyunsaturated fats; whole grains and fiber; vitamins and minerals from well-washed fruits and vegetables; and good hydration with water as well as pasteurized fruit juices. Small snacks of energy-dense foods (that might not typically be considered "healthy") may be needed to provide extra calories. Also, their son should avoid snacks that may make treatment-related side effects worse. If diarrhea is a problem, for example, avoid popcorn and raw fruits and vegetables. If mucositis is a problem, their son should avoid dry, coarse, or acidic foods. He should increase the amount of fiber he eats if constipation is an issue. In addition, taste can change with treatment. Some things that were formerly considered delicious may not appeal and vice versa. Getting enough protein may be a problem with a strict vegetarian diet. The parents may be willing to modify their child's eating practices to allow more variety during treatment and the early days of recovery (American Cancer Society 2014).

> **Case Vignette**
> A 17-year-old boy is starting treatment for stage IV B Hodgkin's disease. The parents ask about using probiotics.

Probiotics are a heterogeneous group of live nonpathogenic strains of microorganisms that can be taken as foods (sea kelp, algae, yogurt) or supplements to modify gut microbial ecology, leading to beneficial structural and functional changes. Of all the gut microbiota, *Lactobacilli* and *Bifidobacteria* are considered the most important to maintaining good health. Because chemotherapy and radiation therapy target rapidly dividing neoplastic cells, they also affect rapidly dividing cell populations throughout the body. As a result, the epithelia of the GI tract are particularly susceptible, leading to the development of mucositis. It appears that intestinal damage is due both to increased apoptosis and to the activity of pro-inflammatory cytokines (Wardill et al. 2012). Most probiotic preparations available over-the-counter are heterogeneous. However, achieving the potentially beneficial effects of probiotic treatment appears to require a high degree of species and strain specificity (Prisciandaro et al. 2011).

Probiotics are classified as "generally regarded as safe" with most safety concerns related to risk of infection caused by the probiotic bacteria and transfer of antibiotic resistance. However, the antibiotic resistance is intrinsic and so nontransmissible. This resistance may benefit patients if their intestinal flora has become unbalanced due to the administration of multiple antimicrobial agents. On the negative side, some strains carry potentially transmissible plasmid-encoded antibiotic resistance genes that could be transferred to endogenous flora producing a new antibiotic-resistant pathogen. This risk is increased in immunocompromised hosts. Overall, despite a substantial number of publications, findings from the current literature are inconclusive about the use of probiotic interventions during treatment (Mego et al. 2013). Lastly, virtually all studies have been conducted in adults, and although the patient presented here might possibly fall into that physiological category, his risk is not fully represented by the data available.

Dietary Supplements

> **Case Vignette**
> A 7-year-old girl is undergoing treatment for ALL with vincristine, doxorubicin, cytarabine, 6-mercaptopurine, methotrexate, cyclophosphamide, and prednisone. Her parents ask if she can use coenzyme Q10 during treatment.

There are three primary concerns about the use of dietary supplements in pediatric cancer patients: (1) the paucity of evidence-based data to help guide safe use, (2) low rates of disclosure creating risk of unwanted drug–herb interactions; and (3) selected supplements high in antioxidant activity interfering with commonly used chemotherapies that act against cancer cells by generating free radicals.

Many patients have questions about coenzyme Q10, which is synthesized in the body and present in most tissues (e.g., heart, liver, kidneys, and pancreas). It has an active role as a carrier of electrons and protons in mitochondrial ATP synthesis and in its reduced form (ubiquinol), acts as an antioxidant, protecting cells from damage due to free radicals (Ernster and Forsmark-Andree 1993).

Coenzyme Q10 deficiency was correlated with certain cancers in the early 1960s, and interest remains high in its potential use in treatment due to its role in energy production, positive effect on the immune system (Folkers et al. 1982, 1991), and antioxidant properties that stabilize cell membranes and protect against free radical damage to tissue (National Cancer Institute 2014b). However, other studies raised concern that the free radical scavenging action of coenzyme Q10 may interfere with the efficacy of some cancer treatments, such as radiation therapy (Lund et al. 1998).

Studies of coenzyme Q10 as either primary or adjuvant therapy in humans are limited, with mixed results. Other common antioxidants, such as vitamin C, vitamin E, and lycopene, have similarly limited evidence for use in cancer prevention or treatment, especially in pediatrics (van Dalen et al. 2008; Greenwald et al. 2007; Fortmann et al. 2013).

A comprehensive review of antioxidant supplementation by Ladas and Kelly (2010) concludes that insufficient evidence exists to broadly recommend antioxidant therapies. Current NCI recommendations urge caution in the use of any antioxidant supplement during cancer treatment. However, ingestion of normal amounts of antioxidants in foods is not contraindicated (National Cancer Institute 2014a).

Case Vignette
A 3-year-old boy with ALL is being discharged after hospitalization for fever and neutropenia. His father asks if the boy can take elderberry syrup as an immune booster.

Black elderberry extract has an excellent safety profile and has been shown to have strong antiviral properties, especially against some strains of influenza. Small studies have also investigated its potential to activate a healthy immune system by increasing cytokine production. One study in 12 healthy adult volunteers using black elderberry extract demonstrated increased production of inflammatory cytokines, especially TNF-alpha, compared to controls (Barak et al. 2001). However, similar studies on the immunostimulating properties of elderberry, or other natural immune stimulants, are lacking in immunocompromised children making it difficult to recommend using the supplement. Simple supportive measures (e.g., adequate sleep/good nutrition) are low risk and may provide benefit.

Case Vignette
A 10-year-old girl has significant anticipatory nausea and vomiting associated with chemotherapy. Her parents ask if she may use ginger as an antiemetic.

Ginger has been shown to be safe and effective in clinical trials for motion sickness and postoperative vomiting and in pregnancy. Although some studies have shown promise and low risk for the use of ginger in anticipatory nausea and vomiting in cancer treatment, results have been limited by variable study design and quality issues. Randomized, double-blind, placebo-controlled trials are underway in adults; similar studies are needed in children (Marx et al. 2014). Interest in the use of other approaches, for example, antinausea lollipops, is high; however, there are currently no evidence-based recommendations for the use of other dietary supplements in pediatric anticipatory nausea and vomiting. Research is ongoing in this area (Gottschling et al. 2014).

Case Vignette
A 5-year-old girl with ALL has developed chemotherapy-related hepatotoxicity. Is milk thistle a viable treatment option?

Milk thistle (*Silybum marianum*) has historically been used to treat hepatic and biliary disorders and in detoxification of hepatic toxins (Greenlee et al. 2007; Tamayo and Diamond 2007). A double-blind study of 50 children with ALL and hepatic toxicity given a 28-day course of milk thistle showed a significantly lower AST level and a trend toward a lower ALT level in the treatment group at day 56. No evidence of interference with treatment was observed (Ladas et al. 2010a, b).

These brief vignettes demonstrate the complexity of dietary supplement use in pediatric oncology and reinforce the importance of having an organized approach to researching the dietary supplement in question. A systematic review of articles examining the prevalence of CT use in pediatric cancer patients identified 28 studies ($n=3526$ patients with varied cancer diagnoses). Herbal remedies were the most commonly used modality and occurred in up to 48 % of patients. *Only 50 % of patients disclosed use of the dietary supplement or botanical to their doctor* (Ndao et al. 2013).

A five-step approach to dietary supplement use in pediatric oncology:

1. Encourage open, nonjudgmental discussion of supplement use, at every visit.
2. Verify product name and examine the label if possible.
3. Establish safety, efficacy, and potential side effects using a reputable resource.
4. Consult with a colleague trained in integrative oncology.
5. When in doubt, err on the side of caution.

Counteracting Nondisclosure

To help counteract high rates of nondisclosure of dietary supplement use, providers should create an atmosphere of receptive listening and openness so a thoughtful risk–benefit analysis can take place (Girard and Vohra 2011). To help facilitate the discussion, the Society of Integrative Oncology Clinical Practice Committee (2014) developed a list of ten of the most commonly used supplements in oncology patients, including mechanism of action in cancer, safety and side effects, dosage recommendations, drug interactions, and cautions. Because there are so little data on children, recommendations are largely extrapolated from adult studies (Frenkel et al. 2013).

Mind–Body Medicine

Mind–body medicine is the deliberate harnessing of positive interactions between thought, emotion, and physiology for the specific purpose of enhancing health. In a 2007 US population study, mind–body therapies were identified as the second most common CT used by people <18 years old (Birdee et al. 2010). Mind–body therapies are also used to address caretaker stress and distress (Kanitz et al. 2013; Elkins et al. 2010). The need for more effective interventions to reduce pain and stress has increased with better understanding of the detrimental physiologic effects of chronic pain and stress in children (Garner et al. 2012; Zempsky 2008; Kennedy et al. 2008).

Some of the best studied mind–body modalities in pediatrics include:

Clinical hypnosis Guided imagery Meditation, mindfulness	Massage therapy Yoga	Creative arts/ Expressive therapy (McClafferty 2011) Biofeedback, EEG Neurofeedback

Case Vignette
A 14-year-old girl with ALL was learning about yoga in gym class. She wonders if she should do some poses to help her relax.

Yoga can be a gentle, safe approach to stress management and physical fitness. A study of 286 young-adult cancer survivors showed 32.8 % had practiced yoga from their initial diagnosis to promote relaxation and maintain flexibility. Average length of practice was 25 months, with a mean of 7 hours of practice/month. Positive benefit was noted, and no adverse outcomes were reported (Park et al. 2013). Studies have shown improvement in gross motor function and QOL (Geyer et al. 2011) and significant improvement in flexibility and fitness (Wurz et al. 2014).

Special considerations in oncology patients participating in any movement therapy such as yoga, tai chi, or Qigong include physician approval, verifying teacher credentialing, avoiding any pose that causes pain or discomfort, and attention to wounds or indwelling catheters.

Other Frequently Used Mind–Body Therapies

Hypnosis and Imagery

Clinical hypnosis, which often includes imagery, is a state of focused relaxation. Beneficial effects were reported in the early 1980s in studies comparing hypnotic versus non-hypnotic techniques for management of procedural pain in children (Olness 1981; Zeltzer and LeBaron 1982). Clinical hypnosis also helps improve anticipatory anxiety, nausea, and vomiting (Kanitz et al. 2013; Accardi and Milling 2009).

Caveats regarding the use of hypnosis or imagery include the importance of using only fully trained practitioners and early referral or consultation with a mental health professional for any child with a history of abuse or preexisting mental illness. Hypnosis training for licensed professionals is available through the American Society of Clinical Hypnosis www.asch.net. Pediatric-specific training for licensed professionals is available through the National Pediatric Hypnosis Training Institute http://www.nphti.net/.

Meditation and Mindfulness

Meditation and mindfulness are the focus of active research inquiry in medicine to help address stress, sleep disorders, fear, anxiety, and other challenging emotions (Jones et al. 2013). Mindfulness-based stress reduction (MBSR) is a structured approach to mindfulness involving breath work, relaxation exercises, meditation, and movement exercises developed by Kabat-Zinn (1982). Although there are no large studies of the use of MBSR in pediatric oncology, multiple randomized controlled trials (RCTs) in adults with cancer confirm positive effects on QOL, mood, stress, immune function, and sleep (Carlson et al. 2003; Henderson et al. 2013; Anderson et al. 2013; Wurtzen et al. 2013; Zainal et al. 2013; Post-White et al. 2009). Contraindications to the use of mindfulness are highly individualized and may include prior history of mental illness or trauma. Mindfulness has also been used to help prevent burnout in pediatric oncology staff (Moody et al. 2013). Training in this area remains variable; some programs may use the standardized MBSR curriculum developed by Kabat-Zinn.

Case Vignette
A 12-year-old girl with rhabdomyosarcoma of the pelvis asks if she can have massage therapy to help relieve her back pain.

Massage therapy is the systematic stroking, rubbing, or kneading of the skin, underlying muscle, and other tissues to promote physical and psychological relief, improved circulation, relaxation of sore muscles, and other therapeutic effects (National Center for Complementary and Alternative Medicine (NCCAM) 2014).

The gate control theory suggests that massage may provide stimulation that helps to block pain signals sent to the brain. Massage can release endorphins and serotonin, which can positively affect mood. Small RCTs have shown reduced anxiety and improvement in overall feeling of well-being in children in various stages of cancer treatment with no reported adverse effects (Post-White et al. 2009; Mehling et al. 2012). Massage has also been combined with aromatherapy with positive effect (Fellowes et al. 2004).

The massage technique often used in oncology is Swedish massage characterized by gentle, long rhythmic strokes. *Tapotement* (percussion) and *petrissage* (kneading or knuckling) should be avoided. Other precautions include avoiding deep pressure or trigger point massage techniques, especially near lesions or enlarged lymph nodes, surgical sites or medical devices, or radiation fields. Patients with bleeding tendencies should receive very gentle massage to avoid bruising.

Massage therapy is generally safe when given by a credentialed practitioner trained to work with oncology patients, especially children. Serious adverse events have been associated with exotic types of massage or inexperienced practitioners (Deng et al. 2009). For children who do not like to be touched by strangers, caregivers can be taught simple techniques to massage hands, feet, arms, shoulders, or other noninvolved areas. Studies have shown that massage has relaxation benefits for both the person receiving as well as the person providing the massage. This can be a critical addition to the care plan that allows caregivers to participate directly in alleviating pain and discomfort in their child.

Case Vignette
Nurses on the pediatric oncology unit would like to provide Reiki to all patients.

Reiki therapy uses spiritual, or universal, energy to assist the healing process through the "laying on of hands" in specific positions on or above the patient's body. The origins of Reiki trace back to Buddhist healing practices. It is one of several energy or biofield therapies that include therapeutic touch and healing touch. Common assumptions in considering biofield therapies include the following: (1) The human body is an energy system that extends beyond the body; (2) the normal self-healing properties of the body are supported by the free, balanced flow of energy throughout the system; and (3) disease or disorder can be detected in the energy system and can be affected therapeutically by the conscious healing intent and compassion of the practitioner.

Reiki is understood to be present in every healing encounter. It can be offered as a whole treatment of 60–90 min or as a brief encounter to provide comfort. The energy that is transferred from the practitioner to the recipient can be used as needed. Several hundred thousand nurses have been trained in energy therapy. The Leonard P. Zakim Center at the Dana-Farber Cancer Institute has offered Reiki since the early 2000s without any negative side effects. Patients report feeling peaceful and relaxed, less anxious, able to sleep better, and able to have decreased pain (Potter 2013).

Reiki can be used with patients of all ages. The *Reiki Handbook for Kids and All Ages* by Sara McGrath includes the history of Reiki, meditation and visualization exercises, and hand positions for self-treatment and to treat others. *Reiki for Children: A Reiki Kids Handbook* by Kytka Hilmar-Jezek was written to help children learn about their bodies, inner spirit, personal power, and connection to the universal life force, which is love. Although Reiki has been shown to be gentle and effective, some patients or families may be resistant or skeptical due to the novel nature of the treatment.

Clinicians should be open and respectful of family concerns and treatment preferences.

Creative Arts/Expressive Therapy

Case Vignette
A 15-year-old reserved girl is reticent to engage verbally while undergoing stem cell transplant for relapsed leukemia. The parents ask for psychological help for her.

Times of crisis are the least opportune for learning new interpersonal skills. If anything, behaviors tend to regress and become more childlike. If someone has typically found it difficult to express worries, concerns, or fears, it is unlikely that she will suddenly be able to verbalize feelings during a new crisis. Health care providers tend to be verbal; thus, working with someone that finds verbal self-expression difficult can be frustrating.

Sustained stress (including depression and anxiety) can cause suffering that has significant negative effects on health and well-being as noted in the Institute of Medicine report, "Cancer Care for the Whole Patient"(National Academy of Sciences and National Institutes of Health 2008). Expressive therapies (e.g., music, art, dance, creative writing/journaling) are considered mind–body modalities. Extensive research has shown that they can reduce anxiety, mood disturbance, and pain and improve QOL by reinforcing a sense of control. They have been widely accepted by child life specialists as especially useful in reducing procedural pain (Klassen et al. 2008).

Although many patients are eager to talk about their feelings and will benefit from supportive counseling or cognitive behavioral therapy, some patients, especially children and teens, are less adept in expressing themselves verbally. Indirect expression by composing a song, drawing a picture, or writing a poem that they then share and discuss with a trained therapist can reveal concerns and feelings to which they have not yet assigned a specific word. The use of an expressive therapy should be considered risk-free even if a session leads to distress as the patient comes to grips with what is bothersome but has been repressed.

Music therapy is a branch of health care designed to aid physical and emotional health through the use of music, either through listening, songwriting, performing, or lyric analysis and is provided by a trained therapist with an agreed-upon goal for the session, such as relaxation or symptom reduction. Music therapy has a robust evidence base in pediatric oncology and is used extensively for self-calming and to inspire creativity, facilitate adjustment, and enhance self-image (Robb et al. 2008; Hilliard 2006; O'Callaghan et al. 2012, 2013). Research exploring the science of music therapy is revealing the highly complex nature of the positive effect of music on the neurohormonal and immune systems and its links to pain perception and emotional processing (Leardi et al. 2007). Functional neuroimaging (fMRI) examining the mechanism of action indicates that emotions evoked by music appear to modulate limbic areas of the brain (Koelsch 2010). Research into the effect of music therapy in neuroplasticity and auditory–motor coupling in stroke victims (Rodriguez-Fornells et al. 2012) raises intriguing questions about its possible application in children suffering from neurocognitive deficits after tumor resection or radiation therapy.

Biofeedback

Biofeedback is the use of an external instrument or monitor that helps an individual to learn how psychological state (anxiety, depression, relaxation) affects physiological activity. With practice, the individual learns how changing thinking or emotional state can improve health and performance. Examples of physiologic functions that can be monitored and "fed back" to the individual include brainwaves, muscle tone, skin conductance, finger temperature, heart rate, and respiratory rate. Biofeedback is widely used in children with headache or other pain. One recent study on preprocedural distress in 12 children with cancer showed the benefit of teaching effective relaxation techniques using biofeedback in a four-session intervention (Shockey et al. 2013). A relatively new area of research is the use of neurofeedback (i.e., EEG biofeedback) to improve function in children suffering neurocognitive decline after cancer therapy by training patients to focus on and enhance specific brain wave activity that aids attention, concentration, and organization (de Ruiter et al. 2012).

Traditional Chinese Medicine/ Acupuncture

> **Case Vignette**
> A 15-year-old girl is receiving cisplatin and has been vomiting 10–12 times/day. The parents ask about acupressure as adjunctive therapy to antiemetics.

Traditional Chinese medicine including acupuncture and herbal medicine is commonly used in cancer treatment in China (Li et al. 2013). The search for the active components of these traditional treatments has been increasing (Mohd et al. 2013; Gundeti et al. 2012). Available studies primarily focus on the use of acupuncture (Jindal et al. 2008). Small studies have shown benefit in reduction of chemotherapy-related nausea and vomiting (Gottschling et al. 2008).

In addition to possible needle phobia, another potential concern about acupuncture treatment in oncology patients is bleeding due to thrombocytopenia. This issue was studied retrospectively in 32 pediatric patients who underwent 237 acupuncture treatments by highly trained acupuncturists in an academic pediatric oncology center. Platelet counts ranged from ≤20,000/uL to ≥100,000/uL. Twenty percent of sessions were done in patients with severe thrombocytopenia, 8 % with moderate thrombocytopenia, 19 % with mild thrombocytopenia, and 53 % in those with normal platelet counts. No acute or serious side effects were recorded in any acupuncture session. This small study is reassuring and lays the groundwork for larger prospective studies (Ladas et al. 2010b).

Another option is acupressure applied to acupuncture point P6 using wristbands. Small pediatric studies have shown it to be well tolerated, but no more effective than placebo (Jones et al. 2008). Findings have been more positive in adult studies (Shin et al. 2004).

Case Vignette
The mother of a 2-year-old boy with neuroblastoma would like to use lavender oil in an aromatherapy diffuser to help him sleep better.

Aromatherapy uses plant-based essential oils to treat a wide variety of health issues and can be administered via inhalation or topically, often in conjunction with massage (Lv et al. 2013; Fellowes et al. 2004).

The use of aromatherapy dates back thousands of years and has a wide safety margin, although occasional topical irritation or allergy can be seen, and ingestion is contraindicated – especially in children. Inhalation aromatherapy studies specifically in pediatric oncology patients are sparse. For example, one randomized placebo-controlled study by Ndao et al. found a small (yet not statistically significant) benefit to bergamot aromatherapy for anxiety and pain in pediatric stem cell infusion (Ndao et al. 2012).

However, lavender has a long history of use to promote relaxation and sleep. Lavender aromatherapy has been shown to aid sleep in adult patients in hospice (Soden et al. 2004) and has been used safely with massage in infants with colic (Cetinkaya and Basbakkal 2012) and in bath oil to promote infant relaxation, suggesting a reassuring safety profile in children (Field et al. 2008). Individual preference has a significant influence on aromatherapy. Cancer treatment may alter olfactory and taste preferences.

Other measures to improve sleep in and out of the hospital might include age-appropriate relaxation techniques (breath work, music therapy, progressive muscle relaxation, white noise), implementing a soothing bedtime ritual, minimizing sleep interruptions, reduced lighting at night, and daytime exposure to natural light if feasible (Tamrat et al. 2014).

Clinical Pearls

- Encourage open, nonjudgmental discussion of use of integrative therapies, especially dietary supplements at every visit to help avoid undesirable interactions.
- Consider the addition of mind–body therapies such as clinical hypnosis and guided imagery to help address fear, pain, and anxiety in children and their families.

Where can providers and patients find reliable Web-based information about complementary therapies?

SAFE is an appropriate acronym to use when judging information found on the Internet.

S – *Staff*. Who created the site? Usually, there is an "About this site" page stating who developed or maintains it, the board of directors or a history of the site. What are their credentials? If none are listed, they should explain who they are.

A – *Address*. If the domain in the URL address is .org, it is run by an organization, probably not for profit. .edu or .gov are reliable sites. Be wary of .com or .net.

F – *Fit*. How "fit" is this site? Do several links lead to "page not found?" One or two dead ends may be tolerable, but more indicates the site is missing reasonable fitness goals. Are dates listed for the material and are these current? If a page in a health-related site has not been updated in 2 years, be skeptical about the information.

E – *Evidence*. Is the content well referenced? Are medical journal articles and book chapters cited or does the site consist primarily of individual opinions and biases? If there are references, how old are they? In most cases, research is expanding so rapidly that currency is crucial. Online support groups, consisting of other families' experiences, may be useful, as long as readers are aware that the material is of personal opinion.

PubMed

The *subject filter* "complementary medicine" will yield hundreds of terms referring to modalities as well as herbs/supplements. The subject filter "dietary supplements" also includes vitamins. Using the *Medical Subject Heading (MeSH)*, "complementary therapies" is not as inclusive as the filter, but can offer different results. Other possible MeSH headings include "dietary supplements," "functional food," "plants, medicinal" or "herbal medicine."

http://www.nccam.nih.gov

NCCAM contains video lectures/other resources for professionals, herbal/dietary supplement information, grants/funding opportunities, definitions of and the evidence for various complementary therapies, literature reviews in PubMed, and practice guidelines. It also includes information for patients.

http://cam.cancer.gov

The NCI Web site has a section from its Office of Cancer Complementary and Alternative Medicine, OCCAM.

http://www.integrativeonc.org

The Society for Integrative Oncology is composed of professionals from different backgrounds who promote the evidence base for integrative approaches to patient care. The Society's practice guidelines are located here.

http://www.medlineplus.gov

MedlinePlus, geared toward consumers, is a one-stop, high-quality Web site from the National Library of Medicine. It features background material on herbs and dietary supplements (most originating from Natural Medicines Comprehensive Database or NCCAM). Most links in the topic areas are to government agencies, patient organizations, or professional organizations.

http://www.mskcc.org/cancer-care/integrative-medicine/about-herbs-botanicals-other-products

Memorial Sloan Kettering Cancer Center offers free information on herbs and plants. Explanations are well referenced and managed by their Integrative Medicine Service.

http://www.mdanderson.org/patient-and-cancer-information/care-centers-and-clinics/specialty-and-treatment-centers/integrative-medicine-center/videos/index.html

MD Anderson's Integrative Medicine Center Web pages include audios and videos with such titles as "Music Therapy Inspires Cancer Patients" and "Laughter is Good Therapy."

http://www.cancer.org/treatment/treatmentsandsideeffects/complementaryandalternativemedicine/complementary-and-alternative-medicine-landing

The American Cancer Society's index page for complementary and alternative medicine.

http://www2.aap.org/sections/chim/default.cfm

The American Academy of Pediatrics has a Section on Integrative Medicine, which lists resources for parents as well as clinicians.

Subscription Databases

AMED, the Alternative and Complementary Medicine Database, is produced by the British Library and tends to index journals from European sources.

MANTIS (Manual, Alternative, and Natural Therapy Index System) includes journals on chiropractic, osteopathy, manual medicine, and homeopathy.

Natural Medicines Comprehensive Database is an evidence-based compendium on herbs and supplements, compiled by the Therapeutic Research Center. Search herbs or supplements by name or search by disease.

Natural Standard includes sections on food/herbs/dietary supplements, health/wellness, comparative effectiveness, genomics/proteomics, and brands/manufacturers.

References

Accardi MC, Milling LS (2009) The effectiveness of hypnosis for reducing procedure-related pain in children and adolescents: a comprehensive methodological review. J Behav Med 32:328–339

American Cancer Society (2014) Nutrition for the person with cancer during treatment. www [On-line].

Available: http://www.cancer.org/treatment/survivorshipduringandaftertreatment/nutritionforpeoplewithcancer/nutritionforthepersonwithcancer/nutrition-for-the-person-with-cancer-during-treatment-toc

Anderson SR, Wurtzen H, Steding-Jessen M, Christensen J, Andersen KK, Flyger H et al (2013) Effect of mindfulness-based stress reduction on sleep quality: results of a randomized trial among Danish breast cancer patients. Acta Oncol 52:336–344

Barak V, Halperin T, Kalickman I (2001) The effect of Sambucol, a black elderberry-based, natural product, on the production of human cytokines: I. Inflammatory cytokines. Eur Cytokine Netw 12:290–296

Bauer J, Jurgens H, Fruhwald MC (2011) Important aspects of nutrition in children with cancer. Adv Nutr 2:67–77

Birdee GS, Phillips RS, Davis RB, Gardiner P (2010) Factors associated with pediatric use of complementary and alternative medicine. Pediatrics 125: 249–256

Briggs JP, Killen J (2013) Perspectives on complementary and alternative medicine research. JAMA 310:691–692

Brinksma A, Huizinga G, Sulkers E, Kamps W, Roodbol P, Tissing W (2012) Malnutrition in childhood cancer patients: a review on its prevalence and possible causes. Crit Rev Oncol Hematol 83:249–275

Carlson EA, Sampson MC, Sroufe LA (2003) Implications of attachment theory and research for developmental-behavioral pediatrics. J Dev Behav Pediatr 24:364–379

Cetinkaya B, Basbakkal Z (2012) The effectiveness of aromatherapy massage using lavender oil as a treatment for infantile colic. Int J Nurs Pract 18:164–169

de Ruiter MA, Schouten-Van Meeteren AY, van Mourik R, Janssen TW, Greidanus JE, Oosterlaan J et al (2012) Neurofeedback to improve neurocognitive functioning of children treated for a brain tumor: design of a randomized controlled double-blind trial. BMC Cancer 12:581

Deng GE, Frenkel M, Cohen L, Cassileth BR, Abrams DI, Capodice JL et al (2009) Evidence-based clinical practice guidelines for integrative oncology: complementary therapies and botanicals. J Soc Integr Oncol 7:85–120

Doyle C, Kushi LH, Byers T, Courneya KS, Demark-Wahnefried W, Grant B et al (2006) Nutrition and physical activity during and after cancer treatment: an American Cancer Society guide for informed choice. CA Cancer J Clin 56:323–353

Elkins G, Fisher W, Johnson A (2010) Mind-body therapies in integrative oncology. Curr Treat Options Oncol 11:128–140

Ernster L, Forsmark-Andree P (1993) Ubiquinol: an endogenous antioxidant in aerobic organisms. Clin Investing 71:S60–S65

Fellowes D, Barnes K, Wilkinson S (2004) Aromatherapy and massage for symptom relief in patients with cancer. Cochrane Database Syst Rev (2):CD002287

Field T, Field T, Cullen C, Largie S, Diego M, Schanberg S et al (2008) Lavender bath oil reduces stress and crying and enhances sleep in very young infants. Early Hum Dev 84:399–401

Folkers K, Shizukuishi S, Takemura K, Drzewoski J, Richardson P, Ellis J et al (1982) Increase in levels of IgG in serum of patients treated with coenzyme Q10. Res Commun Chem Pathol Pharmacol 38:335–338

Folkers K, Hanioka T, Xia LJ, McRee JT Jr, Langsjoen P (1991) Coenzyme Q10 increase T4/T8 ratios of lymphocytes in ordinary subjects and relevance to patients having the AIDS related complex. Biochem Biophys Res Commun 176:786–791

Fortmann SP, Burda BU, Senger CA, Lin JS, Whitlock EP (2013) Vitamin and mineral supplements in the primary prevention of cardiovascular disease and cancer: an updated systematic evidence review for the U.S. Preventive Services Task Force. Ann Intern Med 159:824–834

Frenkel M, Abrams DI, Ladas EJ, Deng G, Hardy M, Capodice JL et al (2013) Integrating dietary supplements into cancer care. Integr Cancer Ther 12:369–384

Garner AS, Shonkoff JP, Committee on Psychosocial Aspects of Child and Family Health, Committee on Early Childhood, A. a. D. C., & Section on Developmental and Behavioral Pediatrics (2012) Early chidhood adversity, toxic stress, and the role of the pediatrician: translating developmental science into lifelong health. Pediatrics 129:e224–e231

Geyer R, Lyons A, Amazeen L, Alishio L, Cooks L (2011) Feasibility study: the effect of therapeutic yoga on quality of life in children hospitalized with cancer. Pediatr Phys Ther 23:375–379

Gilmour J, Harrison C, Asadi L, Cohen MH, Vohra S (2011a) Referrals and shared or collaborative care: managing relationships with complementary and alternative medicine practitioners. Pediatrics 128:S181–S186

Gilmour J, Harrison C, Cohen MH, Vohra S (2011b) Pediatric use of complementary and alternative medicine: legal, ethical, and clinical issues in decision-making. Pediatrics 128:S149–S154

Girard L, Vohra S (2011) Ethics of using herbal medicine as primary or adjunct treatment and issues of drug-herb interaction. In: Benzie IFF, Watchtel-Galor S (eds) Herbal medicine: biomolecular and clinical aspects, 2nd edn. CRC Press, Boca Raton

Gottschling S, Reindl TK, Meyer S, Berrang J, Henze G, Graeber S et al (2008) Acupuncture to alleviate chemotherapy-induced nausea and vomiting in pediatric oncology – a randomized multicenter crossover pilot trial. Klin Padiatr 220:365–370

Gottschling S, Meyer S, Langler A, Scharifi G, Ebinger F, Gronwald B (2014) Differences in use of complementary and alternative medicine between children and adolescents with cancer in Germany: a population based survey. Pediatr Blood Cancer 61:488–492

Greenlee H, Abascal K, Yarnell E, Ladas E (2007) Clinical applications of Silybum marianum in oncology. Integr Cancer Ther 6:158–165

Greenwald P, Anderson D, Nelson SA, Taylor PR (2007) Clinical trials of vitamin and mineral supplements for cancer prevention. Am J Clin Nutr 85:314S–317S

Gundeti MS, Sisodia BS, Marlewar S, Reddy RG (2012) Consultative workshop on integrative approach to cancer. J Ayurveda Integr Med 3:230–231

Henderson VP, Massion AO, Clemow L, Hurley TG, Druker S, Hebert JR (2013) A randomized controlled trial of mindfulness-based stress reduction for women with early-stage breast cancer receiving radiotherapy. Integr Cancer Ther 12:404–413

Hilliard RE (2006) Music therapy in pediatric oncology: a review of the literature. J Soc Integr Oncol 4:75–78

Jindal V, Ge A, Mansky PJ (2008) Safety and efficacy of acupuncture in children: a review of the evidence. J Pediatr Hematol Oncol 30:431–442

Jones E, Isom S, Kemper KJ, McLean TW (2008) Acupressure for chemotherapy-associated nausea and vomiting in children. J Soc Integr Oncol 6:141–145

Jones P, Blunda M, Biegel G, Carlson LE, Biel M, Wiener L (2013) Can mindfulness-based interventions help adolescents with cancer? Psychooncology 22:2148–2151

Kabat-Zin J (1982) An outpatient program in behavioral medicine for chronic pain patients based on the practice of mindfulness meditation: theoretical considerations and preliminary results. Gen Hosp Psychiatry 4:33–47

Kanitz JL, Camus ME, Seifert G (2013) Keeping the balance – an overview of mind-body therapies in pediatric oncology. Complement Ther Med (21 Suppl 1):S20–S25

Kennedy RM, Luhmann J, Zempsky WT (2008) Clinical implications of unmanaged needle-insertion pain and distress in children. Pediatrics 122:S130–S133

Klassen JA, Liang Y, Tjosvold L, Klassen TP, Hartling L (2008) Music for pain and anxiety in children undergoing medical procedures: a systematic review of randomized controlled trials. Ambul Pediatr 8:117–128

Koelsch S (2010) Towards a neural basis of music-evoked emotions. Trends Cogn Sci 14:131–137

Ladas E, Kelly KM (2010) The antioxidant debate. Explore (NY) 6:75–85

Ladas EJ, Kroll DJ, Oberlies NH, Cheng B, Ndao DH, Rheingold SR et al (2010a) A randomized, controlled, double-blind, pilot study of milk thistle for the treatment of hepatotoxicity in childhood acute lymphoblastic leukemia (ALL). Cancer 116:506–513

Ladas EJ, Rooney D, Taromina K, Ndao DH, Kelly KM (2010b) The safety of acupuncture in children and adolescents with cancer therapy-related thrombocytopenia. Support Care Cancer 18:1487–1490

Leardi S, Pietroletti R, Angeloni G, Necozione S, Ranalletta G, Del Gusto B (2007) Randomized clinical trial examining the effect of music therapy in stress response to day surgery. Br J Surg 94:943–947

Li X, Yang G, Li X, Zhang Y, Yang J, Chang J et al (2013) Traditional Chinese medicine in cancer care: a review of controlled clinical studies published in Chinese. PLoS One 8, e60338

Lund EL, Quistorff B, Spang-Thomsen M, Kristjanzen PE (1998) Effect of radiation therapy on small-cell lung cancer is reduced by ubiquinone intake. Folia Microbiol 43:505–506

Lv XN, Liu ZJ, Zhang HJ, Tzeng CM (2013) Aromatherapy and the central nerve system (CNS): therapeutic mechanism and its associated genes. Curr Drug Targets 14:872–879

Marx W, McCarthy AL, Ried K, Vitetta L, McKavanagh D, Thomson D et al (2014) Can ginger ameliorate chemotherapy-induced nausea? Protocol of a randomized double blind, placebo-controlled trial. BMC Complement Altern Med 14:134

McClafferty H (2011) Complementary, holistic, and integrative medicine: mind-body medicine. Pediatr Rev 32:201–203

McLean TW, Kemper KJ (2006) Complementary and alternative medical (CAM) therapies in pediatric oncology patients. J Soc Integr Oncol 4:40–45

Mego M, Holec V, Drgona L, Hainova K, Ciernikova S, Zajac V (2013) Probiotic bacteria in cancer patients undergoing chemotherapy and radiation therapy. Complement Ther Med 21:712–723

Mehling WE, Lown EA, Dvorak CC, Cowan MJ, Horn BN, Dunn EA et al (2012) Hematopoietic cell transplant and use of massage for improved symptom management: results from a pilot randomized control trial. Evid Based Complement Alternat Med 2012(450150):1–9

Mohd FF, Koutsoukas A, Lowe R, Joshi K, Fan TP, Glen RC et al (2013) Chemogenomics approaches to rationalizing the mode-of-action of traditional Chinese and Ayurvedic medicines. J Chem Inf Model 53:661–673

Moody K, Kramer D, Santizo RO, Magro L, Wyshogrod D, Ambrosio J et al (2013) Helping the helpers: mindfulness training for burnout in pediatric oncology–a pilot program. J Pediatr Oncol Nurs 30:275–284

Myers C, Stuber ML, Bonamer-Rheingans JL, Zeltzer LK (2005) Complementary therapies and childhood cancer. Cancer Control 12:172–180

National Academy of Sciences & National Institutes of Health (2008) Cancer care for the whole patient: meeting psychosocial health needs. National Academies Press, Washington, DC

National Cancer Institute (2014a) Antioxidants and cancer prevention. www [On-line]. Available: http://www.cancer.gov/cancertopics/factsheet/prevention/antioxidants

National Cancer Institute (2014b) Coenzyme Q10 (PDQ). www [On-line]. Available: http://www.cancer.gov/cancertopics/pdq/cam/coenzymeQ10/HealthProfessional/page1

National Cancer Institute (2014c) Eating hints: before, during, and after cancer treatment. www [On-line]. Available: http://www.cancer.gov/cancertopics/coping/eatinghints/page2

National Center for Complementary and Alternative Medicine (NCCAM) (2014) Massage therapy. www

[On-line]. Available: http://nccam.nih.gov/health/massage

Ndao DH, Ladas EJ, Cheng B, Sands SA, Snyder KT, Garvin JH Jr et al (2012) Inhalation aromatherapy in children and adolescents undergoing stem cell infusion: results of a placebo-controlled double-blind trial. Psychooncology 21:247–254

Ndao DH, Ladas EJ, Bao Y, Cheng B, Nees SN, Levine JM et al (2013) Use of complementary and alternative medicine among children, adolescent, and young adult cancer survivors: a survey study. J Pediatr Hematol Oncol 35:281–288

O'Callaghan C, Barry P, Thompson K (2012) Music's relevance for adolescents and young adults with cancer: a constructivist research approach. Support Care Cancer 20:687–697

O'Callaghan C, Dun B, Baron A, Barry P (2013) Music's relevance for children with cancer: music therapists' qualitative clinical data-mining research. Soc Work Health Care 52:125–143

Olness K (1981) Imagery (self-hypnosis) as adjunct therapy in childhood cancer: clinical experience with 25 patients. Am J Pediatr Hematol Oncol 3:313–321

Park CL, Cho D, Wortmann JH (2013) The impact of yoga upon young adult cancer survivors. Complement Ther Clin Pract 19:77–82

Post-White J, Fitzgerald M, Savik K, Hooke MC, Hannahan AB, Sencer SF (2009) Massage therapy for children with cancer. J Pediatr Oncol Nurs 26:16–28

Potter PJ (2013) Energy therapies in advanced practice oncology: an evidence-informed practice approach. J Adv Pract Oncol 4:139–151

Prisciandaro LD, Geier MS, Butler RN, Cummins AG, Howarth GS (2011) Evidence supporting the use of probiotics for the prevention and treatment of chemotherapy-induced intestinal mucositis. Crit Rev Food Sci Nutr 51:239–247

Robb SL, Clair AA, Watanabe M, Monahan PO, Azzouz F, Stouffer JW et al (2008) A non-randomized [corrected] controlled trial of the active music engagement (AME) intervention on children with cancer. Psychooncology 17:699–708

Rodriguez-Fornells A, Rojo N, Amengual JL, Ripolles P, Altenmuller E, Munte TF (2012) The involvement of audio-motor coupling in the music-supported therapy applied to stroke patients. Ann N Y Acad Sci 1252:282–293

Roth M, Lin J, Kim M, Moody K (2009) Pediatric oncologists' views toward the use of complementary and alternative medicine in children with cancer. J Pediatr Hematol Oncol 31:177–182

Shin YH, Kim TI, Shin MS, Juon H-S (2004) Effect of acupressure on nausea and vomiting during chemotherapy cycle for Korean postoperative stomach cancer patients. Cancer Nurs 27:267–274

Shockey DP, Menzies V, Glick DF, Taylor AG, Boitnott A, Rovnyak V (2013) Preprocedural distress in children with cancer: an intervention using biofeedback and relaxation. J Pediatr Oncol Nurs 30:129–138

Society for Integrative Oncology (2014) www [On-line]. Available: http://www.integrativeonc.org/index.php/about

Soden K, Vincent K, Craske S, Lucas C, Ashley S (2004) A randomized controlled trial of aromatherapy massage in a hospice setting. Palliat Med 18:87–92

Sung L, Zaoutis T, Ullrich NJ, Johnston D, Dupuis L, Ladas E et al (2013) Children's Oncology Group's 2013 blueprint for research: cancer control and supportive care. Pediatr Blood Cancer 60:1027–1030

Tamayo C, Diamond S (2007) Review of clinical trials evaluating safety and efficacy of milk thistle (Silybum marianum [L] Gaertn). Integr Cancer Ther 6:146–157

Tamrat R, Huynh-Le MP, Goyal M (2014) Non-pharmacologic interventions to improve the sleep of hospitalized patients: a systemic review. J Gen Intern Med 29:788–795

Tonorezos ES, Robien K, Eshelman-Kent D, Moskowitz CS, Church TS, Ross R et al (2013) Contribution of diet and physical activity to metabolic parameters among survivors of childhood leukemia. Cancer Causes Control 24:313–321

van Dalen EC, Caron HN, Dickinson HO, Kremer LC (2008) Cardioprotective interventions for cancer patients receiving anthracyclines. Cochrane Database Syst Rev (2):CD003917

Wardill HR, Bowen JM, Gibson RJ (2012) Chemotherapy-induced gut toxicity: are alterations to intestinal tight junctions pivotal? Cancer Chemother Pharmacol 70:627–635

Wurtzen H, Dalton SO, Elsass P, Sumbundu AD, Steding-Jenson M, Karlsen RV et al (2013) Mindfulness significantly reduces self-reported levels of anxiety and depression: results of a randomised controlled trial among 336 Danish women treated for stage I-III breast cancer. Eur J Cancer 49:1365–1373

Wurz A, Chamorro-Vina C, Guilcher GM, Schulte F, Culos-Reed SN (2014) The feasibility and benefits of a 12-week yoga intervention for pediatric cancer outpatients. Pediatr Blood Cancer 61:1828–1834

Zainal NZ, Booth S, Huppert FA (2013) The efficacy of mindfulness-based stress reduction on mental health of breast cancer patients: a meta-analysis. Psychooncology 22:1457–1465

Zeltzer L, LeBaron S (1982) Hypnosis and nonhypnotic techniques for reduction of pain and anxiety during painful procedures in children and adolescents with cancer. J Pediatr 101:1032–1035

Zempsky WT (2008) Optimizing the management of peripheral venous access pain in children: evidence, impact, and implementation. Pediatrics 122:S121–S124

17 Ethics in Pediatric Oncology

Daniel Benedetti and Jennifer C. Kesselheim

Ethical Issues in Informed Consent

For pediatric oncologists the practice of informed consent is so fundamental to oncology care that even the idea of giving chemotherapy without going through the formal informed consent process would feel apocryphal. The process of acquiring consent emerged in the last 60 years, after the legal system deemed failure to obtain consent to be a malpractice violation. The ability to understand informed consent in the pediatric setting hinges on a thorough understanding of the ethical underpinnings of informed consent in adults. Thus, we will first explore informed consent for a competent adult before expanding the discussion to adults without competence and finally to children.

D. Benedetti, MD (✉)
J.C. Kesselheim, MD, MBE, EdM
Department of Pediatric Hematology/Oncology, Dana Farber/Boston Children's Cancer and Blood Disorders Center,
450 Brookline Avenue, Boston, MA 02115, USA
e-mail: Daniel_Benedetti@dfci.harvard.edu; Jennifer_kesselheim@dfci.harvard.edu

Informed Consent for the Competent Adult

The practice of informed consent is a procedural protection for the principle of autonomy, legally conceptualized by the statement: "every human being of adult years and sound mind has a right to determine what shall be done with his body" (Schloendorff v. Society of New York Hospital 1914). There are five recognized components to a valid informed consent: (a) capacity, (b) disclosure, (c) understanding, (d) voluntariness, and (e) decision (Meisel et al. 1977).

Capacity and Competence

Capacity and *competence* are virtually synonymous. Those who make a distinction note that capacity is a medical determination and competence is a legal judgment, while others argue the difference is inconsequential (Appelbaum 2007; Beauchamp and Childress 2013). Here we will consider them together to mean one's ability to cognitively, psychologically, and legally perform the tasks required to make a decision. Being competent is a precondition of providing informed consent; a determination of incompetence makes moot the other components of informed consent. Practically, patients are presumed to be competent in the absence of a compelling reason to question a patient's decision-making (Appelbaum 2007). In addition, courts and scholars note that one's competence may vary based on the task or decision.

A.N. Abrams et al. (eds.), *Pediatric Psychosocial Oncology: Textbook for Multidisciplinary Care*,
DOI 10.1007/978-3-319-21374-3_17

Accordingly, many advocate use of a "sliding-scale" strategy, in which the threshold for judging competence increases as the risk of a particular decision increases (Beauchamp and Childress 2013; Drane 1985; President's Commission for the Study of Ethical Problems in Medicine and Biomedical and Behavioral Research 1982). While there is no accepted tool to assess capacity, Appelbaum suggests four faculties to evaluate: (a) the ability to understand relevant information, (b) the ability to appreciate the situation and its consequences, (c) the ability to manipulate information rationally, and (d) the ability to make and communicate a choice (Appelbaum 2007). Psychosocial clinicians may be called upon to aid in the determination of capacity; however, laws may dictate who has the authority to make that determination. Because statutes vary, providers should be familiar with the laws in their jurisprudence or consult legal counsel if necessary.

Disclosure

Disclosure refers to the provision of information to the patient so she can make a decision. The legal doctrine of informed consent has largely focused on disclosure, because litigation against physicians hinged on the failure to disclose information to patients. Despite this, courts have not adopted consistent standards about what constitutes adequate disclosure. Many standards are described in the literature, and while none is uniformly accepted, there is consensus that certain types of information be included in any disclosure: (a) the nature of the problem, (b) the reason for the intervention, (c) the anticipated benefits, (d) potential risks, and (e) acceptable alternatives.

Understanding

In the ideal consent process, the patient will understand everything the clinician discloses. Yet, faced with the emotions involved in receiving a serious diagnosis, there is reason to expect patients' understanding will be impaired. Misunderstandings appear widespread (Rothberg et al. 2010; Fernandez 2010), so legal precedent has focused on ensuring physician disclosure is adequate. In addition, clinicians must always strive to optimize clarity with their patients.

Voluntariness

Patients must be free to make a choice voluntarily and without unfair constraints (Berg and Appelbaum 2001). When a physician believes one course of action is warranted (e.g., chemotherapy for a favorable-prognosis malignancy), she may persuade the patient to authorize treatment. Whether the physician ought to employ persuasion depends on the likelihood of the desired outcome. While persuasion is morally permissible, coercion is unethical (Berg and Appelbaum 2001; Hawkins and Emanuel 2005; Mandava and Millum 2013). Coercion, which involves the use of intentional and unjustified threats to exert control over another, is generally permissible only where failure to adhere to treatment puts others at significant risk, such as the threat of detainment for a patient refusing therapy for tuberculosis.

Decision

To complete the process of consent, a competent adult must be able to make a decision regarding the proposed intervention. While scholars conceptually agree that consent is more than merely a signature on a piece of paper, in practice the process culminates in formally signing the consent form.

Informed Consent in the Incompetent Patient

Because the law states that individuals under 18 years of age are, by definition, incompetent, we must contemplate how to achieve informed consent for an incompetent patient. For an incapacitated adult, a surrogate or proxy is asked to make medical decisions on her behalf. There are different approaches the surrogate could use to make such decisions. The *substituted judgment standard* asks the surrogate to apply the patient's stated preferences to make the decision she would make if not incapacitated. If no explicit conversation about preferences has taken place, the surrogate must choose based on knowledge of the patient's values. In this context, substituted judgment optimizes patient autonomy, yet surrogates often lack sufficient knowledge to decide just as the patient would. In such cases, they rely on the *best interests standard*, choosing what they believe to be in the patient's best interest.

There are barriers to applying substituted judgment in pediatrics. Because a child has never been legally competent, making choices congruent with her preferences is not possible. Instead, the parent/guardian must apply the best interests standard, which may also pose challenges. Reasonable persons may disagree about what constitutes a child's best interest and conflicting assessments may lead to tension between providers and parents (see dilemmas below).

Informed Consent in Children

In contrast to the adult who has become incompetent and whose prior autonomy we strive to honor, with a child our challenge is to protect emerging autonomy for minors developing decision-making capacity. In such cases, parents generally serve as the proxy, and as stated above, we expect them to use the best interests standard. After applying the best interests standard, parents either will or will not grant parental permission for the proposed medical intervention. While parental permission is not exactly the same as informed consent, in the setting of decision-making for minors, parental permission is a necessary element.

When appropriate, parental permission is bolstered by soliciting the assent of the child. *Assent* refers to a child's expression of approval or agreement to participate in clinical care (Committee on Bioethics and American Academy of Pediatrics 1995). There is no unequivocal age at which a child develops capacity to provide meaningful assent to treatment; however, literature suggests that most children do so by 7 years of age (Diekema 2006; Weithorn 1983). While there are practical challenges in soliciting assent, the American Academy of Pediatrics and Children's Oncology Group provide recommendations to guide providers (Joffe et al. 2006; Committee on Bioethics and American Academy of Pediatrics 1995).

We occasionally make exceptions and grant decision-making capacity to minors. An *emancipated minor* is a minor legally permitted to make decisions as an adult in one of two situations: (a) she lives independently of her parents (i.e., financially independent and living on her own or married), or (b) she has a predetermined health condition (pregnancy, sexual transmitted infection, mental health or substance abuse disorders). Minors who qualify based on independence may make all health-care decisions; however, minors emancipated based on a specific condition may consent for care only related to that condition.

A *mature minor* is a child who does not meet emancipation criteria, yet the state deems to have sufficient capacity to give informed consent for a particular health decision. Not all states have mature minor statutes, and even when satisfied, the child's decisional authority is limited to the specific decision for which it was petitioned. This is not limited to low-risk decisions, as a number of states have allowed minors to refuse lifesaving blood transfusions after finding them to have necessary capacity for such a serious decision (Ellement 1999; Associated Press 2007).

Ethical Dilemmas in Informed Consent

Requests for Nondisclosure of a Cancer Diagnosis

Case Vignette
A 12-year-old boy is diagnosed with Ewing's sarcoma. His mother asks the oncology team to withhold the diagnosis from the boy, because she does not want him upset by the knowledge that he has cancer.

There may be many reasons why a parent would request that the oncology team hide a cancer diagnosis from a child, including cultural or faith-based considerations as well as mental health factors. Clinicians should attempt to clarify a parent's motivation behind this request to better understand the context from which it comes and to figure out how best to proceed. From an ethical standpoint, respecting a child's emerging autonomy means that the child should receive an explanation of why she is sick and what testing and treatment will occur, appropriate for the child's age and development. Also, from a practical standpoint, it will be almost impossible to hide this information from a child who may receive chemotherapy, visit a cancer center, and interact with numerous clinicians whose badges and white coats refer to cancer. Hiding this information from patients is not feasible and attempts to do so may impair trust between the patient and the clinical team, and the patient may experience more fear or sadness knowing that a secret is being kept.

Depending on the child's age and medical circumstances, the child may or may not be present when the diagnosis of cancer is first disclosed. If parents are informed separately, the oncology team should ask for the parents' input into the best way to inform the child, respecting the parents' unique understanding of their child's psychological needs (Mack and Grier 2004). Psychosocial providers may be called upon to help explore a family's rationale for nondisclosure and to help the family and care team plan the best time and way for disclosure to occur.

A Child's Dissent/Refusal of Treatment

Case Vignette

You are called to assess a 16-year-old female to help determine whether she might be depressed. The patient is due to begin chemotherapy for Hodgkin lymphoma but on the day of her first treatment is now refusing her infusion stating she does not want to lose her hair.

Given the side effects and discomforts inherent to cancer care, it is not surprisingly that children frequently object to aspects of their care. And while opposition to research participation is nearly always respected, dissent from conventional diagnosis or therapy is a more challenging dilemma. Persuasion should be used on young children; however, it may be more difficult to persuade adolescents to do something against their will. Some have even run away when parents and physicians have tried to force them to comply with therapy (Ross 2009). Clinicians should assess whether the child might be a mature minor, and if needed, ask for input from psychosocial providers, ethics committees, or attorneys.

Parental Refusal of Recommended Therapy

Case Vignette

Carly is an 8-year-old female with sickle cell disease whose physicians are recommending a packed red blood cell transfusion to treat her acute chest syndrome. Carly's mother states the family's chosen faith is Jehovah's Witness and that Carly may not receive a red blood cell transfusion on the basis of their faith.

There are a growing number of legal cases involving parental refusal of recommended care in oncology (Ridgway 2004). These parents commonly object on religious or cultural grounds, yet the best interests standard and Diekema's *harm principle* suggests we ought to think about these cases from the perspective of the child, regardless of the rationale for refusal. The harm principle, a theoretical framework for deciding when we ought to interfere with parental decision-making, justifies override of parental decisions that put a child at significant risk of serious and imminent harm (Diekema 2004). This threshold is met, and parental authority superseded, if providers transfuse blood to a child against parents' wishes when they are Jehovah's Witnesses.

Clinicians faced with parental refusal should first assess parental capacity. In the unlikely scenario of parental incompetence, a court-appointed surrogate should make the decision on the child's behalf. Assuming parental competence, clinicians have a few options. First, they should attempt to persuade the parents, particularly when the rationale for refusal is based on illogical beliefs or misinformation (Brock and Wartman 1990). Next, if there are concessions they can make that will allow the child to get necessary care with acceptable deviations from the standard of care, they should bargain with the family. The last resort would be to ask a judge to place the child in foster care for the duration of cancer therapy. Before undertaking this adversarial step, clinicians should consider how certain they are of the outcome of therapy. When the likelihood of cure or other benefits is extremely high, judicial involvement is warranted. In contrast, when there is little chance of cure or benefit, providers should be hesitant to ask the court to intervene in order to protect the child from significant psychological stress (Pinnock and Crosthwaite 2005).

Sibling Donors for Hematopoietic Stem Cell Transplant

Case Vignette

Eric is a 6-year-old boy with acute lymphoblastic leukemia. Cytogenetics revealed monosomy 7, and a hematopoietic stem cell transplant is recommended at first remission. Eric's parents ask whether his 2-year-old sister may serve as a stem cell donor.

For children requiring hematopoietic stem cell (HSC) transplantation, HLA-matched, biologically related donors are preferred because of reduced risks of transplant-related complications. Because siblings are the most likely family members to be HLA matched to a patient, issues surrounding sibling donation arise frequently in cancer medicine. Numerous ethical arguments have been made to justify allowing a minor to donate HSC (Kesselheim et al. 2009), and the American Academy of Pediatrics has stated that "minors can ethically participate as hematopoietic stem cell donors" (Committee on Bioethics and American Academy of Pediatrics 2010), based on risk/benefit calculations that take into account the well-being of the donor as it relates to the survival of the recipient (see Table 17.1). Exceptional cases may occur, in particular where the patient and the potential donor sibling have

Table 17.1 Conditions under which a minor may donate hematopoietic stem cells

Condition	Explanation
There is no medically equivalent histocompatible adult relative who is willing and able to donate	An adult will be better able to understand the rationale for donation, the procedural details of donation, and its risks and benefits, more closely approximating ideal informed consent
There is a strong personal and emotionally positive relationship between the donor and recipient	This increases the likelihood that the donor will experience psychological benefits from donation
There is some likelihood that the recipient will benefit from transplantation	If the chance of successful transplantation are below some minimum threshold (not defined), the donor should not be exposed to the medical and psychological risks of donation[a]
The clinical, emotional, and psychosocial risks to the donor are minimized and are reasonable in relation to the benefits expected to accrue to t he donor and to the recipient	This ensures that parents consider the benefits and burdens of sibling donation from the independent perspectives of the donor and recipient
Parental permission and, where appropriate, child assent have been obtained	As with all informed consent, this respects patient autonomy We must acknowledge the conflicts of interest unique to sibling HSC donation[a]: Parents face the tension of exposing their healthy child to modest risks, with the hope of saving the life of their child who is ill Transplant teams primary responsibility is to the recipient; however, the same providers may participate in the evaluation, consent, and treatment of the donor

Adapted from Committee on Bioethics and American Academy of Pediatrics (2010)

[a]A donor advocate (or similar mechanism) may be used to aid in this assessment

no personal relationship, due to adoption or other circumstances. Some well-meaning providers may perform HLA typing on biological siblings, without considering whether there is a positive personal relationship between the potential donor and recipient; however, ethicists agree that this may be inappropriate (Kesselheim et al. 2009; Committee on Bioethics and American Academy of Pediatrics 2010). In at least one case, the legal system has supported this belief, with the 1990 Illinois Supreme Court ruling that "an existing close relationship between the donor and recipient must be present for the donation to be permissible" (Curran v. Bosze 1990).

Ethical Issues in Human Subjects Research

Progress in the field of pediatric oncology is often touted as the archetype of the improved health outcomes attainable through coordinated research efforts of clinicians and scientists around the world (O'Leary et al. 2008). Indeed, ever since Sidney Farber first induced remission in a child with acute lymphoblastic leukemia (ALL) using aminopterin (Farber and Diamond 1948), advances in cancer care now give us greater than 85 % chance of cure for pediatric ALL (Howlader et al. 2014). Despite this success and the promise research offers, the scientific community faces numerous ethical dilemmas in their efforts to cure pediatric cancer.

Historical Background

For more than a century, scholars have advocated for the need to protect children as a vulnerable population who could fall victim to unethical research (Bercovici 1921; Grodin and Glantz 1994). Yet it was not until after World War II, when Nazi experimentation on prisoners was revealed, that the scientific community began to codify ethical standards for medical research, in what is known as the Nuremberg Code (International Military 1949). Without explicitly mentioning children, its emphasis on informed consent provided some guidance until subsequent codes did. In 1964 the World Medical Association's Declaration of Helsinki outlined additional ethical research principles beyond informed consent, such as the concept that the "interests of the subject must always prevail over the interest of science and society" (World Medical Association 1997).

In 1974, as details of the controversial Syphilis Study at Tuskegee emerged, the US Congress created the National Commission for the Protection of Human Subjects of Biomedical and Behavioral Research. The Commission published the Belmont Report, outlining three basic ethical principles, *respect for persons*, *beneficence*, and *justice*, which form the framework for ethical discourse in biomedical research and practice (National Commission for the Protection of Human Subjects of Biomedical and Behavioral Research 1978). Respect for persons embodies the concept of autonomy, requiring that one's preferences be respected. A corollary is that "persons with diminished autonomy [e.g., children] are entitled to protection." Beneficence is defined as an obligation to carry out actions that "(1) do not harm and (2) maximize possible benefits and minimize possible harms." Lastly, justice encompasses the concept that risks and benefits ought to be distributed fairly and equally and that no individual be denied benefits to which they are entitled or forced to shoulder undue burden (Beauchamp and Childress 2013). The report outlined the processes of informed consent, risk/benefit assessment, and fair selection of subjects as procedural safeguards to these principles.

The terms "research" and "human subject" are best defined by the Code of Federal Regulations regarding human subjects research. *Research* is "a systematic investigation designed to develop or contribute to generalizable knowledge," and a *human subject* is "a living individual about whom an investigator conducting research obtains: (1) data through intervention or interaction with the individual, or (2) identifiable private information" (Office for Protection from Research Risks 1983). The regulations include the requirement that an Institutional Review Board (IRB) reviews all research activities. However, members of the scientific community itself have worked to articulate a comprehensive rubric to determine whether research protocols are ethical (Table 17.2).

Table 17.2 Requirements for determining whether human subjects research is ethical

Principle	Explanation
Social or scientific value	Research evaluates a treatment, intervention, or theory with the potential to improve health, well-being, or scientific understanding
Scientific validity	Uses accepted scientific methods likely to produce a valid answer to the study question
Fair subject selection	Recruitment and eligibility of subjects are based on science and risk, not vulnerability or privilege
Favorable risk/benefit ratio	Risks are minimized to the extent possible within the scientific objectives of the study; potential benefits are maximized Risks to subjects are justified by the sum of benefits to the subjects and to society
Independent review	Study design and procedures must be reviewed and evaluated by individuals who are unaffiliated with the research
Informed consent	Information must be provided to subjects about the nature of the research, benefits, risks, and alternatives; subjects must be able to make voluntary and reasoned decisions about enrolling In pediatric research, principles of surrogate permission and assent are applicable
Respect for subjects	Investigators must: Protect subjects' welfare Safeguard subjects' privacy Allow withdrawal from the research Inform subjects of newly acquired information about risks, benefits, or alternatives Notify subjects of study results

Adapted from Emanuel et al. (2000)

Special Requirements for Research in Children

In 1977, the Commission addressed the ethical issues surrounding the use of children as research subjects (National Commission for the Protection of Human Subjects of Biomedical and Behavioral Research 1977). It recognized children as a particularly vulnerable population whose interests warrant additional safeguards yet acknowledged the tension between protecting children and excluding them from research altogether, precluding them from reaping the benefits of research. Shortly thereafter, the Code of Federal Regulations added Subpart D, outlining categories of research involving children that are permissible (Office for Protection from Research Risks 1983).

For nearly all research, parental permission is required, and the process "should be identical to that of informed consent" (Diekema 2006). In addition, the IRB determines when assent is required based on child participants' capacity to provide it, using factors such as age, maturity, and psychological state. There is consensus that a capable child's dissent ought to be respected, with one exception: when the research offers the prospect of direct benefit and is unavailable outside of the research context (Office for Protection from Research Risks 1983).

Prominent Ethical Dilemmas in Research

Phase I Trials

Case Vignette

A 7-year-old boy has recurrent and refractory metastatic rhabdomyosarcoma. Despite radiation and numerous chemotherapy regimens, his disease is progressing. You meet with the patient and his parents to discuss involvement of pediatric hospice services to optimize palliative care. During the meeting, the patient's parents ask whether their son might be eligible for a new phase I trial opening in another state.

The goal of a typical phase I trial is to document the safety of a new intervention, most commonly by determining the dose-limiting toxicity (DLT) and maximum tolerated dose (MTD) of a novel drug. Critics contend that a phase I trial's objective is to learn about safety, without therapeutic intent, raising the important question – can phase I trials offer the prospect of benefit to a child with cancer? (Miller and Joffe

2008; Agrawal and Emanuel 2003). By virtue of the animal data required to justify a phase I trial, the drug must show promise for patient subjects. And indeed, some studies suggest approximately 10 % of subjects have a partial or complete response (Lee et al. 2005). Moreover, many investigators insist that participants receive psychological benefits by contributing to future knowledge and by maintaining hope (Kodish et al. 1992). Once we accept that a trial offers the prospect of direct benefit, it must satisfy other regulatory criteria: (1) the risks of exposing a child to a novel intervention is justified by the anticipated benefit, and (2) the relation of anticipated benefit to risk is at least as favorable as that available with alternative approaches (Office for Protection from Research Risks 1983).

The final ethical concern we will address is that of informed consent. Critics contend that parents' desperation for a cure makes them vulnerable. Available data demonstrates that participants enroll in phase I trials largely for personal benefit (Daugherty et al. 2000), that they overestimate the likelihood of benefit (Miller 2000), and that they have a poor understanding of the primary dose-finding objective of these studies (Cousino et al. 2012). While there is a dearth of quality data to attribute this to inadequate disclosure or instead to optimism, it is clear that a requisite component of any phase I trial is a transparent and forthright consent process.

Randomized Controlled Trials

Case Vignette

A 17-year-old young man recently diagnosed with a testicular tumor, and his family is considering a clinical trial in which subjects are randomly assigned to receive either standard chemotherapy or an alternate chemotherapy regimen that may have less toxicity. The patient is frustrated because he prefers the experimental regimen, but nobody can ensure this will be his regimen. He asks "why should I let a computer make decisions for me?"

Randomized controlled trials (RCTs) are the gold standard of biomedical research, allowing investigators to directly compare two interventions while controlling for factors that confound data generated by other study designs. In a typical oncology RCT, each subject is assigned, by chance, to one of two study groups. Subjects in the control group receive standard therapy, while those in the intervention group receive the treatment of interest. The classic ethical justification for such studies revolves around the concept of *equipoise*. Equipoise refers to "a state of professional uncertainty about [the] relative therapeutic merits" of the two interventions being studied (Miller and Joffe 2011). Put simply, if one of the two options is known to be better, we cannot justify randomly condemning half of the study population to receive the lesser therapy. Moreover, there is no need to conduct the study if we are certain which treatment is better. Conversely, most investigational therapies do not make it to a RCT unless there is evidence to suggest efficacy, so for a disease with poor therapeutic options, the presence of promising preliminary data might move expert opinion in favor of the novel drug, despite the lack of rigorous supporting data.

There are a host of criticisms of the concept of equipoise, and its use as the rationale for the appropriateness of RCTs (Miller and Brody 2003). Firstly, most patients expect their physician to weigh evidence, patient characteristics, and physician experience to determine the best therapeutic option. Equipoise assumes that patients will accept having that decision randomly assigned instead. Additionally, patients themselves may have a preference between treatments, even if the medical community does not. Thirdly, once a study begins, there may reach a point at which preliminary data favors one treatment over another. At this point equipoise, by definition, would be disturbed, and continuing the trial would be considered unethical. Data-monitoring committees are a part of most RCTs, and based on interim, data must either allow a study to continue or halt the study based on predefined stopping rules.

Therapeutic Misconception

Case Vignette
The parents of a 12-year-old female with newly diagnosed leukemia are considering whether to enroll their daughter in a clinical trial. As you meet with them, the patient's mother says "I think we should do the trial. The doctors would not have offered it if they did not think it was the best thing for our daughter."

The National Bioethics Advisory Commission defines the *therapeutic misconception* as "the belief that the purpose of a clinical trial is to benefit the individual patient rather than to gather data for the purpose of contributing to scientific knowledge" (National Bioethics Advisory Commission 2001). This concept is similar to the discussion of informed consent in phase I trials; however, it is also pertinent to RCTs such as the one described above. Despite clinicians' best intentions, a significant percent of parents choosing the RCT will mistakenly believe that the clinician will select the treatment based on her judgment of which option is the best fit for the child (Kodish et al. 2004). There is increasing evidence that this type of misunderstanding is widespread, leading to calls for new approaches to trial enrollment, such as preventing clinicians from being the ones to present study details and offer enrollment (Eder et al. 2007; Appelbaum et al. 2012; Flory and Emanuel 2004).

Ethical Issues at the End of Life

Decision-Making about Life-Sustaining Treatments

When approaching decisions about life-sustaining therapies, parents of dying children often prioritize quality of life, likelihood of improvement, and perceptions of their child's pain (Meyer et al. 2002). Similarly, physicians' recommendations are guided by patient preferences about life support and prognostic factors, such as the likelihood of survival and the likely functional outcome (Cook et al. 2003). To support health-care providers who counsel families of patients who are dying, recommendations regarding limitation of life-sustaining treatments were advanced as early as 1983 by the President's Commission for the Study of Ethical Problems in Medicine and Biomedical and Behavioral Research (President's Commission for the Study of Ethical Problems in Medicine and Biomedical and Behavioral Research 1983). Published guidelines of this kind also reflect lessons learned through paradigm cases (Table 17.3).

Sedatives and Analgesics in the Care of the Dying

Health-care providers have an undeniable moral duty to treat the pain and suffering of terminally ill patients. Yet this imperative may also raise ethical questions if treating the pain and suffering could possibly hasten a patient's death. Although empirical evidence suggests that the use of opioids and sedatives to relieve symptoms at the end of life in no way shortens life, theoretical concern remains (Macauley 2012; López-Saca et al. 2013). The ethical principle relevant to this question is the Doctrine of Double Effect (May 1978). The Doctrine states that when an action has two effects, one of which is inherently good and the other inherently bad, it can be justified if certain conditions are met:

1. The action in itself must be good or at least morally indifferent.
2. The clinician must intend only the good effect and not the bad effect. For example, the clinician must intend only the relief of the patient's suffering by administering an opioid medication. The hastening of death due to respiratory depression may be foreseeable, but is not the clinician's objective.
3. The bad effect cannot be a means to the good effect. For example, the clinician may not administer a poison instead of morphine because doing so allows the bad effect (death) to be the means to the good effect (relief from suffering).
4. The good intended must outweigh the potential bad outcome.

Table 17.3 Paradigm cases involving life-sustaining treatment decisions

Case	Facts of the case	Legal outcome	Relevance for ethical decision-making
Baby Doe 1982–84, Indiana (Lantos 1987; Pless 1983)	Baby Doe was an infant with Down syndrome and tracheoesophageal fistula Parents declined corrective surgery stating that he would never achieve a "minimally acceptable quality of life" New federal regulations were proposed to protect infants with disabilities from having care withheld	Baby Doe law passed requiring all states to create a regulatory system to investigate cases where medically indicated treatment is withheld from handicapped infants	Relevance limited by the use of ambiguous terms not easily applied to actual cases Directed at state agencies, not individual health-care providers Not useful to clinicians making decisions regarding infants at the end of life
Baby K Early 1990s, Virginia (Lo and Jonsen 1980; Post 1995; Annas 1994)	Baby K was an infant with anencephaly Mother demanded mechanical ventilation during multiple hospitalizations Clinicians refused, stating that mechanical ventilation could not reverse her malformation and therefore was not indicated	A federal appeals court ruled in favor of Baby K's mother, arguing that the hospital was required to provide any emergent care, according to the Emergency Medical Treatment and Active Labor Act (EMTALA)	The court did not opine as to how futility enters into medical decisions Decision based on EMTALA rather than on the merits of the futility argument Case does not answer the key question: Can patients and families demand clinical care of providers who believe it will not be beneficial?
Karen Ann Quinlan 1975, New Jersey (McFadden 1985)	Karen Ann Quinlan fell into a coma due to a combination of alcohol and sedative medications Parents requested the ventilator keeping her alive be discontinued Physicians refused the family's request to let her die, a decision supported in the Superior Court of Morristown, N.J. Did not die for 9 more years when the ventilator was ultimately stopped	After a long legal battle, the Supreme Court decided 7–0 to support the parents in March 1976 Court justified their decision based on the patients right to privacy Stated that the patient's father, not physicians, should make decisions of this kind	Provides an ethical argument for unwanted life-sustaining technologies to be considered unethical if requests to discontinue are not honored The clear medical assessment that recovery for the patient was not possible was essential to the case Decision-making absent clear prognostic data is even more challenging
Nancy Cruzan 1990, Missouri, US Supreme Court (Annas 1990; Orentlicher 1990)	Cruzan was an adult patient involved in an automobile accident which left her in a "persistent vegetative state" She was sustained for 7 years with gastrostomy tube feedings	In a 5–4 decision, the Supreme Court ruled there was not enough evidence that Cruzan would have wanted the feeding tube removed	Parents and guardians must act in the best interests of children and incompetent adults Whether a particular intervention indeed reflects best interests can be controversial The US Supreme Court stated that there is no legal difference between withholding and withdrawing life-sustaining therapies

The moral reasoning outlined above remains controversial for a few reasons. First, according to the Doctrine, the moral justification for a clinician's practice hinges on his intention, something that is impossible to know with certainty. In addition, critics believe that the only morally relevant consideration is the informed consent of the patient (or appropriate proxy), which is not explicitly considered in the Doctrine (Quill et al. 1997; Truog et al. 2012).

Medical Futility

Questions of futility arise in cancer medicine when patients or family members request care, such as chemotherapy, that is unlikely to be beneficial. Such requests may be motivated by unrealistic expectations of benefit if, for example, the likelihood that a treatment will improve symptoms or slow the pace of the disease is overestimated. In addition, requests for futile treatments may occur when an individual does not want to be viewed as "giving up" or "losing hope" (Khatcheressian et al. 2008). Disagreements between clinicians, patients, and family members about whether a particular treatment should be offered or continued may result in conflict. Resolving these conflicts hinges on high-quality communication, careful and honest counseling, and compassion on the part of all involved.

The concept and definition of futility has been debated for decades, most publicly in the Baby K case (Table 17.3). In general, proposed definitions lack an empirical basis, expert consensus, or societal endorsement (Burns and Truog 2007). Seeking a definition implies futility in an objective concept, while in reality, controversy around futility often centers on subjective preferences and values. Whether a treatment is valuable, what constitutes benefit, and whether preserving life is "better" than allowing death will remain the subject of ongoing debate.

Guidelines for Decision-Making

How should clinicians approach decisions for and with patients approaching the end of life (Fig. 17.1) In 1983 the President's Commission proposed a useful and frequently cited construct for defining the best interests of a child approaching the end of life (President's Commission for the Study of Ethical Problems in Medicine and Biomedical and Behavioral Research 1983). With these five considerations in mind, the clinician places a proposed treatment or intervention into one of three categories to define the potential benefit for the dying patient. The Commission advises on the best course of action for the patient, considering both the clinician assessment above and the preferences of the patients and parents. In general, when parents prefer to forego life-sustaining therapies that the clinician considers to have ambiguous/uncertain benefit or to be clearly not beneficial, then the clinician should withdraw life-sustaining therapy (Fig. 17.1).

Prominent Ethical Dilemmas at the End of Life

Palliative Sedation

Case Vignette
A 10-year-old with a relapsed and refractory tumor of the brain experiences intractable seizures. The patient and family are intensely disturbed by the seizures and express their primary goal of halting the seizure activity. Doing so requires large doses of sedating medications such that the patient is no longer conscious. The medical team plans to decrease the medications in 48 h to "see how the patient will do," but the family requests the medications continue, stating, "this is the only way our son can have peace."

A rarely used approach to sedation and analgesia at the end of life is palliative sedation, wherein a child must be sedated to the point of unconsciousness in order to be comfortable (Truog et al. 1992; Cowan and Walsh 2001; Postovsky et al. 2007). This practice should be considered, with consent, when all other methods of controlling the patient's suffering have failed (National Ethics Committee 2006). After the patient loses consciousness, hydration and nutrition stop and no attempt is typically made to restore the patient to consciousness. Patients typically die after several days from dehydration or a complication of the treatment.

The US Supreme Court implicitly endorsed palliative sedation, citing the technique as an

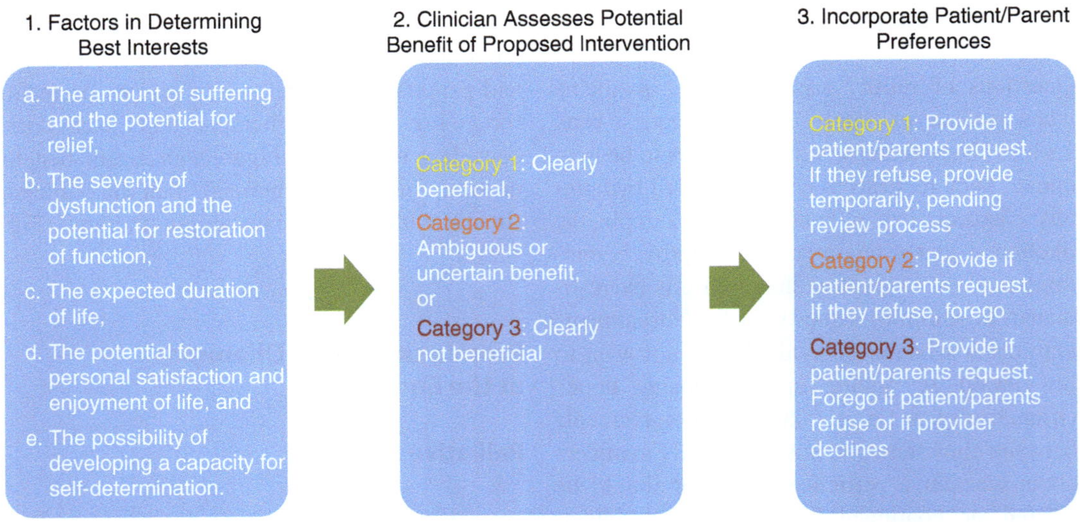

Fig. 17.1 Approach to decision-making at the end of life

alternative to physician-assisted suicide that could, in theory, assure that no patient should die with "untreatable" pain (McStay 2003). At least in part because of this legal endorsement, palliative sedation has become more widely practiced, although its ethical justification remains controversial (Schüklenk et al. 2011; Kiman et al. 2011; Goldstein et al. 2012).

Withholding or Withdrawal of Medical Nutrition and Hydration

Case Vignette

A 14-year-old female has a large intra-abdominal tumor compressing her bowel. Despite numerous chemotherapy regimens, the tumor has progressed. The patient is no longer receiving cancer-directed therapy and both she and her family realize that she will likely die from this cancer. The patient is admitted to the hospital with vomiting and inability to tolerate her nasogastric feeds. The tumor has caused an obstruction in her bowel. The team recommends surgery to alleviate the obstruction, but the patient requests that nasogastric feeds simply be discontinued.

The decision to withhold or withdraw medical nutrition and hydration should be made after weighing the burdens and benefits of therapy for that patient. Such decisions are morally equivalent to those pertaining to mechanical ventilation and other life-sustaining interventions (Levi 2003; Diekema and Botkin 2009; Nelson 1987); however, they can be controversial since many consider nutrition and hydration to be basic supports for ongoing life, without which human dignity is compromised. Some argue that decisions to forego medical nutrition and hydration can constitute patient abandonment. Despite these concerns, courts have ruled that they are medical interventions and may be discontinued on the same grounds as any other medical treatment (Table 17.3).

Ethical Issues in Genetic Testing and Diagnosis

Rapid advances in biomedical technology have increased the accessibility of genetic testing. These evaluations are now an intrinsic component of clinical practice, and in the research context, genetic testing is even more prevalent. Although the intent of such testing is to elucidate genetic mutations underlying a particular tumor, incidental findings may have wider implications for the patient and family, raising new ethical questions (Presidential Commission for the Study of Bioethical Issues 2012).

Information gleaned from genetic testing may be of pivotal importance to the care of a child with cancer. Genetic tests performed on the tumor can reveal details that may influence treatment decisions. In many cases, these tests may be considered standard of care and new research opportunities related to this testing are increasingly common. Other genetic testing performed on the patient may reveal whether a cancer is likely a random event or possibly part of an inherited predisposition to cancer. In this way, results of testing performed for a single patient may be of consequence for that patient's family members, many of whom are not included in decision-making about the tests. Another complexity is that the data obtained from any of these genetic tests may be difficult to interpret. Results are often of unclear significance, stated in terms of risk or probability of affecting the patient in a meaningful way. Because both risk and probability can be challenging for patients and clinicians to understand clearly, these results may generate confusion and distress, an additional psychological risk of genetic testing.

Prominent Ethical Dilemmas in Genetics and Genomics

Cancer Predisposition Testing

Case Vignette
A 40-year-old female with sarcoma was diagnosed with Li-Fraumeni syndrome, an inherited condition that increases her risk of several cancers. She has two children, ages 10 and 16, and requests that the children be tested immediately for the genetic mutation causing Li-Fraumeni.

How ought clinicians decide whether to offer genetic testing to explore whether a child has a cancer predisposition syndrome? Whenever possible these decisions should be made in conjunction with pretest counseling. Through one or even several meetings with a genetic counselor, patients will have ample opportunity to comprehend the risks and benefits of genetic testing, allowing for informed consent to occur (Ross et al. 2013). In addition, decision-making can be aided by the American Society of Clinical Oncology guidelines, relevant to adults, which advise that whether to test depends on if (a) the individual's personal or family history suggests genetic susceptibility, (b) the test is likely to yield interpretable data, or (c) the results will alter management recommendations for the patient and/or family (Robson et al. 2010). Psychosocial consultation may also be useful when there are complex family dynamics or preexisting emotional concerns.

For children, ethicists and genetics experts agree that testing should be postponed until adulthood, when possible. Genetic testing may be ethically permissible for pediatric patients whose potential risk of cancer would be present during childhood or for whom a potentially effective intervention (such as an evidence-based screening regimen) may be advisable before the patient would become a legal adult (Ross et al. 2013).

Incidental Findings

Case Vignette
Your hospital now has the capacity to perform detailed genetic sequencing on newly resected pediatric tumors. The father of a patient calls very concerned because the report from his child's kidney tumor reveals the child may be at risk for diabetes in the future.

Modern sequencing technologies create the challenge of findings unrelated to the original reasons testing was done (Presidential Commission for the Study of Bioethical Issues 2013). Testing, performed most commonly on the tumor, may uncover abnormalities in germline DNA, indicating inherited mutations, rather than anomalies acquired solely within the cancer cells (Bombard et al. 2013). In oncology, pathological examination of tumors will increasingly incorporate sequencing in hopes of elucidating potential targets for therapy. Sequencing may be limited to panels of known cancer-relevant genes or may extend to whole exomes or genomes. As testing becomes more broad, the risk of these incidental or secondary findings increases.

The Use of Genomic Testing in Research

The opportunities for children to participate in research involving genomic testing have multiplied rapidly in recent years (Caulfield et al. 2008). While scientifically exciting, this is also fraught with novel ethical dilemmas, which have not yet been reconciled within the scientific or ethics communities. For example, genetic material from research subjects, including children too young to give consent, may be stored in biobanks that yield data sets available to other investigators. While samples are stored without traditional patient identifiers, each individual's genetic composition is its own source of identification, raising important questions about whether anonymity in such a setting is truly possible (Gymrek et al. 2013; Gurwitz et al. 2009).

Another question is whether to return individual results to research subjects (Wolf et al. 2008; Presidential Commission for the Study of Bioethical Issues 2013). Sharing results with a research subject shows respect for the participant but could also cause harm by burdening the individual with personal genetic data that she may not truly desire. In general, investigators pursue the return of individual genetic test results only if (a) the finding has significant health implications substantiated with clear evidence, (b) there are established and potentially effective interventions, (c) the test is valid, and (d) the individual has chosen to receive his or her results (Fabsitz et al. 2010).

Professionalism

Professionalism is the basis of organized medicine's contract with society. This contract can only exist if the public trusts health professionals and believes in their integrity. For example, patients and families trust that health providers will place patients' interests and needs above their own, that they will respect patient privacy, and that they will practice with compassion and empathy. The American Board of Pediatrics defines professionalism as the ability to demonstrate excellence, humanism, accountability, and altruism in addition to competence in clinical care, communication, and ethics (American Board of Pediatrics Program Directors Committee 2008). The American Psychological Association's ethical principles and code of conduct include obligations to practice competently and honestly while maintaining appropriate relationships with patients and respect for proper boundaries (American Psychological Association 2002).

Privacy and Confidentiality

Confidentiality has always been a central aspect of medical care. The Hippocratic Oath promises that "Whatsoever in the course of practice I see or hear…that ought never to be published abroad, I will not divulge, but consider such things to be holy secrets" (Roter et al. 1998). Despite this acknowledged obligation, new technologies like social media and the electronic medical record can threaten patient privacy if utilized improperly.

A commitment to maintaining patient privacy is an expression of the principle of respect for persons. A patient who is not assured of confidentiality cannot speak freely with the healthcare provider and therefore is deprived of the full benefits of the therapeutic alliance. In such a setting, patients may hesitate to seek care or reveal important information to providers, either of which can have serious health consequences (Beauchamp and Childress 2013).

The Health Insurance Portability and Accountability Act (HIPAA) defines much of the standards for confidentiality in health care (Office for Civil Rights 2002). HIPAA applies to protected health information (PHI) that could be used to identify a particular individual. Healthcare professionals may not disclose PHI without written authorization by the parent/guardian.

Nevertheless, obligations of confidentiality can be overridden for three broad reasons: avoiding harm to others, benefiting the patient, and preserving public health for the benefit of others (Beauchamp and Childress 2013). The best-known legal precedent is the case of Tatiana Tarasoff, who was murdered by Prosenjit Poddar. Prior to the murder, Poddar admitted his intention to harm Tarasoff to a counselor, who alerted law enforcement, but not Tarasoff herself. When the victim's parents took legal action against the counselor, the court determined that breaching patient confidentiality would have been appropriate because there was a credible threat to the well-being of another person (Tarasoff v. Regents of University of California 1976). Health-care providers may be obliged to violate confidentiality in scenarios of child abuse and elder abuse and of communicable disease which threaten public health (Burkle and Cascino 2011).

Specific Dilemmas Involving Privacy and Confidentiality

Case Vignette
A patient confides in a social worker during a clinic visit but then says, "Please don't tell the doctors I said that!"

As this example demonstrates, there are also less grave situations where providers may have a duty to break confidentiality. Requests for secrets to be kept between clinicians should be approached with caution, as even seemingly trivial pieces of information could be important for medical management, and transparency and communication throughout the interprofessional team are essential for good care.

Case Vignette
A nurse is upset by the relapse of a patient and posts online "My heart is breaking for Samuel and his parents tonight!"

In the contemporary setting, a modern threat to confidentiality is the widespread use of social media, and the frequency with which providers participate in the online world (see Chapter 19 on Social Media). Social media has the potential to enhance patient education, therapeutic alliance, the clinician-patient relationship, and even accrual to research studies. Adolescents and young adults are avid social media users who may reach out to providers in the electronic space. At this point, individual clinicians may choose how to respond to this contact, unless their institutions have created policy to guide such behavior. Regardless, discourse on social media must not threaten patient confidentiality. Individual patient identifiers like names, ages, diseases, photos, or hospital units should not be shared via social media.

Conflict of Interest

Case Vignette
A study's principal investigator is having trouble accruing subjects into his clinical trial for medulloblastoma. The institution may close the study if more patients do not choose to enroll. Although the next patient diagnosed with medulloblastoma is not an optimal candidate for the trial, the investigator, who is also a pediatric oncologist, strongly encourages the patient's parents to enroll their child.

The complexities of the health-care arena often cause providers to take on more than one role. A physician may also serve as a consultant to a pharmaceutical company. A psychologist may also conduct a research study. A nurse practitioner may become close friends with a patient's mother. While none of these is inherently unethical, each poses a risk for a conflict of interest (COI) to develop. COI exists when these roles have discordant interests, jeopardizing the integrity of the individual's primary role as a clinician.

Conflicts of interest may undermine professional judgment, thereby compromising the public's trust in health-care professionals. Cases in which the integrity of a clinician's work was compromised by a COI have eroded public confidence in our field (Liang and Mackey 2010; Wilson 2010). To mitigate this tension, health-care providers are expected to identify, disclose, and manage potential COI. Much of the attention from the media and public policy standpoints hovers around financial conflicts of interest. However, nonfinancial COI, as demonstrated by this example, also pose a threat to professionalism that must be resolved by the individual clinician. In this case, the physician/investigator, the other members of the multidiscliplinary care team, and the Institutional Review Board must be assured that decisions about eligibility and the informed consent process are free of conflicts of interest. For example, it may be preferable to involve an additional, less conflicted, individual in the consent process. Such a strategy can avoid patients ill suited to a trial being enrolled as result of the physician-investigator's COI. In some situations, consultation with the ethics committee may be indicated to resolve conflicts of interest.

Boundaries in the Patient-Provider Relationship

Many clinicians choose pediatric oncology as their specialty in part because of the unique relationships between providers and their patients. Cancer medicine offers longitudinal care as well as emotional intensity. The close relationships that emerge between clinicians, patients, and parents usually fortify the therapeutic alliance and enhance patient care. However, it can be challenging to recognize when a relationship crosses professional boundaries and becomes an impediment to good care (Hartlage 2012). A boundary has been violated when a clinician crosses the "limits" of the patient or family member. These "limits" may be emotional, physical, spiritual, or sexual in nature (Washington State Department of Health 2014). Preserving proper boundaries is the ethical duty of the clinician (American Board of Pediatrics Program Directors Committee 2008), not the patient, and thus, clinicians should refrain from seeking out patient information, either during the clinic visit or from alternate sources like the internet, unless necessary for clinical purposes. Keeping separate the private and personal lives of patients and clinicians is essential for productive and professional care.

Conclusion

As demonstrated above, providing medical care for children with cancer is a complex enterprise that raises many moral and ethical questions. All health-care professionals, including psychosocial clinicians, should be familiar with the ethical principles and interests that may be at odds throughout a child's illness. Providers will invariably encounter some of the more common challenges discussed in this chapter. Some will feel comfortable navigating these situations by themselves; others may need the support of colleagues or providers with experience dealing with such challenges. Most institutions have at least one mechanism in place to provide ethical analysis and guidance when requested. The two most common resources are ethics committees and ethics consultants.

An ethics committee is a group that often serves an advisory role to a hospital or institution. In some ways it is similar to an IRB, except that it typically handles dilemmas involving clinical care, and not research. It may be comprised of physicians, nurses, attorneys, administrators, psychosocial and spiritual care providers, and community members, among others. The committee meets to hear about specific ethical concerns that are raised in the course of the clinical care provided at that institution. Providers, and sometimes patients or families, may be invited to present and discuss their concerns with the committee, so that its members can understand the circumstances and pertinent ethical facts, and provide guidance or recommendations. Some ethics committees may also create or evaluate hospital policies regarding delicate or controversial clinical situations, such as when it might be permissible or appropriate to withhold cardiopulmonary resuscitation (CPR) from a dying patient. Additionally, some ethics committees may offer educational programs, such as grand rounds or unit-based ethics rounds, to disseminate information and provide education and support regarding important ethical topics.

The second resource that is frequently available is the ethics consultant. Consultants may be physicians or attorneys or have doctoral degrees in bioethics, and most are formally trained clinical bioethicists. A consultant will meet with the involved parties, provide an analysis of the ethical issues, and, when appropriate, make recommendations. The ethics consultant may discuss the case with colleagues or the ethics committee and will leave a consultation note in the patient's medical record. By utilizing the expertise of ethics consultants and ethics committees, healthcare providers should feel more comfortable handling particularly challenging situations. And while these are the most common support mechanisms, institutions may have others, so each provider should familiarize herself with the available resources.

Clinical Pearls

- The multidisciplinary practice of pediatric oncology involves ethical tensions that providers must be prepared to navigate.
- Ethical analysis requires weighing the principles of autonomy, beneficence, and justice.
- Ethical challenges typically fall into the areas of informed consent, research, genetic results, end-of-life care, and professionalism.
- A major pediatric-specific ethical challenge is protecting the emerging autonomy of the minor who is in the constant process of developing decision-making capacity.
- Ethics consultants and hospital or institutional ethics committees are resources that can provide assistance and guidance to providers struggling with a particular issue.

References

Agrawal M, Emanuel EJ (2003) Ethics of phase 1 oncology studies: reexamining the arguments and data. JAMA 290(8):1075–1082. doi:10.1001/jama.290.8.1075

American Board of Pediatrics Program Directors Committee (2008) Teaching and assessing professionalism: a program Director's guide. American Board of Pediatrics Foundation, Chapel Hill

American Psychological Association (2002) Ethical principles of psychologists and code of conduct. Am Psychol 57:1060–1073

Annas GJ (1990) Nancy Cruzan and the right to die. N Engl J Med 323(10):670–673. doi:10.1056/NEJM199009063231010

Annas GJ (1994) Asking the courts to set the standard of emergency care–the case of Baby K. N Engl J Med 330(21):1542–1545. doi:10.1056/NEJM199405263302120

Appelbaum PS (2007) Clinical practice. Assessment of patients' competence to consent to treatment. N Engl J Med 357(18):1834–1840. doi:10.1056/NEJMcp074045

Appelbaum PS, Anatchkova M, Albert K, Dunn LB, Lidz CW (2012) Therapeutic misconception in research subjects: development and validation of a measure. Clin Trials 9(6):748–761. doi:10.1177/1740774512456455

Associated Press (2007) Boy dies after refusing transfusion over religion. NBC News. http://www.nbcnews.com/id/22032266/ns/health-health_care/t/boy-dies-after-refusing-transfusion-over-religion/#.U--42aPFj65I. Accessed 24 Aug 2014

Beauchamp TL, Childress JF (2013) Principles of biomedical ethics, 7th edn. Oxford University Press, New York

Bercovici K (1921) Orphans as guinea pigs. The Nation 112(2921):911–913

Berg JW, Appelbaum PS (2001) Informed consent : legal theory and clinical practice, 2nd edn. Oxford University Press, Oxford

Bombard Y, Robson M, Offit K (2013) Revealing the incidentalome when targeting the tumor genome. JAMA 310(8):795–796. doi:10.1001/jama.2013.276573

Brock DW, Wartman SA (1990) When competent patients make irrational choices. N Engl J Med 322(22):1595–1599. doi:10.1056/NEJM199005313222209

Burkle CM, Cascino GD (2011) Medicine and the media: balancing the public's right to know with the privacy of the patient. Mayo Clin Proc 86(12):1192–1196. doi:10.4065/mcp.2011.0520

Burns JP, Truog RD (2007) Futility: a concept in evolution. Chest 132(6):1987–1993. doi:10.1378/chest.07-1441

Caulfield T, McGuire AL, Cho M, Buchanan JA, Burgess MM, Danilczyk U, Diaz CM, Fryer-Edwards K, Green SK, Hodosh MA, Juengst ET, Kaye J, Kedes L, Knoppers BM, Lemmens T, Meslin EM, Murphy J, Nussbaum RL, Otlowski M, Pullman D, Ray PN, Sugarman J, Timmons M (2008) Research ethics recommendations for whole-genome research: consensus statement. PLoS Biol 6(3), e73. doi:10.1371/journal.pbio.0060073

Committee on Bioethics, American Academy of Pediatrics (1995) Informed consent, parental permission, and assent in pediatric practice. Pediatrics 95(2):314–317

Committee on Bioethics, American Academy of Pediatrics (2010) Children as hematopoietic stem cell donors. Pediatrics 125(2):392–404. doi:10.1542/peds.2009-3078

Cook D, Rocker G, Marshall J, Sjokvist P, Dodek P, Griffith L, Freitag A, Varon J, Bradley C, Levy M, Finfer S, Hamielec C, McMullin J, Weaver B, Walter S, Guyatt G, Level of Care Study Investigators and the Canadian Critical Care Trials Group (2003) Withdrawal of mechanical ventilation in anticipation of death in the intensive care unit. N Engl J Med 349(12):1123–1132. doi:10.1056/NEJMoa030083

Cousino MK, Zyzanski SJ, Yamokoski AD, Hazen RA, Baker JN, Noll RB, Rheingold SR, Geyer JR, Alexander SC, Drotar D, Kodish ED (2012) Communicating and understanding the purpose of pediatric phase I cancer trials. J Clin Oncol 30(35):4367–4372. doi:10.1200/JCO.2012.42.3004

Cowan JD, Walsh D (2001) Terminal sedation in palliative medicine–definition and review of the literature. Support Care Cancer 9(6):403–407

Curran v. Bosze (1990) NE 2d, vol 566. Ill: Supreme Court

Daugherty CK, Banik DM, Janish L, Ratain MJ (2000) Quantitative analysis of ethical issues in phase I trials: a survey interview of 144 advanced cancer patients. IRB 22(3):6–14

Diekema DS (2004) Parental refusals of medical treatment: the harm principle as threshold for state intervention. Theor Med Bioeth 25(4):243–264

Diekema DS (2006) Conducting ethical research in pediatrics: a brief historical overview and review of pediatric regulations. J Pediatr 149(1 Suppl):S3–S11. doi:10.1016/j.jpeds.2006.04.043

Diekema DS, Botkin JR (2009) Forgoing medically provided nutrition and hydration in children. Pediatrics 124(2):813–822. doi:10.1542/peds.2009-1299

Drane JF (1985) The many faces of competency. Hastings Cent Rep 15(2):17–21

Eder ML, Yamokoski AD, Wittmann PW, Kodish ED (2007) Improving informed consent: suggestions from parents of children with leukemia. Pediatrics 119(4):e849–e859. doi:10.1542/peds.2006-2208

Ellement J (1999) Ruling clarifies minors' rights; court gives weight to medical wishes. The Boston Globe, Boston, MA, p B1

Emanuel EJ, Wendler D, Grady C (2000) What makes clinical research ethical? JAMA 283(20):2701–2711

Fabsitz RR, McGuire A, Sharp RR, Puggal M, Beskow LM, Biesecker LG, Bookman E, Burke W, Burchard EG, Church G, Clayton EW, Eckfeldt JH, Fernandez CV, Fisher R, Fullerton SM, Gabriel S, Gachupin F, James C, Jarvik GP, Kittles R, Leib JR, O'Donnell C, O'Rourke PP, Rodriguez LL, Schully SD, Shuldiner AR, Sze RK, Thakuria JV, Wolf SM, Burke GL, National Heart Ln, and Blood Institute Working Group (2010) Ethical and practical guidelines for reporting genetic research results to study participants: updated guidelines from a National Heart, Lung, and Blood Institute working group. Circ Cardiovasc Genet 3(6):574–580. doi:10.1161/CIRCGENETICS.110.958827

Farber S, Diamond LK (1948) Temporary remissions in acute leukemia in children produced by folic acid antagonist, 4-aminopteroyl-glutamic acid. N Engl J Med 238(23):787–793. doi:10.1056/NEJM194806032382301

Fernandez A (2010) Improving the quality of informed consent: it is not all about the risks. Ann Intern Med 153(5):342–343. doi:10.7326/0003-4819-153-5-201009070-00011

Flory J, Emanuel E (2004) Interventions to improve research participants' understanding in informed consent for research: a systematic review. JAMA 292(13):1593–1601. doi:10.1001/jama.292.13.1593

Goldstein NE, Cohen LM, Arnold RM, Goy E, Arons S, Ganzini L (2012) Prevalence of formal accusations of murder and euthanasia against physicians. J Palliat Med 15(3):334–339. doi:10.1089/jpm.2011.0234

Grodin MA, Glantz LH (1994) Children as research subjects : science, ethics, and law. Oxford University Press, New York

Gurwitz D, Fortier I, Lunshof JE, Knoppers BM (2009) Research ethics. Children and population biobanks. Science 325(5942):818–819. doi:10.1126/science.1173284

Gymrek M, McGuire AL, Golan D, Halperin E, Erlich Y (2013) Identifying personal genomes by surname inference. Science 339(6117):321–324. doi:10.1126/science.1229566

Hartlage HN (2012) Exploring boundaries in pediatric oncology nursing. J Pediatr Oncol Nurs 29(2):109–112. doi:10.1177/1043454212438965

Hawkins JS, Emanuel EJ (2005) Clarifying confusions about coercion. Hastings Cent Rep 35(5):16–19

Howlader N, Noone AM, Krapcho M, Garshell J, Miller D, Altekruse SF, Kosary CL, Yu M, Ruhl J, Tatalovich Z, Mariotto A, Lewis DR, Chen HS, Feuer EJ, Cronin KA (2014) SEER cancer statistics review, 1975–2011. National Cancer Institute, Bethesda, pp 1975–2011

International Military Tribunal (1949) Trials of war criminals before the Nuernberg Military Tribunals under Control Council law no. 10; Nuremberg, Oct 1946–Apr 1949

Joffe S, Fernandez CV, Pentz RD, Ungar DR, Mathew NA, Turner CW, Alessandri AJ, Woodman CL, Singer DA, Kodish E (2006) Involving children with cancer in decision-making about research participation. J Pediatr 149(6):862–868. doi:10.1016/j.jpeds.2006.08.027

Kesselheim JC, Lehmann LE, Styron NF, Joffe S (2009) Is blood thicker than water?: ethics of hematopoietic stem cell donation by biological siblings of adopted children. Arch Pediatr Adolesc Med 163(5):413–416. doi:10.1001/archpediatrics.2009.43

Khatcheressian J, Harrington SB, Lyckholm LJ, Smith TJ (2008) 'Futile care': what to do when your patient insists on chemotherapy that likely won't help.

Oncology (Williston Park) 22(8):881–888; discussion 893, 896, 898

Kiman R, Wuiloud AC, Requena ML (2011) End of life care sedation for children. Curr Opin Support Palliat Care 5(3):285–290. doi:10.1097/SPC.0b013e3283492aba

Kodish E, Stocking C, Ratain MJ, Kohrman A, Siegler M (1992) Ethical issues in phase I oncology research: a comparison of investigators and institutional review board chairpersons. J Clin Oncol 10(11):1810–1816

Kodish E, Eder M, Noll RB, Ruccione K, Lange B, Angiolillo A, Pentz R, Zyzanski S, Siminoff LA, Drotar D (2004) Communication of randomization in childhood leukemia trials. JAMA 291(4):470–475. doi:10.1001/jama.291.4.470

Lantos J (1987) Baby Doe five years later. Implications for child health. N Engl J Med 317(7):444–447. doi:10.1056/NEJM198708133170709

Lee DP, Skolnik JM, Adamson PC (2005) Pediatric phase I trials in oncology: an analysis of study conduct efficiency. J Clin Oncol 23(33):8431–8441. doi: 10.1200/JCO.2005.02.1568

Levi BH (2003) Withdrawing nutrition and hydration from children: legal, ethical, and professional issues. Clin Pediatr 42(2):139–145

Liang BA, Mackey T (2010) Confronting conflict: addressing institutional conflicts of interest in academic medical centers. Am J Law Med 36(1):136–187

Lo B, Jonsen AR (1980) Clinical decisions to limit treatment. Ann Intern Med 93(5):764–768

López-Saca JM, Guzmán JL, Centeno C (2013) A systematic review of the influence of opioids on advanced cancer patient survival. Curr Opin Support Palliat Care 7(4):424–430. doi:10.1097/SPC.0b013e328365763a

Macauley R (2012) The role of the principle of double effect in ethics education at US medical schools and its potential impact on pain management at the end of life. J Med Ethics 38(3):174–178. doi:10.1136/medethics-2011-100105

Mack JW, Grier HE (2004) The day one talk. J Clin Oncol 22(3):563–566. doi:10.1200/JCO.2004.04.078

Mandava A, Millum J (2013) Manipulation in the enrollment of research participants. Hastings Cent Rep 43(2):38–47. doi:10.1002/hast.144

May WF (1978) Double effect. In: Reich WT (ed) Encyclopedia of bioethics. Free Press, New York, pp 316–320

McFadden RD (1985) Karen Ann Quinlan, 31, dies; Focus of'76 right to die case. The New York Times, 12 June 1985

McStay R (2003) Terminal sedation: palliative care for intractable pain, post Glucksberg and Quill. Am J Law Med 29(1):45–76

Meisel A, Roth LH, Lidz CW (1977) Toward a model of the legal doctrine of informed consent. Am J Psychiatry 134(3):285–289

Meyer EC, Burns JP, Griffith JL, Truog RD (2002) Parental perspectives on end-of-life care in the pediatric intensive care unit. Crit Care Med 30(1):226–231

Miller M (2000) Phase I cancer trials. A collusion of misunderstanding. Hastings Cent Rep 30(4):34–43

Miller FG, Brody H (2003) A critique of clinical equipoise. Therapeutic misconception in the ethics of clinical trials. Hastings Cent Rep 33(3):19–28

Miller FG, Joffe S (2008) Benefit in phase 1 oncology trials: therapeutic misconception or reasonable treatment option? Clin Trials 5(6):617–623. doi:10.1177/1740774508097576

Miller FG, Joffe S (2011) Equipoise and the dilemma of randomized clinical trials. N Engl J Med 364(5):476–480. doi:10.1056/NEJMsb1011301

National Bioethics Advisory Commission (2001) Ethical and policy issues in international research: clinical trials in developing countries, vol 1. United States, National Bioethics Advisory Commission. http://bioethics.georgetown.edu/nbac/clinical/Vol1.pdf

National Commission for the Protection of Human Subjects of Biomedical and Behavioral Research (1977) Research involving children: report and recommendations. DHEW publication, vol no (OS) 77-0004. United States, National Commission for the Protection of Human Subjects of Biomedical and Behavioral Research, Bethesda

National Commission for the Protection of Human Subjects of Biomedical and Behavioral Research (1978) The Belmont report: ethical principles and guidelines for the protection of human subjects of research. DHEW Publication, vol no (OS) 78-0012. United States, Government Printing Office, Bethesda/Washington, DC

National Ethics Committee VHA (2006) The ethics of palliative sedation as a therapy of last resort. Am J Hosp Palliat Care 23(6):483–491. doi:10.1177/1049909106294883

Nelson LJ (1987) Foregoing nutrition and hydration. Clin Ethics Rep 1(1):1–7

O'Leary M, Krailo M, Anderson JR, Reaman GH, Children's Oncology Group (2008) Progress in childhood cancer: 50 years of research collaboration, a report from the Children's Oncology Group. Semin Oncol 35(5):484–493. doi:10.1053/j.seminoncol.2008.07.008

Office for Civil Rights, Health and Human Services (2002) Standards for privacy of individually identifiable health information. Final rule. Fed Regist 67(157):53181–53273

Office for Protection from Research Risks (1983) Protection of human subjects. Code of federal regulations, vol 45 CFR 46, Rev. as of 8 Mar 1983, edn. National Institutes of Health (U.S.), Bethesda

Orentlicher D (1990) From the office of the General Counsel. The right to die after Cruzan. JAMA 264(18):2444–2446

Pinnock R, Crosthwaite J (2005) When parents refuse consent to treatment for children and young persons. J Paediatr Child Health 41(7):369–373. doi:10.1111/j.1440-1754.2005.00643.x

Pless JE (1983) The story of Baby Doe. N Engl J Med 309(11):664. doi:10.1056/NEJM198309153091111

Post SG (1995) Baby K: medical futility and the free exercise of religion. J Law Med Ethics 23(1):20–26

Postovsky S, Moaed B, Krivoy E, Ofir R, Ben Arush MW (2007) Practice of palliative sedation in

children with brain tumors and sarcomas at the end of life. Pediatr Hematol Oncol 24(6):409–415. doi:10.1080/08880010701451079, 781393138 [pii]
President's Commission for the Study of Ethical Problems in Medicine and Biomedical and Behavioral Research (1982) Making health care decisions: a report on the ethical and legal implications of informed consent in the patient-practitioner relationship. U.S. Government Printing Office, Washington, DC
President's Commission for the Study of Ethical Problems in Medicine and Biomedical and Behavioral Research (1983) Deciding to forego life-sustaining treatments. U.S. Government Printing Office, Washington, DC
Presidential Commission for the Study of Bioethical Issues (2012) Privacy and progress in whole genome sequencing. United States, Presidential Commission for the Study of Bioethical Issues, Washington, DC
Presidential Commission for the Study of Bioethical Issues (2013) Anticipate and communicate: ethical management of incidental and secondary findings in the clinical, research, and direct-to-consumer contexts. United States, Presidential Commission for the Study of Bioethical Issues, Washington, DC
Quill TE, Dresser R, Brock DW (1997) The rule of double effect–a critique of its role in end-of-life decision making. N Engl J Med 337(24):1768–1771. doi:10.1056/NEJM199712113372413
Ridgway D (2004) Court-mediated disputes between physicians and families over the medical care of children. Arch Pediatr Adolesc Med 158(9):891–896. doi:10.1001/archpedi.158.9.891
Robson ME, Storm CD, Weitzel J, Wollins DS, Offit K, American Society of Clinical Oncology (2010) American Society of Clinical Oncology policy statement update: genetic and genomic testing for cancer susceptibility. J Clin Oncol 28(5):893–901. doi:10.1200/JCO.2009.27.0660
Ross LF (2009) Against the tide: arguments against respecting a minor's refusal of efficacious life-saving treatment. Camb Q Healthc Ethics 18(3):302–315. doi:10.1017/S0963180109090471; discussion 315–322
Ross LF, Saal HM, David KL, Anderson RR, American Academy of Pediatrics, American College of Medical Genetics and Genomics (2013) Technical report: ethical and policy issues in genetic testing and screening of children. Genet Med 15(3):234–245. doi:10.1038/gim.2012.176
Roter DL, Hall JA, Merisca R, Nordstrom B, Cretin D, Svarstad B (1998) Effectiveness of interventions to improve patient compliance: a meta-analysis. Med Care 36(8):1138–1161
Rothberg MB, Sivalingam SK, Ashraf J, Visintainer P, Joelson J, Kleppel R, Vallurupalli N, Schweiger MJ (2010) Patients' and cardiologists' perceptions of the benefits of percutaneous coronary intervention for stable coronary disease. Ann Intern Med 153(5):307–313. doi:10.7326/0003-4819-153-5-201009070-00005
Schloendorff v. Society of New York Hospital (1914) 211 N.Y. 125, 105 N.E. 92. NY: Court of Appeals
Schüklenk U, van Delden JJ, Downie J, McLean SA, Upshur R, Weinstock D (2011) End-of-life decision-making in Canada: the report by the Royal Society of Canada expert panel on end-of-life decision-making. Bioethics 25(Suppl 1):1–73. doi:10.1111/j.1467-8519.2011.01939.x
Tarasoff v. Regents of University of California (1976) P. 2d, vol 551. Cal: Supreme Court
Truog RD, Berde CB, Mitchell C, Grier HE (1992) Barbiturates in the care of the terminally ill. N Engl J Med 327(23):1678–1682. doi:10.1056/NEJM199212033272311
Truog RD, Brock DW, White DB (2012) Should patients receive general anesthesia prior to extubation at the end of life? Crit Care Med 40(2):631–633. doi:10.1097/CCM.0b013e3182413b8a
Washington State Department of Health, Medical Quality Assurance Commission (2014) Professionalism and Electronic Media. http://www.doh.wa.gov/Portals/1/Documents/3000/MD2014-02January2014.pdf. Accessed 20 Aug 2014
Weithorn LA (1983) Children's capacities to decide about participation in research. IRB 5(2):1–5
Wilson RF (2010) The death of Jesse Gelsinger: new evidence of the influence of money and prestige in human research. Am J Law Med 36(2–3):295–325
Wolf SM, Lawrenz FP, Nelson CA, Kahn JP, Cho MK, Clayton EW, Fletcher JG, Georgieff MK, Hammerschmidt D, Hudson K, Illes J, Kapur V, Keane MA, Koenig BA, Leroy BS, McFarland EG, Paradise J, Parker LS, Terry SF, Van Ness B, Wilfond BS (2008) Managing incidental findings in human subjects research: analysis and recommendations. J Law Med Ethics 36(2):219–248. doi:10.1111/j.1748-720X.2008.00266.x, 211
World Medical Association (1997) Declaration of Helsinki. Recommendations guiding physicians in biomedical research involving human subjects. JAMA 277(11):925–926

Spiritual Care in Pediatric Oncology

18

Reverend Kathleen Ennis-Durstine
and Reverend Mark Brown

What is religious? What is spiritual? And why should we pay attention to these issues in healthcare?

There have been many efforts to define the two concepts of religion and spirituality. For instance, Harold Koenig defines religion as "an organized system of beliefs, practices, rituals, and symbols designed to facilitate closeness to the sacred or transcendent" (Koenig et al. 2001). The Oxford English Dictionary begins with this focus on structure as well: "The belief in and worship of a superhuman controlling power, especially a personal God or gods; a particular system of faith and worship." This is often associated with an organized community where "worship" includes historic and/or traditional practices and beliefs and which has in common, with other organized communities, an authoritative text or narrative. Interestingly, there is a third definition that departs from this structuralism: "A pursuit or interest to which someone ascribes supreme importance." When defining spirituality, Koenig suggests that it is "the personal quest for understanding answers to ultimate questions about life, about meaning, and about relationship with the sacred or transcendent, which may (or may not) lead to or arise from the development of religious rituals and the formation of community" (Koenig et al. 2001). The Oxford English Dictionary similarly states: "Of, relating to, or affecting the human spirit or soul as opposed to material or physical things." Many of us in the work of providing spiritual and/or religious care to those who are ill or dying have our own idiosyncratic connotations, which typically revolve around the search for meaning, feeling to the world, to others, connected to something "greater than one's self."

R.K. Ennis-Durstine, MDiv, BCC (✉)
Department of Family Services, Children's National Health System, 111 Michigan Ave., NW, Washington, DC 20010, USA
e-mail: kennisdu@childrensnational.org

R.M. Brown, MDiv., BCC
Department of Chaplain Services, St. Jude Children's Research Hospital, 262 Danny Thomas Place, Mail Stop 141, Memphis, TN 38105, USA
e-mail: mark.brown@stjude.org

Most believe that human beings are much more than merely the sum of their parts. We seek to find some meaning in who we are, to understand the relationships between our experienced reality and ultimate purpose. We want to "bind together" (the meaning of the Latin root word for religion) and "breathe" (the meaning of the Latin root word for spirituality) life and meaning into existence. On any ordinary day, we may be more or less concerned with these implications and more or less connected to our spirituality and religion. But when our vitality and health are diminished or threatened, the quest for meaning and understanding becomes much more an intrinsic part of our lives.

A.N. Abrams et al. (eds.), *Pediatric Psychosocial Oncology: Textbook for Multidisciplinary Care*,
DOI 10.1007/978-3-319-21374-3_18

Religion and Spirituality in Medical Settings

By 2010, more than 326 quantitative, peer-reviewed studies have examined the relationship of religion and spirituality with medical care. Of those, nearly 80 % found a significant positive association between religion and spirituality and well-being (Koenig et al. 2001). One important paper reported that nearly half of the persons who wished to have a discussion about their spiritual concerns with a healthcare provider were denied that experience (Williams et al. 2011). Another landmark longitudinal study with 444 hospitalized medical patients found an association between religious (spiritual) items patients struggle with and an increase in mortality, independent of physical and mental health (Barnes et al. 2000). The items are listed in Table 18.1.

Overall, the research supports the importance of religion and spirituality on several fronts: (1) Many patients and families are religious and/or spiritual and would like their faith addressed in their healthcare; (2) many patients and families have religious and/or spiritual needs related to illness that could affect mental health, but go unmet; (3) patients and families, during times of hospitalization, are frequently isolated from their supporting communities; (4) religious and spiritual beliefs affect medical decision making and may conflict with treatments; and (5) religion and spirituality influence healthcare in the community. Additionally, the Joint Commission expects religious and spiritual needs and desires to *not* be ignored in the healthcare setting (The Joint Commission, Standard R1.01.01.01).

Table 18.1 Patients Expressed These Concerns with Regard to Connections Between Their Illness and Their Faith/Spirituality

Wondered whether God had abandoned me [felt abandoned]
Felt punished by God for my lack of devotion [felt responsible for own predicament]
Wondered what I did for God to punish me [felt responsible for own predicament]
Questioned God's love for me [questioned lovability and worth/value]
Wondered whether my church had abandoned me [felt abandoned by or outside caring community]
Decided the Devil made this happen [attributed evilness of situation to outside influence]
Questioned the power of God [questioned concept of providence]

Religion and Spirituality in Pediatric Settings

An article in pediatrics titled *Spirituality, Religion, and Pediatrics: Intersecting Worlds of Healing* reported that religion and spirituality play important roles in shaping the way families live their lives and therefore may have broader implications for children's health (Barnes et al. 2000). This may impact everything from how parents seek healthcare for their children or turn to religious and spiritual healing therapies, to specific ways that children cope with multiple aspects of their health and illness or loss. Yet the paper noted that pediatricians and other healthcare providers may be uncomfortable addressing what they assess to be negative aspects of religion or spirituality affecting the health of a child, rather than the important and varied role religion and spirituality play in the ongoing well-being of a child and their family (Barnes et al. 2000). In a paper by Purow et al. (2011), it is noted that spiritual beliefs play an important role in providing comfort and support for children with cancer and their families.

Guidelines for integrating spiritual and religious resources into pediatric practice are listed in Table 18.2:

Children as Spiritual and Religious Beings

Most of the tools used to explore what is significantly spiritual or religious in a person's life are adult models. Children frequently experience their spirituality and religion both physically

Table 18.2 Guidelines for integrating spirituality and religious resources into pediatric settings (Barnes et al. 2000)

Anticipate the presence of religious and spiritual concerns
Develop self-awareness of your own spiritual history and perspectives
Become broadly familiar with the religious worldviews of the cultural groups in your patient population
Allow families and children to be your teachers about the specifics
Build strategic interviewing skills and ask questions over time
Develop a relationship with available chaplaincy services
Build a network of local consultants
Refer to family-preferred spiritual care providers
Listen for understanding rather than for agreement or disagreement

and temporally; for them, this is not so much a cognitive construct or a rational explanation of the irrational as it is purely experiential. Children will respond to their experiences from within their developmental capacity. Spirituality at every age can be transforming as well. Therefore, it is important to have some basic understanding of what the basic developmental tasks, strengths, and distresses are of each major age group.

The Spiritual Life of Young Children

For preschoolers (ages 3–6), awe and trust remain a large part of their experience, but storytelling is becoming compelling for them. They begin to take some responsibility for family rituals such as prayers at meal or bedtime; they will initiate them, remind elders when they haven't been observed, and are very intrigued with creating their own rituals. If they are learning the stories of their family's faith system, or the stories of meaning as the family makes meaning, they are able to retell the story, insert themselves in it, and change it to make sense of their particular world.

Case Vignfoette

Christopher, a 4-year-old boy with a brain tumor, wanted the chaplain to read the story of David and Goliath every time she visited. For several days she simply read the story and observed that Christopher became calm and focused during and after hearing the story. His mother was very anxious and afraid to take a strong role in giving her son medications or helping with his mouth care. Christopher had learned his regimen and saw to it that it was followed. He appeared to percevie himself as David facing the Goliath of his disease. Not only did he "live" this story, he was able to articulate it when the chaplain asked him what he liked most about it. "David was very brave, even when other people were afraid [perhaps like his mother?]. He said to Goliath, 'you can't beat me' and he believed it."

The Spiritual Life of School-Age Children

When ill or hospitalized, the young school-age child (6–10-year-olds) can feel the sense of letting one's team down, one's parents down, and one's self down. A child also may come to feel that he or she has let down his or her religious and spiritual community. For example, some faith traditions place heavy obligations on members for their own healing ("If you have enough faith, you will be healed"), are intolerant of sincere expressions of fear or doubt ("You aren't supposed to question God," or fixate on a higher power that is overly punitive. This may compound a child's feelings of shame and guilt.

The child may live in two separate worlds. One is a logical, "schooled" world of work, organized play, and peer involvement. The other is a private world of imagination, which is still largely mythical and analogical. These worlds are not contradictory for school-age children; rather they are examples of how children experiment with both sides of their brain as they seek a way for logic and myth to be combined and recombined. They use stories to gather and shape their fantasies.

Case Vignette
A chaplain was visiting with Steven a 7-year-old boy with Ewing sarcoma and they talked about the story of Jonah and the Big Fish. As they speculated about Jonah's thoughts and feelings, Steven made connections to his own experiences. He understood what it felt like to be in a scary, isolated place. He recognized the fear that goes with being carried along on a journey he did not choose, the outcome of which is uncertain. He knew that, in a situation like Jonah's, one might just wonder what God is up to.

For the later elementary to middle school-age child (11–13 years old), this is a time for rites of passage: for example, first communion, confirmation, youth group, and bar/bat mitzvahs. In addition, the symbols of the faith community have real power and majesty: the ark, the Cross, and the Qur'an. Children use these symbols and turn them over, not only in their hands but also in their psyches, looking for meaning and/or imbuing them with special authority and effectiveness as the following case illustrates.

Case Vignette
In the oncology playroom, Robert, a 12-year-old Christian boy with sarcoma, was fashioning popsicle sticks into an "X" shape on top of a square piece of foam. The chaplain said,
"Hi, Robert. What are you making today?"

"Don't you know what this is? It's a God-thing!"

"A God-thing?"

"Yes. Where they put Jesus and he died."

"Oh, a cross."

"Yeah. He died."

"That's true."

"They put nails in him."

"That's true, too. It must have hurt a lot."

"Nope! He could get away anytime he wanted!"

Prayers, rituals, blessings, and even cursing can be very powerful for school-age children. Salma, an 11-year-old Muslim girl with rhabdomyosarcoma, was in the hospital during Ramadan. Although younger than the required age for fasting, she wanted to participate in the daily fast. It was a spiritual discipline that she felt deepened her relationship with Allah and increased her potential for healing. Nutrition services were concerned about her health and did not want her to fast. The chaplain met with Salma and her parents and nutritionist to create a plan that would honor her religious beliefs while meeting her nutritional requirements. The team agreed that if Salma was willing to take liquids during the day, she could eat a meal before dawn and after dusk and still meet her nutritional needs.

School-age children judge very quickly and may want people to be punished for breaking the rules of justice as they perceive them. This plays out spiritually when a child feels that God isn't playing fair and should be held accountable. It is important for spiritual caregivers to listen to the questions and comments of the ill or dying child. It is often more vital to listen than to talk. Children in this age group will ask questions about matters they want to understand. They are not necessarily "comforted" by being put off or given "nice" answers. They can also have "unfinished business." It may be as simple as a school project or as complex as making up for some real or imagined fault. These are all spiritual tasks.

The Spiritual Life of Adolescents

Decision-making is based on what the adolescent considers important. This is very much a part of their spiritual character and struggle. There is a great deal happening in an adolescent's life including navigating family, friends, school, society, media, and technology and perhaps religion and spirituality. If spirituality and faith are going to have meaning for the adolescent, it needs to be in a way that helps them organize their worldview and establish their own identity.

Often, the experience in personal relationships drives how adolescents perceive unifying values. Teenagers will often be drawn into faith and spiritual groups because of defining values which seem utopian to the adolescent or, if not utopian, certainly pervasive and "true." The lure of cults can be very powerful during this developmental stage. These values simply "are" to the adolescent and they frequently do not examine them closely or reflect upon how they "work" or do not "work" in their lives or in the world. Teenagers develop ideologies they may hold to with determination. When they disagree with the values of another, it is often perceived as a difference in the sort of person one is and not based on a difference of ideas. Adolescents will identify and adhere to authority that they deem to have personal worth or is valued by their peers. A spiritual challenge faced at this age is that the expectations and evaluations of others, the values themselves, and the traditions either from the past or created specifically to meet adolescents' needs and desires can become so internalized, even made sacred, that their personal autonomy, judgment, and drive to act might be jeopardized. Also, any betrayal by a "worthy" authority or peer can lead to despair.

Physical changes that result from illness or injury can also lead to profound spiritual distress, though the underlying spiritual issue may be masked by an obvious physical concern. Adolescents receiving chemotherapy are often traumatized by the physical changes they anticipate and undergo. Teenage girls frequently voice special concerns about hair loss. This may be for them a spiritual dilemma as well as a physical one. A fear of feeling "different" or "embarrassed" in front of peers is real enough. But sometimes the distress is rooted in spiritual questions: "Am I still the same person I was before this change occurred?" "Am I more than my body?" "To what degree has the love and acceptance I've known been related to my appearance?" As they anticipate hair loss, many adolescent girls seek out natural-looking wigs; at the time certain they will never allow themselves to be caught without it. But later, many girls lay the wigs aside to walk proudly, and baldly, into the world. Perhaps the underlying spiritual questions have been answered. "I am a loved and valued person because of who I am and not because of how I look." "I have supportive and loving people in my life, no matter what."

Even during times of spiritual dissonance, seriously ill adolescents can survive with strength and purpose. This is particularly true if they have a sense of personal power that they have some control over things that are occurring, a sense of purpose that life has meaning, and a sense of optimism regarding their own future. Adolescents may be very interested in providing some sort of legacy, not only for their families but for the "world." One teenager organized an art show on her inpatient unit and arranged for hospital leadership to come and judge the art in several categories. The projects were sold and the patient arranged for the proceeds to fund a juried art show every year on her birthday. Teenagers want to know that their life matters and that they are able to accomplish something and can make a difference in the world. These are human needs, but they are also spiritual needs. Faith and spirituality give us a sense of place and purpose not only as individuals but as participants in something much larger and much more eternal than ourselves.

We have several tasks as caregivers. One is to participate and legitimate the adolescent's search for meaning and not to tell them what it is. Another is to respect the struggles, the ideas, and the hard work in which adolescents are engaged. And a third is to empower adolescents to find and use their own voice. It is our task, as well, to assist adolescents in developing spiritual health. We are able to do this one on one with the adolescent and within the teenager's community. We can offer a variety of ideas for consideration as well as share doubt, particularly when cure is no longer possible.

Adolescents have a much more adult understanding of death and dying in terms of what occurs biologically and how living and dying are interwoven. But they may be confused about it theologically, emotionally, and socially. Some of their understanding and lack of understanding come from prior experiences with death as well as the teaching in their family and community.

As adolescents approach end of life, they often need supportive listeners who will sit patiently while they grieve the lives they will never have. In contrast to older adults at end of life, adolescents mourn not only the relationships and experiences they leave behind (both good and bad); they mourn a future that will not be realized. Teenagers often voice deep sorrow that they will miss opportunities to graduate from high school or college, engage in romantic or sexual relationships, experience the adult world of work, or become parents and grandparents themselves. One adolescent said of his life, "There are so many things I haven't done. I don't feel whole."

It is important for adolescents who confront their own mortality to identify connections with their own family's faith stories, if they have them, especially if doing so can facilitate a feeling of peace or reassurance. At the same time, they must be allowed to voice the questions for which there are no easy answers, no matter how uncomfortable they are to hear.

Some adolescents who are dying will want to spend as much time as possible with their peers and it may be their friends who participate in discussions with them about dying and about what the adolescent believes and hopes.

Models of Children's Spirituality and Religious Consciousness

Children express their spirituality and religious consciousness very naturally. Often we see instances of this in their day to day lives through their actions and their narratives and in their sense of belonging to family, community, God, and the world. Children show us or tell us how they feel thankful and the ways in which they feel safe and loved. Through their rituals (either formally or personally), we learn that they believe they have what they need to live and that there is, or is not, someone who cares for them. Sometimes, children will want to be very active and demonstrative in the ways they contribute to the goodness of the world such as sharing a special toy with a friend who may be ill or participating in a fundraiser for their specific type of cancer. Often times, children express their specific understanding of their own spirituality and religious consciousness.

Case Vignette

Upon learning of his diagnosis, Lucas, a bright, articulate, and faith-knowledgeable 7-year-old boy with osteosarcoma, asks to see the chaplain. Lucas wants to know why God would let something so horrible happen to him. Over several days the chaplain visited Lucas and they talked about many things, including God. Together, they explored the God Lucas had come to know and believe in. One afternoon Lucas was able to express his own answer. He told the chaplain that God must have been very busy the day Lucas got sick – maybe holding up an elephant in one hand. If God had to drop the elephant in order to prevent Lucas' bones from getting sick, then the elephant could have been seriously hurt. God had a hard decision to make and God must have known that Lucas and his family were going to be all right but the elephant would have died if he dropped him.

Lucas was expressing not only his own belief in a God who is complex but operates in a meaningful system of love, trust, and care. Often through a child's play or stories, we see children's strength in their spirituality and religious consciousness, as well as in the way they demonstrate hope and perceive the future and their own and the world's future (Yust and Roehlkepartain 2009).

Mark Tobin published a book called *The Secret Spiritual World of Children*. Along with his theoretical discussion, he collected stories about children who wonder, who listen to wisdom, who are deeply embedded in relationships and the "lovingness" between themselves and another, who are curious, and who see beyond the physical to the spiritual planes (Tobin 2003). In his chapter regarding wonder, he begins with this story: A man and his 8-year-old daughter were at the beach where he watched her for over an hour as she just stood in the water up to her waist, swaying gently in the surf. It was nearly an hour and a half before she came out of the water, absolutely glowing and peaceful. She sat down next to him without a word. After a few minutes, he managed to gently ask what she had been doing. "I was the water," she said softly. "The water?" he repeated. "Yeah, it was amazing. I was the water. I love it and it loves me. I don't know how else to say it." They sat quietly until she hopped up to dig in the sand a few minutes later. "Somehow I felt completely overwhelmed, like I had witnessed grace," the father said.

Many things influence the development of spiritual and religious consciousness in children. Foremost are family and community, what is taught and what is expected. We cannot make assumptions or judgments about how children will develop their religious and spiritual identities. Children in great need may seek meaning and purpose in different ways. Each child must be approached as a unique being.

Joyce Ann Mercer, a professor of pastoral theology, proposes four categories of children's spirituality: mystic, activist, sage, and holy fool (Mercer 2006). The *mystic* child is one who seems deeply in touch with the numinous and who describes encounters and memories of being with and connected to their Holy One. They understand that the world is mysterious, there are possibilities far beyond anyone's ability to comprehend, and the boundaries between "real" and mystical are fluid and permeable. *Activist* children live out what they believe either through their social awareness or kinesthetically. An activist child may be involved in helping endeavors with school or family, visiting the elderly, and giving away items either of their own or collected on behalf of others. These children may also feel most alive and connected when engaged in physical activity.

The *sage* is the wise-beyond-one's-years child. They practice deep compassion and make connections between other's stories, their own story, and Holy stories. They do not hesitate to say what they perceive or experience and frequently take for granted how exceptional their insights are. Emma, a 4-year-old, was one such sage. One afternoon, when Will, her 2-year-old brother was within a few days of dying from a brain tumor, Emma sat with the chaplain to read books and paint. The chaplain said to Emma, "I wonder what you know about what is happening with Will." Emma, who had been mostly quiet during the encounter, said "Look." Taking a sheet of paper, she planted a fat dot of red paint in a corner. "This is Will." Next to that, she painted a circle. "This is God. And God is dreaming of Will." Even at 4, Emma felt reassured by her belief that there was a Will-shaped space in God and that Will and God were somehow connected in a relationship of dreaming and wonder.

Last, in Mercer's metaphorical categories, is the *Holy Fool*. They are the children who speak the truth lovingly – but truth it is. Others may simply perceive these children as "cute," but they are much more. For example, Melissa, a 6-year-old with ALL, was being teased at Sunday school about the loss of her blond curly hair. Melissa remained calm and said to the other children "my hair will grow back because it is a gift from God." When the Sunday school teacher laughed at her "cute" response, Melissa was surprised and said "but you are the teacher and you should know about God" (Mercer 2006).

Another model for children's spiritual and religious consciousness describes four dimensions of relationship: God/transcendence, others, world, and self. These point us "to spirituality as concerned with the deepest levels of human experiencing, the places of ultimacy, value, and deepest meaning in and for our lives"(Hay and Nye 2006).

Children have an intuitiveness that helps them connect on the subliminal level. Many psychosocial clinicians will describe some of the children they have worked with as "old souls." Some children display this characteristic more deeply than others, but we believe all have the potential for accessing wisdom that is beyond their years.

Thinking about Spiritual Interventions with Children

It is the work of the entire care team to respond not only with the best physical care for children but also with sensitive emotional, spiritual, and religious care. It is important to discover the child's own unique religious and spiritual consciousness and also to provide opportunities to grow and nurture that consciousness. Children intuitively feel awe and delight. We can observe it in the newborn who catches sight of sun and shadows playing tag on the wall. As children develop, they see, hear, and experience mystery in their relationship to nature, to others, and to themselves. As they grow, learn, imagine, and practice what it is like being themselves as distinct, unique individuals in a world with other unique, distinct individuals (as well as a few inanimate, animal, and mythic realities), their concept of the numinous becomes healthier and more universal. It is important for the psychosocial clinician to remember that for children the world is bigger than a particular event or illness and usual children's pleasures such as laughing and playing still exist. Helping a child remember, plan, and enjoy what is possible is a spiritual endeavor.

Children will sometimes declare that they have had conversations or connections with God. For example, one young child shared, "God just talked to me! It was so wonderful; quiet and warm. It felt like being wrapped up in my fleece blanket – only I wasn't hot. We held hands – he said even if I was very afraid of my medicine and treatments that sometimes he would know, and would be near to help take care of me." Older school-age children often experience transcendence and awe very kinesthetically, as noted earlier in the story of the child standing in the ocean "becoming" the water.

Table 18.3 Ways to explore what the child with cancer wonders about

I am going to draw a picture of something that makes me feel safe; can you draw one, too?
How long is time?
Tell me about one good thing
Tell me about one scary thing
Who do you feel blesses you?
How do you bless others?
If God, Jesus, Allah, etc., were sitting here with us, what do you think he or she would say to you? What would you say to him or her?
I'd really like to know what you think heaven is like
What is the most wonderful thing in the world?
What is perfect?
Can you describe yourself just with colors? (then – what part of you is red/black?)
I like the sound of or don't like the sound of.... What sound do you like, or don't like?
Do you have a special word you like? How does it make you feel?
Would you like to have someone pray with you?
If you could go one place right this minute, where would it be? Why?
When I feel sad, I cry or go off by myself. What do you do when you feel sad?
Can you tell me one thing you feel sorry about?
Sometimes I get really mad because.... Do you ever get really mad?
What is your favorite book, movie, etc.? (Then explore the spiritual themes in it)

When we are attempting to help children and adolescents nurture and articulate their religious and spiritual consciousness, psychosocial clinicians must be attentive to being with the child and not merely visiting or carrying clipboards with a research questionnaires or screening forms. This "being with" is important so that we may differentiate the child's religious and spiritual consciousness from that of their parents and family. The values, beliefs, and needs of each may be very different. Table 18.3 provides ways to open conversations about spiritual matters. When you are considering how to bring to the surface a child's thoughts about faith, or blessing, or one of the other spiritual categories, conversation starters listed in Table 18.3 may be of help.

We can assist children in talking about what they find awful by being patient and by asking open-ended questions and statements, bringing pictures or books, and watching videos or movies. There is a godly talk opportunity about almost anything in which a child has some interest.

Case Vignette

A chaplain, watching the movie "Neverending Story" with a young patient receiving treatment for leukemia commented on how extraordinary the author's imagination was and how sad a world it would be if imagination disappeared. The child responded "That would never happen – people will always imagine wonderful, good, sometimes bad, things; they will search, because they need to, for different ways to tell us the same stories about how evil almost overcomes good, but that good always triumphs in the end. And besides, God gave us freewill."

Sometimes children will want to talk about their relationship with the one they call God, or Allah, or Yahweh, or another deity. Patience and the willingness to listen without correcting or questioning too directly can give us significant insight into how children experience the values and teaching of family and community and what they understand, accept, and reject. It is not our job to fix what we may hear as a faulty theology; rather it is our job to listen to the child's theology and words and stories. If the child is troubled, it may be important for them to share their questions and their philosophic explorations with a family member or compassionate leader of their community.

Children can tell us about what they feel, or have experienced, as good and bad and how those are balanced in their lives; they can tell us when they feel as if they have some control or no control. It is important to explore with a child their locus of control. If it is all external (e.g., God, parents, family, and doctors), they may feel helpless and anxious. However, a locus of control that is primarily internal, that is, that the child typically has a sense of being powerful and in charge, can also lead to feelings of helplessness when they are unable to change their circumstances.

As caregivers, we also need to examine our perceptions and expectations about our relationship with the universe. If we are unclear, it will be considerably more difficult for us to open ourselves to the unique ways children express their religious/spiritual consciousness.

Several other spiritual and religious consciousness components are also valuable to consider: faith, gratefulness, repentance, communion, and vocation (Pruyser 1976). Faith is both the ability children have to describe certain precepts of what they believe about God, life, and death and rules for living and their ability to communicate to us whether they feel that life has some intrinsic value. Does living and the experiences garnered in life mean something? Does it mean something to someone or something greater than one's self? Do they perceive life as an "adventure" or as a commodity to hoard? Both are spiritual responses; the spiritual is never merely the positive side of one's experiences or perceptions. What is spiritual, and/or religious, in our lives either opens up possibilities or closes them to us. When we work with seriously ill children, we need to gain an understanding of where they are on this continuum. Our work may be to draw them closer to the open end of spiritual/religious experiences and perceptions, or it may be to stay with them exactly where they are and help to make their closed life experience more tenable.

Human beings of any age typically wish to feel blessed and that they are a blessing to others, in other words: they wish to experience gratefulness. Certainly this is true of children who are sick. They want to know they are loved and that they deserve being loved even if they are not perfect. Children who can accept that they are agents in their own lives, even creating some of those things they dislike, are typically more open to seeing how they are and are not responsible for their current situation.

An important work of spiritual consciousness for children of all ages that becomes increasingly significant during adolescence is the ability to gain insight into one's own shortcomings, misdeeds, and hurtful impulses. Caregivers often must prompt young children to consider the negative impact of words or actions and remind them to "say sorry." Teenagers often do not need prompting to feel regret for the ways they have hurt other people, but may brood over feelings of shame or guilt in silence.

Case Vignette

Philip, a 19-year-old with a terminal brain tumor, had spent much of the previous 5 years incarcerated in a juvenile facility for gang-related activity. Reflecting on his life, Philip was grief stricken by the damage his early and persistent involvement with a gang had done to himself, to his family, and to many others who crossed his path. He expressed his shame and sorrow to his chaplain. He was sorry he had disappointed his mother, had not been able to have a close relationship with younger siblings, had bullied other young people at the juvenile facility, and had "wasted" his life. He did not believe that God could forgive him. He expressed little hope for finding peace before he died. Through spiritual support and counseling, Philip was able to participate in a ritual of repentance, naming explicitly the causes of his sorrow and accepting the forgiveness offered him by his family and by his faith. The process helped Philip move, in his final months, from feeling helpless before his human failings to a position of hopefulness and even joy in relationships restored.

Communion and vocation are the experiences children have of being a part of a community, having a role to play, feeling that they are part of the "circle of life," and how they participate in those roles. All of these concepts are intertwined in myriad ways. We are engaging children and adolescents around the ideas of being involved or uninvolved, of seeing mostly possibility and safety or mostly negation and danger, of having purpose or being out of control, and of continuity or discontinuity with all life, all meaning, all purpose – and everything along these continua. When children are seriously ill, these are extraordinarily important aspects of their ability to understand what is happening, to be able to describe for themselves why it is happening, and to feel that they can have some choices that matter desperately to them.

Conclusion

Each member of the psychosocial team has a role to fill in meeting the spiritual and religious needs of children who are diagnosed with cancer. Employing critical thinking and one's own unique skills, combined with openness and curiosity as well as deep regard for what children perceive and believe, is the starting point. Physical and psychosocial development and spiritual development are often established along similar trajectories. However, with children who are seriously ill, spiritual development frequently progresses more dramatically.

Clinical Pearls

- Many patients and families are religious and/or spiritual and would like their faith addressed in their healthcare.
- Many pediatric patients and families have religious and/or spiritual needs related to illness that could affect their mental health, but go unmet.
- Patients and families, during times of hospitalization, are frequently isolated from their supporting communities. Religious/spiritual beliefs affect medical decision making and may conflict with treatments.

References

Barnes L, Plotnikoff G, Fox K, Pendleton S (2000) Spirituality, religion, and pediatrics: intersecting worlds of healing. Pediatrics 106:899

Hay D, Nye R (2006) The Spirit of the Child. Jessica Kingsley Pub, London

Koenig H, McCullough M, Larson D (2001) Handbook of Religion and Health, 1st edn. Oxford University Press, New York
Mercer J (2006) Children as mystics, activists, sages, and holy fools: understanding the spirituality of children and its significance for clinical work. Pastoral Psychology. doi:10.1007/s11089-005-0013-y
Pruyser P (1976) The Minister as Diagnostician: Personal Problems in Pastoral Perspective. Westminster John Knox Press, Kentucky
Purow B et al (2011) Spirituality and pediatric cancer. Southern Medical Journal 104(4):299–302
The Joint Commission. Patient-Centered Communication Standards & EPs – Hospital Accreditation Program. R1.01.01.01. http://www.imiaweb.org/uploads/pages/275.pdf
Tobin H (2003) The Secret Spiritual World of Children. Inner Ocean Publishing, Inc., Makawao, Maui, HI
Williams JA et al (2011) Attention to inpatients' religious and spiritual concerns: predictors and association with patient satisfaction. J Gen Intern Med 26(11):1265–71. doi:10.1007/s11606-011-1781-y
Yust K, Roehlkepartain E (2009) Real kids, real faith: practices for nurturing children's spiritual lives. Jossey-Bass., San Francisco

Social Media Use in Pediatric Oncology: Tweets, Blogs, and Boundaries

19

Sima Zadeh and Rachel Tunick

Tweets, Blogs, and Boundaries: Social Media Use in Pediatric Oncology

At its start, the Internet was primarily a forum where people could search for and read information. Over the years, particularly in the last decade, advances in technology have transformed and popularized the Internet in substantial and wide-reaching ways, and at present the Internet has become integrated into virtually every facet of human life. According to Internet World (2014) 87 % of the US population are Internet users. The development of social media, and the growth and dissemination of these forms of technologies, has played a significant role in this "digital revolution." Social media have transformed the Internet into a participatory space where people can create, contribute, and interact with countless others (Colineau and Paris 2010). The Internet has become a place where people may not only nurture their existing, "real-life" social networks but also forge new "virtual" relationships by forming or joining communities of interest. Within the realm of healthcare, these developments have created a wide range of opportunities for both patients and providers. However, along with these possible benefits come a host of potentially adverse consequences.

Given the vast and pervasive use of social media by pediatric oncology patients and their families (as well as by providers in our field), it is our responsibility as psychosocial providers to be aware of the why's and how's of social media use in the context of matters of health. This chapter will first outline the various types of social media available, and how these different media tend to be used. With this framework in place, we can better appreciate both the opportunities and challenges presented to psychosocial providers by these technological advances.

Defining Social Media

Social media are broadly defined as a range of electronic communication (i.e., websites, applications) through which users may create online communities to share information, ideas, personal messages, and other content. As a unifying

S. Zadeh, PsyD (✉)
Pediatric Oncology Branch, National Institutes of Health, National Cancer Institute, 10 Center Drive, Bldg. 10, 1H-PEDS, Room 1-5460, Bethesda, MD 20892, USA
e-mail: zadehsl@mail.nih.gov

R. Tunick, PhD
Boston Children's Primary Care at Longwood, Boston Children's Hospital, Hunnewell GF 300 Longwood Avenue, Boston, MA 02115, USA
e-mail: rachel.tunick@childrens.harvard.edu

A.N. Abrams et al. (eds.), *Pediatric Psychosocial Oncology: Textbook for Multidisciplinary Care*,
DOI 10.1007/978-3-319-21374-3_19

theme, social media consist of user-generated, interactive materials. There are many categories of social media, with the most popular and relevant forms presented in Table. 19.1. These various forms of social media are becoming increasingly central to the lives of many, and for many, including adolescents and young adults, social media represent the primary means of communication, establishment and maintenance of relationships, and self-expression (Lehavot et al. 2010).

Social Networks

Social networks are websites or online services that facilitate communication among friends, colleagues, or other users. These networks allow users to establish a personal profile with which they may readily connect with others. Some examples of popular social networking sites include Facebook and LinkedIn. Facebook is a free social networking website through which registered users may create profiles, share media (photos, video), send messages, and generally keep in touch with friends, family, and colleagues. LinkedIn is a business-oriented service primarily used for professional networking. User profiles tend to focus on career-related matters, with access to employment opportunities, news, and networks related to one's stated job interests.

Table. 19.1 Categories of social media

Categories of social media	Example
Social networks	Facebook LinkedIn
Weblogs/microblogs	Twitter CaringBridge CaringPages
Content communities	YouTube Pinterest Instagram
Collaborative projects	Wikipedia
Podcasts	Cancer. Net CDC Cancer
Forum/message boards	Yahoo! Answers

Weblogs and Microblogs

Weblogs ("blogs") are websites on which users maintain electronic journals comprising material such as personal opinions, activities, and experiences. Content may be organized chronologically or by category, and readers may post comments in response to user entries. Users may also create video blogs ("vlogs") featuring shared or homemade videos.

Microblogs feature short (as opposed to journal-style) posts. Users are typically restricted to posting only a few lines of text, or uploading individual images or videos. Microblogging is particularly common for posting quick updates and widely distributing content via mobile devices. Twitter, a popular form of microblog, is an online social networking service that enables users to send and read short (140-character) messages called "tweets," which are distributed to all of the user's registered followers. For example, a sample tweet by an adolescent oncology patient may read: "getting hooked up to my last chemo today—good-bye cancer!" Registered users can both read and post tweets, but unregistered users can only read them.

Oftentimes, users on social media platforms such as Twitter, Instagram, or Facebook will use "hashtags," denoted using the # symbol followed by a phrase (e.g., #lastchemo), to categorize a post or photo. This practice allows for users to easily search for all media related to a certain topic of interest. For example, if an individual wanted to search Twitter for all posts pertaining to cancer, they could enter the search term: #cancer.

Content Communities

Content communities (also known as multimedia sharing) are websites that allow users to share and comment about varying forms of content, including images and videos. The most widely used content communities at present include Pinterest, Instagram, and YouTube. Pinterest is an online service that promotes the sharing of images through social networking. For example, a Pinterest user could create a Pinterest board on ways to creatively wear hats, scarves, and other accessories during chemotherapy, displaying examples that have been posted by other users and adding their own contributions as well.

Instagram is an online mobile photo-sharing, video-sharing, and social networking service that enables users to take pictures and videos and share them across a variety of social networking platforms. YouTube is a video-sharing site which hosts an immense variety of video content including television clips, music videos, educational material, and video blogs.

Collaborative Projects

Collaborative projects allow for the joint and simultaneous creation of content by many users. A prominent example of a collaborative project is Wikipedia, a free, open content online encyclopedia created through the collaborative effort of a community of users known as Wikipedians. Anyone registered on the site can create an article for publication; however, registration is not required in order to make edits to existing entries, and as such, accuracy of material on such sites may not be guaranteed.

Podcasts

Podcasts are audio and video files available through subscription services such as Apple iTunes, which may be downloaded or streamed to a computer or mobile device. Podcasts can include audio or video of digital radio, novels, educational series, or WebTV.

Internet Forums/Message Boards

An Internet forum is an online discussion site where users participate in conversations in the form of posted messages. Similarly, message boards are sites where messages (usually about a specific topic or area of interest) may be posted, read, and responded to. Forums and message boards represent a wide range of topics and content, including specific health issues.

Uses and Benefits of Social Media by Pediatric Oncology Patients and Families

Social media have irrevocably transformed the experience of illness and its treatment for pediatric oncology patients and families. These technologies afford a variety of opportunities including enhanced access to interpersonal and social support, community development, distribution of health-related information, education, treatment guidance, and clinical trial recruitment.

Obtaining Health-Related Information

Case Vignette
After being diagnosed with osteosarcoma, Shawna begins to research her disease and treatment options online. She comes across a weblog of a young adult who has recently undergone a limb-sparing procedure and has subsequently gone into remission. When Shawna next meets with her healthcare provider, she has several questions about her own options to undergo a limb-sparing procedure versus an amputation, and whether the limb-sparing procedure might afford her better chances for remission.

Given the wealth of health-related information that is readily available on the Internet, it has become a routinely used resource for patients and families in their quest to better understand and plan around their illness and its treatment. An estimated 72 % of Internet users report searching for online health information within the past year (Fox and Dugan 2013). Patients and families may turn to social media in order to learn more about their diagnoses, search for guidance and treatment options, or obtain information regarding the management of treatment side effects. Additionally, these technologies may be pursued in efforts to access information on opportunities for clinical trials, second opinions, and relevant scientific research, and as such patients today often present at their health appointments in a highly informed manner.

Patients have reported that they access online health information because they want to be thoroughly informed to ensure understanding, identify questions, and be certain that information they receive from their doctors is comprehensive (Colineau and Paris 2010). Access to online healthcare information shifts the locus of control to the patient and his or her family, such that one-on-one encounters with providers are not substituted by social media use, but rather allow for richer engagement and deeper doctor-patient relationships. Greater access to cancer-related information has been associated with decreased levels of anxiety, depression, and negative self-esteem in children and adolescents undergoing cancer treatment (Last and Van Veldhuizen 1996).

Facilitation of Communication and Support for Patients and Families

No matter one's age, coping during stressful times depends heavily on the nature and quality of one's support systems, with stronger supports associated with more optimal adjustment and better quality of life (Treadgold and Kuperberg 2010). As such, one of the chief benefits of social media, particularly in the health-related domain, relates to its emphasis on the provision of social support. Social media use allows individuals to share information about their medical journeys with others undergoing similar experiences, thereby allowing users to better understand their condition, share stories, and get advice (Johnson and Ambrose 2006). The more connected people perceive themselves to be, regardless of the nature of the connection, the greater the benefit of perceived support (Nabi et al. 2013).

The various forms of social media can help to facilitate and promote efficient communication across a wide network of friends and family, which can be particularly beneficial for those managing taxing and stressful medical circumstances. Additionally, social media facilitate communication to help overcome barriers due to location, isolation, physical difficulties (i.e., neutropenia, mobility issues, fatigue), scheduling challenges, cost, and limited resources, while also providing anonymity and support when desired (Treadgold and Kuperberg 2010). In recent years, patients and their families have turned to social media as a way to share and disseminate information about their (or their child's) illness to a large support network. For example, websites such as CarePages and CaringBridge are designed specifically for people experiencing medical illness and provide platforms which allow users to maintain blogs for updating family and friends through journal entries or to coordinate everyday support. If families prefer to have a social media means of organizing care and support but are not interested in maintaining a blog, websites like Lotsa Helping Hands may be useful. Such sites permit members of the user's online community to leave supportive messages, in addition to providing a forum for efficient organization and delegation around pragmatic tasks (such as meals for the family, visits, and rides to the hospital). It is often helpful for families to delegate the task of updating these sites to another family or community member so as to minimize stress on the parent.

Using social media allows patients and families to access ongoing support across an extensive network of friends and family, without having to contact each person individually, thereby reducing the burden of an otherwise time-consuming and emotionally exhaustive task. Utilizing social media, patients or family members can provide updates when they are ready and available to discuss their experiences, and "visitors" can leave supportive messages of their own. In this regard social media provides opportunities for patients and families to receive ongoing emotional and practical support, as well as "virtual" visitation from loved ones.

Additionally, utilization of social media can serve as a fundraising mechanism where patients and families can, among many things, ask for donations to help with costly medical care, raise awareness about a diagnosis, or engage in blood or bone marrow drives. For bereaved families, or those whose children are nearing end of life, social media can provide a therapeutic means to document and preserve memories of their child, as well as celebrate and honor them (Tunick and Brand In Press).

Development of Virtual Support Networks and Communities

Case Vignette

Dwayne, a 17-year-old with leukemia, has been hospitalized at a research hospital far from home and will be on isolation precautions for a month. He is accompanied by his mother who has significant anxiety about her son's disease and treatment, further complicating his ability to access social support. Dwayne decides to search the web for support from other teenagers undergoing similar treatments. He locates an online support community through which he can both message and video chat with others who have shared his experience and are able to provide comfort and advice.

Illness and invasive treatments can place individuals at risk for disruption of normal development and significantly impact ones access to social support. This is particularly true for adolescents and young adults (AYA) who rely on peer relationships and social acceptance to formulate an identity and foster independence (Suris et al. 2004). AYAs with chronic illness often have a significant number of school absences or are homeschooled during more intensive treatments. Research indicates that peer support is invaluable in helping AYAs cope with their illness (Hollis and Morgan 2001; Treadgold and Kuperberg 2010). In fact, AYAs rank the availability of peer support as the top priority among various aspects of the cancer experience (Zebrack 2008), further validating the benefits of virtual support networks and communities.

While many forms of social media are developed to maintain existing relationships, other platforms serve as a means for people to develop new connections. In the health realm, this is especially important as patients value the shared experience of connecting with others who are undergoing (or have undergone) a similar illness or treatment course. Such a community can often provide a level of empathy and understanding that doctors, nurses, or even close friends or family cannot (Colineau and Paris 2010). Social media also benefit patients because it provides a mechanism for contact when individuals are remotely located or when physical contact must be limited. Shirky (2008) noted that each year, thousands of online communities are formed for access to information and to gain emotional support for being sick.

The formation and use of virtual support networks is particularly helpful in pediatric cancer, as many types of childhood cancer are quite rare. Online support communities allow families undergoing similar experiences to become closely connected, regardless of geographical location. Families around the country (and even more broadly around the world) can connect via social media to build relationships and exchange support with others undergoing similar experiences, therefore helping them feel less isolated in their own journeys. Not only do virtual communities break the barrier of geographic location, they allow access to information and support on an individual's own time frame and at their own pace, which can be particularly important for parents who are highly stressed or who have unpredictable schedules.

The need for peer support and acceptance may be further complicated in pediatric cancer by the feeling that non-ill peers may not understand or accept the affected child. Many adolescents and young adults have such a profound wish for normalcy that they keep their cancer experience separate from their healthy peers (Suzuki and Kato 2003). Furthermore, parents often communicate the need to remain cheerful and optimistic, indirectly leading youth to feel unable to express their fears with them (Treadgold and Kuperberg 2010). Given such circumstances, a virtual community of support can provide a unique opportunity for patients to discuss stressors and fears with those who genuinely can understand and share their experiences. Given ill patients often have limited access to peers with a shared diagnosis or close location, online forums for this type of support are increasingly relevant and important. Interestingly, surveyed users of online health communities indicated that they do not consider the people they meet in online health communities to be strangers, but rather as peers or trusted people whom they consider friends (Colineau and Paris 2010). Given the critical importance of peer relationships, it is essential that providers pay close attention to AYA capacity to access peer support networks when undergoing treatment.

Uses and Benefits of Social Media by Pediatric Oncology Providers

In recent years, these technologies have also become predominant in both the personal and professional lives of those working in the field of pediatric oncology. A recent survey suggested that a growing majority of those in the field of medicine (93 % of medical students, 79 % of medical residents, and 42 % of practicing physicians) use social media on a regular basis (Bosslet et al. 2011); similarly, students across various health-related disciplines (e.g., nursing, occupational therapy) reported a preference for online media as their chief source of information (Giordano and Giordano 2011). Relative to other medical subspecialists, those in the field of oncology are three times more likely to communicate with their patients in an online format (Hede 2012).

In the personal domain, those working in the field of pediatric oncology may turn to social media as an outlet or distraction from a stressful and taxing professional life. Social media may help to support non-work-related interests and hobbies and promote connectivity with friends and family. In this regard social media participation may potentially encourage a healthy work-life balance, minimize stress, or even help to offset compassion fatigue or burnout in those engaged in this challenging work (Tunick and Brand In Press).

In the professional domain, social media offers many opportunities for providers in the field to enhance their clinical and professional repertoire. For example, via social media, providers may engage in continuing education or connect with other professionals for consultation or collaboration, either individually or via a broader "community of practice" founded upon common professional interests (McKenna and D'Alessandro 2011). An example of such a site that has been established for professionals in the field of pediatric psycho-oncology is http://pediatrics.cancer.gov/psycho-oncology/index.asp. Via social media and related technologies such as patient portals, professionals may readily be in touch with patients and their families around matters pertaining to clinical care, and social media may also be employed for broader public health messaging (Dizon et al. 2012). Social media are also widely used as a "method of mass communication" within the field of medicine more broadly and among oncology providers in particular. For example, information regarding newly published research findings may be widely broadcast via Twitter (Terry 2009). This medium has also recently been widely used in the context of professional conferences as a resource both for on-site attendees and for others not present at the forum (Chaudhry et al. 2012).

Ethical and Professional Challenges

While social media undoubtedly affords a wide range of opportunities and benefits for children with cancer and their families, these technologies are also associated with a range of personal, ethical, and professional risks and challenges. It is important for clinicians in the field to understand and anticipate these potential dilemmas in order to most effectively offset possible deleterious effects. Such threats may arise in the context of social media use by patients and their families, by providers themselves, and/or by the intersection of use by both parties. Professional and ethical threats related to social media use span a number of broad domains including privacy and confidentiality, scope and content of online information, professional boundaries, patient care, professional reputations, and work-life balance.

Privacy/Confidentiality Threats

Families and patients (particularly while consumed by the stressful circumstances of their child's illness) may not fully appreciate the ease with which countless strangers may view their site's content or the relative permanency of information posted online and the degree to which, once posted, that material is no longer under their personal control (e.g., future prospective employers may be able to access personal details regarding an applicant's medical history by conducting a Google search and locating their old CaringBridge blog). This may lead to potential compromises around the patient's and/or family's privacy. Additionally, because adolescents may have their own ideas about what they are comfortable sharing publically, parents should be advised to talk with adolescents about their preferences to avoid violating their teen's sense of personal privacy. This can be a concern even for teens who themselves are very open online, but who may prefer that their parents not share information for them.

Similarly, within the community of pediatric oncology patients and family members, it is not uncommon to encounter families who include identifying and personal material (such as full names, photographs, and medical information) about other patients on their own or their child's social media site. For example, families may discuss important social connections that they've forged with other families facing similar medical challenges and circumstances. However, in cases where such postings are made without the knowledge or consent of the named individuals, complicated situations around privacy and confidentiality matters of these other patients and families may arise. Such concerns may become particularly salient in the context of complex medical courses and in the unfortunate event of the death of a child within one's social network.

Confidentiality and privacy breaches may also arise when medical providers or personnel share information about their professional world on their own social media sites. If viewed by readers outside of one's intended personal social circle, online material has the potential to be linked to a particular patient or family, and threats to confidentiality and privacy may ensue.

Threats around Information Overload, Misinformation, and Scope of Information

The amount of online information pertaining to the field of pediatric oncology is simply staggering. Laypeople (such as families of children facing an oncology diagnosis) may not have the requisite knowledge to cull through this inexhaustible stream of online material and differentiate accurate useful information from that which is misleading, erroneous, or not pertinent to their own (child's) situation. This can be potentially very overwhelming, frightening, or otherwise harmful and of particular concern for adolescent and young adult patients, who may browse the Web independently in order to learn more information about their medical condition, but lack the background and expertise required to effectively filter material that they encounter.

Patients and families may also become distressed from unanticipated content posted on their social media sites, such as when visitors offer unsolicited feedback or are critical regarding treatment decisions, or when others criticize a medical provider toward whom the family has a great deal of trust. On a similar note, online language and behavior may be easier to misinterpret compared to face-to-face interactions. Readers may have difficulty deciphering the intended tone or emotion in someone's posts on a social media site, and this may result in conflict and distress. Such difficulties may also arise in the context of an interactive online forum that lacks a trained facilitator or moderator.

Blurring of Professional and Therapeutic Boundaries

Case Vignette
A pediatric oncology social worker decides to search Facebook for one of his adolescent patients, Jessica, without her knowledge. Although he does not typically view social media sites of his patients, he has had particular difficulty forming a therapeutic connection with this patient and hopes to glean more information about her with the goal of strengthening their clinical relationship. In reviewing recent posts on Jessica's Facebook page, he sees a photo from the previous weekend depicting Jessica drinking alcohol, a substance that should not be mixed with her current treatment. He is left feeling very uneasy and uncertain about his follow-up course of action.

"Virtual" encounters between patients and families with clinicians, such as online chatting, viewing each other's photos and status updates on Facebook, or corresponding via a CarePages blog, may blur the therapeutic boundaries that serve as a cornerstone of the patient-provider relationship. Such contact via social media or other related technologies, which occurs outside of the traditional in-person context, may be construed within the framework of a dual relationship and has the potential (either subtly or more overtly) to alter the nature of the professional relationship. Ultimately this may affect the quality of care that is delivered.

Boundary blurring due to virtual encounters may arise in unexpected ways. For example, patients may Google their providers and (particularly in the case when providers have not established conservative privacy settings on their social media sites) subsequently learn intimate information pertaining to their personal lives (Guseh et al. 2009). Unintended self-disclosure of this nature may have implications regarding matters of personal responsibility, integrity, and role modeling that are inherent in the professional relationship. Similarly, when a provider chooses to pursue online information about a patient or family under their care, such as viewing social media activity of a patient or Googling the parent of a youngster in one's caseload, he or she may acquire information that otherwise might not have been known. This has potential implications regarding the quality and content of the professional relationship and around matters of trust, confidence, and respect (Tunick et al. 2011). Professionals may be uncertain about how to proceed when faced with a potentially boundary-blurring situation, such as if they receive a Facebook "friend request" from the parent of a patient or former patient (particularly if one's home institution or discipline has not established specific guidelines to help guide one's decision-making around such matters); see Wiener et al. (2012) for further discussion about such matters and suggestions around appropriate action steps.

Threats to Patient Care

Case Vignette
Mrs. Smith, the young mother of four-year-old Oscar (a pediatric oncology patient), has become "Facebook friends" with several of the clinic nurses at her son's care facility and regularly exchanges messages with them via their Facebook pages. One weekend, Oscar begins experiencing symptoms that could be potential side effects to a new medication. Recognizing that this might be a problem, Mrs. Smith messages one of her son's nurses on Facebook and waits for a response.

Threats regarding patient care have the potential to arise when patients and families become accustomed to communicating with providers through social media sites, and clear expectations have not been established regarding appropriate means of medical communication, especially in the event of an emergency. For example, such concerns might ensue if the parent of a sick patient posted a question after-hours (directed to one of the child's providers) pertaining to acute clinical symptoms requiring swift follow-up action, but the intended viewer is not online and does not see the message until later the following day. Additionally, when communication is done through social media, rather than the appropriate designated means of the institution (such as through a patient portal), documentation of these reports can be much more difficult and are not confidential. Many medical institutions have set up electronic patient portals in order to prevent problems of this nature.

Similarly, challenging ethical situations posing threats to patient care may arise when clinicians view patient social media sites without having transparently discussed this practice with their patient in advance. For example, if a clinician were to view concerning information (such as around acute medical problems or other safety concerns, as in the case of suicidal ideation (Lehavot et al. 2012)) on a patient's social media site, his or her follow-up course of action is less clear than if that material had been learned in a face-to-face interaction.

Threats to Professional Reputation

Case Vignette
Tyler's oncologist has heard that his parents have been maintaining a blog on CarePages, documenting their son's medical journey. She decides to view the blog to read more about the family's perspectives about this challenging illness course. In reviewing the blog, the oncologist discovers that Tyler's mother discusses several complaints she has with clinical staff, whom she names directly, at the care facility where Tyler is undergoing his treatment. To the oncologist's knowledge, such concerns have not been shared directly by the family with any of the medical staff.

It is not uncommon for patients and families in the pediatric oncology setting to provide detailed commentary on their social media sites regarding the nuances and details of their medical journey, and this may include names or other identifying information regarding providers involved in the child's care. Although much of this material may be positive in valence, providers may learn of or view material about themselves that is less than favorable, or even at times disparaging. Such circumstances may lead to unease and distress on the part of providers (and in more extreme cases, fears regarding potential legal ramifications, and/or reluctance to continue to care for the child). Named individuals also may have concerns regarding the impact of such material on their professional reputation (Hurley and Smith 2007; Tunick and Mednick 2008).

Threats to Work-Life Balance

Another concern regarding the use of social media in the pediatric oncology context involves potential threats to the work-life balance of those working in the field. Social media and related technologies make it possible for clinicians to connect with patients and families and monitor their medical updates at any hour of the day or night. While such practices undoubtedly may be beneficial, they also may lead to increased compassion, fatigue, or burnout (Wiener et al. 2012). Please refer to the Self Care chapter (21) in this textbook for further discussion as well as specific recommendations around managing such concerns.

Summary

Within the field of pediatric oncology, social media afford a vast range of benefits and opportunities including community development, interpersonal connection, clinical trial recruitment, and dissemination of health-related information for patients, families, and providers alike. However, with these advantages come a host of associated challenges and risks to which providers should be mindful and proactive, both for themselves and for the patients and families with whom they work. This is especially pertinent given that advances in technology and social media undoubtedly will continue to evolve at a rapid pace.

Clinical Pearls

Recommendations Regarding Patient and Family Use of Social Media

- Provide psychoeducation to patients and families regarding the use, benefits, and risks of social media in the context of their child's oncology treatment.
- Remain informed about accurate and trustworthy websites and social media resources. Connect with colleagues to share and disseminate information about reliable and reputable resources and check them out yourself.
- Initiate discussions with patients and their families about the specific social media they use or visit and integrate this into discussions of disease and treatment education. This will allow the provider to assure reliable sources are being accessed and also encourage patients and their families to share the information they find online with their care providers, thereby enhancing the care provider relationship.

Recommendations Regarding Care Provider Use of Social Media

- Be mindful of the implications of both your personal and professional social media use. Consider the benefits and risks associated with online activity.
- Remain transparent and proactive with patients and families about your institution's social media policy, recognizing that policies may differ between disciplines.

References

Bosslet GT, Torke AM, Terry CL, Helft PR (2011) The patient–doctor relationship and online social networks: results of a national survey. J Gen Intern Med 26(10):1168–1174

Chaudhry A, Glode LM, Gillman M, Miller RS (2012) Trends in twitter use by physicians at the american society of clinical oncology annual meeting, 2010 and 2011. J Oncol Pract 8(3):173–178

Colineau N, Paris C (2010) Talking about your health to strangers: understanding the use of online social networks by patients. New Rev Hypermedia Multimedia J 16(1–2):141–160

Dizon DS, Graham D, Thompson MA et al (2012) Practical guidance: the use of social media in oncology practice. J Oncol Pract 8(5):e114–e124

Fox S, Dugan M (2013) Health online 2013. Pew Internet and American Life Project. www.pewInternet.org/reports/2013/Health-Online. Accessed 10 Sep 2014

Giordano C, Giordano C (2011) Health professions students' use of social media. J Allied Health 40(2):78–81

Guseh JS, Brendel RW, Brendel DH (2009) Medical professionalism in the age of online social networking. J Med Ethics 35:584–586

Hede K (2012) Online networks present challenges, opportunities for Oncology. J Natl Cancer Inst 104(15):1115–1116

Hollis R, Morgan S (2001) The adolescent with cancer: at the edge of no man's land. Lancet 2:43–48

Hurley M, Smith C (2007) Patients' blogs: do doctors have anything to fear? BMJ 335:645–646

Internet World Stats (2014) The Internet big picture: world Internet users and population stats. Available via http://www.Internetworldstats.com/stats.htm. Accessed 10 Sep 2014

Johnson GJ, Ambrose PJ (2006) Neo-tribes: the power and potential of online communities in health care. Commun ACM 49(1):107–113

Last B, Van Veldhuizen A (1996) Information about diagnosis and prognosis related to anxiety and depression in children with cancer aged 8–16 years. Eur J Cancer Care 32(2):290–294

Lehavot K, Ben-Zeev D, Neville RE (2012) Ethical considerations and social media: a case of suicidal postings on Facebook. J Dual Diag 8(4):341–346

Lehavot K, Barnett JE, Powers D (2010) Psychotherapy, professional relationships, and ethical considerations in the MySpace generation. Prof Psychol Res Pr 41(2):160–166

McKenna MP, D'Alessandro D (2011) Social networks and the practice of medicine: harnessing powerful opportunities. J Pediatr 158(1):1–2

Nabi RL, Prestin A, So J (2013) Facebook friends with (health) benefits? Exploring social network site use and perceptions of social support, stress and well-being. Cyberpsychol Behav Soc Netw 16(10):721–728

Shirky C (2008) "Here comes health" in keynote speeach at the Health 2.0 Conference: User-Generated Healthcare, San Francisco, 22 Oct 2008. Available via: http://health2con.com/2009/07/19/clay-shirky-keynote-here-comes-health/. Accessed 10 Sep 2014

Suris JC, Michaud PA, Viner R (2004) The adolescent with a chronic condition: part 1. Developmental issues. Arch Dis Child 89:938–942

Suzuki LK, Kato PM (2003) Psychosocial support for patients in pediatric oncology: the influences of parents, school, peers and technology. J Pediatr Oncol Nurs 20:159–174

Terry M (2009) Twittering healthcare: social media and medicine. Telemed J E Health 15(6):507–510

Treadgold CL, Kuperberg A (2010) Been there, done that, wrote the blog: the choices and challenges of supporting adolescents and young adults with cancer. J Clin Oncol 28(32):4842–4849

Tunick RA, Brand, SR (2015) Social media. In: Quick reference for pediatric oncology clinicians: the psychiatric and psychological dimensions of pediatric cancer symptom management, 2nd edn 2015:345–356

Tunick RA, Mednick L (2008) Commentary: electronic communication in the pediatric setting - dilemmas associated with patient blogs. J Pediatr Psychol 34(5):585–587

Tunick RA, Mednick L, Conroy C (2011) A snapshot of child psychologists' social media activity: professional and ethical practice implications and recommendations. Prof Psychol Res Pract 42(6):440–447

Wiener L, Crum C, Grady C, Merchant M (2012) To friend or not to friend: the use of social media in clinical oncology. J Oncol Pract 8(2):103–106

Zebrack B (2008) Information and service needs for young adult cancer patients. Support Care Cancer 16:1353–1360

eHealth and mHealth in Pediatric Oncology

20

Cynthia W. Karlson and Tonya M. Palermo

Introduction

Use of the Internet and mobile phones (including use of apps and social media) is now widespread across individuals of all ages and ethnicities. The ubiquitous availability presents tremendous opportunities for clinicians and researchers to assess and treat cancer-related symptoms and to deliver education and supportive interventions. While the term eHealth is widely used in many fields of medicine, the precise definition varies among clinicians and researchers (Oh et al. 2005). In this chapter, we define eHealth as the use of information technology (e.g., Internet, virtual reality) in the promotion, prevention, treatment, and maintenance of healthcare for children with cancer. Related, mHealth refers specifically to the use of mobile and wireless applications including text messaging, apps, wearable devices, and the use of social media such as Facebook and Twitter to deliver healthcare.

A growing number of eHealth and mHealth interventions and applications have been developed and evaluated in various pediatric populations, e.g., chronic pain, traumatic brain injury, asthma, and arthritis (Palermo et al. 2009; Ritterband et al. 2003; Wade et al. 2006). Commonly described benefits include addressing barriers to access of in-person health and behavioral services, reducing costs such as family travel-related expenses and clinician time and the ability to tailor information to the individual needs of children and families (Cushing and Steele 2010; Cushing et al. 2011; Palermo and Wilson 2009). Because information technology allows for the use of personalization and tailoring based on such factors as individual characteristics (e.g., age, sex), preferences (e.g., text messages vs e-mail), and treatment regimens (e.g., different medications), these forms of intervention may also be better able to match the evolving nature of individuals' needs while coping with a chronic condition such as cancer.

Although the literature base is relatively less developed in pediatric oncology, this is a rapidly growing area with multiple examples of formative work. In this chapter, we review eHealth and mHealth applications in pediatric oncology that have been used in assessment, health promotion, and treatment delivery. We limit our discussion to eHealth and mHealth that interacts with the

C.W. Karlson, PhD (✉)
Department of Pediatrics, Division of Hematology/Oncology, University of Mississippi Medical Center, 2500 North State Street, Jackson, MS 39216, USA
e-mail: ckarlson@umc.edu

T.M. Palermo, PhD
Department of Anesthesiology and Pain Medicine, University of Washington and Seattle Children's Research Institute, Seattle Children's Hospital Research Institute, M/S CW8-6, 5371, Seattle, WA 98145-5005, USA
e-mail: tonya.palermo@seattlechildrens.org

A.N. Abrams et al. (eds.), *Pediatric Psychosocial Oncology: Textbook for Multidisciplinary Care*,
DOI 10.1007/978-3-319-21374-3_20

patient and family. Technologies that are internal to healthcare systems, such as electronic medical records and in-hospital communication systems, are beyond the scope of this chapter. Telemedicine is also not reviewed in this chapter, as these systems primarily facilitate communication between providers and patients within a healthcare system. We organize the chapter by reviewing the eHealth and mHealth literature base for (1) electronic monitoring, (2) Internet education and interventions (during diagnosis and early treatment, treatment and maintenance therapy, and long-term survivorship), and (3) virtual reality interventions. Tables 20.1, 20.2, and 20.4 provide a summary of the discussed research studies investigating eHealth and mHealth apps and interventions, while Table 20.3 provides a summary of selected Internet websites and mobile apps available for use in pediatric oncology.

Electronic Monitoring

Monitoring behaviors using the Internet and smartphone applications (apps) can assist children, adolescents, and parents in identifying patterns of behavior and help them achieve behavioral goals (Carels et al. 2005). There are several areas (medication adherence, physical activity, and nutrition) that have been targeted for electronic monitoring in pediatric cancer. Please see Table 20.1.

Medication Adherence and Safety

As home medication use increases, patients and families must manage the administration of many medications for cancer. Medication errors have been found to be common in children receiving medications at home (Walsh, et al. 2013), making the safety of medication administration an important priority. Moreover, adherence to cancer treatment regimens is an important clinical concern, as recent studies show that nonadherence with oral chemotherapy agents leads to significantly higher relapse rates (Bhatia et al. 2012, 2014). Technology may be used to help safely organize medications, monitor their use, and provide behavioral interventions to address barriers to adherence. Electronic monitoring of medication adherence has the advantage of providing real-time objective data from patients and there are several published examples of this application. In one study, Rohan et al. (2013) used electronic monitoring to describe patterns of adherence to

Table. 20.1 Summary of research studies investigating education and intervention eHealth and mHealth technologies in pediatric oncology

Areas of use	Authors	Year	Benefits	Limitations
Adherence	1. Rohan et al. 2. Kato et al.	2013 2008	Improves medication adherence Provides real-time objective data Assists family with organizing medications May improve safety of medication regimen May improve self-efficacy for following medication regimen	Few applications have been designed for children and adolescents Free applications have not been examined in research
Physical activity	None		May increase physical activity levels	No research to date
Nutrition	None		May improve diet and nutritional intake	No research to date
Pain	Stinson et al.	2013	Feasible and acceptable to children, publicly available app	Lack of data on whether it improves pain management

Table. 20.2 Summary of research studies investigating electronic monitoring eHealth or mHealth technologies in pediatric oncology

Areas of use	Authors	Year	Benefits	Limitations
Cancer education	1. Ewing et al. 2. Goodenough et al. 3. Jones et al. 4. Sigurdardottir et al. 5. Stinson et al. 6. Stinson et al.	2009 2004 2010 2014 2011 2014	Quality websites provide valuable medical content May improve communication with providers May increase internal locus of control	Research is limited by small sample sizes Many websites are poor quality Many websites use a high reading level Families may not access the website
Coping	1. Askins et al. 2. Bensink 3. Cantrell et al. 4. Mayer 5. O'Conner-Von	2009 2008 2008 2010 2009	Supplements in-person support Families rate information as valuable A variety of technologies can be utilized (phone, Internet, CD-ROM) May improve problem-solving skills and increase feelings of support and hope	Research is limited by small sample sizes Few randomized trials Research is primarily qualitative
Online support groups	1. Coulson et al.	2012	May provide emotional, informational, and esteem support, as well as tangible assistance Easily accessible; convenient Not limited by geographic location	Groups are not generally monitored by a professional Group members may not respond Difficulty maintaining relationships outside of online group
Social Networks	1. Anderson et al. 2. Holden et al. 3. Lewis et al.	2011 2002 2005	May provide information and psychological support Convenient	Research is limited by small sample sizes Greater benefit for women and spiritual individuals
Cognitive Rehabilitation	1. Hardy et al. 2. Hardy et al. 3. Kesler et al.	2011 2013 2011	May improve cognitive abilities on functional outcome measures May increase brain activity in certain brain regions	Research is limited by small sample sizes Few randomized controlled trials Study results may not generalize to academic setting
Survivorship smoking	1. Emmons et al. 2. Emmons et al.	2009 2013	May decrease smoking cessation rates compared to self-help Similar cessation rates as in-person counseling	Users may not access website or utilize other support services (online chat)
Survivorship physical activity	1. Rabin et al. 2. Valle et al.	2011 2013	Increases levels of physical activity May improve mood and other psychosocial outcomes May promote weight loss	Professional not available to monitor engagement and safety

(continued)

Table. 20.2 (continued)

Areas of use	Authors	Year	Benefits	Limitations
Survivorship care plan	1. Blaauwbroek et al. 2. Poplack et al.	2012 2014	May improve provider-patient communication May facilitate family doctor communication and follow-up Promotes adherence to national survivorship recommendations	Logistical limitations of coordination with local family doctors

Table. 20.3 Summary of research studies investigating virtual reality eHealth technologies in pediatric oncology

Areas of use	Authors	Year	Benefits	Limitations
Acute pain	1. Gershon 2. Nilsson 3. Windich-Biermeier	2004 2009 2007	Patients report qualitative positive experience and distraction from pain Reduces observed pain via nurse report May reduce anxiety as measured by pulse rate	Does not reduce pain, fear, or distress via patient or parent report Technology is not easy to disseminate
Distress	1. Li et al. 2. Schneider et al.	2011 2000	May reduce distress during outpatient chemotherapy May increase play behaviors during hospitalization May decrease risk for depressive symptoms during hospitalization	Limited research to date Technology is not easy to disseminate

early maintenance phase therapy for acute lymphoblastic leukemia and lymphoblastic lymphoma. Another adherence electronic monitoring tool is the action-adventure game Re-Mission created by Kato and colleagues (2008). Re-Mission was used in a randomized trial to increase children's adherence to their chemotherapy regimen and those children who used the game reported a threefold increase in self-efficacy to manage their illness.

A number of other adherence enhancing apps are available to manage medication regimens for both Apple and Android devices, such as MyMedSchedule (www.medactionplan.com), MyMeds (www.my-meds.com), and MangoHealth (www.mangohealth.com) (Dayer et al. 2003; Gephart and Effken 2013). MyMedSchedule allows health professionals to input simple or complex medication regimens using existing medication databases that can then be uploaded to patients' mobile devices (Dayer et al. 2003). Patients and providers can enable reminders, indicate missed dosages, and modify medication regimens as needed. MyMedSchedule stores medication regimens on a Health Insurance Portability and Accountability Act (HIPAA) compliant cloud server that can then be accessed online from any device. Such medication adherence apps have not yet been evaluated in pediatric oncology but may be appropriate for adolescent and young adult oncology patients.

Physical Activity and Nutrition

The number of personal activity monitoring apps and nutrition monitoring apps has grown exponentially during the past decade. More than half a million apps have become available since 2008 and more than half of these relate to physical activity (33 %) or nutrition (20 %) (West et al. 2012). Some electronic personal fitness monitors have expanded capabilities and include programs to monitor sleep, connect to the Internet, and interface with social networks. Nutrition apps are often combined with personal fitness apps and provide food tracking and nutrition analyses. While apps such as MyFitnessPal (www.myfitnesspal.com) have been promoted for young breast cancer survivors, at this time, there are no empirical data to indicate usefulness or patient perceived benefit. Research is in the initial phases of development and evaluation of physical fitness and nutrition apps for childhood cancer patients and survivors.

Electronic Reporting of Pain and Other Symptoms

Pain related to the disease process and from ongoing treatment is a very common experience of children with cancer (Van Cleve et al. 2004, 2012). Careful and systematic assessment and documentation of pain are required for pain to be adequately managed, especially in the home environment. Electronic pain diaries (e.g., smartphones and personal digital assistants) have become increasingly used in children and adolescents to document acute and chronic pain and are beginning to emerge in the cancer field. For example, Stinson and colleagues (2013) developed an iPhone application with a law enforcement theme called Pain Squad to collect data on pain intensity, duration, location, and impact (and encourage adherence with monitoring) in adolescents (ages 8–18 years) with cancer. The exciting potential use of mHealth technologies for monitoring pain is to facilitate communication with healthcare providers. Information that children enter into an app about pain and other symptoms could be transmitted to the healthcare team and subsequently lead to more timely and effective pain management.

Case Vignette

Molly is an 11-year-old female with acute lymphoblastic leukemia who is in the maintenance phase of treatment. She has been reporting frequent headaches, limb and back pain, fatigue, and sleep problems. Molly's medical team is not sure whether her symptoms are related to chemotherapy treatment only or whether there are other modifiable behavioral and social factors that might be contributing. Molly's oncologist asks her about her preferences for using technology in her healthcare. Molly has an iPhone and is a frequent user of the Internet. She and her mom are interested in learning about apps that may help her. Her oncologist shows her the Pain Squad app on her iPhone and discusses how it might be useful to track her pain and other symptoms. After 3 weeks, Molly returns to clinic and her oncologist reviews her symptoms on Pain Squad. He notes that Molly is reporting pain almost every day and is experiencing significant distress with fatigue and sleep. They discuss additional strategies to help with her daily pain, and to reduce fatigue, and address nighttime sleep difficulties.

Internet Education and Interventions

As described in Chapter 6 on psychotherapeutic modalities, supportive psychosocial interventions have been developed for children with cancer and their parents to address high levels of stress at the time of diagnosis and throughout the course of treatment and recovery. The majority of psychosocial interventions are delivered in person; however, research on in-person interventions has been limited by relatively low rates of enrollment and low retention of parents and children (Peek and Melnyk 2010; Stehl et al. 2009). Barriers to research enrollment and traditional in-person interventions include participants' feeling overwhelmed during the time of their child's cancer treatment and being unwilling to commit the time necessary for structured interventions (Stehl et al. 2009). eHealth and mHealth may aid clinicians in providing evidence-based psychosocial intervention in more accessible formats through the course of treatment and survivorship. Please see Tables 20.1.

Internet Education and Coping Interventions

Diagnosis and Early Treatment

Pediatric Cancer Education

Providing children and caregivers with education about the child's cancer diagnosis and planned medical regimen is a critical component in the care of children with cancer. Families are often overwhelmed at the time of diagnosis and unfamiliar with medical terminology, making initial patient and caregiver education difficult. Educational websites that compile relevant information on pediatric cancer may be able to address these concerns. As one example, the cooperative clinical trials of the Children's Oncology Group, the world's largest organization devoted to childhood and adolescent cancer research (www.childrensoncologygroup.org), makes medical information, research trials information, and information on coping with pediatric cancer available to patients and families. Other leading organizations such as the National Cancer Institute also distribute similar educational information (www.cancer.gov). There are dozens of other educational websites targeting parents and children or adolescents with cancer (Stinson et al. 2011). Unfortunately, the overall quality of many pediatric cancer educational websites is poor, with low desirability ratings and a reading level too high for most parents and adolescents to understand. Please see Table 20.3 and the Resources chapter 25 for a list of high-quality websites.

Several evidence-based web educational programs have been developed and evaluated by medical professionals and researchers. Earlier studies utilized CD-ROM technology to disseminate evidence-based programs and demonstrated good acceptability of these programs (Goodenough and Cohn 2004; Jones et al. 2010). More recent studies have turned to web-based programs. One group evaluated the favorability and impact on quality of life of a web-based educational and support intervention for families of children with cancer (Sigurdardottir et al. 2014). In this study, all participants (15 mothers, 12 fathers, and 11 children) rated the new website as favorable overall and mothers reported slightly improved cancer communication after the intervention as compared with baseline. Another study that evaluated the usability of a bilingual (English and French) Internet-based self-management program for adolescents with cancer and their parents found that the information presented on the website was appropriate, credible, and relevant (Stinson et al. 2014). Participants reported that having the program would have been extremely helpful when they were first diagnosed with cancer.

Despite patient and parent reported satisfaction with the various educational programs, studies have shown none or only modest improvements in communication or well-being for the families who utilized the programs. Further, all of the studies are limited by small sample sizes such that satisfaction and use of eHealth education programs may not generalize to the larger pediatric oncology population. For instance, Ewing et al. (2009) developed a web-based resource for children newly diagnosed with cancer and their families to provide psychosocial support but found that very few families accessed the website. The timing of when and how interventions are introduced may be critical in their utilization.

Coping

Studies show that patient and parent distress tends to be highest at the time of cancer diagnosis and during the initial stages of treatment (Myers et al. 2014). The need for psychological support and social resources may be greatest during this period of uncertainty and adjustment. Because in-person pediatric cancer support groups tend to be poorly attended during the initial stages of cancer diagnosis and treatment (Stehl et al. 2009), eHealth technologies provide an alternative modality for administering child and parent coping interventions and providing support.

A variety of eHealth interventions, from telephone support calls to interactive web-based programs, have been developed to promote coping in parents as well as patients (Bensink et al. 2008; Mayer et al. 2010; O'Conner-Von 2009). Technology such as the Apple Facetime app integrates the ease of telephone calls with videoconferencing through built-in phone and computer cameras and is available for download to a number of electronic devices. The Facetime app may provide advantages in pediatric oncology care regarding visual confirmation of reported symptoms and real-time multimedia communication between medical providers and families. However, some individuals may not be as comfortable with videoconferencing and thus individual preferences will likely dictate future use of this technology.

There have been a few examples in pediatric oncology of delivery of psychosocial interventions using information technology. Sahler et al.'s (2005) 8-session in-person problem-solving intervention (Bright IDEAS), designed to reduce distress in mothers of children with cancer, has been supplemented with handheld personal digital assistants (PDA) (Askins et al. 2009). In Askins et al. trial, both Spanish-speaking and English-speaking mothers ($n = 197$) of children with newly diagnosed cancer were randomized to traditional problem-solving therapy or problem-solving therapy + PDA programs. PDA devices were designed to provide a brief review of the problem-solving process, practice the five elements of the Bright IDEAS problem-solving approach, prompt the use of problem-solving skills, and record a daily log to record problems confronted as well as solutions. Their findings demonstrated significant positive change over time on psychosocial measures in Spanish- and English-speaking mothers in both groups.

Another web-based program, entitled the Hope Intervention Program (HIP), is an 8-week program designed to promote hope in childhood cancer survivors and was pilot tested with 6 female young adult survivors (Cantrell and Conte 2008). The intervention was delivered online with the use of educational software that included Web cameras and voice and text chat. Participants qualitatively rated the program as feasible, valuable, and promoting feelings of hope; however, no quantitative outcome data was available. Mayer and colleagues (2010) report developing an eHealth system that integrates psychosocial services for parents of children receiving hematopoietic stem cell transplant. The program entitled the Hematopoietic Stem Cell Transplantation-Comprehensive Health Enhancement Support System (HSCT-CHESS) includes information about stem cell transplant basics, caring for your child, working with healthcare providers, taking care of yourself, managing the household, as well as addressing family life, work, insurance, money, and legal issues. Currently, an ongoing randomized multisite controlled trial is evaluating the impact of this system on both parent and child HSCT recipients' quality of life.

Despite the usability and feasibility data being promising on these web-based programs, the lack of published research, limited number of completed randomized trials, and small sample sizes precludes drawing conclusions on their potential benefit. There is a critical need for rigorous evaluation of web-based programs to promote child and family coping. The development and evaluation of psychosocial interventions using eHealth and mHealth platforms in pediatric cancer is only in its formative stages.

Internet and Support Networks

Treatment and Maintenance Therapy

Online Support Groups

The number of online support groups for pediatric cancer patients and their families has grown tremendously in recent years. Several online support websites are available for children and adolescents including 2bMe (www.2bme.org), Beyond the Cure (www.beyondthecure.org), Group Loop (www.grouploop.org), and Stupid Cancer (http://stupidcancer.com). These online support websites offer educational information on cancer-related topics ranging from appearance to nutrition to late effects of cancer and treatment. Most websites are designed for adolescents and some offer online chats and/or a monitored forum for adolescents to post personal stories and message with other adolescents. Professionally monitored forums and professionally facilitated online support groups like those offered on Group Loop are recommended, particularly for young adolescents, as professional monitoring can limit hostile exchanges, limit inaccurate or misleading medical information, and ensure timely responses to posts.

One online support website SuperSibs! (http://www.alexslemonade.org/campaign/supersibs) is designed to support 4-to 18-year-old brothers and sisters of children diagnosed with cancer. The SuperSibs website provides therapeutic tools (e.g., activities, words of support, home resources) to help siblings during and after their sibling's cancer treatment. One study examined support-intended communication for three online support groups aimed at family members of children with cancer (Coulson and Greenwood 2012). Results revealed five types of social support contained within the online messages: emotional, informational, esteem support, and tangible assistance. A few disadvantages of the online support groups were also identified including a lack of response from group members and difficulty maintaining relationships outside the online group context.

Case Vignette

Casey is a 14-year-old female who underwent a total resection of a juvenile pilocytic astrocytoma 18 months ago. At a routine follow-up visit, Casey and her mother meet with the clinic social worker and report concerns about friendships. Casey states that she wants to have more friends, but often feels socially isolated. Mom and Casey do not report any concerns about her mood or school performance. The social worker invites her to a teen support group for cancer survivors, but Casey lives 2 hours away from the clinic and it is not feasible for her to attend. Given the distance issues, her social worker discusses online resources including online support groups. Casey has an iPad and she and her mother express interest in learning more about an online support group that would meet Casey's needs. She is provided with a list of teen-friendly support websites including Group Loop which is a monitored online support group for teenagers. At her next appointment, Casey reports that it has been helpful to read other teenagers' stories on the online support websites and likes being able to chat online with other teenagers who have had cancer.

Social Networking

A social network is a social structure made of individuals or organizations that share one or more types of interdependency, such as friendship, common interests, work, knowledge, prestige, etc. (Masic et al. 2012). Global public social networks such as Facebook and Twitter are among the most popular social networks (see Social media Chapter 19 for more information). More than half of Americans who investigate health problems on the Internet get information about their treatment or medical condition via the Internet, and more than one third of Americans use social networks to obtain day-to-day information and support (Kuehn 2011). Given the popularity of social network websites, these websites have been used to target adolescents for cancer prevention and tobacco control initiatives (Struik et al. 2012), as well as provide forums for sharing personal stories. Unfortunately, the information made available on social networks is not regularly monitored and the quality and reliability are often questionable. There are several medical social network websites freely available to patients and their families including DailyStrength, CaringBridge, and CarePages (Masic et al. 2012). These social network websites allow patients and families to obtain information, create a profile to share stories, and make medical updates readily available to family and friends.

There are also social network sites designed specifically for teens and young adults with cancer or those who have recently completed therapy such as Teens Living With Cancer (www.teenslivingwithcancer.org), Teenage Cancer Trust (www.teenagecancertrust.org), and Planet Cancer (http://myplanet.planetcancer.org) (Elliot et al. 2013). Starbright World (www.starbrightworld.org) is a private, interactive social network that offers teenagers and young adults ages 13–20 who have a serious illness or injury the opportunity to connect with others via videoconferencing, instant messaging, chat rooms, bulletin boards, and e-mail (Holden et al. 2002). Starbright World provides a professional "chat host" to monitor online chat rooms and ensure adherence to community rules. Siblings ages 13–20 are also welcome on Starbright World. Please see the Resources Chapter 25.

Little research has investigated how social networks are used in cancer care (Koskan et al. 2014). Research has been predominately descriptive in nature and focused on adults. For example, Anderson and colleagues (2011) conducted a survey with 1035 adults who set up personalized CaringBridge web pages due to hospitalization, serious illness, or other reasons. Four primary benefits were found including providing information, receiving encouragement through messages, convenience, and psychological support. Analyses indicated that women and individuals with higher spirituality/religiosity received the greatest benefit. A few other online education and social network systems have been developed by medical professionals such as Caring Connection (Lewis et al. 2005). While these online social support networks have the advantage of being developed by medical professionals, they often are pilot tested with only a small sample of families and lack data on generalizability. Overall, online social support networks may offer families and children with cancer a useful resource for seeking emotional and informational support, yet further evaluation is needed to understand their specific benefits and limitations.

Computer, Internet, and Social Network Intervention Programs

Long-Term Survivorship

Computerized Cognitive Rehabilitation

As discussed in Chapter 15, survivors of pediatric brain tumors and acute lymphoblastic leukemia (ALL) are at particular increased risk for neurocognitive deficits in areas of attention and concentration, executive function, and memory (e.g., Campbell et al. 2007; Nathan et al. 2007; de Ruiter et al. 2013). Yet, few empirically supported treatment options exist for these neurocognitive late effects. Computer-based cognitive training programs have been a focus of recent research efforts to provide intervention to survivors and mitigate neurocognitive damage caused by cancer and its treatment (e.g., Hardy et al. 2011, 2013; Kesler et al. 2011). Hardy and colleagues (2013) examined the feasibility and preliminary efficacy of *CogmedRM*, a home-based, computerized training program for survivors of brain tumors or ALL ($n = 20$). The *CogmedRM* program, also discussed in Chapter 10 on neurocognitive issues, consists of twelve visual exercises that target visuo-spatial and auditory working memory skills that are completed in 25 training sessions at home, with weekly, phone-based support. In a small randomized controlled trial of the program, after controlling for baseline intellectual functioning, survivors who completed the *CogmedRM* intervention program evidenced post-training improvements in their visual working memory and in parent-rated learning problems compared with those children in the control group. Children with higher intellectual functioning at baseline appeared to benefit more from the training.

Another pilot study of a computerized executive function cognitive rehabilitation curriculum conducted with 23 pediatric cancer survivors aged 7–19 showed high rates of compliance (83 %), as well as improvements in neurocognitive outcomes including increased processing speed, cognitive flexibility, and increased verbal and visual declarative memory scores after completion of the program (Kesler et al. 2011). This cognitive rehabilitation curriculum is now commercially available on the Internet via Lumos Labs, Inc. (San Francisco, CA) as *Lumosity* (www.lumosity.com). While such computer programs tend to show an improvement in study-related outcomes after training, limitations in the research to date include small sample sizes and lack of randomized controlled trials. This allows for limited conclusions about the efficacy of computer-based neurocognitive interventions. Furthermore, research results do not always generalize to academic achievement and real-world cognitive skills (Butler et al. 2008). The sustainability of improvements over time remains unclear.

Smoking

Smoking among cancer survivors increases the risk of second cancers and late effects from treatment, e.g., cardiovascular disease and pulmonary conditions (Mertens et al. 2002; Oeffinger et al. 2006). To address this concern, several web-based interventions, such as the Partnership for Health-2 smoking prevention program (PFH-2), have been developed for childhood cancer survivors (Emmons et al. 2009; Emmons et al. 2013). Emmons and colleagues (2013) conducted a multi-site randomized controlled trial of the web-based PFH-2 program compared to the previous print-based program. The website provided new content at each log-on and a peer counselor moderated a forum/chat feature. For the 374 young adult childhood cancer survivors, there were similar rates of smoking cessation in the two arms (print = 15 %, Web = 6 %) at 15-month follow-up, and quit rates were equivalent compared to the previous telephone counseling intervention. Thus web-based smoking cessation programs may be a feasible option for childhood cancer survivors who do not have access to in-person counseling.

Physical Activity

Childhood cancer survivors are at increased risk of obesity and deconditioning following cancer therapy (Gocha Marchese et al. 2003; Withycombe et al. 2009). Web-based physical activity interventions are being developed and tested in childhood cancer survivors to facilitate the adoption of physical activity and improve long-term health outcomes. One pilot study recruited 18 young adults aged 18–39 diagnosed with cancer in the past 10 years to complete an Internet-based physical activity intervention (Rabin et al. 2011). Young adult participants were randomized to receive access to the physical activity website for 12 weeks or receive information about cancer. Results indicated medium effect size improvements in physical activity outcomes and large effect size improvements in mood and other psychosocial outcomes at 12 weeks. Another study evaluated the feasibility and preliminary efficacy of a 12-week, Facebook-based intervention (FITNET) aimed at increasing moderate-to-vigorous intensity physical activity compared to a Facebook-based self-help comparison condition (Valle et al. 2013). Young adult cancer survivors ($n = 86$) were randomly assigned to the FITNET group or the self-help group. Over 12 weeks, both groups significantly increased on self-reported weekly minutes of moderate-to-vigorous physical activity. The FITNET group had a greater increase in light physical activity and more weight loss over time than the self-help group. Such Internet-based physical activity programs appear to be feasible, well-accepted, and potentially beneficial to improve physical activity and other health-related outcomes.

Web-Based Cancer Survivor Care Plans

Young adult childhood cancer survivors report wanting more information about late effects (McClellan et al. 2013). Passport For Care (www.passportforcare.org) is a web-based tool that provides childhood cancer survivors and their healthcare providers with summaries of the patient's cancer history and treatment in a user-friendly format (Horowitz et al. 2009). Passport For Care uses algorithms to produce individualized monitoring and management recommendations derived from the Children's Oncology Group long-term follow-up guidelines. In 2014, Passport For Care had been implemented in over half of the almost 200 pediatric cancer clinics affiliated with the Children's Oncology Group (Poplack et al. 2014). Clinicians report that Passport For Care is well integrated into their clinic workflow and that it fosters improved communication with survivors about potential late effects, recommended screenings, and behavioral interventions for improved health. Clinicians also report that they adhere more closely to follow-up care guidelines when using Passport For Care.

Another group developed a similar website, the Survivor Care Plan, for adult survivors and their family doctors (Blaauwbroek et al. 2012). This website is designed to facilitate family doctor-driven follow-up for adult childhood cancer survivors and includes data on diagnosis, treatment, and potential risks as well as recommendations for follow-up. In the Blaauwbroek and colleagues study, 69 (96 %) of 72 family doctors returned data and 83 % of these family doctors reported fully adhering to the recommended medical tests. Thus web-based survivor care plans appear to facilitate improved communication between childhood cancer survivors and medical providers, as well as facilitate dissemination of long-term follow-up medical recommendations.

Case Vignette

Bradley is a 17-year-old male with a history of Wilms tumor at the age of 8. His treatment included surgical resection of the tumor and chemotherapy. He has not had any major health problems since his cancer treatment and has not seen his pediatric oncologist for several years. He did well in high school and is moving out of state for college. Bradley and his mother returned to his pediatric oncologist to ask about recommendations for Bradley as he enters adulthood and moves away from his parents. Bradley's pediatric cancer center uses the Passport For Care survivorship tool. His oncologist reviews Bradley's medical history and discusses current long-term follow-up recommendations including common fertility questions and possible late effects of chemotherapy with Bradley and his parents. She encourages Bradley to stay physically active and find a primary care physician at college for annual exams. Bradley is provided with a printed summary of his diagnosis, treatment, and long-term follow-up recommendations.

Virtual Reality

Virtual reality has primarily been utilized for acute pain management in children with cancer who are undergoing painful medical procedures (Gershon et al. 2004; Nilsson et al. 2009; Windich-Biermeier et al. 2007). Virtual reality uses computer-based technology to simulate the real world or an imaginary world, providing interaction with the computer system and engrossing the users' senses away from painful stimuli (Nilsson et al. 2009).

Several pilot studies have found that the use of virtual reality during subcutaneous venous port access, venipuncture, and lumbar puncture procedures may reduce anxiety and pain as observed by nurses; however, virtual reality does not tend to reduce pain on patient or parent report (Gershon et al. 2004; Nilsson et al. 2009; Windich-Biermeier et al. 2007). Please see Table 20.4. In the largest virtual reality study to date, Li and colleagues observed that 52 children age 8–16 years who completed a virtual reality computer game reported significantly fewer

Table. 20.4 Selected eHealth and mHealth websites and applications for pediatric oncology

Area of use	Title	Website	Download
Adherence	MyMedSchedule	http://mymedschedule.co	Apple Store; Google Play
	MyMeds	http://my-meds.com/	Apple Store; Google Play
	Mango Health	http://www.mangohealth.com	Apple Store; Google Play
Pain management	Pain Squad	http://campaignpage.ca/sickkidsapp	
Nutrition	Cure4Kids Jr.	https://www.cure4kids.org/ums/kids/app/	
Cancer education	Children's Oncology Group	http://www.childrensoncologygroup.org	
	National Cancer Institute	http://www.cancer.gov/	
	Macmillian Cancer	http://www.click4tic.org.uk	
	Macmillian Cancer for Teens and Young Adults	http://www.click4tic.org.uk	
	Cure Search	www.curesearch.org	
	Cancer. Net	www.cancer.net	
Online support	2bMe	http://www.2bme.org	
	Beyond the Cure	http://www.beyondthecure.org	
	Group Loop	http://www.grouploop.org	
	Stupid Cancer	http://stupidcancer.com	
	SuperSibs!	http://www.supersibs.org	
Social networks	Caring Bridge	http://www.caringbridge.org/	
	DailyStrength	http://www.dailystrength.org/	
	CarePages	https://www.carepages.com/	
	Starbright World	https://www.starbrightworld.org	
Survivorship	Passport For Care	https://www.passportforcare.org/	

Note: additional eHealth and mHealth resources are listed in the resources Chapter 25

symptoms of depression on day 7 of inpatient hospitalization compared to children in a standard care control group (Li et al. 2011). Virtual reality may reduce immediate distress during outpatient chemotherapy administration in newly diagnosed pediatric cancer patients (Schneider and Workman 2000); however, these gains do not appear to be sustained. Further studies using larger sample sizes are needed to determine whether virtual reality confers any benefits over and above other distraction and behavioral activation interventions for reducing acute pain, anxiety, and distress. The settings and context in which virtual reality may be helpful in pediatric oncology remain to be explored and serve as promising new areas of eHealth and mHealth research in pediatric oncology.

Conclusions

Technology is readily available to children and families. In the 2013 Pew Internet Survey on Teens, 93 % of teens had a computer or access to one at home and 78 % of teens had a cell phone. Studies in urban, minority populations indicate comparable rates of access to the Internet and even higher rates of cell phone ownership among youth. Parents are also regular users of the Internet and particularly use it to search for health information. Thus, technology provides unparalleled opportunity to reach broad populations of children with cancer and their families to provide education, support, assessment, and treatment of cancer-related symptoms. At this time, the evidence base is too small to make any definitive conclusions about the efficacy of this mode of assessment and intervention in children with cancer. However, we anticipate that given the rapid development of this field that in several years there will be large-scale evaluations of eHealth and mHealth interventions in pediatric cancer available. This area has enormous opportunity for improving the clinical care of children with cancer.

eHealth and mHealth technologies are becoming a more central part of the armamentarium of resources that can be offered to pediatric oncology patients and their families. Clinicians can talk with children and families to understand preferences for the use of technology in their cancer care and use available resources at their discretion. There is an important opportunity to learn from children and families which eHealth and mHealth resources families have used (e.g., medication adherence apps), whether they find them helpful (e.g., pediatric oncology education websites, online support groups), and how providers can provide support to families in this area (e.g., patient training and follow-up on use of mobile apps and websites). Technology will be more effective if clinicians are engaged and involved in monitoring patient response.

Clinical Pearls

- Consider individual child and parent preferences for mode of communication (e.g., text, e-mail, phone, in person). Patient preferences should guide the introduction and use of technology in care. While some patients will readily accept and prefer the use of mHealth technologies for monitoring pain and other cancer-related symptoms and for communication with healthcare providers, other patients may prefer more traditional forms of in-person communication.
- Assess parent and child socioeconomic and emotional resources and risk factors. Individual child and parent risk factors are important to consider in the potential uptake of technology-delivered interventions. Stress at the time of diagnosis or a high level of parent or family ongoing distress may limit engagement in technology. Screening for psychosocial and family distress can help guide decisions about the level and intensity of intervention needed.
- Consider a stepped care approach with technology-based interventions. Technology interventions are low-cost and easily accessible and may be disseminated broadly to patients. However, the clinician should be prepared to "step up" care by assessing response to the technology intervention and augmenting care with additional resources (e.g., in person) for those families who need it.

References

Anderson IK (2011) The uses and gratifications of online care pages: a study of CaringBridge. Health Commun 26:546–559

Askins MA, Sahler OJ, Sherman SA et al (2009) Report from a multi-institutional randomized controlled trial examining computer-assisted problem-solving skills training for English- and Spanish-speaking mothers of children with newly diagnosed cancer. J Pediatr Psychol 34:551–563

Bensink M, Armfiel N, Irving H et al (2008) A pilot study of videotelephone-based support for newly diagnosed paediatric oncology patients and their families. J Telemed Telecare 14:315–321

Bhatia S, Landier W, Shangguan M et al (2012) Nonadherence to oral mercaptopurine and risk of relapse in Hispanic and non-Hispanic white children with acute lymphoblastic leukemia: a report from the children's oncology group. J Clin Oncol 30: 2094–2101

Bhatia S, Landier W, Hageman L et al (2014) 6MP adherence in a multiracial cohort of children with acute lymphoblastic leukemia: a Children's Oncology Group study. Blood 124:2345–2353

Blaauwbroek R, Barf HA, Groenier KH et al (2012) Family doctor-driven follow-up for adult childhood cancer survivors supported by a web-based survivor care plan. J Cancer Surviv 6:163–171

Butler RW, Sahler OJ, Askins MA et al (2008) Interventions to improve neuropsychological functioning in childhood cancer survivors. Dev Disabil Res Rev 14:251–258

Campbell LK, Scaduto M, Sharp W et al (2007) A meta-analysis of the neurocognitive sequelae of treatment for childhood acute lymphocytic leukemia. Pediatr Blood Cancer 49:65–73

Cantrell MA, Conte T (2008) Enhancing hope among early female survivors of childhood cancer via the internet: a feasibility study. Cancer Nurs 31:370–379

Carels RA, Darby LA, Rydin S et al (2005) The relationship between self-monitoring, outcome expectancies, difficulties with eating and exercise, and physical activity and weight loss treatment outcomes. Ann Behav Med 30:182–190

Coulson NS, Greenwood N (2012) Families affected by childhood cancer: an analysis of the provision of social support within online support groups. Child Care Health Dev 38:870–877

Cushing CC, Steele RG (2010) A meta-analytic review of eHealth interventions for pediatric health promoting and maintaining behaviors. J Pediatr Psychol 35:937–949

Cushing CC, Jensen CD, Steele RG (2011) An evaluation of a personal electronic device to enhance self-monitoring adherence in a pediatric weight management program using a multiple baseline design. J Pediatr Psychol 36:301–307

Dayer L, Heldenbrand S, Anderson P et al (2003) Smartphone medication adherence apps: potential benefits to patients and providers. J Am Pharm Assoc 53:172–181

de Ruiter MA, van Mourik R, Schouten-van Meeteren AY et al (2013) Neurocognitive consequences of a paediatric brain tumour and its treatment: a meta-analysis. Dev Med Child Neurol 55:408–417

Elliot DL, Lindemulder SJ, Goldberg L et al (2013) Health promotion for adolescent childhood leukemia survivors: building on prevention science and ehealth. Pediatr Blood Cancer 60:905–910

Emmons KM, Puleo E, Mertens A et al (2009) Long-term smoking cessation outcomes among childhood cancer survivors in the Partnership for Health Study. J Clin Oncol 27:52–60

Emmons KM, Puleo E, Sprunck-Harrild K et al (2013) Partnership for health-2, a web-based versus print smoking cessation intervention for childhood and young adult cancer survivors: randomized comparative effectiveness study. J Med Internet Res 15, e218

Ewing LJ, Long K, Rotondi A et al (2009) Brief report: a pilot study of a web-based resource for families of children with cancer. J Pediatr Psychol 34:523–529

Gephart S, Effken J (2013) Using health information technology to engage patients in their care. Online J Nurs Inform 17:1–6

Gershon J, Zimand E, Pickering M et al (2004) A pilot and feasibility study of virtual reality as a distraction for children with cancer. J Am Acad Child Adolesc Psychiatry 43:1243–1249

Gocha Marchese V, Chiarello LA, Lange BJ (2003) Strength and functional mobility in children with acute lymphoblastic leukemia. Med Pediatr Oncol 40:230–232

Goodenough B, Cohn RJ (2004) Parent attitudes to audio/visual telecommunications in childhood cancer: an Australian study. Telemed J E Health 10(Suppl 2):S-15–S-25

Hardy KK, Willard VW, Bonner MJ (2011) Computerized cognitive training in survivors of childhood cancer: a pilot study. J Pediatr Oncol Nurs 28:27–33

Hardy KK, Willard VW, Allen TM et al (2013) Working memory training in survivors of pediatric cancer: a randomized pilot study. Psychooncology 22:1856–1865

Holden G, Bearison DJ, Rode DC et al (2002) The impact of a computer network on pediatric pain and anxiety: a randomized controlled clinical trial. Soc Work Health Care 36:21–33

Horowitz ME, Fordis M, Krause S et al (2009) Passport for care: implementing the survivorship care plan. J Oncol Pract 5:110–112

Jones JK, Kamani SA, Bush PJ et al (2010) Development and evaluation of an educational interactive CD-ROM for teens with cancer. Pediatr Blood Cancer 55:512–519

Kato PM, Cole SW, Bradlyn AS et al (2008) A video game improves behavioral outcomes in adolescents and young adults with cancer: a randomized trial. Pediatrics 122:e305–e317

Kesler SR, Lacayo NJ, Jo B (2011) A pilot study of an online cognitive rehabilitation program for executive function skills in children with cancer-related brain injury. Brain Inj 25:101–112

Koskan A, Klasko L, Davis SN et al (2014) Use and taxonomy of social media in cancer-related research: a systematic review. Am J Public Health 104:e20–e37

Kuehn BM (2011) Patients go online seeking support, practical advice on health conditions. JAMA 305:1644–1645

Lewis D, Gunawardena S, El Saadawi G (2005) Caring connection: developing an Internet resource for family caregivers of children with cancer. Comput Inform Nurs 23:265–274

Li WH, Chung JO, Ho EK (2011) The effectiveness of therapeutic play, using virtual reality computer games, in promoting the psychological well-being of children hospitalised with cancer. J Clin Nurs 20:2135–2143

Masic I, Sivic S, Toromanovic S et al (2012) Social networks in improvement of health care. Mater Sociomed 24:48–53

Mayer DK, Ratichek S, Berhe H et al (2010) Development of a health-related website for parents of children receiving hematopoietic stem cell transplant: HSCT-CHESS. J Cancer Surviv 4:67–73

McClellan W, Klemp JR, Krebill H et al (2013) Understanding the functional late effects and informational needs of adult survivors of childhood cancer. Oncol Nurs Forum 3:254–262

Mertens AC, Yasui Y, Liu Y et al (2002) Pulmonary complications in survivors of childhood and adolescent

cancer: a report from the Childhood Cancer Survivor Study. Cancer 95:2431–2441
Myers RM, Balsamo L, Lu X et al (2014) A prospective study of anxiety, depression, and behavioral changes in the first year after a diagnosis of childhood acute lymphoblastic leukemia: a report from the Children's Oncology Group. Cancer 120:1417–1425
Nathan PC, Patel SK, Dilley K et al (2007) Guidelines for identification of, advocacy for, and intervention in neurocognitive problems in survivors of childhood cancer: a report from the Children's Oncology Group. Arch Pediatr Adolesc Med 161:798–806
Nilsson S, Finnström B, Kokinsky E et al (2009) The use of virtual reality for needle-related procedural pain and distress in children and adolescents in a paediatric oncology unit. Eur J Oncol Nurs 13:102–109
O'Conner-Von S (2009) Coping with cancer: a web-based educational program for early and middle adolescents. J Pediatr Oncol Nurs 26:230–241
Oeffinger KC, Mertens AC, Sklar CA et al (2006) Chronic health conditions in adult survivors of childhood cancer. N Engl J Med 355:1572–1582
Oh H, Rizo C, Enkin M et al (2005) What is ehealth (3): a systematic review of published definitions. J Med Internet Res 7(1):e1
Palermo TM, Wilson AC (2009) eHealth applications in pediatric psychology. In: Roberts M, Steele R (eds) Handbook of Pediatric Psychology, 4th edn. Guilford Press, New York, pp 227–237
Palermo TM, Wilson AC, Peters M et al (2009) Randomized controlled trial of an Internet-delivered family cognitive-behavioral therapy intervention for children and adolescents with chronic pain. Pain 146:205–213
Peek G, Melnyk B (2010) Coping interventions for parents of children with newly diagnosed cancer: an evidence review with implications for clinical practice and future research. Pediatr Nurs 36:306–313
Poplack DG, Fordis M, Landier W et al (2014) Childhood cancer survivor care: development of the passport for care. Nat Rev Clin Oncol 11:740–750
Rabin C, Dunsiger S, Kirsten K et al (2011) Internet-based physical activity intervention targeting young adult cancer survivors. J Adolesc Young Adult Oncol 1:188–194
Ritterband LM, Cox DJ, Walker LS et al (2003) An internet intervention as adjunctive therapy for pediatric encopresis. J Consult Clin Psychol 71:910–917
Rohan JM, Drotar D, Alderfer M et al (2013) Electronic monitoring of medication adherence in early maintenance phase treatment for pediatric leukemia and lymphoma: identifying patters of nonadherence. J Pediatr Psychol 40:75–84. doi:10.1093/jpepsy/jst093
Sahler OJ, Fairclough DL, Phipps S et al (2005) Using problem-solving skills training to reduce negative affectivity in mothers of children with newly diagnosed cancer: report of a multisite randomized trial. J Consult Clin Psychol 73:272–283
Schneider SM, Workman ML (2000) Virtual reality as a distraction intervention for older children receiving chemotherapy. Pediatr Nurs 26:593–597
Sigurdardottir AO, Svavarsdottir EK, Rayens MK et al (2014) Impact of a web-based educational and support intervention on parents' perception of their children's cancer quality of life: an exploratory study. J Pediatr Oncol Nurs 31:154–165
Stehl ML, Kazak AE, Alderfer MA et al (2009) Conducting a randomized clinical trial of an psychological intervention for parents/caregivers of children with cancer shortly after diagnosis. J Pediatr Psychol 34:803–816
Stinson JN, White M, Breakey V et al (2011) Perspectives on quality and content of information on the internet for adolescents with cancer. Pediatr Blood Cancer 57:97–104
Stinson JN, Jibb LA, Nguyen C et al (2013) Development and testing of a multidimensional iphone pain assessment application for adolescents with cancer. J Med Internet Res 15, e51
Stinson J, Gupta A, Dupuis F et al (2014) Usability testing of an online self-management program for adolescents with cancer. J Pediatr Oncol Nurs. 32:70–82
Struik LL, Bottorff JL, Jung M et al (2012) Reaching adolescent girls through social networking: a new avenue for smoking prevention messages. Nurs Res 44:84–103
Valle CG, Tate DF, Mayer DK et al (2013) A randomized trial of a Facebook-based physical activity intervention for young adult cancer survivors. J Cancer Surviv 7:355–368
Van Cleve L, Bossert E, Beecroft P et al (2004) The pain experience of children with leukemia during the first year after diagnosis. Nurs Res 53:1–10
Van Cleve L, Muñoz CE, Riggs ML et al (2012) Pain experience in children with advanced cancer. J Pediatr Oncol Nurs 29:28–36
Wade SL, Carey J, Wolfe CR (2006) An online family intervention to reduce parental distress following pediatric brain injury. J Consult Clin Psychol 74:445–454
Walsh KE, Roblin DW, Weingart SN, Houlahan KE, Degar B, Billett A, Keuker C, Biggins C, Li J, Wasilewski K, Mazor KM (2013) Medication errors in the home: a multisite study of children with cancer. Pediatrics 131:e1405–e1414
West JH, Hall PC, Hanson CL et al (2012) There's an app for that: content analysis of paid health and fitness apps. J Med Internet Res 14, e72
Windich-Biermeier A, Sjoberg I, Dale JC et al (2007) Effects of distraction on pain, fear, and distress during venous port access and venipuncture in children and adolescents with cancer. J Pediatr Oncol Nurs 24:8–19
Withycombe JS, Post-White JE, Meza JL et al (2009) Weight patterns in children with higher risk ALL: a report from the Children's Oncology Group (COG) for CCG 1961. Pediatr Blood Cancer 53:1249–1254

Self-Care and Sustainability for Pediatric Oncology Providers

21

Barbara L. Jones and Stacy S. Remke

Self-Care for the Pediatric Oncology Practitioner

There are many reasons to celebrate the astonishing strides in pediatric cancer care in recent decades. Survival rates have increased, supportive and palliative approaches have relieved some of the burdens of cancer treatment, and financial relief assistance for families has been established through many programs and philanthropy. Yet some hard facts remain. Families present with a wide array of compelling, sometimes intractable psychosocial challenges and social disparities. Treatment requires many painful and burdensome medical interventions that result in suffering for children and their families even when cure is attained, and up to 20 % of children with a cancer diagnosis still die. It is inescapable that those who care for children with cancer and their families will witness a great deal of suffering. This poses a potential risk for pediatric providers. Psychosocial providers who care for children with cancer are vulnerable to emotional and psychological reactions including burnout, compassion fatigue, secondary traumatic stress, and vicarious trauma simply given the nature of the work (Rourke 2007; Robins et al. 2009; Pearlman and McKay 2008). Secondary traumatic stress is an "occupational hazard" for all practitioners working in pediatric oncology services (Beck 2011). There is limited information in the literature specifically about *pediatric psychosocial oncology* professionals; therefore, this chapter focuses on the existing literature in the following populations: adult and pediatric oncology professionals, pediatric palliative care professionals, and psychosocial professionals. Implications from existing studies will be drawn together to inform how we help pediatric psychosocial oncology professionals take care of themselves professionally.

B.L. Jones, PhD, MSW (✉)
School of Social Work, The University of Texas at Austin, 1925 San Jacinto Blvd, Mail Stop D3500, Austin, TX 78712, USA
e-mail: barbarajones@mail.utexas.edu

S.S. Remke, MSW, LICSW, ACHP-SW
School of Social Work, University of Minnesota, Peters Hall 105, 1404 Gortner Avenue St, Paul, MN 55108, USA
e-mail: remke005@umn.edu

Case Vignette
Louise, a pediatric oncology social worker, has been in her job for 8 years. She begins her day with multidisciplinary patient care rounds where the 22 patients on the floor and the additional 25 patients who will be seen in clinic that day are discussed. With too many patients to discuss in great detail, the team identifies new diagnoses and

A.N. Abrams et al. (eds.), *Pediatric Psychosocial Oncology: Textbook for Multidisciplinary Care*,
DOI 10.1007/978-3-319-21374-3_21

patients who are having issues with either their medical course or psychosocial situation. Also children who are in deteriorating health, or entering the dying phase, are identified and reviewed. Usually, the focus during this meeting is the medical situation, next steps, and who on the team would do what that day. Louise learns that three patients she had followed over the past couple of years were being admitted for various reasons. Alice, 14 years old, has a suspected relapse of her osteosarcoma that had previously responded well to treatment. Her family had been there every step of the way and always said they were "fighters." This would be a rough piece of news for them. Danny, a 7 year old with ALL, was being readmitted for a resistant infection. He had been receiving intensive antibiotic therapy, was very weak, and seemed to be "running out of gas." Danny was severely immunocompromised and his infection placed him in a precarious situation. Louise knew his single mother was quite exhausted too. She made a mental note to check in with her. This mom had a tendency to become more depressed when Danny's medical situation took a downturn. Fatima, a 17 year old with AML, was being admitted for a pre-bone marrow transplant (BMT) workup. A BMT was her best chance for cure, but Louise knew the team was very concerned due to her poor general health status. Her mother and father were originally from Senegal and were very unfamiliar with the road that lay ahead for them with transplant. There was also significant marital conflict that tended to get worse when they were under stress. They had many questions about medical insurance, transportation, and how they could afford to take off work to be at the hospital with Fatima. As she left the meeting, Louise was relieved to see it was only 10:30 am as she wanted to attend the 11:00 am memorial service for Billy, a 3-year-old boy and long-time patient, who had died the previous week from neuroblastoma.

Chronic Exposure to Stress

Practitioners who value the work that they do and who find meaning in their profession might not notice the slow and creeping effects of exposure to the suffering of patients and their families. Like the proverbial frog who adapts to gently boiling water until it becomes too hot and he boils to death, practitioners are in danger of becoming overwhelmed before they know it. The process of learning and performing an important role with skill leads to greater capacity. Over time, the experience of performing that role without respite becomes burdensome. What might at first seem emotionally overwhelming becomes something that one adjusts to and can sometimes become numb to. Avoidance, irritability, impatience, cynicism, and feelings of helplessness or hopelessness can arise (Dane and Chachkes 2001; van Dernoot Lipsky and Burk 2009). The constant exposure to the suffering and hardship of others erodes resilience in ways that are insidious and potentially damaging to the practitioner. The demands on pediatric oncology providers are high and often relentless; there are always more children being diagnosed, needing treatment, dying, or facing new challenges in survivorship. Practitioners in this field observe the struggles and pain first hand and for extended periods of time.

Serious, life-threatening illness is a traumatic event (Dane and Chachkes 2001). This is especially true when such illness occurs in childhood. Secondary traumatic stress can occur in those who are important to the survivor's life: family, friends, community, and professional caregivers. Proximity to those experiencing trauma and those suffering puts practitioners at risk for the development of symptoms like those experienced in post-traumatic stress disorder. The only difference is that the exposure is indirect: it is not personally experienced; it is produced through the lens of another person's experience. This pattern can confound one's ability to notice or acknowledge developing secondary traumatic stress. It is easy to minimize concerns or feel confused by reactions when the precipitants are in fact unclear, indirect, and perhaps not even tied to a single event. The cumulative effect of these exposures is one of the major determinants in the development of secondary traumatic stress and related conditions.

Compassion Fatigue, Burnout, Secondary Traumatic Stress, and Compassion Satisfaction

Recent studies have shed light on the role that compassion fatigue, burnout, and vicarious trauma or secondary traumatic stress can play in the work lives of professionals who witness suffering and trauma. These concepts are sometimes conflicting and overlapping but can offer insights into work in stressful healthcare contexts (van Dernoot Lipsky and Burk 2009; Rossi et al. 2012). Additionally, these terms are commonly used interchangeably. While there is some overlap in the concepts of burnout, compassion fatigue, and secondary or vicarious trauma, they are best understood as distinct phenomena.

Burnout is a state of emotional, physical, and psychological exhaustion, coupled with a reduced sense of accomplishment that develops over time. Burnout is also associated with the experience of an unsupportive work environment, a reaction to high workloads, conflict with colleagues, and unresponsive administration among other factors (Ellwood et al. 2011). In contrast, vicarious trauma or secondary traumatic stress is the natural by-product of bearing witness to and empathetic engagement with those who suffer trauma. It is the *cumulative effect* of exposure to the suffering of others. This exposure leads to changes in worldview, psychological, spiritual, and physical well-being. Over time, these changes can become permanent. Secondary traumatic stress refers to the "cumulative, transformative effect" of working with those who are traumatized (Pearlman and McKay 2008). In secondary traumatic stress, the practitioner adapts to the suffering of others and in that process adjusts their identity, worldview, and engagement with others. The effects of secondary traumatic stress or vicarious stress can become permanent, altering the manner in which the practitioner engages and interprets the world (Rossi et al. 2012; Robins et al. 2009; Sinclair and Hamill 2007; Pearlman and McKay 2008).

Studies have shown that exposure to the pain and suffering of children is particularly provocative for caregivers. Researchers report that the most frequently reported triggers of compassion fatigue were seeing painful procedures done to children, too much sadness, and too many deaths of children suffering with chronic illness (Maytum et al. 2004; Figley 1995; Najjar et al. 2009). Pediatric oncology physicians also feel sadness related to patient deaths and may experience periods of crying, irritability, disrupted home lives, and a sense of personal loss (Granek et al. 2015). Clearly repeated exposure to childhood deaths poses risks to all practitioners in this field.

To avoid vicarious trauma and its effects, it is helpful to recognize that those who work closely with those who suffer are vulnerable to it. There are clear warning signs that have been identified. Being alert to these signs in one's self and one's colleagues can help practitioners identify and address the factors that contribute to vicarious trauma and also those factors that contribute to resilience in the context of work with children who have cancer.

Warning Signs of Secondary Trauma Exposure/Response

Adapted from L. van Dernoot Lipsky and C. Burk, 2009

- Feeling helpless
- Sense of hopelessness
- Hypervigilance
- Diminished creativity
- Inability to embrace complexity
- Minimizing
- Chronic exhaustion, physical ailments
- Inability to listen, deliberate avoidance
- Dissociative moments, intrusive thoughts
- Sense of persecution
- Guilt
- Fear
- Anger and cynicism
- Inability to empathize, numbing
- Addictions
- Grandiosity: empathize, numbing thoughts

Secondary traumatic stress occurs through a number of interacting dynamics. There are aspects of the individual practitioner that may cause them to be more vulnerable (personality, prior history of trauma, boundary practices, and perceptions), aspects of the team (culture, conflict, mutuality of support, and other dynamics), as well as aspects of the organizational and administrative structure (supervision, adequate resources, responsiveness, manageable workloads, continuing education resources) that contribute to exacerbation or minimization of risks. Each of these dimensions requires consideration.

It is important to acknowledge the importance of compassion satisfaction, the reason many are drawn to and sustained in this work. The rewards from serving children and families in need and participating in an often dynamic and challenging team context are many. Studies have indicated that there is an inverse relationship between compassion satisfaction and compassion fatigue or secondary traumatic stress: the higher the degree of secondary traumatic stress, the lower the perceived compassion satisfaction. In order to sustain compassion satisfaction, it is important to acknowledge and attend to the risks and burdens of caring for others. This is not an "either/or" proposition but rather requires a "both/and" emphasis.

The Role of Empathy

Empathy in psychosocial oncology care can serve as both a risk and protective factor for secondary traumatic stress disorder. There is an essential paradox within the clinical relationship: empathy is crucial for the work and also potentially dangerous to providers (Crumpei and Dafinoiu 2011). It is essentially a double-edged sword. Empathic professionals have better results in outcomes and patient satisfaction. Emotional involvement could in fact put providers at higher risk of secondary traumatic stress (Figley 1995). It is important to note the difference between affective empathy (which increases risk) and cognitive empathy (which tends to be protective). Figley argues that those who feel and express empathy are at greater risk of secondary traumatic stress (Figley 1995). The development of awareness, reflective skills, and a cognitive frame for interactions with patients and families is essential for practitioner wellness.

Prevention Strategies

A combination of investigative studies, practice reports, systematic reviews, and anecdotal reports points toward continuing education, professional and personal supports, organizational structures, interdisciplinary teamwork, mentoring, wellness sessions, retreats, each of which focuses on meaning and perspective, maintaining balance and self-management strategies as potential tools to prevent vicarious trauma and compassion fatigue in psychosocial oncology professionals (Aycock and Boyle 2009; Emanuel et al. 2011; Rohan and Bausch 2009; Zadeh et al. 2012).

In recent systematic reviews, studies have offered specific recommendations for preventing and ameliorating secondary traumatic stress among nurses and social workers. Beck (2011) found seven studies that looked at secondary traumatic stress among nurses. The studies recommended continuing education about the vulnerability to and symptoms of secondary traumatic stress (Beck 2011; Ting et al. 2006) and peer support for nurses (Townsend and Campbell 2009). Rourke (2007) identified three tiers of strategies for preventing secondary traumatic stress and compassion fatigue in nurses: personal, professional, and organizational. Aycock and Boyle (2009) found interventions to manage compassion fatigue among nurses fell into three categories: on-site professional resources (EAP programs, staff counselor or mental health professionals, support groups, and employee wellness programs), educational programs, and specialized retreats. Other identified institutional supports included working in interdisciplinary teams, having mentorship, adequate staffing, memorial services, and monthly rounds like Schwartz Center Rounds (www.theschwartzcenter.org) to facilitate open reflection and enhance compassionate caregiving (Aycock and

Boyle 2009). Flexible scheduling and time away from direct patient care responsibilities, undertaking activities like quality improvement projects, resource development and research, or writing projects have also been described as helpful (Rohan and Bausch 2009).

In a qualitative study of pediatric oncology social workers, the findings highlighted the importance of vigilant and purposeful self-care (Jones 2004). Examples included "Take care of yourself or you won't be able to help anyone!"; "Be in touch with their (your patients) feelings and utilize supervision, every death is different and there is no correct way, no matter how effective you are, you can't take away the pain;" and "Know when you need time for yourself, it is okay to cry with a family when appropriate…we are humans too." (Jones 2004). The social worker participants spoke of creating a balance between work and home responsibilities and the importance of professional and personal supports. In this study, professional supports were mentioned much more frequently than personal supports. Professional supports include good relationships with colleagues: "I have excellent relationships with my colleagues in the social work profession as well as with other disciplines." Formal mechanisms for support were also mentioned: "we started a monthly staff support time to talk about the work we do. I allow myself to process the loss and then let it go." Focusing on personal relationships of all kinds was also very important. Forming strong personal relationships inside and outside of work can facilitate one's self-care as well, "finding support through people close to me (family, friends, church)

Pediatric oncology social workers report using a variety of methods for self-care which include but are not limited to personal interests and activities, self-nurturance, and spiritual/contemplative practices (Jones 2004). Similarly, oncology nurses have benefitted from renewal strategies such as spiritual faith, art and music, attending to their own physical health, creating professional and personal balance, and renewing their commitment to the profession (Aycock and Boyle 2009). In a study by Rohan and Bausch (2009), oncology physicians, nurses, and social workers reported a need for replenishing themselves to sustain the work. They did so by seeking refuge, using spiritual practices and rituals, adjusting expectations of success, perceiving work differently over time, and reorganizing career and work (Rohan and Bausch 2009).

Case Vignette

Alison, a pediatric oncology psychologist, noticed that she felt out of sorts and distressed when a patient that she followed died. When she went home to her own family and kids, she was expected to just get on with her day. It was hard to know what to do with her feelings. After reflecting upon this and talking with friends at work, she realized that she needed a way to make the transition between work and home smoother, especially after a loss had occurred. It was important to her to be authentic to her own spiritual life. She resonated with nature, though she was not particularly religious. She decided that after a child she worked with died, she would walk to the park by the river, find a special stone, and think about all the things she remembered about that child. She allowed herself to feel whatever feelings emerged and then would throw the stone into the river as she said goodbye to that person. In this way, she found closure and a way to separate her work life from her home life more effectively.

Personal Strategies

When considering personal strategies to address or prevent compassion fatigue, a few exemplars stand out:

- Meaning making/remembering
- Facilitated compassion fatigue training
- Mindfulness-based interventions

Making Meaning and Benefit Finding

Despite the struggles, oncology practitioners report finding "abundant rewards" in the work, particularly by easing suffering and receiving patient gratitude, having intimate emotional connections, being inspired by the human spirit, and gaining wisdom or perspective (Rohan and Bausch 2009). The majority of clinicians interviewed in Rohan and Bausch's study described having their outlook on life changed by their oncology work. While some loss of innocence was reported, for most, the work served as a reminder of what is important in life (Rohan and Bausch 2009). In a recently published study, physicians reported that their experiences with patient deaths encouraged positive insights, including a deepening appreciation for life (Granek 2015).

Pediatric oncology social workers report that constructing personal meaning out of the losses faced enhanced their personal philosophy of life and loss (Jones 2006). In the aforementioned study, many pediatric oncology social workers described the relationship with the child and family as a gift that they have gratitude for: "I am thankful for the gifts of these families—the children I have known. I am thankful for having been able to be part of their lives at such an important time in their family history." Another respondent summed up what many expressed: "Knowing I have made a difference in the lives of these patients and families" (Jones 2006).

For pediatric oncology social workers, remembering what the patients taught them in their lives was helpful (Jones 2006): "I feel like in every loss there is a gift the child and family give, something that teaches me about life. I try to give thanks for that and honor the time I have been given with that child and family, attaching that certain quality like parents of a young child who were so patient. I then focus on the gift of patience, visualize them, and then tuck it in my heart." Not every social worker indicated that they did "make meaning" out of the losses. Some respondents focused instead on helping the family find meaning: "I don't think I 'make meaning' out of the losses. I just try and help families come to terms with the loss and help them 'make meaning.' If I can do that, then that gives my work meaning." Perhaps it is not important or possible to have the work make sense as one respondent states: "Letting go of the need to have it 'make sense'—recognize that certain things happen which we may never understand."

Compassion-Focused and Mindfulness-Based Interventions

In addition to meaning-focused reflections, the Accelerated Recovery Program (ARP), a five-session compassion fatigue intervention, has been found to be helpful and effective in addressing symptoms of compassion fatigue and burnout in professional caregivers (Gentry 2002). Certified Compassion Fatigue Specialist Training (CCFST) for caregivers was developed to train caregivers in compassion fatigue interventions (Gentry 2002). CCFST helped participants cope with compassion fatigue in themselves as well as in other participants (Gentry et al. 2002). In addition to CCFST, Aycock and Boyle (2009) found only one intervention in the literature that helped nurses directly with the costs of caring: a compassion fatigue nurse support group led by a social worker who was a compassion fatigue therapist has been reported to help nurses directly with the costs of caring.

Another set of promising strategies for compassion fatigue and vicarious traumatization are mindfulness-based interventions. Mindfulness can be defined as the process by which we "examine who we are, questioning our view of the world and our place in it, and cultivate some appreciation for the fullness of each moment we are alive" (Kabat-Zinn 1994). Mindfulness is a dimension of awareness that can be developed through instruction and practice. In the *Precious Necessity of Compassion,* Joan Halifax states:

> Mindful and compassionate caregiving entails listening with full attention, emotional awareness and self-regulation while caregiving, and positive regard for self and other, the ability to prioritize and be attuned to one's surroundings, and bringing compassion and nonjudgmental acceptance to interactions. (Halifax 2011)

Clinical and research interest in mindfulness has grown tremendously in part because of mindfulness-based stress reduction (MBSR), an evidence-based intervention developed by Kabat-Zinn and colleagues. MBSR was developed to address and decrease emotional and physical pain in patients suffering from chronic illness, while observing the connection between the mind and body (Kabat-Zinn 1994, 2003). Anxiety and worry about past and future events can damage both physical and psychological health by increasing levels of stress. Thus, the MBSR program aims to bring focus to the present moment (Kabat-Zinn 2003). Its main goal is to bring awareness to different manifestations of stress, in order to detect first signs of anxiety and to act voluntarily and willingly to correct usual patterns of response. Thus, the anxiety and depression that often accompany stress can be targeted quickly, in order to achieve general well-being and peace of mind (Kabat-Zinn 2003).

Mindfulness-based stress reduction (MBSR) has been shown to reduce stress, increase coping, and even increase empathy in healthcare practitioners (Beach 2013; Fortney 2013; Praissman 2008; Moody et al. 2013). Recent studies of physicians and nurse practitioners in primary care found that mindfulness-based interventions eased their burden and reduced burnout (Beach 2013; Chen 2013; Fortney et al. 2013; Moody et al. 2013). The more mindful practitioners were more patient centered and efficient. This increased efficiency may further decrease the stress of their work (Beach 2013; Chen 2013).

Enhancing Resilience

Resilience in pediatric oncology practitioners can be fostered and strengthened. Researchers have identified attributes of the resilient or "stress-proof" professional. When one has concerns about vicarious stress, the first step is to take a break from the situation that stimulates the reaction: reduce exposure (van Dernoot and Burk 2009). Taking vacations, continuing education pursuits, and undertaking alternative work duties are some common strategies. As practitioners address vulnerabilities to vicarious stress, and plan for reducing the impact of it, they can simultaneously develop strategies that promote resilience as practitioners.

Key Components of Resilience Include

- Physical resilience: physical "toughening" and "tempering," good health habits
- Psychological resilience: "situations viewed as challenges, not threats," general psychological health and flexibility
- Activation of social networks including confiding relationships
- Adequate external supports
- Challenging one's self
- Adequate preparation and training for the job
- Looking for meaning through involvement
- Continued education, learning, and openness (Hellerstein 2011; Figley et al. 2013)

Countertransference

It is important for clinicians to be aware of the dynamics of countertransference, or one's emotional entanglement with a patient, and how important it is to reflect on the needs and emotions of the patient and family. Psychosocial or mental health practitioners are generally trained and more attuned to these phenomena and have skills for dealing with them. However, other multidisciplinary practitioners deeply engaged with patients may also experience countertransference and remain unaware of it. Educating colleagues about these phenomena, developing reflective skills—as individuals and as a team—and creating strategies for supportive feedback can contribute to good patient care and not hinder professional effectiveness (Katz and Johnson 2006). Good supervision is essential when providing psychosocial care to children with cancer and their families (Joubert et al. 2013).

Organizational Issues and Opportunities

While it is important for individual practitioners to address their own needs for well-being and self-care, it is also crucial to note that individual strategies alone are not enough to prevent burnout and vicarious trauma. Structural elements in how staffing is planned, how provisions for adequate resources to do the job are made available, flexibility with work schedules, continuing education opportunities, and time off are additional elements that foster positive coping with challenging roles. "Organizational burnout" is a term coined by William White that describes this dilemma. The failures of organizations to plan adequately for the demands of a role or job end up creating unsustainable tensions for the individual worker or team to manage. A practitioner's perception of organizational support has important implications for work satisfaction (White 1997; Ellwood et al. 2011).

Many pediatric oncology programs operate as closed systems: members interface frequently with each other and do not interact much with others outside the field. Dedicated staff become highly specialized and focused. Their work is intense and complex. Stakes for performance are high. In this context, a culture of trust and interdependence is highly desirable. The system becomes vulnerable when secondary traumatic stress asserts itself because trust can erode, resources for care provision become stretched, and conflicts can erupt. This kind of stress can permeate the oncology system of care and act as a "contagion": when one member of the team becomes "infected" by this level of stress, it has a tendency to spread and impact the entire system (Figley 1995), with serious implications for team and program effectiveness, as well as practitioner job satisfaction. Therefore, the whole team must be attuned to the needs for balance and resilience of individual team members. When approached with awareness and sensitivity, within a culture of respect and concern, indicators of secondary traumatic stress or vicarious stress can be identified, addressed, and contained. Alternatively, when not addressed, these symptoms in an individual can be interpreted as personal limitations or failures, and the solution is seen as needing to change or oust the "difficult" person (White 1997). The individual may experience this situation as a personal failure, and yet there are unrealistic expectations and inadequate resources to do the job. The team may therefore lose perspective of the real threat, which is the constant exposure to high degrees of suffering, and to which any member of the team may be vulnerable.

Organizational dynamics can be helpful in identifying appropriate benchmarks, priorities, and expectations for job performance (White 1997).

Case Vignette

Joanne, a pediatric oncology social worker, was experiencing burnout and recognized the need for some time off from work. After she returned, she attended a team meeting where a colleague was discussing a case plan and need for the team's intervention. The oncologist, who she respected and trusted, stated afterwards, "I would have asked you to do it, but I know you are not really committed to this team…" Joanne was shocked and hurt by this characterization.

Team culture and expectations can have a strong influence on how behaviors are interpreted. As Joanne's case demonstrates, when a team member attends to personal wellness in a way that is not understood or sanctioned by the team, disappointments and misunderstandings can occur. If these needs and recommendations had been openly discussed, and norms established for self-care and mutual support, Joanne's experiences and insights may have contributed to positive changes for the whole team. Well-functioning interprofessional teams that display mutual support and respect may provide a protective factor against the difficulty of psychosocial oncology care (Rohan and Bausch 2009).

A number of researchers and theorists have identified the important role that teamwork, structures, and expectations within an organizational culture can play to reduce or exacerbate conditions that lead to burnout, secondary traumatic stress, as well as contribute to work or care satisfaction as the following quotes illustrate (Rohan and Bausch 2009; Li et al. 2014):

> Part of what we all use each other for is, you know, the camaraderie.
> We all enjoy what we do, and it's nice to kind of share some of the experiences together and also to deal with the problems together. – Oncologist, quoted in Rohan and Bausch 2009, p. 97
> So the stress (of the work) is more the emotional sadness and the intensity… When (the team) works, it absorbs the stress….. You can quote me on that. – Oncology social worker, quoted in Rohan and Bausch 2009, p. 98

One's ability to cognitively frame experiences with insight and awareness, access peer support and validation, as well as manage exposure has important implications for preventing or reducing secondary traumatic stress and burnout (van Dernoot and Burk 2009; Li et al. 2014). High case loads, complex and demanding cases, lack of perceived organizational support, and inadequate staffing are among stressors described as contributing to secondary traumatic stress (Li et al. 2014; Rohan and Bausch 2009). Organizations that are sensitive to the needs of practitioners can offer resources and supports that minimize the negative impact of exposure to trauma and high stress.

Organizational Strategies to Enhance Sustainability

Hospitals and healthcare organizations can play a distinct role in the prevention of secondary traumatic stress and in fostering resilience in their pediatric oncology providers. One set of strategies that have the potential to improve self-care include provision of a structured orientation, ongoing continuing education about vicarious and secondary traumatic stress, and the provision of specific professional support to address compassion fatigue as it arises (Aycock and Boyle 2009; Zanders et al. 2013). Both formal and informal supports are frequently mentioned in the research as helpful tools in preventing compassion fatigue. This means that hospitals and clinics must foster an environment that is conducive to true interprofessional teamwork, collaboration, mentoring, and supervision and the permission to express vulnerability and sorrow in the face of suffering (Aycock and Boyle 2009; Joubert et al. 2013; Zanders et al. 2013).

Another important tool for the mental health of providers is adequate and flexible staffing (Zanders et al. 2013). Reflection, meaning making, and mindfulness interventions all have the power to enhance well-being of psycho-oncology staff and can be included as organizational strategies (Beach et al. 2013; Fortney et al. 2013; Zanders et al. 2013). When considering intervention planning to enhance the well-being of psychosocial oncology professionals, institutions can ask the following questions first suggested by Brown (2006):

- What needs to change in our setting to enhance a more healing environment?
- Would you feel rested or comfortable if you were one of our patients?
- Should we have a quiet space for breaks?
- Do you find yourself tensed or relaxed when you work?
- Does the environment create a relaxed or technological aura?

Conclusion

Working with children with cancer and their families exposes the pediatric oncology professional to the tremendous suffering and distress of children and parents. Empathy and personal strength are required in order to remain emotionally present. Deep caring is essential to the work and can also lead to the practitioner's personal distress, compassion fatigue, and secondary traumatic stress. In this way, empathy is both a potentially protective factor and risk for the pediatric oncology professional. Both personal and organizational strategies can ameliorate this trauma and allow practitioners to continue to do the work that many describe as a "calling." Mental health providers will continue to care deeply for children and families but must also care for themselves in order to continue to provide psychosocial services. Psychosocial providers bear witness not only to the suffering and challenges children with cancer and their families face, but also to the incredible resilience of the human spirit in the face of these challenges. It is the latter that provides many with a sense of privilege in being able to provide this care and the capacity to remain fully engaged in the work.

Clinical Pearls

- Pediatric psychosocial oncology professionals face extreme suffering in children and families dealing with cancer and are at risk for vicarious traumatization, secondary traumatic stress, and compassion fatigue.
- The constant exposure to the suffering and hardship of others erodes resilience in ways that are insidious and potentially damaging to the practitioner.
- Personal strategies to prevent and ameliorate vicarious trauma include but are not limited to work-life balance, opportunities for reflection and professional growth, and mindfulness and compassion-based interventions.
- Adequate staffing, structured support, and an ongoing awareness and education about compassion fatigue and secondary traumatic stress responses are useful interventions and support sustainability within the pediatric oncology setting.
- A well-functioning interprofessional team can offer protection against secondary trauma if professionals feel that they are able to openly discuss, share, and receive support for the distress that they witness daily.

References

Aycock N, Boyle D (2009) Interventions to manage compassion fatigue in oncology nursing. Clinical Journal of Oncology Nursing 13(2):183–191

Beach MC, Roter D, Korthuis PT, Epstein RM, Sharp V, Ratanawongsa N, Cohn J, Eggly S, Sankar A, Moore RD, Saha S (2013) A multicenter study of physician mindfulness and health care quality. Annals of Family Medicine 11(5):428

Beck CT (2011) Secondary trauma stress in nurses: a systematic review. Archives of Psychiatric Nursing 25(1):1–10

Brown C (2006) Promoting self-caring and healing in your workplace. American Nurse Today 1(12):54–55

Chen PW (2013, September 26). Easing doctor burnout with mindfulness. The New York Times. Retrieved from www.nytimes.com

Crumpei I, Dafinoiu I (2011) The relation of clinical empathy to secondary traumatic stress. Procedia: Social and Behavioral Sciences 33:438–442

Dane B, Chachkes E (2001) The cost of caring for patients with an illness: contagion to the social worker. Social Work in Health Care 33(2):31–51

Ellwood L, Mott J, Lohr J, Galovski J (2011) Secondary trauma symptoms in clinicians: a critical review of the construct, specificity and implications for trauma focused treatment. Clinical Psychology Review 31:25–36

Emanuel L, Ferris FD, von Gunten CF, Von Roenn JH (2011) Combating compassion fatigue and burnout in cancer care. Excerpted from EPEC-O: education in palliative and end-of-life care for oncology (Module 15: Cancer Doctors and Burnout). Accessed on 21 Nov 2014 at www.medscape.com/viewarticle/742941

Figley C (1995) Compassion fatigue as secondary traumatic stress disorder: an overview. In: Figley C (ed) Compassion fatigue: coping with secondary traumatic stress disorder in those who treat the traumatized. Psychological stress, vol 23. Brunner Mazel, Philadelphia, pp 1–20

Figley C, Huggard C, Rees CE (2013) First do no self harm: understanding and promoting physician stress resilience. Oxford University Press, New York

Fortney L, Luchterhand C, Zakletskaia L, Zgierska A, Rakel D (2013) Abbreviated mindfulness intervention for job satisfaction, quality of life, and compassion in primary care clinicians: a pilot study. Annals of Family Medicine 11(5):412–420

Granek L, Bartels U, Scheinemann K, Labrecque M, Barrera M (2015) Grief reactions and impact of patient death on pediatric oncologists. Pediatr Blood Cancer 62(1): 134–142. doi:10.1002/pbc.25228, Epub 2014 Sep 11

Gentry J, Baranowsky A, Dunning K (2002) The accelerated recovery program for compassion fatigue. In: Figley C (ed) Treating compassion fatigue. Routledge, New York, pp 123–137

Halifax J (2011) The precious necessity of compassion. Journal of Pain and Symptom Management 41(1):146–153

Hellerstein D (2011) How can I become more resilient? In: Heal your brain: exploring the new neuropsychiatry. Psychology Today. Retrieved 12/12/14. http://www.psychologytoday.com/blog/heal-your-brain/201108/how-can-i-become-more-resilient

Jones B (2004) "Tucked in My Heart": The role of social work in pediatric palliative and end-of-life care. A mixed methodology study. (Doctoral dissertation). Available from ProQuestDissertations and Theses database. (Document ID 3132861). University of Texas at Austin

Jones B (2006) Tucked in my heart: the use of ethnopoetry to represent the meaning-making of social workers in pediatric palliative care. Journal of Palliative Medicine 9(3):789–790

Joubert L, Hocking A, Hampson R (2013) Social work in oncology-managing vicarious trauma- the positive impact of professional supervision. Social Work in Health Care 52(2-3):296–310

Kabat-Zinn J (1994) Wherever you go, there you are: mindfulness meditation in everyday life. Hyperion, New York: NY

Kabat-Zinn J (2003) Mindfulness-based interventions in context: past, present, and future. Clinical psychology: Science and practice 10(2):144–156

Katz R, Johnson T (2006) When professionals weep: emotional and countertransference responses in end of life care. Routledge, New York

Li A, Early S, Mahrer N, Klaristenfeld K, Gold J (2014) Group cohesion and organizational commitment: protective factors for nurse residents' job satisfaction, compassion fatigue, compassion satisfaction and burnout. Professional Nursing 30:89–99

Maytum J, Bielski-Heiman M, Garwick A (2004) Compassion fatigue and burnout in nurses who work with children with chronic conditions and their families. Journal of Pediatric Health Care 18:171–179

Moody K, Kramer D, Santizo R, Magro L, Wyshogrod D, Ambrosio J, Castillo C, Lieberman R, Stein J (2013) Helping the helpers: mindfulness training for burnout in pediatric oncology- a pilot program. Journal of Pediatric Oncology Nursing 30:275–284

Najjar N, Davis LW, Beck-Coon K, Doebbeling CC (2009) Compassion fatigue: a review of the research to date and relevance to cancer care providers. Journal of Health Psychology 14(2):267–277

Pearlman L, McKay L (2008) Understanding and addressing vicarious Trauma. Headington Institute. Retrieved 12/12/14: http://www.headington-institute.org/files/vicarious-trauma-handout_85433.pdf

Praissman S (2008) Mindfulness-based stress reduction: a literature review and clinician's guide. Journal of American Academy of Nurse Practitioners 20:212–216

Robins P, Meltzer L, Zelikovsky N (2009) The experience of secondary traumatic stress upon care providers working within a children's hospital. Journal of Pediatric Nursing 24(4):270–279

Rohan E, Bausch J (2009) Climbing Everest: oncology work as an expedition in caring. Journal of Psychosocial Oncology 27(1):84–118

Rossi A, Cetrano G, Pertile R, Rabbi L, Donisi V, Grigoletti L, Curtolo C, Tansella M, Thornicroft G, Amaddeo F (2012) Burnout, compassion fatigue, and compassion satisfaction among staff in community-based mental health services. Psychiatry Research 200(2012):933–938

Rourke M (2007) Compassion fatigue in pediatric palliative care providers. Pediatric Clinics of North America 54(2007):631–644

Sinclair H, Hamill C (2007) Does vicarious traumatization affect oncology nurses? A literature review European Journal of Oncology Nursing 11:348–356

Ting L, Sanders S, Jacobson JM, Power J (2006) Dealing with the aftermath: a qualitative analysis of mental health social workers' reactions after a client suicide. Social Work 51:329–341

Townsend SM, Campbell R (2009) Organizational correlates of secondary traumatic stress and burnout among sexual assault nurse examiners. Journal of Forensic Nursing 5:97–106

Van Dernoot Lipsy L, Burk C (2009) Trauma stewardship: an everyday guide to caring for self while caring for others. Berrett-Koehler Publishers, San Francisco

White W (1997) The incestuous workplace: stress and distress in the organizational family. Hazelden, Center City

Zadeh S et al (2012) Taking care of care providers: a wellness program for pediatric nurses. Journal of Pediatric Oncology Nursing 29(5):294–299

Zanders M, Hutton A, King L (2013) Exploring resilience in paediatric oncology nursing staff. Collegian 20:17–25

Parents' Perspective on the Role of Psychosocial Care in Pediatric Oncology

22

Victoria A. Sardi-Brown and Peter J. Brown

Introduction

It is well understood that cancer is the worldwide leading cause of death by disease (World Health Organization 2014). However, in our society, it is much more common for people to know adults who have been diagnosed with cancer rather than children. Children are not supposed to contract life-threatening illnesses and potentially die before their parents. This goes against the natural order of life. On a daily basis, we are inundated with news and exposed to crises and tragedies both nationally and internationally through the media. People seem intrigued to view all sorts of other news and videos online but shy away from those associated with childhood cancer. These visuals stimulate parents' worst fears and therefore in order to cope with such painful realities, sometimes parents of healthy children rationalize childhood cancer away by saying, "this couldn't possibly happen to my child."

Each year, 15,700 families in the United States hear, "your child has cancer" (CureSearch 2014). It is hard to imagine how four little words can transform your life, but they do in a very surreal way. Almost as if you are a bystander in a car crash and you are watching it happen in slow motion. In slow motion, because with childhood cancer, it is not just the one time diagnosis that is tragic and overwhelming, but instead, the cancer journey is a series of significant losses. As a parent, you long for the life you left behind and yet you are cognizant that things will never be the same again.

When a child is diagnosed with cancer, parents are faced with a multitude of pervasive stressors such as the burden of adhering to a complicated treatment regiment (Pai et al. 2007) and significant medical side effects (Bryant 2003; Pai et al. 2007), but "childhood cancer is not just about the medicine" (Mattie Miracle Cancer Foundation 2014). The common factor that unites all children and families together is the psychological and social concerns, fears, and day-to-day management of the disease. The whole family is affected and forever changed (Alderfer and Kazak 2006; Varni et al. 1996; Wallander et al. 1992). Childhood cancer is as much a psychological disease as it is a physical one in which children and families need help managing the day-to-day isolation, pain, treatment challenges, and the consequences on their daily life. Childhood cancer threatens every aspect of the family's life and the possibility of a future, which is why optimal cancer treatment must include psychosocial care services (Institute of Medicine 2008).

V.A. Sardi-Brown, PhD, LPC (✉)
P.J. Brown, MBA
Mattie Miracle Cancer Foundation,
6485, Arlington, VA 22206, USA
e-mail: vicki@mattiemiracle.com;
pbrown@mattiemiracle.com

A.N. Abrams et al. (eds.), *Pediatric Psychosocial Oncology: Textbook for Multidisciplinary Care*,
DOI 10.1007/978-3-319-21374-3_22

This chapter is written by two parent advocates who give voice to their son, Mattie, and his courageous journey with osteosarcoma. We discuss our perspectives on the role of psychosocial care along the cancer continuum from the time of diagnosis to end-of-life care, highlighting conversations and approaches that were learned along the journey. Finally, the collaboration between parent advocates and leading health-care providers that is underway to develop national psychosocial standards of care for childhood cancer is described.

Mattie Brown and The Mattie Miracle Cancer Foundation

Mattie was born on April 4, 2002. Mattie was a precocious child who demonstrated many strengths, such as a sense of humor, observational skills, ability to understand how things worked (at the tender age of two he was disassembling and reassembling his hot wheel cars with a screwdriver), and empathy beyond his years. He had a vivacious and voracious need to have fun, and he convinced others to participate in his antics. In July of 2008, when Mattie was 6 years old and attending a tennis camp, he complained of pain in his right arm. When the symptoms got worse, his pediatrician ordered an x-ray, which revealed a mass suggestive of osteosarcoma in Mattie's right humerus. CT, MRI, PET scans, and a biopsy confirmed four primary tumor sites: (1) right humerus, (2) left humerus, (3) right femur, and (4) left radius. We were informed that our only child had multifocal synchronous osteosarcoma.

Sixteen days after diagnosis, Mattie began 14 months of treatment including high-dosage chemotherapies with doxorubicin, cisplatin, methotrexate, ifosfamide, and etoposide. He underwent three limb-salvaging surgeries and a bone graft. Eleven months after his diagnosis, Mattie had a sternotomy, to remove the nine tumors found in his lungs.

What we, as Mattie's parents and our family members, observed was his struggle to learn how to cope with the profound functional impact of his surgeries and the change in his daily life due to his treatments. He could no longer walk, run, dress, or toilet himself. Within months of his second surgery, Mattie began working with a child psychiatrist who diagnosed him with clinical depression, anxiety, and medical post-traumatic stress disorder. He was started on Celexa and Klonopin to reduce his significant sadness and anxiety.

In August of 2009, only 6 weeks off of chemotherapy, scan results revealed that Mattie's cancer had spread to his lungs and liver. Conversations with Mattie's medical team turned from curative intent to end-of-life care. We had to face our worst fears: the reality that our child was dying and the stressful and frightening medical decisions associated with this reality. Mattie died on September 8, 2009.

The devastation of losing a child to cancer is both unimaginable and indescribable for parents. Such a death symbolizes a reversal of the natural order of life and it erases the dreams and hopes that parents have for their child and for themselves (Alam et al. 2012). Parents may continue to grieve long after the death of their child (Kreichbergs et al. 2004; Wing et al. 2001). Such chronic grief has been associated with many psychological (e.g., depression and anxiety) and somatic symptoms (e.g., loss of appetite, sleep disturbances, and fatigue), including increased mortality risk (Alam et al. 2012; Li et al. 2003; Wing et al. 2001; Znoj and Keller 2002). In November of 2009, two months after Mattie's death, we created the Mattie Miracle Cancer Foundation, a 501(c)(3) tax-exempt public charity. Mattie Miracle is headquartered in Washington, DC, and is dedicated to addressing the psychosocial needs of children and families living with childhood cancer as well as educating health-care providers on the impact of such a diagnosis on children and their families. The foundation enhances awareness, advocacy, and access to psychosocial support on both the local and national levels.

Psychosocial Care along the Continuum

The provision of psychosocial care has been shown to yield better management of common disease-related symptoms and adverse effects of treatment such as pain and fatigue (Jaaniste et al. 2007; Jacobsen et al. 2012; Kazak 2005). Within the first few days and weeks of a diagnosis, parents immediately seek out information and supportive resources to reduce the chaos they are experiencing (Björk et al. 2005). However, the strain of such a diagnosis can send parents into shock (McGrath et al. 2007) making it difficult to recall and process medical information under stress (Jedlicka-Köhler et al. 1996). Parents are learning medical terminology, understanding the nature of their child's disease and treatment plan, maintaining their child's day-to-day care, figuring out how a hospital works and the hierarchy of the personnel within it, and of course doing all of these while potentially trying to maintain a job and the rest of their family's obligations.

Establishing a therapeutic alliance between psychosocial professionals and children/parents is a vital aspect of pooling resources together toward a common goal (Masera et al. 1998). Though parents need the support, guidance, and resources that their psychosocial care team provides, it is important for clinicians to approach families right from the beginning with the attitude that they are an integral part of the treatment team. Parents have an expert understanding of their own children and clinicians need to respect these insights. This is critically important for parents who feel vulnerable and powerless over their child's disease (Holm et al. 2003) and the uncertainty surrounding their child's treatment outcome.

Diagnosis: Fight Mode

After Mattie was diagnosed with cancer, we went into a mental fight mode, in which we became hypervigilant about his care and sought out vast amounts of medical information about osteosarcoma. Though we understood Mattie had a poor prognosis, we did not want to give up hope. In fact, the fight mode kept us very focused on Mattie's care and empowered us to help him cope with cancer. Mattie was a sensitive and intuitive child, and like many children, he took his cues from us, his parents. If Mattie had sensed our fears about his treatment, it would have negatively impacted his outlook on his cancer care. It is imperative for psychosocial providers to respect the significance of this fight mode and understand that trying to discuss emotionally laden issues at this point in time may be counterproductive, particularly if parents are in the same room as their child.

As Mattie's parents, it was very hard for us to accept that he had cancer and even harder to come to terms with all the doctors and professionals who entered our world on a daily basis. It was a huge adjustment to move from our home into a hospital for months on end, leaving behind life as we knew it. We also were conflicted because on the one hand, we wanted to do what was in Mattie's best interest, but on the other hand, we did not want to be in a hospital, have Mattie deal with childhood cancer, or have conversations with psychosocial staff members on how cancer was going to impact our son, our marriage, and our lives. Clinicians need to be aware that some parents may not want to hear this information upfront and may be hesitant to receiving advice on how their child is coping. After all, parents have served their role for years prior to meeting psychosocial providers, and it can be very difficult to receive guidance and insights from someone, who, until very recently, has been unfamiliar with one's child and family.

As an example, when Mattie was undergoing his first round of chemotherapy, his psychosocial care providers told us they were concerned about how we were managing and coping with his diagnosis. They were particularly concerned that we were spending 24 hours a day in Mattie's room and not emoting our feelings about his diagnosis. They felt we needed a reprieve from the hospital and went so far as to check us into the on-campus hotel. Despite their efforts, we never used the hotel room or left Mattie's side. What was not assessed was our family's dynamics and structure prior to Mattie developing cancer. If this was assessed, then it would have been understood that we had a very close family bond and connection. Mattie was never left unsupervised even when healthy, so most certainly when undergoing chemotherapy, he would not have been left by himself at the hospital to manage this alone.

It took time for us to build a relationship with the oncology team and to experience that we were working as a team, toward the same goal. Providing too much or too little information can cause anxiety in parents (McGrath et al. 2007), but the key is for clinicians to be able to read parent cues and when uncertain about the quantity of information, simply ask parents for feedback. Additionally, taking the time to learn about the family is advantageous to both the family and the professional. Asking about the family's functioning prior to a cancer diagnosis helps to build trust and rapport and is a comfortable way to collect information about the child and to learn about family resources, coping mechanisms, and strategies that will help along the cancer journey.

The Hospital

One of the most surprising things to all children and parents undergoing treatment for the first time is being in a hospital. It is an absolutely foreign culture, with its own language, time schedule, people, and chain of commands, regulations, and food. Arming families with knowledge helps them feel more in control and able to cope and manage their needs more effectively. Prior to being admitted, parents should be introduced to where treatment will be administered, what patient rooms look like, what kind of storage space exists in these rooms, whether families have to share bathrooms, and how to access food, laundry, and other resources in the hospital or in the vicinity. Like the analogy of an immigrant moving into a foreign land, when parents become inpatient in a pediatric unit, they learn to acculturate into the medical world while bringing with them aspects of their "home" culture. This may be subtle (decorations, music, celebrations), but these traditions are important to the family, and they help to provide a sense of normalcy.

Treatment

Mattie's treatment was primarily done on an inpatient basis. We spent very little time at home as a family. Vicki, Mattie's mom, gave up her professional obligations to oversee Mattie's care and though Peter, Mattie's dad, continued to work so the family had health benefits, he slept at the hospital every night with the family. Therefore, the hospital became our second home. In the beginning of treatment, when Peter would go to work in the morning, Vicki was left to manage Mattie's care alone. Vicki found it daunting and was not sure she could handle it by herself. Since there were crises at every turn, big decisions were always being made regarding Mattie's care, and the days were extremely long and tedious.

Mattie's dad was torn each day between leaving his family at the hospital and going to work. The conflict and stress of leaving the ones you love behind made his daily existence simply unbearable. Most people at work avoided asking how Peter was doing or how Mattie was, as it made them uncomfortable. Everyone could see the emotional pain Peter was going through, but few had the courage to ask him how he was doing. Having no outlet and shuttling between work and "home" (i.e., the hospital) left Peter feeling as if he was only a partial participant in both worlds, leaving him emotionally isolated and professionally alienated.

Two examples will illustrate the need for early comprehensive psychosocial assessments. We were constant advocates for Mattie's needs and encouraged his oncologist and treatment team to consider sedating him for all scans. Given that we knew Mattie's history with sensory integration issues prior to his cancer diagnosis, we understood that he was highly sensitive to sound, tight spaces, and being confined in any way. However, we were consistently told that PET and CT scans were short and noninvasive, and for safety reasons, it would be better for Mattie to manage without sedation. The team believed that with staff, family reassurance, and some distractions, Mattie could manage the scans. It was not until the head of pediatric sedation nursing and the child life specialist observed the terror Mattie experienced when attempting a CT scan without sedation that a new scanning strategy was implemented. Information about his sensory issues and coping abilities obtained up front could have potentially avoided the additional anxiety, stress, fear, and trauma Mattie experienced by being required to stay still in the scanner. Moreover, this stress carried over into all treatments he perceived as invasive, and as a result despite our best efforts, we were left feeling as if we failed to protect our child.

The second example pertains to the delivery of scan results. When Mattie had his first MRI scan, we were in the pediatric inpatient unit and can vividly remember a team of ten people walking down the hallway to deliver the news. The team was comprised of medical staff, psychosocial providers, and the chaplain. We knew immediately what we were about to hear. We encouraged Mattie to go into his room with his child life specialist, so we could protect him from this news until we could digest the information for ourselves. Psychosocial providers are our advocates, and having a strategy in place that reflects parents' coping needs and learning style, including which professionals would be helpful to have present when scan results are received, would help empower families and give them a better sense of control.

End of Life

Hope, as we knew it, died the day we learned Mattie's cancer metastasized, when all treatment options were exhausted, and the conversation turned to "making him comfortable." Mattie's physicians never used the word death or dying with us. It was Mattie's nurses who were very direct and told us that Mattie was dying. Once this reality was disclosed, his physicians began talking to us about Do Not Resuscitate orders and other directives. Perhaps the medical team was so invested in saving Mattie's life, facing his death and accepting the limits of medicine were exceptionally challenging to address with us directly.

When Mattie died, we not only lost our son, our only child, but all that came with our roles as a parent such as the prospect of a wonderful life watching Mattie grow and flourish, holidays and making our own traditions and memories, and the new adventures and rewarding experiences that come with raising a child and being a parent. Although subtle at first, new types of losses continued after Mattie's death. The house became more quiet than a place of worship, summer vacations were no longer child friendly, there were no graduations to look forward to, or weekend children's birthday parties and holidays did not seem as festive anymore. With the death of our only child, we lost our purpose and direction in life, we lost our social circle, as this was largely comprised of parents of Mattie's friends, we had no more parental milestones or "firsts" to look forward to, and no more chances to see the world through our child's eyes.

We came to the hospital as three and on the day Mattie died, we left as two. That was a profound loss, which was compounded by the fact that we also had to say goodbye to our daily support network at the hospital, a network who had been with us through a 14-month cancer journey. Leaving the hospital and trying to reintegrate back into the world was and continues to be hard for both of us, especially for Mattie's mom, who has not returned to her previous professional role. In the first month after Mattie's death, friends told her she needed counseling, they wanted her "fixed" so she could go back to being the person she was. So Vicki went to talk with Mattie's social worker. The advice she received remains with her always and has carried her forward. The advice was, "who is the counseling for, you or for your friends?" Though well intentioned, friends and even some family members are not always sure how to help grieving parents and in the process can make one feel like they are not grieving and coping the "right" way. Psychosocial providers need to remind parents there is no right way to grieve. There is no timeline, there are no quick fixes, and importantly, parents need to be prepared with this information before being discharged from the care of the psychosocial team.

For some parents, advocacy can be an antidote to overwhelming helplessness or grief. Yet, for the grieving parent, there can also be loneliness with that experience. When Mattie died, we also discovered that we no longer fit into the cancer world, since we did not have a child fighting for a cure or one who was in survivorship mode. This has left us in a very precarious position, as we are still trying to figure out our place in the world. We may look childless to most people now, but the fact of the matter is in our hearts we will always be parents and we were also parents to a child who had cancer. As providers of psychosocial care, you must remember the importance of the role you play and the support you deliver as this will help parents in their new reality of living a life without their child.

The Psychosocial Standards of Care Project for Childhood Cancer

Given the growing recognition that psychosocial care is an important component of comprehensive care for people diagnosed with cancer (IOM 2008), there is a demand for accountability and outcome-driven, cost-effective models for this care. Psychosocial clinicians are being challenged to standardize their approach and evaluate the efficacy of their clinical efforts (Noll et al. 2013; Wiener et al. 2014).

We have tried to find meaning and perspective from Mattie's suffering by advocating for the development of National Psychosocial Standards of Care to support children and their families along the cancer continuum. Based upon our experiences, we believe that psychosocial care is an essential component to the treatment and care of childhood cancer and began advocating on Capitol Hill in 2010 for these issues. We initiated the effort for national psychosocial standards of care so that all children and families living with childhood cancer receive a minimum level of psychosocial care from time of diagnosis through survivorship or end-of-life care.

The Psychosocial Standards of Care Project for Childhood Care (PSCPCC) was initiated in 2012. The Project involves over four dozen researchers and clinicians representing the fields of psychology, psychiatry, hematology/oncology, nursing, social work, child life, and parent advocates. The project's standards, containing recommendations and guidelines built on evidence-based research and consensus, will be published as a Special Issue in the journal *Pediatric Blood and Cancer, in press*. The project is committed to creating and disseminating a twenty-first century, widely applicable blueprint to support universally available psychosocial services (Wiener et al. 2015).

References

Alam R, Barrera M, D'Agostino N, Nicholas DB, Schneiderman G (2012) Bereavement experiences of mothers and fathers over time after the death of a child due to cancer. Death Stud 36(1):1–22

Alderfer M, Kazak AE (2006) Family issues when a child is on treatment for cancer. In: Brown RT (ed) Comprehensive handbook of childhood cancer and sickle cell disease. Oxford University Press, New York, pp 53–75

Björk M, Wiebe T, Hallström I (2005) Striving to survive: families' lived experiences when a child is diagnosed with cancer. J Pediatr Oncol Nurs 22:265–275

Bryant R (2003) Managing side effects of childhood cancer treatment. J Pediatr Nurs 18:113–125

CureSearch for Children's Cancer (2014) Childhood cancer statistics. Retrieved from http://www.curesearch.org/Childhood-Cancer-Statistics/

Holm KE, Patterson JM, Gurney JG (2003) Parental involvement and family-centered care in the diagnostic and treatment phases of childhood cancer: results from a qualitative study. J Pediatr Oncol Nurs 20(6):301–313

Institute of Medicine of the National Academies (2008) Cancer care for the whole patient: meeting psychosocial health needs. National Academies Press, Washington, DC

Jaaniste T, Hayes B, von Baeyer CL (2007) Providing children with Information about forthcoming medical procedures: a review and synthesis. Clin Psychol Sci Pract 14:124–143

Jacobsen PB, Holland JC, Steensma DP (2012) Caring for the whole patient: the science of psychosocial care. J Clin Oncol 30(11):1151–1153

Jedlicka-Köhler I, Götz M, Eichler I (1996) Parents' recollection of the initial communication of the diagnosis of cystic fibrosis. Pediatrics 97:204–209

Kazak A (2005) Evidence-based interventions for survivors of childhood cancer and their families. J Pediatr Psychol 30(1):29–39

Kreichbergs U, Valdimarsdottir U, Onelov E, Henter JI, Steineck G (2004) Talking about death with children who have severe malignant disease. N Engl J Med 351:1175–1186

Li J, Precht DH, Mortensen PB, Olsen J (2003) Mortality in parents after death of a child in Denmark: a nationwide follow-up study. Lancet 361:363–367

Masera G, Spinetta JJ, Jankovic M, Ablin AR, Buchwall I, Van Dongen-Melman J, Eden T, Epelman C, Green DM, Kosmidis HV, Yoheved S, Martins AG, Mor W, Oppenheim D, Petrilli AS, Schuler D, Topf R, Wilbur JR, Chesler MA (1998) Guidelines for a therapeutic alliance between families and staff: a report of the SIOP working committee on psychosocial issues in pediatric oncology. Med Pediatr Oncol 30:183–186

Mattie Miracle Cancer Foundation (2014) Retrieved from http://www.mattiemiracle.com/

McGrath P, Kail-Buckley S, Philips E (2007) Learning a new language. Informational issues for parents of children treated for acute lymphoblastic leukaemia. Aust Asian J Cancer 6:205–212

Noll RB, Patel SK, Embry L, Hardy KK, Pelletier W, Annett RD, Patenaude A, Lown EA, Sands SA, Barakat LP (2013) Children's Oncology Group's 2013 blueprint for research: behavioral science. Pediatr Blood Cancer 60:1048–1054

Pai ALH, Greenley RN, Lewandowski A, Drotar D, Youngstrom E, Peterson CC (2007) A meta-analytic review of the influence of pediatric cancer on parent and family functioning. J Fam Psychol 21(3):407–415

Varni JW, Katz ER, Colegrove R, Dolgin M (1996) Family functioning predictors of adjustment in children with newly diagnosed cancer: a prospective analysis. J Child Psychol Psychiatr 37: 321–328

Wallander JL, Varni JW, Babani L, Banis HT, Wilcox KT (1992) Family resources as resistance factors for psychological maladjustment in chronically ill and handicapped children. In: Roberts MC, Wallander JC (eds) Family issues in pediatric psychology. Lawrence Erlbaum Associates, Hillsdale, pp 129–145

Wiener L, Viola A, Koretski J, Perper ED, Patenaude AF (2015) Pediatric psycho-oncology care: standards, guidelines, and consensus reports. Psychooncology. 24(2):204-11doi:10.1002/pon.3589

Wing DG, Clance PR, Burge-Callaway K, Armistead L (2001) Understanding gender differences in bereavement following the death of an infant: implications for treatment. Psychotherapy 38:60–73

World Health Organization (2014) Cancer Fact Sheet. Retrieved from http://www.who.int/mediacentre/factsheets/fs297/en/

Znoj HJ, Keller D (2002) Mourning parents: considering safeguards and their relationship to health. Death Stud 26:545–565

In Their Own Voices: Experiences of Children and Adolescents with Cancer

23

Michael H. Tang

> I guess [cancer] is going to affect everybody differently. It all depends on what's going on in your life. – Scott (Tang 2013)

In 2000, I was a 20-year-old college junior, 10 years removed from completing cancer treatment. Both for academic interest and to place my own experience in a larger context, for my undergraduate thesis in sociology, I wanted to interview cancer survivors from diverse ethnic and socioeconomic backgrounds. This project was approved both by my college and the hospital where all the interviewees were treated for cancer (see study methodology below). To encourage them to speak freely, none of the interviewees knew during the main portion of the interview that I had cancer as a child. Below are some of the topics they described.

> The predominant theme that I'm trying to get at is that I had a normal life before [cancer], I wanted to keep the normal life during, and now I want to continue with the normal life—normal being life outside cancer. – Roberto

The word "normal" was used by the vast majority of those I interviewed. It was used to refer to three main types of "normal": a physical normal (such as having hair after being bald from chemotherapy), a social normal (such as attending school after being hospitalized), and an internal normal (including psychologically feeling "fine" despite the disruptions). The quest for a normal life played out in all areas of these children's lives, including at the hospital, home, school, within cancer organizations, and in the media.

M.H. Tang, MD
Department of Pediatrics, The Dimock Center,
55 Dimock Street, Roxbury, MA 02119, USA
e-mail: mhtang@dimock.org

Hospital

At diagnosis, most of the people I spoke with believed cancer was a fatal illness, despite the actual 75 % cure rates for pediatric cancers. Physicians and staff played a major role in communicating that cancer is not "a death sentence," destigmatizing the disease through education, emotional support, and encouraging the maintenance of an age-appropriate routine:

> [The doctors and nurses] just treated you normal, just like they should. You're just another person that they're helping. – Mark

However, several minority and low-income patients reported communication barriers:

> Yeah, the doctors tried to tell me what was going on. But they used those terms that I didn't understand. I was like, "what?" – Dontae

A.N. Abrams et al. (eds.), *Pediatric Psychosocial Oncology: Textbook for Multidisciplinary Care*,
DOI 10.1007/978-3-319-21374-3_23

Another adolescent, whose parents did not graduate from high school, summarized that at diagnosis and throughout treatment:

> My parents didn't have enough education about cancer to know and be able to tell me. I didn't have enough education, no one from my family had that education, so it was hard. We had no knowledge, therefore we didn't know what to expect. Farheen

Home

The support of family was instrumental for those interviewed. I heard stories of parents providing a shoulder to cry on, cleaning up vomit, holding hands before surgeries, and staying with their children overnight in the hospital. Families also held their own views about cancer. Several people suggested that stereotypes of cancer as a fatal disease weighed heavily on their families, making coping more challenging, perhaps particularly among immigrants:

> So people, especially from the Hispanic area, when they would think of cancer, they would think of death. They got that attitude from their parents and they gave the attitude to us… So I thought about death and what would happen after I die. That depressed me a little bit when I was going through cancer. – Manuel

One person described the effect of cancer on his single father, who lost his job after taking too much time off from work to care for his son:

> The bad things of having had cancer? Probably more say with my family. Like my dad had a good job, he was happy, he had a girlfriend, and he lost all that because of me. We lost a lot. A lot of time, a lot of money. There were a lot of negative things that came out of it. – Dave

School

Those interviewed described missing school and facing the challenge of keeping up academically. In an effort to keep cancer patients with their peers, despite not fulfilling all of the academic requirements, several of the survivors reported being socially promoted to the next grade:

> The school was really good. It was at the end of fourth grade when they first found [my cancer]. And my principal told my mom to just pass me. 'Just go on to the fifth grade.' I think that was probably the best thing to do. – Cynthia

Peers at school also provided support:

> [My friends] would sit with me in lunch hour and talk. They'd act like nothing was different. They'd act like I was just anybody else. That was really helpful. – Traci

School also had negative experiences; the vast majority of people described stigmatizing incidences, and about half recounted overt bullying from peers. While Traci had supportive friends, described above, she also faced these experiences:

> There were other kids in the school that were particularly mean. When I came back [to school], I had no hair, so I had to wear a wig. So there would be incidents where the people pulled things off, things like that. They were very traumatic. I'd hide in my locker at lunchtime. I could actually get in my locker and close it from the inside… I just wanted to disappear. – Traci

One person, who attended an urban public school, recounted the stigma of being held back a grade and being ignored by peers:

> I missed a whole year of school, so I actually had to repeat second grade and was a whole year behind. [When I returned to school] nobody wanted to be my friend. They felt like cancer was something they could catch by touching me… Nobody wanted to talk to me, so I kind of lost my identity. – Gloria

While Gloria's school did not educate her classmates about cancer, almost half of the people reported their schools gave formal presentations that helped dispel misinformation and ease the transition back to school. In my school, a counselor met with my 5th grade classmates to explain why I was missing school and losing my hair, and I wonder if this helped minimize stigma from my peers.

Cancer Camp, Organizations, and the Media

Specialized camps provide an opportunity for children who are undergoing or have completed cancer treatment to interact with other survivors.

Of those interviewed, almost half participated in a local camp. Cancer organizations, such as the Make-A-Wish Foundation, often donate computers and tickets to sporting events. The media can also provide unique chances for children to be featured in uplifting local newspapers stories and television broadcasts. Overall, the vast majority of the interviewees were involved with one of these "special opportunities" for children with cancer, through camps, cancer organizations, or the media. While these interviews predated the widespread use of social media and Internet-based cancer support groups, these online forums could play a similar role for children with cancer.

Cancer camps and organizations helped many of those I interviewed adopt a more positive attitude toward their cancer; of those who attended camp, almost all believed it was valuable:

> Those years [at camp], I learned who I was, what I could do, what I was capable of doing. And I came away knowing that I am capable of doing just about anything. I can do anything that a normal person can. – Greg

Several minority and low-income interviewees suggested these positive opportunities particularly benefited them, since they typically could not afford access to these special events, such as premium tickets at a baseball game:

> I was an urban kid; I didn't get skybox seats! When I went to [the stadium], we broke in! – Juan

Through cancer organizations, I attended Chicago Bulls basketball games and received a free computer, which I believe helped make my cancer experience more positive. While I was given the opportunity to attend a cancer camp, I never accepted, partly because as an Asian-American who grew up in a city, my family and I never viewed camping as a recreational activity. And while many people highlighted the positives, these special opportunities can have negative sides, as one person recalled about her time at a camp:

> I didn't like going to camp. I didn't like the bunk beds or the food. And it was kind of depressing, being around kids that—they weren't all survivors. They were still undergoing treatment and such. There were worse cases, like going to camp with people and reading that they just died a month later or things like that. I didn't really enjoy it that much. – Rebecca

As described in a separate account, celebrity portrayals in the media, such as Lance Armstrong, can also influence the attitudes of adolescents with cancer (Tang 2013). For example, Tiffany discussed the impact television had on her as she tried to make sense of her past:

> Just seeing what other people [with cancer] go through, and as an adult looking back and seeing what I've been through [having had cancer]… I've watched a lot of Biography and shows like that. So seeing how my life was and how other people's lives were, I'm like, "my experience really was traumatic." Now I see my life has been—could have been—as traumatic as other people's. They're calling themselves survivors, I guess I am too. That's how I look at it now. – Tiffany

Cancer Narratives

Given the diversity of experiences people had in the hospital, home, school, camps, and cancer organizations, how did cancer affect people overall? While most people I spoke with described their illness in moderate ways—with mostly neutral or positive assessments—these two examples illustrate the full spectrum in which interviewees described their cancer experiences.

Jamilla is an African-American Hodgkin's disease survivor over 30 years old at the time of the interview. She did not graduate from high school and was unemployed. Jamilla recalled her experience during her cancer treatment:

> [It was] hard to get along with kids at school, because they heard the rumor around that I had cancer and they thought if I touched them they'd get it. I really didn't have too many friends then.

There were also communication breakdowns with her oncologist at the hospital:

> [The doctor] said when I would get older it would be a 95 % chance that it would come back.

It is improbable that a pediatric oncologist would inform her of a 95 % chance of recurrence, since, even at the time, Hodgkin's disease was approximately 87 % curable. Since Jamilla believed there was a 95 % chance of recurrence, she suspected her cancer had relapsed:

> I guess I'm supposed to have [cancer] somewhere in my throat. The doctor said he was afraid to do surgery because I would have to take medicines. And I guess he said he didn't want to do it because at the time I wasn't really taking my medicine right. Instead, I just didn't get the surgery done.

Overall, Jamilla thought she was dying of an untreated cancer, so she was applying for welfare and government disability benefits. She also alluded to psychological traumas, when she was asked to define a cancer survivor:

> It's the bad things that you went through while you're sick. That's what it means to me… I don't think about cancer and I try to keep it as far from my mind as possible, because I remember every little thing that happened to me and it emotionally hurts. My mind is still scarred by it.

Jamilla's experiences and perceptions contrasted with Bill, a white survivor of cancer, whose father was a physician. Bill reported receiving excellent support at the hospital:

> It was nice for me because I got the best of everything; my dad knew all the questions to ask. Whereas a lot of other people who are uneducated or overwhelmed with the whole situation, they don't know what kinds of questions to ask. My dad knew everything, so it was a big help to me.

Bill also received get-well cards from his classmates at school and was active in a local cancer camp. Because of this support from his family, friends, teachers, camp, and cancer organizations, Bill believed his illness had only positive effects:

> I don't think having had cancer has affected me negatively at all. It has made me more open, it has made me a better person than I was before. I can't complain about anything. If I had to go through it again, I would definitely go through it again.

Overall Bill spoke about his view toward cancer survivors:

> I think anyone who has had the courage and the strength to beat cancer has really accomplished something. Every kid at that camp is my hero. I think anybody who has beaten cancer, I think they are true heroes.

Hearing the stories of these 32 people and writing my undergraduate thesis became part of my own cancer narrative. I am now a pediatrician, child and adult psychiatrist, and have the opportunity to work with many adults who as children faced illnesses and other obstacles. How does one make sense of his or her experiences? Is a person "scarred" by trauma or does a person perceive oneself as a "hero" who won the war against hardship? These stories taught me that there is no single narrative for being a cancer survivor; each person faces a diversity of positive and negative experiences that are shaped by his or her social context. Both during treatment and for the years after the cure, each survivor strives to build a "new normal," creating his or her own story about life with cancer.

Study Methodology

Using a list of 304 adult survivors of pediatric cancer, an oncologist who knew the patients selected 66 adults without cognitive impairment who were representative of pediatric cancer diagnoses and were oversampled to ensure ethnic and socioeconomic diversity. I was able to reach 40 of these adults within a month of the letters being sent, and 37 agreed to participate, with only 1 person explicitly refusing. While 5 people could not be interviewed due to time constraints, 32 adults (average age of 24 years) with childhood cancer (average age at diagnosis 13 years) were interviewed in person, almost all in their homes. Demographically 9 identified as African-American, 4 as Hispanic, and 1 as "Other"; 9 identified as growing up in single-parent households; and 15 identified having fathers with a high school education or less.

Reference

Tang MH (2013) The Lance Armstrong story: should we find another hero? Pediatr Blood Cancer 60:1071–1072

24 Advocacy: Helping Others Understand What Children with Cancer Need

Sandra E. Smith and Ruth I. Hoffman

Introduction

The word "advocacy" in relation to pediatric oncology may bring a variety of thoughts to mind. In the early 1960s, Dr. Donald Pinkel advocated for aggressive multidrug treatment (Total Therapy) of acute lymphoblastic leukemia at a time when combination drug therapy was considered reckless and cure was not considered possible (Roswell Park Cancer Institute n.d.). More recently, a number of pediatric neuro-oncologists and families of children with diffuse intrinsic pontine glioma (DIPG) have advocated for postmortem tumor tissue donations for the purpose of research; as a result, there is now an increased understanding of DIPG tumor biology (Alabran et al. 2013). This chapter explores the history of childhood cancer advocacy, considers parents as advocates for their children and children as advocates for themselves, and examines childhood cancer advocacy as a cause, including some of its challenges.

S.E. Smith (✉) • R.I. Hoffman, MPH
American Childhood Cancer Organization,
10920 Connecticut Avenue Suite A, Kensington,
MD 20895, USA
e-mail: sews@me.com; rhoffman@acco.org

Childhood Cancer Advocacy in History

In 1953, when three-year-old Robin Bush was diagnosed with leukemia, the doctor advised her parents George and Barbara Bush, "Number one, don't tell anyone." This was the culture of the time (Cunningham n.d.). Cancer in a child was considered a death sentence, and parents were routinely instructed not to speak of it. Families were expected to shoulder the incomprehensible burden alone. Sixteen years later in 1970, six-year-old Danny McGaughy was diagnosed with acute lymphoblastic leukemia. When interviewed in November 2014, Danny's parents Bob and Beverly McGaughy confirmed that they, like the Bush family, were advised not to talk about their child's cancer. However, they were concerned about the small amount of government funding to the National Cancer Institute (NCI), so they convinced their son's doctors to arrange a meeting of parents whose children were being treated for cancer at DC Children's Hospital, now Children's National Medical Center. The initial meeting was held in the basement of the hospital and was attended by 25 parents, a number who were Capitol Hill insiders. Several of the parents were surprised to learn that some of their colleagues also had children with cancer. At a time when families of children with cancer were encouraged not to speak of their plight, this group came together and decided they could no longer be silent.

A.N. Abrams et al. (eds.), *Pediatric Psychosocial Oncology: Textbook for Multidisciplinary Care*,
DOI 10.1007/978-3-319-21374-3_24

Dick Sullivan, chief counsel to the House Public Works Committee, was one of the parents who attended the meeting. Within three or four days of the initial meeting, he arranged for the group to begin meeting more officially in the Rayburn House Office Building. According to the November 2014 interview with the McGaughys, they were advised by a cancer lobbyist who worked for Mary Lasker, to contact the members of the House Appropriations Committee who had jurisdiction over the NCI budget. Dick Sullivan set up meetings for the parents with Congressional staff, and Bob McGaughy set up meetings with the National Cancer Institute. Bob and Beverly McGaughy and Dick and Julie Sullivan, along with other parents in the group, worked with their political, professional, and personal connections to lobby for immediate increased funding, as well as consistent long-term funding, for basic cancer research (Bernstein 2011). In 1970, this group led to the formation of the Candlelighters Foundation, a 501(c) (4), which in 2010 became the American Childhood Cancer Organization (American Childhood Cancer Organization n.d.).

Al Karr and Arnie Weiss, fathers who attended that first meeting, contributed their expertise in journalism and law, respectively (American Childhood Cancer Organization n.d.). Peter Koltnow, another father and Candlelighters' first president, was a Congressional liaison for the Highway Users Federation (Bernstein 2011); he and his wife Dorothy were gifted in communications. Dick Sullivan, Beverly McGaughy, and Grace Ann Monaco, a young attorney and the mother of a toddler with cancer, testified repeatedly on Capitol Hill. The group created position statements, wrote their own testimonies, and told their stories. Monaco said, "We dashed around banging people over the head in nice ways and were very successful in obtaining national research funds for pediatric cancer" (Keene 2001).

Childhood Cancer Advocacy Defined

To advocate is "to support or argue for," according to the Merriam-Webster Dictionary. When parents of children with cancer were asked by the American Childhood Cancer Organization to define the term in 2014, the responses varied. Some parents thought of advocacy in terms of caring for their own child with cancer (Table 24.1).

Others thought of advocacy on a larger scale (Table 24.2).

Table 24.1 Parent comments gathered from Facebook survey conducted by the American Childhood Cancer Organization in October 2014

Individual advocacy
Always expressing my thoughts and feelings to everyone who is involved in any type of care that is provided to my child
Never settling
Putting your own needs aside to aid in the care of another
Fighting to make life better for someone
Making sure the child is heard
Taking a stand
Speaking up and ensuring that your child is getting the best medical care possible
Fighting for what is needed
Being the voice for my child
Helping others to help themselves

Table 24.2 Parent comments gathered from Facebook survey conducted by the American Childhood Cancer Organization in October 2014

Cause advocacy
To take on and believe in a cause
Fighting every day to help all kids with cancer because they can't help themselves
Being strong not only for those who cannot be, but also for those who just don't know how
Stepping up and taking action
Standing strong and realizing you do have the power to change hearts and lives
Making enough noise so that children diagnosed with cancer have a better chance
Working together as a community to see change for children with cancer
Being relentless
Having a national conversation to evoke meaningful change
Finding better treatments and cures

Parents as Advocates

Advocacy is being able to have your child's wishes realized, being able to find someone to answer their questions truthfully, making sure their treatment is handled respectfully and privately, making sure that the child is comfortable at all times, making sure that the care team is all on the same page. – parent of a teen boy who died of brain cancer

When a child is diagnosed with cancer, parents or guardians may be thrust into the role of advocate for their child for the very first time in their lives. While a parent may not have previously questioned their child's physicians, following a cancer diagnosis when their child's life could be in danger, they may feel compelled to question treatment decisions. Parental advocacy comes in many forms: quiet, firm, loud, crass, respectful, and even rude. Pediatric clinicians can choose to view a parent who advocates for a child as an annoyance or a challenge, or they can recognize that the child's cancer diagnosis is almost certainly the most difficult thing the family has ever faced and assume that most parents want what is best for their children, whether it be a second opinion, good quality of life, or a comfortable death. Physicians and psychosocial professionals have the extraordinary opportunity to work with parents to ensure the provision of the best medical and psychosocial care for children with cancer.

Listening to Children: Valuing their Perspective

Advocacy is finding the best words you can to help others understand what is needed. – mother of a child with cancer

Andrea Román's son Riley was diagnosed with cancer at the age of seven. In an October 2014 interview, Andrea revealed that she and Riley worked together to encourage each other in their efforts to advocate for what he needed during his treatment for cancer. Andrea reminded physicians and nurses, "No one knows what Riley's going through better than Riley does!" And if Riley felt that someone was dismissing his mother's concerns, he reminded them, "Well, that's my mom, and she's known me all my life; so if you don't believe me, believe her."

When doctors, nurses, or other professionals asked Andrea questions, she often turned to her son to give him the opportunity to respond. Riley advocated for his own comfort and safety by telling his nurses what worked well for him when they accessed his port. He said that if they counted to three, he was better able to prepare for the poke. If the nurse did not give him a mask, he requested a mask to protect the port site from germs. If a nurse did something that caused more pain than usual, Riley explained the way other nurses had accessed his port successfully, and with less pain, in the past. Similarly, when Riley's medical team felt that he needed a feeding tube, Andrea encouraged Riley to learn about the options. After a couple of outpatient teaching appointments, along with some videos about G-tube surgery and NG-tube placement, Riley eventually chose to try an NG-tube, and he requested to place it himself. Though it was not a request the staff had received in the past, they allowed Riley to place the tube with their guidance, and he was able to place it correctly.

Childhood Cancer Advocacy: The Cause

Advocacy is standing up for what's right—even if you're in a room full of people, and you're the only one standing. Advocacy means never backing down in the face of adversity even when others try to silence you—because it's in moments like these that advocates are truly needed most, and it's in moments like these that the potential for change is greatest. – parent of a child with cancer

Advocacy can be carried out on a personal level or on a broader level. Whether the child advocates for himself or herself, or the parent advocates for the child, personal advocacy can be the first step toward advocacy on a larger scale.

The motive behind advocacy for a cause may or may not be personal. Some parents are involved in this type of advocacy because it may directly benefit their own children, while others are involved because they feel compelled to advocate for all children with cancer. In an October 2014 interview, Deb Fuller, whose daughter Hope died of brain cancer at the age of 12, stated that she believes advocacy is taking her desire to have saved her own child's life to a much larger level in an attempt to save the lives of children who have cancer today or who will be diagnosed with cancer tomorrow. Some parents like Deb, whose children have died of cancer, feel compelled to make a difference because they live every day with the absence of their children, a constant reminder of the urgency of the cause. Others, parents and childhood cancer survivors themselves, live with a different type of reminder—the long-term effects of the treatments that make survival possible.

Unfortunately, advocacy for a cause is often slow to produce results. Less than 10 % of proposed bills become law in the United States, and the process often takes years (Drug Approvals 1999). The Caroline Pryce Walker Conquer Childhood Cancer Act, named to memorialize former Representative Deborah Pryce's daughter Caroline who died at age nine of neuroblastoma, was signed into law in 2008 (Childhood Cancer Caucus n.d.). The purpose of the legislation was to establish a national childhood cancer registry and to advance childhood cancer research and treatments. Though it passed unanimously, it was never fully funded, and there has been a push for reauthorization and expansion of the legislation ever since.

Similarly, it takes an average of twelve years for a drug to make it from the research lab to Federal Drug Administration (FDA) approval. A meager 5 in 5000 drugs advance from preclinical to human testing, and only one of those 5 drugs will be approved (Drug Approvals 1999). If parents and other childhood cancer advocates do not understand the pace of advocacy at this level, they can easily become discouraged and even angry. An adult survivor of childhood cancer articulated it well, "Advocacy is standing up for what is right; striving for change, awareness and action; not giving up until things are better."

In September 2014, the National Institutes of Health announced a new clinical trial for children with advanced cancer. The Molecular Analysis for Therapy Choice Program (MATCH) will enroll children whose cancer has progressed on standard therapy into personalized treatment plans based on the tumor's unique fingerprint (Childhood Cancer Caucus 2014). In a November 2014 interview, Peter Adamson, chair of Children's Oncology Group, stated, "Advocacy helped lead to a $3 million investment in the MATCH Study for Pediatric Cancer." Multiple childhood cancer organizations came together, coordinated common messaging, utilized social media, and gained community support, leading to the government funding of this important study.

Childhood Cancer Advocacy: The Challenges

While the MATCH study is a positive example of what can happen when people work together to achieve a common goal, advocacy may also be misdirected. A family, a physician, or even an organization may push for something that is not in the best interest of the child. A family may get caught up in a treatment they believe offers hope, when in reality it does not. Parents may think they are advocating for research that will benefit their own child, but it may be years before that research directly benefits patients.

Advocating for childhood cancer awareness and research is complicated by the existence of a number of groups who do not all use the same statistics to convey the burden of childhood cancer. Many foundations are started to honor a specific child or to focus on a specific cancer. One of the main challenges of collaboration on the cause level is that individual organizations are reluctant to give up their own identities, or ownership of a particular cause, to embrace the larger cause. On the other hand, there are more opportunities for collaboration today because of the Internet, and the opportunity for awareness is magnified through social media.

Good intentions do not always lead to constructive action or to favorable results; and ineffective advocacy may actually hurt the cause. Bob and Beverly McGaughy, along with the other early parent advocates, realized that Members of Congress did not want to be perceived by the public as insensitive to the need for increased funding of cancer research. The parents' approach, which included building positive relationships with their government representatives, rather than publicly shaming them, led to an overwhelmingly successful 20 % increase in government funding of the NCI in 1970, during the first year of their advocacy efforts, according to a November 2014 interview with Bob and Beverly McGaughy. Working with a collaborative spirit, respect for each other's strengths, and passion for a cause that had impacted each of their lives, the original parent advocates transformed the government funding of cancer research by bringing attention and focus to the cause.

Conclusion

While the advocacy efforts of a small group of parents in the 1970s did not lead to new treatments that saved their own children's lives, it is because of their tireless work that there are children today who survive cancer. Similarly, the efforts of today's advocates will have an impact on the unique needs of children who will be diagnosed with cancer tomorrow.

Clinical Pearls

- It may be beneficial to find creative ways to connect the families of children newly diagnosed with cancer to veteran families. There is wisdom in experience, and many families find comfort in knowing that they are not alone.
- Medical professionals have the opportunity to engage childhood cancer community advocates in ways that will help them to gain both the knowledge and the skills needed to advocate for childhood cancer research and funding. Interactions should include taking opportunities to educate, to build relationships, and to continue regular dialogue.
- Families can benefit from information about opportunities to participate in advocacy events such as those sponsored by the Alliance for Childhood Cancer (http://www.allianceforchildhoodcancer.org/), to attend the annual Childhood Cancer Summit hosted by the Congressional Childhood Cancer Caucus, and to take part in meetings such as the Pediatric Cancer Nanocourse started by Charles Keller of the Children's Cancer Therapy Development Institute (http://www.cc-tdi.org/).
- Parents should be encouraged to advocate for the best medical care for their children. This may include pursuing second opinions or exploring the range of possible treatment options.
- With the best of intentions, a family may advocate sincerely for a treatment that will not help their child. Providers need to keep these good intentions in mind as they support parents in making medical decisions.

References

Alabran JL, Hooper JE, Hill M et al (2013) Overcoming autopsy barriers in pediatric cancer research. Pediatr Blood Cancer 60(2):204–209, Available from: http://www.ncbi.nlm.nih.gov/pubmed/23015377. [31 Oct. 2014]

American Childhood Cancer Organization (n.d.) History of American Childhood Cancer Organization. Available from: http://www.acco.org/about/history/. Accessed 21 Feb 2015.

Bernstein A (2011) 'Peter G. Koltnow, advocacy group leader'. The Washington Post 8 December. Available from: http://www.washingtonpost.com/local/obituaries/peter-g-koltnow-advocacy-group-leader/2011/12/08/gIQAb1zHgO_story.html. Accessed 7 Nov 2014.

Congressional Childhood Cancer Caucus (2014) NCI announces a pediatric MATCH trial for childhood cancer, Available from: http://childhoodcancer-mccaul.house.gov/press-release/nciannounces-pediatric-match-trial-childhood-cancer. Accessed 14 Nov 2014.

Congressional Childhood Cancer Caucus (n.d.) Caroline Pryce Walker Childhood Cancer Reauthorization Act. Available from: https://childhoodcancer-mccaul.house.gov/issue/carolinepryce-walker-conquer-childhood-cancer-act-0. Accessed 31 Oct 2014.

Cunningham A (n.d.) Good-bye to Robin: interview with Barbara Bush. Available from: http://chatteringmind.com/articles/barbarabush.html. Accessed 31 Oct 2014.

Drug approvals – from invention to market (1999) Available from: http://www.medicinenet.com/script/main/art.asp?articlekey=9877. Accessed 31 Oct 2014.

Keene N (2001) Meet activist Grace Ann Monaco. Available from: http://www.oreilly.com/onconurse/news/activist_monaco.html. Accessed 31 Oct 2014.

Roswell Park Cancer Institute (n.d.) A sense of urgency: Donald Pinkel and the quest to cure ALL. Available from: https://www.roswellpark.org/donaldpinkel. Accessed 31 Oct 2014.

Resources Chapter 25

Sima Zadeh, Mitch Golant, Farya Phillips, and Barbara L. Jones

Families facing a cancer diagnosis can gather information and find supportive resources in numerous ways. Organizations dedicated to specific cancer diagnoses can be a useful resource to increase a family's initial understanding of the disease. Books and videos geared toward each member of the family are also widely available and useful for providing information or support in a developmentally appropriate and sensitive manner. When working with pediatric oncology patients and their families, guiding them through the many ways in which they can access information on disease and treatment options, supportive services, financial assistance, survivorship, and end-of-life care can be invaluable.

*While we tried to include all potentially useful resources, this list is not exhaustive. New and additional resources may be available.

Books/Articles for Children with Cancer and Their Families

Children

Because…Someone I Love Has Cancer (American Cancer Society) Kids' activity book

Chemo, Craziness, and Comfort: My Book About Childhood Cancer by Nancy Keene, Candlelighters Childhood Cancer Foundation, 2002

Dear Bruno by Alice Trillin, New Press, 1996.

Franklin Goes To The Hospital by Paulette Bourgeois. Scholastic, 2011

Healing Images for Children: Teaching Relaxation and Guided Imagery to Children Facing Cancer and Other Serious Illnesses by Nancy C. Klein. Inner Coaching, 2001

Kathy's Hats: A Story of Hope by Trudy Krisher, Nadine Bernard Westcott (illustrator). Albert Whitman and Company, 1992

S. Zadeh, PsyD (✉)
Pediatric Oncology Branch, National Institutes of Health, National Cancer Institute,
10 Center Drive, Bldg. 10, 1H-PEDS, Room 1-5460, Bethesda, MD 20892, USA
e-mail: zadehsl@mail.nih.gov

M. Golant, PhD
Cancer Support Community,
1050 17th Street NW, Suite 500, Washington, DC 20036, USA
e-mail: mitch@cancersupportcommunity.org

F. Phillips, PhD, CCLS
School of Social Work, The University of Texas at Austin, 1925 San Jacinto, D3500, Austin, TX 78712, USA
e-mail: Farya@utexas.edu

B.L. Jones, PhD, MSW
School of Social Work, University of Texas at Austin, 1925 San Jacinto Blvd, Mail Stop D3500, Austin, TX 78712, USA
e-mail: barbarajones@mail.utexas.edu

A.N. Abrams et al. (eds.), *Pediatric Psychosocial Oncology: Textbook for Multidisciplinary Care*, DOI 10.1007/978-3-319-21374-3_25

Little Tree: A Story for Children with Serious Medical Problems by Joyce C. Mills, Magination Press, 2003

Living Well With My Serious Illness by Marge Eaton Heegaard. Fairview Press, 2003

My Body Needs Help by Annette Abrams, Tenley Circle Press, 2011

The Amazing Hannah, Look at Everything I Can Do! by Amy Klett, Candlelighters Childhood Cancer Foundation, 2002

The Hospital Scares Me by Paula Z. Hogan and Kirk Hogan, Raintree Steck-Vaughn Publishers, 1995

The Sandbox King by Susanne M. Swanson, Writer's Press, 1995

The Jester Has Lost His Jingle by David Saltzman. Jester Books, 1995

This is My World (workbook) by Sima Zadeh and Lori Wiener. National Cancer Institute and the National Institute of Mental Health, 2010 https://ccr.cancer.gov/Pediatric-Oncology-Branch-psychosocial-education

What About Me? When Brothers and Sisters Get Sick by Allan Peterkin, Magination Press, 1992

Teens

It's Not About the Bike: My Journey Back to Life by Lance Armstrong and Sally Jenkins. Berkley Trade, 2001

Teens with the Courage to Give: Young People Who Triumphed Over Tragedy and Volunteered to Make a Difference by Jackie Waldman and Steven A. Culbertson. Conari Press, 2000

The Bald-Headed Princess: Cancer, Chemo, and Courage by Maribeth Ditmars. Magination Press, 2010

Parents/Adults

Caregiver's Guide for Bone Marrow/Stem Cell Transplant (Practical Perspectives) by Melanie Goldish, 2003

Childhood Brain & Spinal Cord Tumors: A Guide for Families, Friends and Caregivers by Shiminski-Maher, Cullen, Sansalone, O'Reilly & Associates, 2002

Children Diagnosed with Cancer: Returning to school. The American Cancer Society, 2011

Children with Cancer: Effects and Educational Implications by Sarah McDougal, 1997

Educating the Child with Cancer: A Guide for Parents and Teachers by Nancy Keene, American Childhood Cancer Organization, 2003

Learning and living with cancer: Advocating for your child's educational needs, Leukemia and Lymphoma Society, 2005.

Living With Childhood Cancer: A Practical Guide to Help Families Cope by Leigh A. Woznick and Carol D. Goodheart. American Psychological Association, 2001.

Shelter from the Storm: Caring for a Child with a Life-Threatening Condition by Joanne Hilden and Daniel Tobin, with Karen Lindsey. Perseus Publishing, 2002

The Human Side of Cancer: Living with Hope, Coping with Uncertainty by Jimmie Holland and Sheldon Lewis. Harper Perennial, 2001

Therapeutic Activities for Children and Teens Coping with Health Issues by Robyn Hart and Judy Rollins. Wiley, 2011

Young People with Cancer. A Handbook for Parents. NIH/NCI, 2001

Siblings

Brothers and Sisters Together: A workbook for siblings of siblings who are sick by Lori Wiener, 2006 (Also available in Spanish) https://ccr.cancer.gov/Pediatric-Oncology-Branch-psychosocial-education

Drums, Girls and Dangerous Pie by Jordan Sonnenblick. DayBue Publishing, 2004 (fiction)

Hey, What about Me?: A Personal Journal for Teens Whose Brother or Sister Has Cancer by Pam Ganz, SuperSibs!

Oliver's Story: For 'sibs' of kids with cancer by Michael Dodd, Candlelighters Childhood Cancer Foundation, 2004

SuperSibs! Parent Guide for Siblings of Children with Cancer, SuperSibs!

When Your Brother or Sister Has Cancer: A Guide for Teens Paperback by The National Cancer Institute, 2012

Books to Share with Other Students in the Classroom

Jacob has Cancer: His Friends Want to Help by Heather Cooper, American Cancer Society, 2012

The Famous Hat by Kate Gaynor, Special Stories, 2008

Taking Cancer to School by Kim Gosselin, JayJo Books, 2001

The Amazing Hannah, Look at Everything I Can Do! by Amy Klett, Candlelighters Childhood Cancer Foundation, 2002

The Long and Short of It: A Tale About Hair by Barbara Meyers and Lydia Criss Mays, American Cancer Society, 2011

Why, Charlie Brown, Why by Charlie Schultz, Ballentine Books, 2002

Resources for Teachers

Cancervive Teacher's Guide for Kids with Cancer by Susan Nessim & Ernie Katz, Cancervive, 2000

Children with Cancer in the Classroom by Virginia Peckman, Teaching Exceptional Children, 1993

Pupils with Cancer: A Guide for Teachers. The Royal Marsden NHS Foundation Trust and the Specialist Schools and Academies Trust, 2008

Dealing with cancer in the classroom: The teacher's role and responsibilities by C. Spinnelli, Teaching Exceptional Children, 2004

Cancer Survivors

Can Survive: Reclaiming Your Life After Cancer by Susan Nessim & Judith Ellis, Houghton Mifflin, 2000

Childhood Cancer Survivors: A Practical Guide to Your Future, 2nd Edition, by Kathy Ruccione, Nancy Keene, & Wendy Hobbie, O'Reilly Media, Inc, 2006

Childhood Cancer Survivorship: Improving Care and Quality of Life by the Institute of Medicine, National Cancer Policy Board, National Academies Press, 2003

Grief and Loss

Am I Still a Sister? by Alicia M Sims, Big A & Company, 1986

Gentle Willow: A Story for Children About Dying by Joyce C. Mills, Magination Press, 2003

Helping Teens Work Through Grief, 2nd Edition, by Mary Kelly Perschy, Routledge, 2004

Someday Heaven by Larry Libby, Multnomah Publishers, Inc., 2001

The Grieving Teen: A Guide for Teenagers and Their Friends by Helen Fitzgerald, Fireside, 2000

Waterbugs and Dragonflies by Doris Stickney, The Pilgrim Press, 1982

Videos/Websites

Better than a Spoonful of Sugar: How to Swallow Pills A training video for teaching pill swallowing. www.ucalgary.ca/research4kids/pillswallowing

Get Empowered: Life, Living & Follow-Up Care After Childhood Cancer A video education series for childhood cancer patients and survivors by Robert H. Lurie Comprehensive Cancer Center, http://cancer.northwestern.edu/empowered/index.cfm

The Trish Greene Back-to-School Program for Children with Cancer by Leukemia & Lymphoma Society, www.leukemia-lymphoma.org

This is Awkward: Fertility Preservation for Boys with Cancer by the Children's Hospital of Philadelphia, http://www.chop.edu/video/oncology/fertility-preservation-boys.html

Cancer.Net Videos provides patient-friendly videos developed by ASCO http://www.cancer.net/multimedia/videos

Cancer Camps in North America

American Cancer Society (ACS): www.cancer.org
Arizona Camp Sunrise and Sidekicks, Arizona: www.azcampsunrise.org
Camp Boggy Creek: www.boggycreek.org
Camp Make-A-Dream: www.campdream.org
Camp Oochigeas: www.ooch.org
Camp Quality, throughout the United States: www.campqualityusa.org
Camp Rap-A-Hope, Alabama: www.camprapahope.org
Camp Simcha:: www.chailifeline.org
Camp Smile-A-Mile (SAM): www.campsam.org
Camp Sunshine: www.campsunshine.org
Camp Sunshine, Georgia: www.mycampsunshine.com
Children's Oncology Camping Association: www.cocai.org
Double H Ranch: www.doublehranch.org
First Descents: www.firstdescents.org
One Step at a Time Camp: www.onestepcamp.org
The Hole in the Wall Gang Camp: www.holeinthewallgang.org
Special Love, Inc. (Camp Fantastic): www.speciallove.org
Sunshine Kids: www.sunshinekids.org
For additional camp listings by state, please visit: www.ped-onc.org/cfissues/camps.html

Scholarship Information

National Scholarships in the U.S.
American Cancer Society: www.cancer.org
Andre Sobel River of Life Foundation: www.andreriveroflife.org
Anne Ford Scholarship: www.ncld.org
Austin Sunshine Camps: www.sunshinecamps.org/scholarship
Beyond the Cure: www.beyondthecure.org
Cancer for College: www.cancerforcollege.org
Cancer Survivors Fund: www.cancersurvivorsfund.org
Friends for Michael Foundation:www.friends4michael.org
Friends of Scott Foundation: www.friendsofscott.org
Hydrocephalus Association: www.hydroassoc.org
Hyundai Hope on Wheels: www.hopeonwheels.com
Kyle Lee Foundation: www.kylelee28.com/Kyle
National Amputation Foundation: http://nationalamputation.org/scholar1.html
National Collegiate Cancer Foundation: www.collegiatecancer.org
The National Grace Foundation: www.Graceamerica.org
Patient Advocate Foundation: www.patientadvocate.org
The Pacific West Cancer Fund Scholarships: www.pacificwestcancerfund.org
Pediatric Brain Tumor Foundation: www.curethekids.org
Ronald McDonald House Charities: www.rmhc.org
Stephen T. Marchello Scholarship Foundation: www.stmfoundation.org
Surviving and Moving Forward: www.thesamfund.org
The Ulman Fund-Scholarship: http://ulmanfund.org/gethelp/support-programs-resources/scholarships/
Working Against Cancer: www.workingagainstcancer.org

Scholarships for Siblings

SuperSibs
Website: http://www.alexslemonade.org/campaign/supersibs

Organizations in the U.S. Providing Information and Education

All Cancers

American Cancer Society (ACS)
Nationwide community-based voluntary health organization dedicated to preventing cancer, saving lives, and diminishing suffering from

cancer, through research, education, advocacy, and service. www.cancer.org

Brave Kids

Serves children with disabilities and chronic/life-threatening illnesses by providing a support community, information, and resources on numerous medical conditions. Has a "Just for Kids" tab on the website to guide children through their disability or illness. www.bravekids.org

Childhood Cancer Guides

Serves the childhood cancer community by providing explanations of the various types of childhood cancer, descriptions of treatments, emotional support for every member of the family, and access to helpful resources. www.childhoodcancerguides.org

The Children's Cause for Cancer Advocacy (CCCA)

Nonprofit organization that works to stimulate drug discovery and development for childhood cancers; to expand resources for research and treatment, advocacy, and policy change; and to address the needs and concerns of survivors.www.childrenscause.org

CureSearch

The Children's Oncology Group and the National Childhood Cancer Foundation unite to offer information about types of childhood cancer and treatments. Available in Spanish. www.curesearch.org

Hope Portal

Developed by Children's Hospital Los Angeles as a clearinghouse for finding resources and information about childhood cancer and other conditions. http://searchhope.chla.org/

Livestrong

Offers support and resources to help patients and their families through the entire cancer experience. www.livestrong.org

Prepare to Live

Provides resources for young adults coping with cancer. www.preparetolive.org

Oncolink – Pediatric Cancers

Comprehensive website with cancer-related information for childhood cancers. www.oncolink.org

SurvivorLink

Website designed to help survivors of childhood cancer communicate with their doctors and nurses. www.cancersurvivorlink.org

Sarcomas

GIST Support International

Provides education, news, resources, and support for patients affected by gastrointestinal stromal tumor and their families and friends. www.gistsupport.org

Sarcoma Foundation of America

The website offers patients information and support, informational links, clinical trials, and a public forum. www.curesarcoma.org

Leukemia and Lymphoma

Children's Leukemia Research Association

Offers a patient aid program to help pay for leukemia medication not covered by insurance. Also funds research grants. www.childrens-leukemia.org

Childhood Leukemia Foundation

Offers a wide range of free services designed to provide emotional, financial, social, educational, and recovery support to children and families touched by cancer. www.clf4kids.org

Leukemia and Lymphoma Society of America

Offers family support group programs, referrals to local sources of help, education, patient aid, and research funding. Focuses on leukemia, lymphomas, myeloma, and Hodgkin's disease. www.lls.org

Brain & Spinal Cord Cancers

American Brain Tumor Association

Offers free publications about brain tumors, support group lists, referral information, a pen pal program, and research support. www.abta.org

The Childhood Brain Tumor Foundation

Volunteer-based organization that helps educate families whose children have been diagnosed with brain tumors. www.childhoodbraintumor.org

The Children's Brain Tumor Foundation

Provides research, support, education, and advocacy to families and survivors to improve the treatment, quality of life, and the long-term outlook for children with brain and spinal cord tumors. www.cbtf.org

Neuroblastoma

Children's Neuroblastoma Cancer Foundation
CNCF provides a forum for patients with neuroblastoma and their family members. www.cncfhope.org

The Neuroblastoma Children's Cancer Society
An organization that advocates for children with neuroblastoma and serves as a support center for their families. www.neuroblastomacancer.org

Retinoblastoma

Retinoblastoma International
Committed to supporting education, clinical care, research, early diagnosis, and awareness.
www.retinoblastoma.net

Rare Cancers

Memorial Sloan-Kettering Rare Cancer Page
Provides short descriptions of a variety of rare cancers with links to MSK Cancer Center physicians who treat a particular cancer. www.mskcc.org

National Institutes of Health (NIH)
The primary Federal agency for conducting and supporting medical research. Composed of 27 Institutes and Centers, NIH provides extensive research on clinical trials.
www.nih.gov; www.clinicaltrials.gov

National Cancer Institute, Pediatric Oncology Branch, NIH
Lists active treatment protocols for a variety of pediatric malignancies. Children with newly diagnosed or recurrent malignancies may be eligible for treatments. http://pediatrics.cancer.gov/

Survivors

Cancer Survivors Network
http://csn.cancer.org

Livestrong
www.livestrong.org

National Cancer Institute: Office of Cancer Survivorship
http://dccps.nci.nih.gov/ocs

National Cancer Survivors Day Foundation
www.ncsdf.org

National Coalition for Cancer Survivorship
www.canceradvocacy.org

OncoLink: LiveSTRONG™ Care Plan
www.oncolink.org/oncolife

Pediatric Oncology Resource Center
www.acor.org/ped-onc

Planet Cancer for Young Adults (A LiveSTRONG™ Initiative)
http://myplanet.planetcancer.org/

Support Organizations

American Psychosocial Oncology Society Helpline
Toll-free helpline to obtain referrals for local counseling and support services.
http://ce.apos-society.org/survivors/helpline/helpline.aspx

Cancer Care, Inc.
Provides free professional help to people with all cancers through counseling, education, information, referral, and direct financial assistance. www.cancercare.org

Cancer FAQ
Online information about cancer resources. www.faqs.org/faqs/medicine/cancer-faq/

Cancer Support Community
Provides free emotional support, education, and hope for people with cancer and their loved ones. www.cancersupportcommunity.org

CarePages & Caring Bridge
Free sites that help family and friends communicate when a loved one is receiving care.
www.carepages.com; www.caringbridge.org

Chemo Angels
Children can apply to be "adopted" by a Chemo Angel who will provide support and encouragement throughout treatment with cards, notes, and small gifts. www.chemoangels.net

ChemoDuck
An organization that provides cancer patients with a Chemo Duck, a play therapy tool to

help alleviate fears and anxiety. http://chemoduck.org

CURE Childhood Cancer

Provides funding for cancer research and support to patients and their families.
www.curechildhoodcancer.org

Family Voices

Resources, tips, brochures, and a newsletter offering advocacy for children's health care needs. www.familyvoices.org

Lotsa Helping Hands

A web-based calendar resource that allows parents to produce a Help Calendar, where members of their family or community can schedule and sign up for tasks that provide caregiver support, including meals for the family, rides to medical appointments, and visits. www.lotsahelpinghands.com

Pediatric Oncology Resource Center

A place for parents, friends, and families of children who have or had childhood cancer. This site was created by and for people who know young people who are recovering from cancer. www.ped-onc.org

Padres Contra El Cáncer

Organization committed to improving the quality of life for Latino children with cancer and their families through case management, family educational programs, crisis intervention, support groups, economic assistance, and quality-of-life events.
www.iamhope.org

Starlight Children's Foundation

Provides entertainment, education, and family activities for seriously ill children in the United States and their families. www.starbright.org

Stop Childhood Cancer Alliance

Hope to be the driving source in increasing awareness of childhood cancer and enhancing the support for the young people fighting this disease. www.stopchildhoodcancer.org

The Father's Network – Washington State

Celebrates and supports fathers and families raising children with special health care needs. Also in Spanish. www.fathersnetwork.org

The Never-Ending Squirrel Tale

Online support, practical tips, and encouragement for parents of children with cancer.
http://neo4u.org/the-never-ending-squirrel-tale/

U.S. Department of Education

Provides information regarding education law in the United States. www.ed.gov

Wrightslaw Special Education Law and Advocacy

Provides accurate, reliable information about special education law, education law, and advocacy for children with disabilities. www.wrightslaw.org

Children

Cancer Kids

Helps children with cancer tell their stories to the world. Offers resources, stories, discussion forums, and helpful tips. www.cancerkids.org

CoachArt

Improves the quality of life for children with chronic and life-threatening illnesses and their siblings by providing free lessons in the arts and athletics. www.coachart.org/

Common Threads

Provides children in low-income families healthy, easy, and cost-effective tips for proper nutrition. www.commonthreads.org

KIDSAID

Specializes in grief and loss; email support groups where peers provide support while also being monitored by a trained therapist and psychiatrist. www.kidsaid.com

KIDSCOPE

Provides help to families and children to better understand the effects from cancer and chemo, including a 16-page color comic book designed to help children cope with cancer and treatment. Website also in Spanish. www.kidscope.org

Kids Konnected

Website information includes 24-Hour Hotline to get answers, share concerns, or just talk; monthly support group meeting and group listings, chat room, online newsletter, database on books about cancer and coping skills; summer camps; and Teddy Bear outreach program for younger kids. www.kidskonnected.org

Kidz with Leukemia: A Space Adventure
CD-ROM video game teaches about leukemia, chemotherapy, and side effects. www.kidz-withleukemia.com

Teens

CanTeen Australia
Australian support organization for young people with cancer (aged 12–24) living with cancer, designed to support, develop, and empower them. www.canteen.org.au

The Children's Cause
A patient advocacy group that is dedicated to empowering and supporting children who had or still are living with cancer. www.children-scause.org

Group Loop: Teens Talk Cancer Online
Provides free professionally facilitated online support groups and moderated discussion boards for teens with cancer to receive support, education, and hope after the diagnosis of cancer. www.grouploop.org

Look Good…Feel Better
A hospital-based public service program that provides resources and programs for teens with cancer to deal with issues related to appearance, health, and social aspects of cancer treatment. http://lookgoodfeelbetter.org/programs/programs-for-teens

Melinda's Home Page for CancerKids
Created by a young girl living with cancer, this site provides information and support to adolescents with cancer and their caregivers. www.monkey-boy.com/melinda

Next Step
This organization for teens and young adults with serious illness offers retreats and workshops around the country. www.nextstepnet.org

Re-Mission by HopeLab
A video game for young people with cancer. www.re-mission.net

Songs of Love
Creates personalized, free songs for chronically ill children and young adults. www.songso-flove.org

Starbright World
Online social network for teens with chronic and life-threatening medical conditions. www.starbrightworld.org

Starlight Children's Foundation Coping with Chemo
Offers individual "webisodes" addressing diagnosis, talking to friends, side effects, and ending treatment. http://chemo.starlight.org

Teenage Cancer Trust
Charity devoted to improving the lives of teenagers and young adults with cancer. www.teen-agecancertrust.org

Teen Impact
Program at Children's Hospital Los Angeles for teens and young adults who have or once had cancer or a blood disease. Open to teens and young adults from any part of the country, hospital, or treatment center. www.teenim-pactprogram.com

Teens Living with Cancer
Provides information for teens living with cancer and has a discussion board and articles written by teens with cancer. Also in Spanish. www.teenslivingwithcancer.com

Siblings

Sibshops
National program dedicated to the interests of brothers and sisters of people with special health and developmental needs. Offers links to "sibshops," resources, and a question and answer section specifically designed to meet the needs of siblings. www.seattlechildrens.org/classes-community/classes-events/sibshops/

Starbright World
An online social network for teens with chronic and life-threatening illness and their siblings. www.starbrightworld.org

Supersibs
Siblings of children diagnosed with cancer are sent welcome packets and periodic packages throughout the year. Comprehensive support guides are also offered to medical staff,

teachers, and parents. http://www.alexslemonade.org/campaign/supersibs

Young Adults

The Ashley Foundation

Provides assistance to teens affected by cancer through educational and supportive programs, such as scholarship money for college and teen resources for hospitals. www.theashleyfoundation.org

Cancer*Care*– Young Adult Program

Offers specialized services for young adults, caregivers, and those who have lost a loved one. www.cancercare.org/tagged/young_adults

Cancer and Careers

Empowers and educates people with cancer to thrive in their workplace by providing expert advice, interactive tools, and educational events. The organization offers career coaching, support groups, and educational seminars

Website: www.cancerandcareers.org

CancerQuest

Provides education on the biology of cancer through visuals and writings. www.cancerquest.org

Critical Mass: The Young Adult Cancer Alliance

A coalition of organizations with the goal of improving survival rates and quality of life for young adults (ages 15–40) with cancer. http://criticalmass.org/

Cryobank

Full service sperm bank in California. Online learning center with links, articles, and glossary of terms. www.cryobank.com

First Descents

Provides whitewater kayaking and other outdoor adventure experiences to promote emotional, psychological, and physical healing for young adults with cancer. www.firstdescents.org

Friends of Jaclyn Organization

Pairs up children with brain tumors and their families with college and high school sports teams who give these children love, support, and friendship. www.friendsofjaclyn.org

Hope for Young Adults with Cancer

Connects young adults with cancer with peers 18–40 in the fight to provide financial support and a social network and outlet for those battling, surviving, and living with cancer. www.hope4yawc.org

Imerman Angels

Provides personalized connections that enable one-on-one support among cancer fighters, survivors, and caregivers by connecting them with a Mentor Angel (someone who is a cancer survivor or survivor's caregiver; around same age, gender, and who has beaten the same type of cancer). www.imermanangels.org

LIVESTRONG Fertility Services

Provides reproductive information, support, and hope to cancer patients and survivors whose medical treatments present the risk of infertility. www.livestrong.org/we-can-help/fertility-services/

National Cancer Institute: Adolescents and Young Adults with Cancer

Continually updated information portal on adolescents and young adults with cancer. www.cancer.gov/cancertopics/aya

Peer to Peer through the Sarcoma Alliance

Facilitates positive relationships between individuals affected by sarcoma so that they may find emotional support, encouragement, and information. http://sarcomaalliance.org/peer-to-peer/

Planet Cancer

A community for young adults with cancer, it is a place to share insights, explore fears, and laugh with others who understand. http://myplanet.planetcancer.org/

Rise Above It (RAI)

Provides support to adolescents and young adults affected by cancer, as well as financial assistance to patients ages 15–39 who are either undergoing or actively pursuing Phase I, II, or III clinical trial treatment options. www.raibenefit.org

Stupid Cancer

Provides individuals under 40 with hundreds of age-appropriate resources and social networks with young adult survivors and caregivers.www.stupidcancer.org

Tracey's Kids

A pediatric program for children with cancer that uses art therapy to engage with young patients, their siblings, and parents so that they can express feelings and reflect on their treatment experiences. www.tracyskids.org

Ulman Cancer Fund for Young Adults

A network that addresses areas of cancer support, advocacy, and education specific to young adults dealing with cancer. www.ulmanfund.org

Young Cancer Spouses

Strives to bring together other spouses to share ideas, lend support, and validate their wide range of feelings and emotions so they can find comfort in an understanding community. www.youngcancerspouses.org

Financial Assistance

Aid to Families with Dependent Children (AFDC)

Offers monthly checks for the care of dependent children who are in financial need. www.acf.hhs.gov/programs/ofa

Andre Sobel River of Life Foundation

Helps with urgent expenses, allowing single parents to stay at their child's bedside during catastrophic illness. www.andreriveroflife.org

American Childhood Cancer Organization (formerly Candlelighters)

Provides information, local and online support groups, and specialized information to families and caregivers of children with cancer. www.acco.org/

Cancer Care

Provides financial assistance to help with some types of costs, including transportation, homecare, childcare, and pain medication. www.cancercare.org

First Hand Foundation

Helps children with health-related needs when insurance and other financial resources have been exhausted. www.firsthandfoundation.org

Insure Kids Now

A national campaign to link the nation's uninsured children (0–18) to free and low-cost health insurance. www.insurekidsnow.gov

Local Department of Human Resources and Social Services

DHR or DSS can assist with rent or monthly payments, moving expenses, utility bills, financial help toward prescriptions, and medical supplies. The phone number of DHR/DSS is in the county government section of one's local telephone directory.

National Children's Cancer Society (NCCS)

Financial and fundraising assistance related to medical treatment, such as lodging and travel.www.thenccs.org/

Ruritan Club

Local clubs help families pay for medical equipment and supplies, prescription medications, and medical transportation. www.ruritan.org

State and Local General Assistance Programs

Designed to provide small amounts of cash assistance to individuals who are not eligible for AFDC or SSI or who are awaiting enrollment in another income subsidy program. Check the county's DHR/DSS to determine if the state or county has a General Assistance Program and where to call or how to apply.

Wishing Organizations and Services

3 Little Birds 4 Life

www.3littlebirds4life.org

The Association of Wish Granting Organizations (AWGO)

www.awgo.org

Believe in Tomorrow Children's Foundation

www.believeintomorrow.org

Chemo Angels

www.chemoangels.com

Children's Hopes and Dreams Foundation

www.childrenswishes.org

Children's Wish Foundation International

www.childrenswish.org

Dream Factory

www.dreamfactoryinc.org

Dream Foundation
www.dreamfoundation.org
Fairygodmother Foundation
www.fairygodmotherfoundation.org
Famous Fone Friends
www.famousfonefriends.org
Jason's Dream for Kids
www.jasonsdreamsforkids.com
Kids Wish Network (USA)
http://kidswishnetwork.org
Make-A-Wish Foundation of America
www.wish.org
Special Wish Foundation
www.spwish.org
Songs of Love
www.songsoflove.org
Starbright Foundation (USA)
www.starbrightfoundation.org
Sunshine Foundation
www.sunshinefoundation.org

Hair and Wig Organizations

ChemoCare HeadWear
http://www.chemocareheadwear.com
Girl on the Go
http://www.girlonthego.biz
Hair Club for Kids
www.hairclub.com/hairclub-for-kids.php
Headcovers Unlimited
www.headcovers.com
Hip Hats with Hair
www.hatswithhair.com
Locks of Love (USA)
www.locksoflove.org
Wigs for Kids (USA)
www.wigsforkids.org

End-of-Life Support and Grief and Bereavement

A Caring Hand: The Billy Esposito Bereavement Center
Provides services to help individuals with their emotional journey and financial assistance to aid their future education. www.acaringhand.org
Association for Death Education and Counseling® (ADEC)
Resources for individuals experiencing a death-related loss or for those seeking to help others. www.adec.org
Cancer Care, Inc.
Provides group, individual, family, and bereavement counseling, referral to local community resources, supplementary financial assistance for home care, transportation, and pain medication. www.cancercare.org
Centering Corporation
Provides guidance as well as pamphlets, books, and videos for families experiencing grief. www.centering.org
Children's Brain Tumor Foundation: Loss, Grief, and Bereavement Program
Provides support groups (peer to peer support, in person, on the phone, and online).
www.cbtf.org/connections/loss-grief-bereavement
Children's Hospice International
Provides hospice referral and information services. www.chionline.org
Compassionate Friends
National network of support groups that focus on assisting siblings and parents who have lost a child of any age, from any cause. www.compassionatefriends.org/home.aspx
Growth House, Inc.
Resources for life-threatening illness and end-of-life care to improve the quality of compassionate care for people who are dying. www.growthhouse.org
Hospice Net
Offers information and links for families facing life-threatening illness. www.hospicenet.org
KidsSaid
An online support program for kids to share and to help each other cope with grief.
www.kidsaid.com/
National Hospice and Palliative Care Organization
An organization committed to improving end-of-life care and expanding access to hospice

care with the goal of profoundly enhancing quality of life for people dying in America and their loved ones. http://nhpco.org/

The Dougy Center

Provides peer support groups, education, and training for children, teens, young adults, and their families who are grieving a death. www.dougy.org

Transportation

Air Care Alliance

www.aircareall.org

Air Charity Network (formerly Angel Flight America)

Arranges free air ambulance flights for patients and families in need.

www.aircharitynetwork.org

American Airlines – Miles for Kids in Need

Provides transportation for children and their families as well as for organizations dedicated to improving the quality of life for children with needs. www.aa.com/kids

Angel Flight

Serves patients needing transportation to or from the heartland region for surgery, chemotherapy, dialysis, and other treatments. www.angelflight.com

Children's Flight of Hope

Provides free air transportation to and from medical facilities for seriously ill or injured children who cannot travel to their destinations by any other method. www.childrensflightofhope.org

Corporate Angel Network

Allows cancer patients to fly free in empty seats on corporate jets. www.corpangelnetwork.org

Delta Air SkyWish at United Way

www.delta.com/skywish

Lifeline Pilots

Facilitates free air transportation through volunteer pilots for financially distressed passengers with medical and humanitarian needs.www.lifelinepilots.org

Mercy Medical Airlift

Provides transportation for financially stressed patients to distant specialized medical centers for evaluation and/or treatment. www.mercymedical.org

National Patient Air Travel

Provides information about all forms of charitable, long-distance medical transportation and provides referrals to all appropriate sources of help available in the national charitable medical transportation network. www.patienttravel.org

TWA Operation Liftoff

Operation Liftoff provides air transportation for children with a life-threatening illness for a treatment trip. www.operationliftoff.com

Professional Organizations and Research Facilities

Academy of Psychosomatic Medicine (APM)

www.apm.org

American Pediatric Society/Society for Pediatric Research (PAS/ASPR)

www.aps-spr.org

American Psychosocial Oncology Society (APOS)

www.apos-society.org

American Academy of Pediatrics (AAP)

www.aap.org

Association of Cancer Online Resources (ACOR)

www.acor.org

American Cancer Society (ACS)

www.cancer.org

American Society of Clinical Oncology

www.cancer.net

Association of Pediatric Hematology/Oncology Nurses (APON)

www.apon.org

British Psychosocial Oncology Society (BPOS)

www.bpos.org

Canadian Association of Psychosocial Oncology (CAPO)

www.capo.ca

Children's Oncology Group (COG)

www.childrensoncologygroup.org

HopeLab

www.hopelab.org

Hope Street Kids
http://neo4u.org/hope-street-kids/
International Psycho-Oncology Society (IPOS)
www.ipos-society.org
Leukemia & Lymphoma Society
www.leukemia-lymphoma.org
National Coalition for Cancer Survivorship (NCCS)
www.canceradvocacy.org
National Institutes of Health (NIH)
www.nih.gov
New Approaches to Neuroblastoma Therapy (NANT)
www.nant.org
Societe Internationale D'Oncologie Pediatrique (International Society of Paediatric Oncology) (SIOP)
www.siop.nl
The Association of Pediatric Oncology Social Workers (APOSW)www.aposw.org

The authors also extend many thanks to Emory Golant for her input to this chapter.

MIX
Papier aus verantwortungsvollen Quellen
Paper from responsible sources
FSC® C105338

If you have any concerns about our products,
you can contact us on
ProductSafety@springernature.com

In case Publisher is established outside the EU,
the EU authorized representative is:
Springer Nature Customer Service Center GmbH
Europaplatz 3, 69115 Heidelberg, Germany

Printed by Libri Plureos GmbH
in Hamburg, Germany